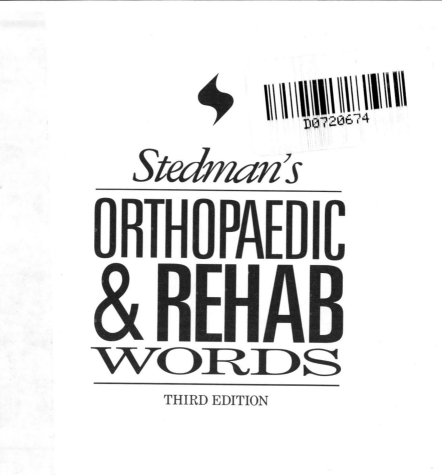

Stedman's

ORTHOPAEDIC & REHAB
WORDS

THIRD EDITION

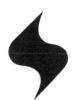

Stedman's
ORTHOPAEDIC
& REHAB
WORDS

THIRD EDITION

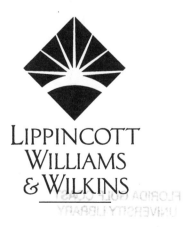

LIPPINCOTT
WILLIAMS
& WILKINS

Series Editor: Maureen Barlow Pugh
Managing Editor: Beverly J. Wolpert
Database Content Editor: Jennifer Schmidt
Art Direction: Jonathan Dimes
Production Manager: Patricia M. Smith
Typesetter: Peirce Graphic Services, Inc.
Printer & Binder: Vicks Lithograph & Printing

Copyright © 1999 Lippincott Williams & Wilkins
351 West Camden Street
Baltimore, Maryland 21201-2436 USA

All rights reserved. This book is protected by copyright. No part of this book may be reproduced in any form or by any means, including photocopying, or utilized by any information storage and retrieval system without written permission from the copyright owner.

Printed in the United States of America

Third Edition, 1999

Library of Congress Cataloging-in-Publication Data

Stedman's orthopaedic & rehab words. – 3rd ed.
    p.cm. – (Stedman's word book series)
    ISBN 0-683-30778-9
    1. Orthopedics Terminology. 2. Physically handicapped - Rehabilitation
Terminology. I. Stedman, Thomas Lathrop, 1853-1938. II. Title: Stedman's
orthopaedic and rehab words. III. Title: Orthopaedic and rehab words. IV.
Series: Stedman's word books.
    (DNLM: 1. Orthopedics Terminology-English. 2. Rehabilitation
    Terminology-English.   WE 15 S812 1999)
    RD723.S74   1999
    616.7'0014— dc21
    DNLM/DLC
    for Library of Congress
                                     99-16399
                                         CIP
                                    00 01
                       3 4 5 6 7 8 9 10

FLORIDA GULF COAST
UNIVERSITY LIBRARY

Contents

Acknowledgments

An important part of our editorial process is the involvement of medical transcriptionists—as advisors, reviewers and/or editors.

We extend special thanks to Ellen Atwood for reviewing, proofreading, and researching questions related to *Stedman's Orthopaedic & Rehab Words, Third Edition.*

We also extend special thanks to Jeanne Bock, CSR, RPR, MT, and to Suzanne Taubert, CMT, for editing the new terms added to *Stedman's Orthopaedic & Rehab Words, Third Edition,* and for helping to resolve many difficult content questions, as well as to Kathryn Mason for contributing much of the material for the appendix sections; Barbara Werner for editing the front matter and appendix sections; Helen Littrell for editing the manuscript and format; and Martha Richards, RRA, for reviewing and proofreading *Stedman's Orthopaedic & Rehab Words, Second Edition.*

Thanks as well to our MT Editorial Advisory Board for *Stedman's Orthopaedic & Rehab Words, Third Edition,* including Rose M. Berry; Patty White; Diane Edgar; Janice Deal, RN, BSN; Darcy Johnson; and Karen Thomas-Bates, CMT. These medical transcriptionists served as important contributors, editors, and advisors.

Other important contributors to this edition include Charmaine Backens; Sheila Hatch, MT; Renée Hentz, RRA; Nicole Peck; Wendy Ryan, ART; Jenifer Walker, MA; and Sandra Wideburg, CMT.

Barb Ferretti played an integral role in the process by reviewing the content files for format, updating the database, and providing a final quality check.

As with all our *Stedman's* word references, this resource incorporates the suggestions and expertise of our many contacts in the medical transcriptionist community. Thanks to all of our advisory board participants, reviewers, and editors; AAMT meeting attendees; and others who have written us with requests and comments—keep talking, and we'll keep listening.

Editor's Preface

As babyboomers grow older and increasingly act on the quest for better physical fitness and healthy, youthful bodies, the practices of orthopaedics, podiatry, chiropractic, occupational therapy, and physical therapy are experiencing parallel booms.

But the babyboomers alone can't account for this explosion. Today, doctors can treat a wide range of disabilities, from correcting congenital conditions and providing augmentations that allow people to participate in activities they might never have dreamed possible, to easing day-to-day pain and discomfort associated with arthritis. The elderly, as well as the young, are now encouraged to keep using their bodies to prevent or to slow down deterioration.

It's no wonder that the language of these specialties continues to change and expand at a daunting pace. The terminology has to grow to accommodate new developments in procedures, treatments, therapies, drugs, and equipment. The vast number of new terms means that an easy-to-use, current reference is now more important than ever.

This collection brings together current terms in orthopaedics, podiatry, chiropractic, occupational therapy, and physical therapy to provide a single reference serving the needs of medical language specialists. Such a collection is the result of collaborative efforts on many levels, but most important, founded on the participation of practicing medical transcriptionists. Working on this project has been an enlightening experience for me, and I can only hope that the resulting reference makes your working lives easier.

Jeanne Bock, CSR, RPR, MT

Publisher's Preface

This third edition of *Stedman's Orthopaedic & Rehab Words* offers an authoritative assurance of quality and exactness to the wordsmiths of the healthcare professions—medical transcriptionists, medical editors, copy editors, health information management personnel, court reporters, and the many other users and producers of medical documentation.

Users will find thousands of words encompassing orthopaedics, rehabilitiation, and chiropractic, in addition to physical therapy, occupational therapy, and podiatry. This collection includes many equipment terms for each of these specialties that, until now, have not been documented in a single word book, especially expanded coverage of surgical equipment and devices.

This compilation of more than 59,000 entries, fully cross-indexed for quick access, was built from a base vocabulary of more than 32,000 medical words, phrases, abbreviations, and acronyms. The extensive A-Z list was developed from the database of *Stedman's Medical Dictionary* and supplemented by terminology found in current medical literature (please see References on page xvi).

We at Lippincott Williams & Wilkins strive to provide you with the most up-to-date and accurate word references available. Your use of this word book will prompt new editions, which we will publish as often as updates and revisions justify. We welcome your suggestions for improvements, changes, corrections, and additions—whatever will make this *Stedman's* product more useful to you. Please complete the postpaid card at the back of this book, and send your recommendations care of "Stedman's" at Lippincott Williams & Wilkins.

Explanatory Notes

Medical transcription is an art as well as a science. Both are needed to interpret correctly the dictation of a physician, whose language is a product of education, training, and experience. This variety in medical language means that there are several acceptable ways, including jargon, to express certain terms. *Stedman's Orthopaedic & Rehab Words, Third Edition* provides variant spellings and phrasings for many terms. These elements, in addition to complete cross-indexing, make *Stedman's Orthopaedic & Rehab Words, Third Edition* a valuable resource for determining the validity of terms as they are encountered.

Alphabetical Organization

Alphabetization of main entries is letter by letter as spelled, ignoring punctuation, spaces, prefixed numbers, Greek letters, or other characters. For example:

acid-fast staining methods
acid formaldehyde hematin
α_1-acid glycoprotein
acid hematin

In subentry alphabetization, the abbreviated singular form or the spelled-out plural form of the noun main entry word is ignored.

Format and Style

All main entries are in **boldface** to expedite locating a sought-after term, to enhance distinction between main entries and subentries, and to relieve the textual density of the pages.

Irregular plurals and variant spellings are shown on the same line as the singular or preferred form of the word. For example:

arthritis, pl. **arthritides**

disk, disc

Hyphenation

As a rule of style, multiple eponyms (e.g., Mears-Rubash approach) are hyphenated. Also, hyphens have been added between a manufacturer and one or more eponyms (e.g., Vital-Metzenbaum dissecting scissors). Please note that hyphenation is a question of style, not of accuracy, and thus is a matter of choice.

Possessives

Possessive forms have been dropped in this reference for the sake of consistency and conformance with the guidelines of the American Association for Medical Transcription (AAMT) and other groups. Please note, however, that retaining the possessive is a question of style, not of accuracy, and thus is a matter of choice.

Cross-indexing

The word list is in an indexlike main entry-subentry format that contains two combined alphabetical listings:

(1) A *noun* main entry-subentry organization, which is typical of the A-Z section of medical dictionaries like **Stedman's:**

orthotic
   Bioflex o.
   Blue Line o.
   DesignLine o.
   Diab-A-Thotics o.
   DressFlex o.

paraplegia
   incomplete p.
   postoperative p
   Pott p.
   spastic p.
   traumatic p.

(2) An *adjective* main entry-subentry organization, which lists words and phrases as you hear them. The main entries are the adjectives or modifiers in a multiword term. The subentries are the nouns around which the terms are constructed and to which the adjectives or modifiers pertain:

Drummond
   D. button
   D. spinal instrumentation

scapulothoraci
   s. arthrodesis
   s. dissociation

| D. spinous wiring technique | s. fusion |
| D. wire | s. joint |

This format provides the user with more than one way to locate and identify a multiword term. For example:

reamer
    acetabular r.

acetabular
    a. reamer

technique
    abduction traction t.
    Ace-Colles frame t.
    bag of bones t.

Ace-Colles
    A.-C. external fixator
    A.-C. fracture frame
    A.-C. frame technique

It also allows the user to see together all terms that contain a particular descriptor, as well as all types, kinds, or variations of a noun entity. For example:

radius
    absent r.
    r. of angulation
    r. of curvature
    distal r.

Wherever possible, abbreviations are separately defined and cross-referenced. For example:

DREZ
    dorsal root entry zone

dorsal
    d. root entry zone (DREZ)

zone
    dorsal root entry z. (DREZ)

References

In addition to the manufacturers' literature we gather at various medical meetings, scientific reports from hospitals, and the lists of our MT Editorial Advisory Board members (from their daily transcription work), we used the following sources for new words for *Stedman's Orthopaedic & Rehab Words, Third Edition:*

Books

Agur AMR, Lee MJ. Grant's atlas of anatomy, 9th ed. Baltimore: Williams & Wilkins, 1991.

Anderson MK, Hall SJ. Fundamentals of sports injury management. Baltimore: Williams & Wilkins, 1997.

Cipriano JJ. Photographic manual of regional orthopaedic and neurological tests, 3rd ed. Baltimore: Williams & Wilkins, 1997.

Dorland's illustrated medical dictionary, 28th ed. Philadelphia: WB Saunders Company, 1994.

Fordney MT, Diehl MO. Medical transcription guide: do's and don'ts, 1st ed. Philadelphia: WB Saunders Company, 1990.

Jonas WB, Levin JS, eds. Essentials of complementary and alternative medicine. Baltimore: Lippincott Williams & Wilkins, 1999.

Lance LL. Quick look drug book. Baltimore: Lippincott Williams & Wilkins, 1999.

Pyle V. Current medical terminology, 5th ed. Modesto, CA: Health Professions Institute, 1994.

Rosenfeld I. Dr. Rosenfeld's guide to alternative medicine. New York: Random House, 1996.

Sloane SB. The medical word book, 3rd ed. Philadelphia: WB Saunders Company, 1991.

Stedman's medical dictionary, 26th ed. Baltimore: Williams & Wilkins, 1995.

Tessier C, ed. The AAMT book of style for medical transcription. Modesto, CA: American Association of Medical Transcription, 1995.

Journals

ACSM's Health & Fitness Journal. Baltimore: Lippincott Williams & Wilkins, 1998–1999.

American Journal of Sports Medicine. Waltham: American Orthopaedic Society for Sports Medicine, 1996–1998.

Chiropractic Products. Torrance, CA: Novicom, 1996-1999.

Chiropractic Technique. Baltimore: Williams & Wilkins, 1996.

Foot and Ankle International. Baltimore: Williams & Wilkins, 1995–1999.

Internal Medicine. Montvale, NJ: Medical Economics, 1995–1999.

Journal of the American Association for Medical Transcription. Modesto: American Association for Medical Transcription, 1995–1999.

Journal of Bone and Joint Surgery. Needham, MA: Journal of Bone and Joint Surgery, Inc., 1996–1999.

Journal of Foot and Ankle Surgery. Baltimore: Data Trace Publishing, 1998.

Journal of Orthopaedic and Sports Physical Therapy. Baltimore: Williams & Wilkins/ American Physical Therapy Association, Orthopaedic and Sports Physical Therapy Sections, 1996–1998.

Journal of Orthopaedic Nursing. Edinburgh: Churchill Livingstone, 1996.

Journal of Sports Chiropractic & Rehabilitation. Baltimore: Williams & Wilkins, 1996.

MT Monthly. Gladstone, MO: Computer Systems Management, 1994–1999.

O & P Almanac. Alexandria, VA: Orthotics & Prosthetics National Office, 1996–1999.

Perspectives on the Medical Transcription Profession. Modesto, CA: Health Professions Institute, 1993–1998.

Physical Therapy. Alexandria, VA: American Physical Therapy Association, 1996–1999.

Podiatric Products. Torrance, CA: Novicom, Inc., 1996–1999.

Podiatry Management. Upper Darby, PA: Kane Communications, 1996.

Stedman's WordWatcher. Baltimore: Williams & Wilkins, 1995–1997.

The Latest Word. Philadelphia: WB Saunders Company, 1994–1999.

Websites

www.http://www.medscape.com

www.medmedia.com/orthoo/1300.htm (the site for Wheeless' textbook of orthopaedics)

www.neoforma.com

www.orthoindustry.com

A
>A pin
>A wave

A1–A4 annular pulley

AA
>active-assistive

AAA
>antigen-extracted allogeneic
>diagnostic arthroscopy, operative
>arthroscopy, and possible operative
>arthrotomy
>>AAA bone
>>AAA bone graft

AAD
>atlantoaxial dislocation

AAI
>activating adjusting instrument

AAL
>ant ax line
>anterior axillary line

AAOS
>American Academy of Orthopaedic
>Surgeons
>>AAOS acetabular abnormalities
>>classification

AARF
>atlantoaxial rotatory fixation

AAROM
>active ankle joint complex range of
>motion

AARP
>American Association of Retired Persons

AAS
>atlantoaxial subluxation

AATB
>American Association of Tissue Banks

AB/AD ratio

ABAQUS modeling program

abatement

Abbe operation

Abbott
>A. brace
>A. gouge
>A. knee approach
>A. method
>A. splint

Abbott-Carpenter posterior approach

Abbott-Fischer-Lucas hip arthrodesis

Abbott-Gill
>A.-G. epiphyseal plate exposure
>A.-G. epiphysiodesis
>A.-G. osteotomy

Abbott-Lucas
>A.-L. arthrodesis
>A.-L. shoulder operation

Abbreviated Injury Scale (AIS)

ABC
>American Board of Certification
>aneurysmal bone cyst

ABD
>abdominal
>abduction
>>ABD pad

abdominal (ABD)
>a. binder
>a. dressing
>a. flap
>a. incision
>a. injury
>a. lap pad
>a. muscle
>a. reflex
>a. syndrome

abduct

abducted thumb

abduction (ABD)
>a. bolster
>a. brace
>a. contracture
>a. cushion
>a. deformity
>a. external rotation test
>a. finger splint
>hinge a.
>hip a.
>a. hip orthosis
>a. humeral splint
>humerothoracic a.
>index finger a.
>a. knee separator
>a. osteotomy
>a. pillow
>a. pillow cover splint
>a. stress test
>a. thumb splint
>a. traction technique
>a. wedge

a-b-duction (as dictated)

abduction-external
>a.-e. rotation (AER)
>a.-e. rotation fracture

abductor
>a. digiti minimi (ADM)
>a. digiti minimi magnus musculus
>a. digiti minimi muscle
>a. digiti minimi nerve
>a. digiti minimi opponensplasty

abductor *(continued)*
    a. digiti minimi pedis musculus
    a. digiti quinti (ADQ)
    a. digiti quinti muscle
    a. digiti quinti opponensplasty
    a. digiti quinti tendon
    a. hallucis muscle
    a. hallucis tendon
    a. insufficiency
    a. lever arm
    a. lurch
    a. lurch gait
    a. mechanism
    a. osteotomy
    a. pollicis brevis muscle
    a. pollicis brevis tendon
    a. pollicis longus muscle
    a. pollicis longus tendon
    side-lying hip a.
abductor/adductor ratio
abductor-plasty
    flexor pollicis longus a.-p.
    Smith flexor pollicis longus a.-p.
abductory
    a. midfoot osteotomy
    a. wedge osteotomy
abductovalgus
    hallux a., hallux abductus valgus
    (HAV)
abductus
    digitus a.
    forefoot a.
    hallux a. (HA)
    metatarsus a.
    midfoot a.
    pes planovalgus a.
    pollex a.
aberration
    hypokinetic a.
abet
abetted
abetting
ABG cement-free hip system
ABI
    acquired brain injury
    ankle-brachial index
ability
    abstracting a.
    bathing and dressing a.
    conceptual a.
    constructional a.
    Porch Index of Communicative A.
    (PICA)
    positive a.
    Scales of Cognitive A.
    squatting a.
ablation
    cartilage a.
    cyst a.
    nerve rootlet a.
    radical nail bed a.
    surgical a.
    Zadik total nail bed a.
ablative
    a. arthroplasty
    a. surgery
Ableware Volumeter
abnormal
    a. fixation
    a. instantaneous axis of rotation
    A. Involuntary Movement Scale
    (AIMS)
    a. posterior talar process
    a. shoe wear
abnormalities
    D'Antonio classification of
    acetabular a.
abnormality
    bony a.
    bulbar a.
    cranial nerve a.
    cytoarchitectonic a.
    dislocation contour a.
    fibropathic a.
    frontal plane growth a.
    sensorineural a.
    soft tissue a.
    sonographic a.
    spinal cord injury without
    radiographic a. (SCIWORA)
    tissue texture a. (TTA)
    torsional a.
ABOS
    American Board of Orthopaedic Surgery
abouna splint
above
    a. elbow
    a. knee (AK)
above-elbow (AE)
    a.-e. amputation
    a.-e. cast
above-knee
    a.-k. amputation (AKA)
    a.-k. prosthesis
    a.-k. suction enhancement system
ABPTS
    American Board of Physical Therapy
    Specialists
abrader
    cartilage a.
**Abraham-Pankovich tendo calcaneus
repair**
Abramson catheter
abrasion
    a. arthroplasty

a. chondroplasty
graft-bony tunnel wall a.
Abrikossoff tumor
ABS
amniotic band syndrome
abscess
arthrifluent a.
bone a.
Brodie metaphyseal a.
button a.
collar-button a.
growth-plate a.
horseshoe a.
intraosseous a.
metaphyseal a.
midpalmar a.
paraspinal a.
paravertebral a.
pelvic a.
posterior pharyngeal a.
psoas a.
retropharyngeal a.
retrosternal a.
spinal a.
subaponeurotic a.
subcutaneous a.
subperiosteal a.
subphrenic a.
subplatysmal a.
subungual a.
suture a.
abscessogram
absence
congenital intercalary limb a.
congenital terminal limb a.
absent
a. patella
a. radius
a. reflex
a. spinous process
a. thumb
a. ulna
absolute
a. refractory period
a. scotomata
absorbable
a. polyparadioxanone pin
Absorbine
A. Antifungal Foot Powder
A. Jock Itch
A. Jr. Antifungal

absorptiometry
dual-energy x-ray a. (DXA)
dual-photon a. (DPA, DPX)
peripheral dual-energy x-ray a.
(pDXA)
absorption
bone a.
bony a.
a. cavity
energy a.
lysosomal a.
shock a.
abstracting ability
abut
abutment
ulnocarpal a.
abutted
abutting
AC
acromioclavicular
AC joint
AC joint separation
ACA
American Chiropractic Association
acanthoma
epidermolytic a.
acanthosis nigricans
acanthotic
ACC
Association of Chiropractic Colleges
acceleration
angular a.
swing-phase a.
tibial a.
acceleration/deceleration injury
accelerator
linear a. (LINAC)
accelerometer
piezoelectric a.
acceptance
weight a.
access
southern a.
accessoria
os carpalia a.
accessorius
talus a.
accessory
a. atlantoaxial ligament
Auto Glide walker a.
a. bone
a. collateral ligament

NOTES

3

accessory *(continued)*
>   a. communicating tendon
>   a. digit
>   Isola spinal implant system a.
>   a. lateral collateral ligament
>   a. motion
>   a. movement technique
>   a. navicular
>   a. navicular cast
>   a. nerve
>   a. nerve injury
>   a. ossicle
>   a. ossification center of calcaneus
>   a. phalanx
>   pneumatic drill a.
>   portal a.
>   a. portion
>   a. sesamoid

AccessTrainer exerciser
accident
>   ATV a.
>   cerebrovascular a. (CVA)
>   compensable a.
>   horseback riding a.
>   motorcycle a. (MCA)
>   motor vehicle a. (MVA)
>   skateboarding a.
>   vascular a.
>   vehicular a.

acclivity
accommodation
>   a. curve
>   a. reflex

accommodative
>   a. brace
>   a. orthosis

Accommodator arch support
accordion test
Accu-Back back support
Accucore II
Accuflate tourniquet
Accu-Flo
>   A.-F. polyethylene bur hole cover
>   A.-F. silicone rubber bur hold cover
>   A.-F. ultrafiltration system

Aculength arthroplasty measuring system
Accu-Line
>   A.-L. dual pivot
>   A.-L. femoral resector
>   A.-L. guide
>   A.-L. knee instrument
>   A.-L. knee instrumentation
>   A.-L. tibial resector

accumulation
>   onset of blood lactate a. (OBLA)

AccuPressure heel cup

Accurate Surgical and Scientific Instruments Corporation (ASSI)
Accusway balance measurement system
Accu-Tron microcurrent machine
Accuvac smoke evacuation attachment
ACDF
>   anterior cervical diskectomy and fusion

Ace
>   A. adherent bandage
>   A. bandage reduction
>   A. intramedullary (AIM)
>   A. intramedullary femoral nail system
>   A. pin
>   A. screw
>   A. Unifix fixation
>   A. Unifix fixation apparatus
>   A. Unifix fixation device
>   A. wrap

Ace-Colles
>   A.-C. external fixator
>   A.-C. fracture frame
>   A.-C. frame technique
>   A.-C. half ring

Ace-Fischer
>   A.-F. external fixator
>   A.-F. fixation
>   A.-F. fracture frame
>   A.-F. ring frame

Ace/Normed osteodistractor
Acephen
ACET
>   aquatic cardiac evaluation and testing
>   ACET system

Aceta
acetabula (*pl. of* acetabulum)
acetabular
>   a. allograft
>   a. angle
>   a. angle of Sharp
>   a. augmentation graft
>   a. cap
>   a. cement compactor
>   a. component
>   a. component loosening
>   a. cup
>   a. cup arthroplasty
>   a. cup holder
>   a. cup peg drill guide
>   a. cup positioner
>   a. cup template
>   a. cyst
>   a. endoprosthesis
>   a. expander
>   a. extensile approach
>   a. gauge
>   a. index
>   a. knife

a. labrum
a. liner
a. osteolysis
a. posterior wall fracture
a. pressurizer
a. prosthesis
a. prosthetic interface
a. prosthetic liner
a. protrusio deformity
a. reamer
a. reconstruction plate
a. rim
a. rim fracture
a. rim syndrome
a. roof
a. seating hole
a. slot
a. spacer
a. trial set
acetabulectomy
acetabuli
ligamentum transversum a.
acetabuloplasty
Albee a.
Pemberton a.
shelf a.
acetabulum, pl. **acetabula**
deep-shelled a.
dysplastic a.
false a.
floor of the a.
intrapelvic protrusio a.
lip of a.
malunited a.
protrusio a.
transverse ligament of a.
true a.
weightbearing dome of a.
acetaminophen
a., aspirin, and caffeine
a. and codeine
a. and dextromethorphan
a. and diphenhydramine
hydrocodone and a.
oxycodone and a.
a. and phenyltoloxamine
propoxyphene and a.
acetate
cortisone a.
Cortone A.
Hydrocortone A.
mafenide a.

methylprednisolone a.
paramethasone a.
triamcinolone a.
acetonide
triamcinolone a.
acetylsalicylic acid (ASA)
ACF
anterior cervical fusion
ache
theater a.
acheiria
aches and pains
achilleo-calcaneal-plantar system
achilleo-calcaneal vascular network
Achilles
A. bulge sign
A. heel pad
A. jerk
A. peritendinitis
A. squeeze test
A. tendinitis
A. tendon (AT)
A. tendon advancement
A. tendon lengthening
A. tendon pain
A. tendon reflex
A. tendon rupture (ATR)
A. tendon shortening
A. tendon test
A. tenotomy
Achillis
tendo A.
achillobursitis
achillodynia
Albert a.
achillorrhaphy
achillotenotomy
Achillotrain
A. active Achilles tendon support
Bauerfeind A.
aching
interscapular a.
a. pain
achondroplasia
achondroplastic dwarfism
achromatopsia
Achromycin Topical
Achterman-Kalamachi fibular hemimelia
acid
acetylsalicylic a. (ASA)
benzoic acid and salicylic a.
bichloracetic a.

NOTES

acid *(continued)*
    essential fatty a.
    fenamic a.
    folic a.
    gadolinium-diethylenetriamine
      pentaacetic a.
    gadolinium-labeled diethylenetriamine
      pentaacetic a.
    gamma aminobutyric a. (GABA)
    indoleacetic a.
    mefenamic a.
    paraaminosalicylic a.
    PhysioLogics Alpha Lipoic A.
    polyglycolic a. (PGA)
    polylactic a.
    poly-L-lactic a. (PLLA)
    salicylic a. and lactic a.
    salicylsalicylic a.
    tranexamic a.
    valproic a.
acid-citrate-dextrose solution
acidosis
    lactic a.
Acinetobacter
    A. anitratus
    A. wolffii
Ackerman criteria for osteomyelitis
ACL
    anterior cruciate ligament
    ACL-deficient knee
    ACL drill
    ACL drill guide
    ACL graft
    ACL graft knife
    ACL reconstruction
    ACL repair
Acland
    A. clamp
    A. clamp-applying forceps
    A. clamp approximator
    A. double-clamp approximator
aclasis
    diaphyseal a.
ACLR
    anterior capsulolabral reconstruction
ACOEM
    American College of Occupational and
    Environmental Medicine
acorn
    Midas Rex a.
    a. reamer
Acor Quikform I, II shoe
acoustic myography
ACP
    anterior cervical plate
acquired
    a. brain injury (ABI)
    a. clubfoot
    a. flatfoot
    a. immunodeficiency syndrome
     (AIDS)
    a. myopathy
    a. torticollis
ACR
    American College of Rheumatology
Acra-Cut wire pass drill
acral lentiginous melanoma
Acrel ganglion
ACRM
    American Congress of Rehabilitation
    Medicine
acrocephalosyndactylism
acrocephalosyndactyly
acrodysesthesia
acrokeratoelastoidosis
acromacria
AcroMed
    A. screw
    A. VSP fixation system
    A. VSP plate
acromegaly
acromial
    a. angle
    a. spur
    a. spur index (ASI)
acromiale
    os a.
acrominonectomy
acromioclavicular (AC)
    a. arthroplasty
    a. articulation
    a. cyst
    a. injury classification
    a. joint
    a. joint dislocation
    a. joint injury
    a. joint repair
    a. ligament
    a. separation
acromioclaviculare
    ligamentum a.
acromiocoracoid ligament
acromiohumeral interval (AHI)
acromion
    nonunion of a.
acromionectomy
    Armstrong a.
acromioplasty
    anterior a.
    arthroscopic a.
    decompressive a.
    McLaughlin a.
    McShane-Leinberry-Fenlin a.
    Neer a.
    Rockwood anterior a.
acroosteosclerosis

acropachy
acropectorovertebral dysplasia
acrosyndactyly
Acrotorque hand engine
acrylic
    a. bar prosthesis
    a. bone cement
    a. cap splint
    a. implant material
    a. orthotic device
    a. template splint
ACS
    anterior compartment syndrome
ACSM
    American College of Sports Medicine
    ACSM Guidelines for Exercise
      Testing and Prescription
Act
    Americans with Disabilities A.
      (ADA)
    A. joint support
    United States Vocational
      Rehabilitation A.
ACTH
    adrenocorticotropic hormone
Acthar
actinic keratosis
actinomycosis
action
    a. current
    double-pendulum a.
    inversion of muscle a.
    A. Jr. wheelchair
    a. line
    a. potential (AP)
    A. Research Arm (ARA)
    A. traction system
    a. tremor
activated partial thromboplastin time
  test (APTT)
activating adjusting instrument (AAI)
activation
    a. force
    latency of a.
    order of a.
activator
    tissue-type plasminogen a.
active
    a. ankle joint complex range of
      motion (AAROM)
    a. bending test
    a. contraction

    a. deformer
    a. electrode
    a. flexion
    a. hip movement
    a. insufficiency
    a. integral range of motion
      (AIROM)
    a. knee extension (AKE)
    a. knee extension test
    a. mobility
    a. motion testing (AMT)
    a. movement testing
    MPO 2000 A.
    a. and passive range of motion
    a. range of motion (AROM)
    a. range of movement
    a. range-of-motion exercises
    a.-release technique (ART)
    a. restraint
    a. sock
    a. treatment
active-assisted
    a.-a. range of motion
    a.-a. range-of-motion exercise
active-assistive (AA)
    a.-a. motion therapy
    a.-a. range of motion
ActiVin
activities of daily living (ADLs)
activity
    a. adaptation
    a. analysis
    biphasic endplate a.
    cingulate gyrus a.
    a. configuration
    discrete a.
    diversional a.
    endplate a.
    functional a.
    a. grading
    a. group
    increased insertional a.
    insertion a.
    involuntary a.
    level of a.
    A. Loss Assessment (ALA)
    mechanoreceptor a.
    monophasic endplate a.
    motion a.
    motor a.
    opsonic a.
    a.-pattern analysis

NOTES

activity *(continued)*
    physical a.
    pivoting and cutting a.
    prolonged insertional a.
    purposeful a.
    push-pull a.
    reduced insertion a.
    spontaneous a.
    sudomotor a.
    a. synthesis
    a. training (AT)
    volitional a.
    voluntary a.
Actron
ActSet
actual leg length test
actuator
    NYU-Hosmer electric elbow and
    prehension a.
ACU-derm wound dressing
AcuDriver osteotome
ACU-dyne antiseptic
Acufex
    A. alignment guide
    A. ankle distractor
    A. arthroscopic instrument
    A. arthroscopic instrumentation
    A. bioabsorbable fixation device
    A. convex rasp
    A. curette
    A. curved basket forceps
    A. distractor pin
    A. double-lumen arthroscopic
    cannula
    A. drill
    A. drill-guide
    A. Edge
    A. gouge
    A. grasper
    A. knee laxity arthrometer
    A. mallet
    A. meniscal basket
    A. microsurgical rear-entry to
    front-entry femoral guide system
    A. microsurgical tendon stripper
    A. MosaicPlasty instrument
    A. nerve hook
    A. osteotome
    A. probe
    A. rotary biting basket forceps
    A. rotary punch
    A. scissors
    A. tensiometer
    A. tibial guide
Acumeter
Acupoint stimulator
acupressure
acupuncture

acute
    a. angular kyphosis
    a. avulsion fracture
    a. foot strain
    a. gout
    a. hematogenous arthritis
    a. hematogenous osteomyelitis
    (AHO)
    a. inflammatory polyradiculopathy
    a. ischemic contracture
    a. low-back syndrome
    a. spinal arthritis
    a. stretch injury
    a. transverse myelitis
    a. traumatic hemarthrosis
    a. traumatic lesion
    a. whiplash
ACUTENS
Acutrak small bone fixation system
acyclovir
ADA
    Americans with Disabilities Act
adactyly, adactylia
Adair
    A. breast clamp
    A. screw compressor
Adalat CC
ADAM
    Amniotic Deformity, Adhesion,
    Mutilation
Adam
    A. and Eve rib belt splint
    A. sign
adamantinoma
Adamkiewicz artery
Adams
    A. forward-bending test
    A. hip operation
    A. position test
    A. procedure
    A. saw
    A. scoliosis test
    A. splint
    A. transmalleolar arthrodesis
    A. view
Adapin
Adapta physical therapy table
adaptation
    activity a.
adapter, adaptor
    Christmas tree a.
    chuck a.
    Collet screwdriver a.
    French a.
    Grace plate 4-hole a.
    Hudson chuck a.
    Jacobs chuck a.
    Lloyd a.

Mayfield a.
SACH foot a.
Smith-Petersen nail with Lloyd a.
Trinkle brace and a.
Trinkle chuck a.

Adapteur multi-functional drill guide

Adaptic

A. crown
A. dressing
A. gauze
A. packing
A. sponge

adaptive equipment

adaptor (*var. of* adapter)

Adcon adhesive control gel

Adcon-L anti-adhesion barrier gel

ADD

adduction

Add-A-Clamp

Hex-Fix A.-A.-C.

Addis test

adduct

adducta

coxa a.

adducted thumb

adduction (ADD)

a. contracture
a. deformity
Edgarton-Grand thumb a.
a. fracture
a. osteotomy
a. stress to finger
a. stress test
a. traction technique

a-d-duction (as dictated)

adduction-internal rotation deformity

adductocavus

metatarsus a.

adductor

a. aponeurosis
a. hallucis longus
a. hallucis tendon
a. hamstring tightness
a. hiatus
a. longus muscle rupture
a. magnus
a. magnus adductor flap
a. muscle group
a. origin
a. pollicis brevis tendon
a. pollicis muscle
a. pollicis paralysis

a. pollicus
a. reflex
a. sweep of thumb
a. tendon and lateral capsular release
a. tenotomy
a. tenotomy and obturator neurectomy (ATON)

adductovarus

a. deformity
forefoot a.
metatarsus a.

adductus

congenital metatarsus a.
dynamic metatarsus a.
forefoot a.
metatarsus a. (MTA)
metatarsus primus a. (MPA)
midfoot a.
pes equinovarus a.
true metatarsus a. (TMA)

A-delta

A.-d. fiber
A.-d. nociceptor ending

adenine arabinoside (ara-a)

adenoma

papillary a.

adenomyosis

adenosine thallium scan

adherent

a. profundus tendon
Tuf-Skin tape a.

adhesion

band-like a.
capsular a.
fibrous a.
filmy a.
a. formation
intraarticular a.
subacromial bursal a.
subdeltoid bursal a.

adhesion/cohesion mechanism

adhesive

APR cement fixation a.
Aron Alpha a.
Biobrane a.
a. capsulitis
Coe-pak paste a.
Coverlet a.
cyanoacrylate a.
fibrin glue a.
Histoacryl glue a.

NOTES

adhesive *(continued)*
> hydroxyapatite a.
> Implast a.
> ligand a.
> LLPS hydroxyapatite a.
> medical a.
> methyl methacrylate a.
> Orthomite II a.
> Palacos cement a.
> Simplex cement a.
> a. strapping
> Superglue a.
> Surfit a.
> T-Stick a.
> Zimmer low viscosity a.

ADI
> atlantodens interval
> atlantodental interval

adiabatic fast passage
adipofascial flap
adipose tissue
adiposis dolorosa
ADJ
> adjustable dynamic joint

Adjective ColorCards
adjoining pedicle
adjunctive screw fixation
Adjustaback wheelchair backrest system
adjustability
> 3D positional a.

adjustable
> A. Advanced Reciprocating Gait
> Orthosis (ARGO)
> a. aiming apparatus
> a. aiming device
> a. angle guide
> a. dynamic joint (ADJ)
> A. Leg and Ankle Repositioning
> Mechanism (ALARM)
> a. nail
> a. pedicle connector
> a. 2-point caliper sensory
> assessment device
> a. postoperative protective prosthetic
> socket (APOPPS)
> a. splint

Adjusta-Wrist
> A.-W. hinge
> A.-W. splint

adjusting
> figure-eight a.

adjustive
> a. art
> a. thrust
> a. treatment

adjustment
> a. of the articulations and adjacent
> tissue

> a. of cervical spine
> chiropractic a.
> a. equipment
> general a.
> a. of lumbar spine
> manual a.
> osseous a.
> set-hold a.
> specific a.
> a. of thoracic spine
> toggle-recoil a.
> vertebral a.

adjuvant chemotherapy
Adkins
> A. spinal fusion
> A. technique spinal arthrodesis

ADL
> adrenoleukodystrophy
> ADL indices

Adlone Injection
ADLs
> activities of daily living
> extended ADLs
> hierarchical scales of ADLs
> indices of ADLs
> instrumental ADLs

ADM
> abductor digiti minimi

Administration
> Occupational Safety and Health A.
> (OSHA)

adolescent
> a. back pain
> a. idiopathic scoliosis (AIS)
> a. kyphosis
> a. scoliosis

Adprin-B
> Extra Strength A.-B.

ADQ
> abductor digiti quinti

adrenal
> a. cortex
> a. disorder

adrenergic vagal function
adrenocorticotropic hormone (ACTH)
adrenogenital syndrome
adrenoleukodystrophy (ADL)
adrenomedullin
Adriamycin
> A. PFS
> A. RDF

ADROM
> ankle dorsiflexion range of motion

Adson
> A. bur
> A. cerebellar retractor
> A. drill guide
> A. drill guide forceps

A. hemilaminectomy retractor
A. hypophyseal forceps
A. laminectomy chisel
A. maneuver
A. periosteal elevator
A. rongeur
A. saw guide
A. sign
A. spiral drill
A. suction tube
A. test
A. twist drill
Adson-Rogers perforating drill
ADT
   anterior drawer test
adult
   a.-acquired flatfoot deformity
   a. gait
   a. respiratory distress syndrome
     (ARDS)
   a. scoliosis
   a. scoliosis patient
   a. scoliosis surgery
advancement
   Achilles tendon a.
   Atasoy V-Y a.
   calcaneonavicular ligament-tibialis
     posterior tendon a.
   Chandler patellar a.
   en bloc a.
   a. flap
   a. flap graft
   heel cord a. (HCA)
   Johnson pronator a.
   Lloyd-Roberts-Swann trochanteric a.
   Maquet a.
   Murphy Achilles tendon a.
   Murphy heel cord a.
   patellar a.
   plantar calcaneonavicular ligament-
     tibialis posterior tendon a.
   profundus a.
   tendon a.
   trochanteric a.
   vastus medialis a. (VMA)
   Wagner profundus a.
   Wagner trochanteric a.
advancer
Advantim knee system
adventitia

adventitial
   a. forceps
   a. scissors
adventitious
   a. bursa
   a. movement
adversive attack
advertising
AE
   above-elbow
   AE amputation
AE1, AE3 antibody
Aebi-Etter-Coscia fixation dens fracture
AEP
   auditory evoked potential
Aequalis
   A. head
   A. reamer
   A. shoulder prosthesis
   A. stem
   A. system
AER
   abduction-external rotation
aerate
aeration
Aeroaid
aerobe
aerobic
   a. bacteria
   a. cellulitis
   a. exercise
   a. infection
   a. walking
AerobiCycle
   Universal A.
Aerodine
aeroplane splint
Aeroplast dressing
Aerosol
   Fluro-Ethyl A.
aeruginosa
   Pseudomonas a.
Aesculap
   A. bipolar cautery
   A. bipolar cautery forceps
   A. clamp
   A. drill
   A. forceps
   A. headholder
   A. saw
**Aesculap-PM noncemented femoral
   prosthesis**

NOTES

aesthesiometer
AF
  antifungal
AFC
  anticipating financial compensation
affection
  patellar a.
afferent
  a. fiber
  a. nerve impulse
AFI total hip replacement prosthesis
AFO
  ankle-foot orthosis
  ankle-foot orthotic
  articulated AFO
  AFO brace sock
  AFO molded
  AFO pediatric brace
  AFO posterior leaf-spring
  sliding AFO
  AFO standard shell
  Type C-50, C-90 AFO
A-frame
  A.-f. notch
  A.-f. orthosis
Aftate
  A. for Athlete's Foot
  A. for Jock Itch
AG
  antigravity
AGC
  anatomically graduated component
  AGC Biomet total knee system
  AGC femoral prosthesis
  AGC knee prosthesis
  AGC tibial prosthesis
AGE
  angle of greatest extension
age
  a.-associated degenerative change
  bone a.
  Greulich-Pyle bone a.
  skeletal a.
Agee
  A. carpal tunnel release system
  A. force-couple splint reduction
  A. 4-pin fixation device
Agee-WristJack
  A.-W. external fixator
  A.-W. fracture reduction system
Agency for Health Care Policy and Research (AHCPR)
agenesis
  Bayne classification of radial a.
  caudal spinal a.
  lumbar a.
  sacral a.
agenetic fracture

agent
  antiosteoclastic a.
  antipyretic a.
  Cara Klenz cleansing a.
  chondroprotective a.
  chymopapain blocking a.
  contrast a.
  fibrinolytic a.
  keratolytic a.
  mechanical a.
  nociceptor a.
  phlogistic a.
  physical a.
  thermal a.
  uricosuric a.
  water-soluble contrast a.
AGF
  angle of greatest flexion
agglomerans
  Enterobacter a.
aggressive
  a. infantile fibromatosis
  a. solitary plasmacytoma
  a. tumor
agility drill
Aging
  American Association of Homes for the A.
agitans
  paralysis a.
Agliette
  A. measurement
  A. supracondylar osteotomy
Agnew splint
agonist-antagonist
agonistic muscle
agonist muscle
AHCPR
  Agency for Health Care Policy and Research
Ahern trochanteric debridement
AHI
  acromiohumeral interval
  Arthritis Helplessness Index
AHO
  acute hematogenous osteomyelitis
AHP
  American Hand Prosthesis
  American Hand Prosthetics
  AHP digital
  AHP digital prosthesis
AHSC
  Arizona Health Science Center
  AHSC elbow prosthesis
AHSC-Volz
  A.-V. elbow prosthesis
  A.-V. hinge
A-hydroCort

Aicardi syndrome
aid
>Carex ambulatory a.
>Compoz Nighttime Sleep A.
>erogenic a.
>Ortho-Turn transfer a.
>sock a.
>Turn-Easy transfer a.

AIDS
>acquired immunodeficiency syndrome

AIIS
>anterior inferior iliac spine
>AIIS avulsion fracture

Aiken osteotomy
AIM
>Ace intramedullary
>AIM continuous passive motion
>AIM CPM
>AIM femoral nail system

aimer
>Arthrotek femoral a.
>tibial a.

aiming bow
AIMS
>Abnormal Involuntary Movement Scale
>Alberta Infant Motor Scale
>Arthritis Impact Measurement Scale

Ainslie acrylic splint
Ainsworth modification of Massie nail
air
>A.-Back spinal system
>a. band
>a. bicycle
>a. contrast
>a. contrast study
>a. cylinder
>a. drill
>a.-driven oscillating saw
>A.-Dyne bicycle
>a. embolism
>a. filter
>a.-flow enclosure
>a. flow mat
>a. inflation system
>a. plasma spray (APS)
>a.-powered cutting drill
>a. pressure splint
>A.-Soft Splint
>a. splint
>a. walker

airborne bacteria

Aircast
>A. Air-Stirrup brace
>A. ankle brace
>A. Cryo Cuff
>A. fracture brace
>A. Knee System
>A. leg brace
>A. pneumatic brace
>A. Swivel-Strap
>A. Swivel-Strap brace
>A. walking brace

Airex
>A. balance pad
>A. mat

Airfoam splint
AirGEL ankle brace
AirLITE support pad
AIROM
>active integral range of motion

airplane
>a. cast
>a. shears
>a. splint
>a. splint orthosis

AirStance pylon
Air-Stirrup
>A.-S. ankle brace
>A.-S. ankle training brace

AIS
>Abbreviated Injury Scale
>adolescent idiopathic scoliosis

AITA modular trauma system
Aitken
>A. classification of epiphyseal
>fracture
>A. epiphyseal fracture classification
>A. femoral deficiency
>A. hip class

AJ
>ankle jerk

AJC
>ankle joint complex

AK
>above knee
>applied kinesiology
>AK prosthesis

AKA
>above-knee amputation

AKE
>active knee extension
>AKE test

NOTES

Akin
- A. bunionectomy
- A. procedure
- A. proximal phalangeal osteotomy

Akne-Mycin Topical

Akros
- A. extended care mattress
- A. pressure mattress

AkroTech mattress

AK-Taine

ALA

Activity Loss Assessment

ala, pl. **alae**
- sacral a.

AlamarBlue osteoblast proliferation assay

Alanson amputation

alar
- a. creaking
- a. crease
- a. dysgenesis
- a. ligament
- a. rim
- a. screw

alaria
- ligamentum a.

ALARM

Adjustable Leg and Ankle Repositioning Mechanism

alarm
- a. cushion
- wandering a.

Albee
- A. acetabuloplasty
- A. bone graft
- A. drill
- A. hip arthrodesis
- A. lumbar spinal fusion
- A. olive-shaped bur
- A. orthopaedic table
- A. osteotome
- A. shelf procedure

Albee-Compere fracture table

Albee-Delbert procedure

Albers-Schönberg disease

Albert
- A. achillodynia
- A. knee operation

Alberta Infant Motor Scale (AIMS)

Albright
- A. hereditary osteodystrophy
- A. syndrome
- A. synovectomy

Albright-Chase
- A.-C. arthroplasty

Albright-McCune-Sternberg syndrome

albumin

Alcaine

Alcock canal

alcohol
- denatured a.
- a. fat embolism syndrome
- a. injection
- polyvinyl a.

Alcon
- A. Closure System
- A. Instrument Delivery System tray

Alden
- A. CDI orthosis
- A. CDI orthotic

aldolase

alendronate

Aleve

Alexander
- A. chisel
- A. costal osteotome
- A. costal periosteotome
- A. gouge
- A. periosteal elevator
- A. rasp
- A. technique
- A. view

Alexander-Farabeuf
- A.-F. periosteotome
- A.-F. rasp

Alexian Brothers overhead frame

alfa
- epoetin a.

alfalfa

Alfenta Injection

alfentanil hydrochloride

Alginate dressing

Algisite Alginate wound dressing

algodystrophy syndrome

algometer

algoneurodystrophy

algorithm
- Clanton-DeLee a.
- injury a.
- Tile polytrauma a.

AliBrite padding

AliCool splint spray

AliCork Foot Orthosis

AliDeep massage cream

AliEdge edge rest cushion

AliFleece gloves

align

aligner
- Charnley femoral inlay a.
- femoral a.
- patellar a.
- tibial a.

alignment
- anatomic a.
- angular a.
- atlantoaxial a.

colinear a.
dynamic a.
extramedullary a.
a. of fracture fragment
a. guide
a. guide rod
a. index
integrity and a.
patellar a.
patellofemoral a.
a. pin
poor a.
a. rod
rotational a.
sagittal anatomic a.
static a.
talocrural a.
tibiofemoral a.
torsional a.
transfemoral a.
transverse plane a.
a. of vertebral bodies

AliMed
A. Conductive Patient Shifter
A. diabetic night splint
A. insert
A. putty
A. turnbuckle elbow splint
A. wrist/thumb support
AliMed-Freedom arthritis support
AliMold stretch cloth
Aliplast
A. blank
A. custom-molded foot orthosis
A. insole
A. pad
Alisoft splinting material
AliStrap
AliTane cushion cover
AliTex cushion cover
Alivium
A. implant metal
A. implant metal prosthesis
alkaline phosphatase
alkaloid
opium a.
Alka-Mints
Alkeran
ALL
anterior longitudinal ligament
all
a.-inside repair

a.-median nerve hand
a. or none law
A. Poly Deltafit keel
a.-polyethylene socket
a.-purpose boot (APB)
A.-Purpose Boot Hi
a.-terrain vehicle (ATV)
Allen
A. arm/hand surgery table
A. arthroscopic elbow positioner
A. arthroscopic knee positioner
A. arthroscopic wrist positioner
A. Diagnostic Module
A. maneuver
A. open reduction of calcaneal fracture
A. reduction
A. shoulder arthroscopy
A. shoulder/wrist arthroscopy traction system
A. sign
A. stirrups
A. test
A. wrench
Allen-Brown prosthesis
Allender vertical laminar flow room
Allen-Ferguson Galveston pelvic fixation
Allen-headed screwdriver
Allen-Kocher clamp
allergenic arthritis
allergy
latex a.
AllerMax Oral
Allevyn
A. Island dressing
A. wound dressing
Allgöwer
A. stitch
A. suture technique
Alliance rehabilitation system
alligator
a. grasping forceps
Allis
A. clamp
A. maneuver
A. sign
A. tissue forceps
Alli test
Allman
A. acromioclavicular injury classification

NOTES

Allman *(continued)*
    A. modification of Evans ankle
      reconstruction
allodynia
Allofix cortical bone pin
allogeneic
    antigen-extracted a. (AAA)
    a. lyophilized bone grafts implan
      material
allogenic bone graft
allogenous bone graft
allograft
    acetabular a.
    bone a.
    bone-tendon-bone a.
    a. bone vise
    a. coronary artery disease
    femoral cortical ring a.
    femoral diaphyseal a.
    fresh frozen a.
    a.-host junction
    a. iliac bone
    intercalary diaphyseal a.
    large composite a.
    a. ligament replacement
    MTE a.
    napkin ring calcar a.
    osteoarticular a.
    osteochondral a.
    a. reconstruction of fibular
      collateral ligament
    Red Cross freeze-dried a.
    shell a.
    tendon-bone a.
    a. transplantation
AlloGrip bone vise
allopathic medicine
alloplastic
    a. graft
    a. material
Allo-Pro hip system
allopurinol
alloy
    cobalt-based a.
    cobalt-chromium a.
    Eligoy metal a.
    stainless steel a.
    Ti-6A1-4V a.
    Ti-Nidium a.
    titanium a.
    Vitallium a.
    Wood a.
Allport retractor
all-purpose
all-ulnar nerve hand
Alm wound retractor

aloe
    A. Grande creme
    a. vera
Alor 5/500
Alora Transdermal
Alouette amputation
ALP
    ankle ligament protector
alpha
    A. Chymar
    a. chymotrypsin
    A. cushion liner
    A. flat sheet
    A. suction attachment block kit
alpha fetoprotein
    maternal serum a. f. (MSAFP)
alphaprodine
alprazolam
ALPS
    anterior locking plate system
    Amset ALPS
Alps
    A. ClearLine silicone suspension
     liner
    A. ClearPro silicone suction socket
    A. CustomPro custom liner
    A. Lock Mod610
ALPSA
    anterior labrum periosteum shoulder
     arthroscopic lesion
    ALPSA lesion
ALRI
    anterolateral rotary instability
    ALRI test
ALS
    amyotrophic lateral sclerosis
    anterolateral sclerosis
alta
    A. cancellous screw
    A. CFX reconstruction od
    A. cortical screw
    A. cross-locking screw
    A. lag screw
    A. modular trauma system
    patella a.
    A. tibial-humeral rod
    A. tibial nail
    A. transverse screw
altered
    a. intervertebral mechanics
    a. regional mechanics
    a. sensation
alternating pressure pad
alternative
    graft material a.
altitudinal anopsia
Altona finger extension device
Alumafoam splint

A

alumina
    a. bioceramic joint replacement
    A. cemented total hip prosthesis
aluminate
    calcium a.
aluminum
    a. bridge splint
    a. contouring template set
    a. fence splint
    a. finger cot splint
    a. foam splint
    a. hand splint
    implant alloy a.
    a. master rod
    a. oxide arthroplasty material
    a. oxide ceramic coating
    a. toxicity
    a. wire splint
Alvarado
    A. collateral ligament protector
    A. knee holder
    A. legholder
    A. Orthopedic Research
Alvar condylar bolt
alvei
    Hafnia a.
alveolar
    a. bone fracture
    a. rhabdomyosarcoma
    a. soft-part sarcoma
ALVO
    anterolateral ventricular opening
**ALZET continuous infusion osmotic
  pump**
amalgam
amantadine
AMBI
    A. compression hip screw system
    A. fixation
    A. hip screw
ambidextrous
Ambien
ambifixation
AMBRI
    atraumatic, multidirectional, bilateral
      instability
    AMBRI procedure
ambulate with assistance
ambulation
    assisted a.
    brace-free a.
    crutch a.

    functional a.
    prosthetic a.
    a. skills
    a. training orthosis
ambulator
    Apex a.
    A. Bio-Rocker sole
    A. Chukka Boot
    A. conform footwear
    A. shoe
ambulatory
    a. function
    a. status
    a. traction
AMC total wrist prosthesis
AMD
    arthroscopic microdiskectomy
    articular motion device
AME
    American Medical Electronics
    Austin Medical Equipment
    AME bone growth stimulator
    AME microcurrent TENS unit
amebiasis
Amefa Flatware
amelanotic
amelia
American
    A. Academy of Orthopaedic
      Surgeons (AAOS)
    A. Academy of Orthopaedic
      Surgeons classification of
      acetabular deficiency
    A. Academy of Orthopaedic
      Surgeons/Hip Society questionnaire
    A. Academy of Orthotists and
      Prosthetists
    A. Association of Homes for the
      Aging
    A. Association of Retired Persons
      (AARP)
    A. Association of Tissue Banks
      (AATB)
    A. Board of Certification (ABC)
    A. Board of Certification of
      Orthotics and Prosthetics
    A. Board of Orthopaedic Surgery
      (ABOS)
    A. Board of Physical Therapy
      Specialists (ABPTS)
    A. Chiropractic Association (ACA)

NOTES

American *(continued)*
A. College of Occupational and Environmental Medicine (ACOEM)
A. College of Rheumatology (ACR)
A. College of Sports Medicine (ACSM)
A. Congress of Rehabilitation Medicine (ACRM)
A. Hand Prosthesis (AHP)
A. Hand Prosthetics (AHP)
A. Heyer-Schulte chin prosthesis
A. Heyer-Schulte-Hinderer malar prosthesis
A. Heyer-Schulte Radovan tissue expander prosthesis
A. Medical Electronics (AME)
A. Musculoskeletal Tumor Society rating scale
A. Nursing Home Association
A. Orthopaedic Foot and Ankle Society (AOFAS)
A. Orthopaedic Society for Sports Medicine
A. Orthotic and Prosthetic Association (AOPA)
A. Physical Therapy Association (APTA)
A. Red Cross Tissue Services
A. Rheumatism Association (ARA)
A. Seating Access-O-Matic bed
A. shoulder and elbow system (ASES)
A. Society of Anesthesiologists physical status classification system
A. Society for Testing and Materials (ASTM)
A.'s with Disabilities Act (ADA)
A-methaPred injection
AMFH
angiomatoid malignant fibrous histiocytoma
Amfit
A. custom orthosis
A. digitizer
A. orthotic
Amico drill
Amigo mechanical wheelchair
amikacin
aminobiphosphonate
aminoglycoside
aminoglycoside-impregnated methyl methacrylate bead
aminohydroxy propylidene diphosphonate
aminophylline
aminoquinoline
Amitone

amitriptyline
AMK
anatomic modular knee
AMK fixed bearing knee system
AMK total knee system
AML
amyotrophic lateral sclerosis
anatomic medullary locking
AML socket
AML Tang femoral prosthesis
AML total hip prosthesis
AML total hip system
AML trial hip component
Ammens foot powder
AM-MI orthopedic table
amnesia
hypnotic a.
amniotic
a. band syndrome (ABS)
A. Deformity, Adhesion, Mutilation (ADAM)
amobarbital and secobarbital
Amoss sign
amphetamine
amphiarthrodial disk
amphiarthrosis
amphotericin B
ampicillin and sulbactam
ampicillin/sulbactam
Amplatz anchor system
amplitude
high velocity/low a.
amplitude-summation
a.-s. interferential current
a.-s. interferential current therapy (ASICT)
Ampoxen sling
amputation
above-elbow a.
above-knee a. (AKA)
AE a.
Alanson a.
Alouette a.
Beclard a.
below-elbow a.
below-knee a. (BKA)
Berger interscapular a.
Bier a.
bilateral a.
border ray a.
Boyd ankle a.
Bunge a.
Burgess below-knee a.
button toe a.
Callander a.
central ray a.
chop a.
Chopart hindfoot a.

circular open a.
circular supracondylar a.
closed a.
closed-flap a.
complete a.
congenital above-elbow a.
congenital below-elbow a.
corporectomy a.
digital a.
disarticular a.
femoral head a.
fingertip a.
fishmouth a.
forearm a.
forefoot digital a.
forequarter a.
Gordon-Taylor hindquarter a.
Gritti-Stokes a.
guillotine a.
hand a.
hindquarter a.
incomplete a.
index-ray a.
interilioabdominal a.
interinnominoabdominal a.
interpelviabdominal a.
interphalangeal a.
interscapular a.
interscapulothoracic a.
Jaboulay a.
King-Steelquist hindquarter a.
Kirk distal thigh a.
a. knife
Lisfranc a.
lower-extremity a. (LEA)
McKittrick transmetatarsal a.
middle-finger a.
midthigh a.
multiple-ray a.
nonreplantable a.
one-stage a.
open a.
Pirogoff a.
ray a.
replantable a.
a. retractor
a. saw
shoulder a.
Sorondo-Ferré hindquarter a.
a. stump
a. stump neuroma
supracondylar a.

supramalleolar open a.
Syme ankle disarticulation a.
tarsal a.
tarsometatarsal a.
through-knee a.
toe a.
transcarpal a.
transcondylar a.
transfemoral a.
transiliac a.
translumbar a.
transmetatarsal a. (TMA)
transpelvic a.
transtibial a.
traumatic a.
two-stage Syme a.
Wagner modification of Syme a.
Wagner two-stage Syme a.

amputee cushion
AMREX
    AMREX muscle stimulator
    AMREX therapeutic ultrasound
AMS
  antimigration system
    AMS intramedullary fixation
Amset
    A. ALPS
    A. ALPS anterior locking plate
      system
    A. R-F fixation system
    A. R-F rod
    A. R-F screw
Amspacher-Messenbaugh
    A.-M. closing wedge osteotomy
    A.-M. technique
Amstutz
    A. cemented hip prosthesis
    A. femoral component
    A. reattachment
    A. resurfacing
    A. resurfacing technique
    A. total hip replacement
Amstutz-Wilson osteotomy
AMT
  active motion testing
amyloid
amyloidosis
amyoplasia congenita
amyotonia congenita
amyotrophic lateral sclerosis (ALS, AML)

NOTES

amyotrophy
Aran-Duchenne a.
Amytal
ANA
antinuclear antibody
anabolic steroid
Anacin
anaerobe
anaerobic
a. bacteria
a. cellulitis
a. exercise
a. infection
a. osteomyelitis
a. threshold (AT)
Anafranil
anal
a. reflex
a. triangle
a. wink
analgesia
patient-controlled a. (PCA)
analog
visual a. scale (VAS)
analogous signal detector
analysis
activity a.
activity-pattern a.
bioelectrical impedance a. (BIA)
biomechanical a.
carbohydrate a.
chiropractic a.
computerized musculoskeletal a.
deformity a.
EMED gait a.
footprint a.
force plate foot a.
Fourier a.
frequency a.
gait a.
a. of gait
high-resolution a.
Kaplan-Meier a.
Khan-Lewis phonological a.
lateral flexion dynamic visual a.
Mann-Whitney a.
muscle a.
occipital-fiber a.
peak-pressure a.
plumb-line a.
postural a.
roentgenstereophotogrammetric a.
spinal a.
three-dimensional a.
trapezius fiber a.
a. of variance (ANOVA)
video-dimensional a. (VDA)
video-gate a.

analyzer
CA-6000 spine motion a.
Futrex body fat a.
Metrecom spinal a.
Nordotrack motion a.
Stride A.
Tanita Professional Body
Composition A.
Anametric
A. total knee prosthesis
A. total knee system
anaphylaxis
latex a.
Anaprox DS
anastomosis, pl. anastomoses
end-to-end a. (EEA)
end-to-side a.
end-weave a.
fishmouth a.
flexor tendon a.
Ma-Griffith end-to-end a.
Ma-Griffith tendon a.
Martin-Gruber a.
microvascular surgical a.
Riche-Cannieu a.
side-to-side a.
anatomic
a. alignment
a. axis
a. barrier
a. fracture reduction principle
a. hook
a. insertion
a. intermetatarsal angle
a. leg length inequality
a. location of fracture
a. medullary locking (AML)
a. medullary locking hip system
a. modular knee (AMK)
a. plane
porous-coated a. (PCA)
a. porous replacement (APR)
A. Precoat hip prosthesis
a. short leg
a. snuffbox
a. surface prosthesis
anatomical
a. classification system of Severin
a. vertical
**anatomically graduated component
(AGC)**
anatomopathological study
anatomy
cervicothoracic pedicle a.
Daseler-Anson classification of
plantaris muscle a.
designed after natural a. (DANA)
dorsalis pedis artery a.

knee a.
neurovascular a.
pedicle a.

Ancef
anchor
BioRoc a.
BioSphere suture a.
E-Z ROC a.
FastIn threaded a.
a. hole
Isola spinal implant system a.
Mitek a.
Panalok absorbable a.
a. plate
Revo suture a.
ROC a.
a. screw
a. splint
suture a.
Tacit threaded a.
Therap-Loop door a.

anchorage-dependent growth
anchoring
a. hole
a. peg
a. point
a. tendon

Anchorlok soft tissue suture anchor
system
anchovy
a. procedure
tensor fasciae latae a.

ancillary muscle group
anconeal
anconeus
anconoid
Anderson
A. acetabular prosthesis
A. ankle fusion
A. distractor
A. fixation apparatus
A. fixation device
A. leg lengthening apparatus
A. leg lengthening device
A. modification of Berndt-Harty
classification
A. screw placement technique
A. splint
A. system
A. tibial pseudarthrosis
classification
A. traction

Anderson-D'Alonzo odontoid fracture
classification
Anderson-Fowler
A.-F. anterior calcaneal osteotomy
pes planus
A.-F. calcaneal displacement
osteotomy
A.-F. procedure
Anderson-Green growth prediction
Anderson-Hutchins
A.-H. technique
A.-H. unstable tibial shaft fracture
andersoni
Dermacentor a.
Anderson-Neivert osteotome
Andersson hip status system
André anatomical hook
Andrews
A. gouge
A. iliotibial band reconstruction
A. iliotibial band tenodesis
A. lateral tenodesis
A. osteotome
A. spinal surgery frame
A. SST-3000 spinal surgery table
A. technique
anecdotal procedure
anemia
blood loss a.
sickle-cell a.
anergy
aneroid gauge
anes
anesthesia
Anestacon
anesthesia (anes)
ankle-block a.
Bier block a.
continuous intravenous regional a.
(CIVRA)
digital-block a.
epidural a.
gauntlet a.
general endotracheal a.
graded spinal a.
hypotensive a.
inhalant a.
inhalation a.
intrathecal a.
intravenous block a.
intravenous regional a. (IVRA)
local a.

NOTES

anesthesia *(continued)*
    lumbar a.
    MAC a.
    Madajet XL local a.
    Mayo block a.
    patient-controlled a. (PCA)
    peripheral nerve block a.
    regional a.
    ring block a.
    saddle-block a.
    short-acting block a. (SAB)
    spinal a.
    supraclavicular brachial block a.
    tactile a.
    thermal a.
    toe-block a.
anesthesiologist
anesthetic
aneurysm
    arterial a.
    brachial artery a.
    Charcot-Bouchard intracerebral a.
    clavicular fracture a.
    false a. (FA)
    mycotic a.
aneurysmal bone cyst (ABC)
Anexsia
Angell
    A. James dissector
    A. James hypophysectomy forceps
angel wing guide
Anghelescu sign
angioblastoma
Angiocath
    14-gauge A.
angiodysplasia
angioendotheliomatosis
angiofibroblastic
    a. hyperplasia tendinosis
    a. proliferation
angiofibroma
angiogram
    biplane a.
angiography
    bypass graft a.
    coronary a.
    digital subtraction a. (DSA)
angiokeratoma
angioleiomyoma
angiolipoma
angioma
    cirsoid a.
    a. serpiginosum
angiomatoid malignant fibrous
  histiocytoma (AMFH)
angiomatosis
    skeletal-extraskeletal a.
angiosarcoma

angiospasm
angiotropic lymphoma
angle
    acetabular a.
    acromial a.
    anatomic intermetatarsal a.
    antegonial a.
    anteroposterior talocalcaneal a.
     (APTC)
    antetorsion a.
    a. of anteversion
    arch a.
    articular facet a.
    Baumann a.
    Beatson combined ankle a.
    bimalleolar a.
    Böhler calcaneal a.
    Böhler lumbosacral a.
    Bowman a.
    C a.
    calcaneal inclination a.
    calcaneal-second metatarsal angle
     inclination a.
    calcaneoplantar a.
    calcaneotibial a.
    capital epiphyseal a.
    capitolunate a.
    carrying a.
    CCD a.
    CE a.
    center-edge a.
    central collodiaphyseal a. (CCD)
    cervicothoracic pedicle a.
    Citelli a.
    Clarke arch a.
    Cobb lumbar a.
    Cobb scoliosis a.
    Codman a.
    condylar a.
    congruence a.
    a. of convergence
    costal a.
    costolumbar a.
    costophrenic a.
    costosternal a.
    costovertebral a. (CVA)
    craniofacial a.
    declination a.
    a. of declination of metatarsal
    distal articular set a. (DASA)
    distal metatarsal articular a.
    a. of divergence
    DMA a.
    dorsoplantar talometatarsal a.
    dorsoplantar talonavicular a.
    Drennan metaphyseal-epiphyseal a.
    Engel a.
    Eulerian a.

facet a.
femoral-trunk a.
femorotibial a. (FTA)
Ferguson sacral base a.
a. finder
first-fifth intermetatarsal a.
first-second intermetatarsal a.
flexion a.
foot a.
foot-progression a.
Fowler-Philip a.
functional intermetatarsal a.
a. of gait
Garden a.
Glissane crucial a.
gonial a.
a. of greatest extension (AGE)
a. of greatest flexion (AGF)
hallux dorsiflexion a. (DFA)
hallux valgus a. (HVA)
hallux valgus interphalangeus a.
Hibbs metatarsocalcaneal a.
Hilgenreiner a.
hip joint a. (HJA)
humeral-ulnar a.
inclination a.
a. of incongruity
increased carrying a.
inferior a.
intermetatarsal a. (IM, IMA)
intermetatarsal a. I or II
intrascaphoid a.
a. isometric testing
Kite a.
Konstram a.
lateral deviation a.
lateral plantar metatarsal a.
lateral talocalcaneal a. (LATC)
lateral tarsometatarsal a.
Laurin a.
Lisfranc articular set a. (LASA)
lumbosacral joint a.
mandibular a.
a. of Mary
Meary metatarsotalar a.
mediolateral rediocarpal a.
Merchant congruence a.
metaphyseal-diaphyseal a.
metaphyseal-epiphyseal a.
metatarsal phalangeal fifth a.
metatarsocalcaneal a.
metatarsotalar a.

metatarsus adductus a.
metatarsus primus a.
Mikulicz a.
navicular to first metatarsal a.
neck-shaft a.
negative congruence a.
neutral a.
occipitocervical a.
Pauwels a.
pedicle axis a.
pelvic a.
pelvic-femoral a.
physeal a.
plantar metatarsal a.
proximal articular facet a.
proximal articular set a. (PASA)
Q a.
quadriceps a. (Q angle)
radiocarpal a.
resting forefoot supination a.
rib-vertebral a.
sacral base a.
sacrofemoral a.
sacrohorizontal a.
sacrovertebral a.
sagittal pedicle a.
salient a.
scapholunate a.
set a.
Sharp acetabular a.
slip a.
Southwick lateral slip a.
spinographic a.
a. splint
sulcus a.
talar axis-first MT base a. (TAMBA)
talar-tilt a.
talocalcaneal a.
talocrural a.
talometatarsal a.
talonavicular a.
tarsometatarsal a.
thigh-foot a.
a. of thoracic inclination
tibiofemoral a. (TFA)
tibiotalar a.
TMA-thigh a.
toe-out a.
Toygar a.
transverse pedicle a.
tuber a.

NOTES

angle *(continued)*
    tuber-joint a.
    ulnar-humeral a.
    valgus a.
    varus MTP a.
    Wiberg center edge a.
    Wiltze a.
angled
    a. arthroscope
    a. awl
    a. bearing insert
    a. blade plate fixation
    a. DeBakey clamp
    a.-down forceps
    a. jaw rongeur
    a. pituitary rongeur
    a. probe
    a. rasp
    a. Scoville curette
    a. showerhead lavage
    a.-up forceps
angular
    a. acceleration
    a. alignment
    a. bone rongeur
    a. deformity
    a. deviation
    a. displacement
    a. momentum
    a. motion
    a. osteotomy
    a. position
    a. process of orbit
    a. tilt
    a. velocity
angulated fracture
angulation
    anterior a.
    apex dorsal a.
    cephalic a.
    a. deformity
    degrees of valgus a.
    degrees of varus a.
    forefoot a.
    a. fracture
    kyphotic a.
    limb length a.
    a. motion
    a. osteotomy
    plantar a.
    posttraumatic a.
    radius of a.
    screw a.
    spinal a.
    valgus a.
    varus-valgus a.
angulatory malunion
Angus-Cowell scale

anhidrosis, anidrosis
anhydrous ethanol
animal beanbag exerciser
anisomelia
anisotropic
anisotropy
anitratus
    Acinetobacter a.
Ank-L-Aid brace
ankle
    a.-arm blood pressure index
    a.-arm ischemic index
    a. arthrodesis
    a. arthroplasty
    autologous reverse graft to a.
    a. block
    a.-block anesthesia
    a. clonus
    a. contracture orthosis
    C Stance a.
    a. dorsiflexion range of motion (ADROM)
    a. dorsiflexion test
    eccentric axis of rotation of the a.
    a. equinus
    a. eversion
    a. exercise machine
    a. exerciser
    football a.
    a. foot orthosis brace sock
    a. fusion
    a.-hindfoot scale
    a. hitch
    a. immobilizer
    a. injury
    instability of the a.
    a. instability
    internal fixation compression arthrodesis of the a.
    a. inversion-eversion range of motion
    a. jerk (AJ)
    a. jerk reflex test
    a. joint complex (AJC)
    a. joint leg-curl
    a. laxity
    a.-level arteriotomy
    A. Ligament protector
    a. ligament protector (ALP)
    a. ligament protector brace
    a. magnet
    medial ligament of a.
    a. mortise
    a. mortise diastasis
    a. mortise fracture
    Multi Axis A.
    Nélaton dislocation of a.
    neuropathic a.

a. orthosis (AO)
pronation-eversion-external rotation
   injury of a.
a. prosthesis
a.-pump exercise
a. reflex
a. rehab pump
R-HAB lighter weight a.
Rincoe human action bionic a. (R-
   HAB)
a. stabilizer
syndesmosis sprain of a.
synthetic graft bypass to a.
a. systolic pressure
tailor's a.
a. traction bandage
transmalleolar a.
USMC multi axis a.
Wiltse osteotomy of a.

ankle-brachial
   a.-b. blood pressure index
   a.-b. index (ABI)
   a.-b. pressure ratio

ankle-foot
   a.-f. orthosis (AFO)
   a.-f. orthotic (AFO)
   a.-f. orthotic splint
   a.-f. plastic orthosis

Ankle-Foot Elgon electrogoniometer
AnkleTough
   A. ankle rehabilitation system
   A. Rehab System

ankylodactyly
ankylose
ankylosing
   a. spinal hyperostosis
   a. spinal stenosis
   a. spondylitis

ankylosis
   bony a.
   carpal bone fracture a.
   extraarticular a.
   extracapsular a.
   false a.
   fibrous a.
   intracapsular a.
   ligamentous a.
   shoulder a.
   spurious a.
   vertebral a.

anlage
   cartilaginous a.

fibular a.
a. a priori
radial head a.
ulnar a.

ANNA-DOTE Positioning Support
Ann Arbor double towel clamp
anneal
annealed
annular, anular
   congenital a. band
   a. constricting band syndrome
   a. fiber
   a. fibrosis
   a. groove
   a. injury
   a. ligament
   a. ligament of radius
   a. periradial recess

annulare
   subcutaneous granuloma a.

annularis
   limbus a.

annulospiral ending of muscle spindle
annulotomy
annulus, anulus
   a. fibrosus

anodal block
anode
Anodynos-DHC
anomalous
   a. fibular nutrient artery
   a. insertion

anomaly
   congenital a.
   facet a.
   hand a.
   Kimerle a.
   root a.

anonychia
anopsia
   altitudinal a.

anoscope
ANOVA
   analysis of variance

anoxia
ANS
   autonomic nervous system

Ansaid Oral
anserine bursitis
anserinus
   pes a.

NOTES

Anspach
  A. Cement Eater
  A. cementome
  A. 65K Universal instrument
    system
  A. power drill
  A. reamer
ant
  anterior
    ant ax line (AAL)
antagonist
  a. muscle
  opiate receptor a.
  reversal of a. (ROA)
antagonistic muscle
antalgic
  a. gait
  a. lean
anteater-nose sign
antebrachial
  a. cutaneous nerve
  a. fascia
  a. fascial graft
antecedent sign
antecubital fossa
antegonial angle
antegrade
  a. method
  a. nailing
antenatal dislocation
antenna procedure
Antense anti-tension device
anterior (ant)
  a. acromioplasty
  a. acromioplasty approach
  a. acute flexion elbow splint
  a. angulation
  a. ankle impingement
  a. aspiration
  a. atlantooccipital membrane
  a. atlantoodontoid interval
  a. axillary approach
  a. axillary line (AAL)
  a. bending moment
  a. calcaneal osteotomy
  a. calcaneal process fracture
  a. capsule
  a. capsulolabral reconstruction
    (ACLR)
  a. cervical body fusion
  a. cervical cord syndrome
  a. cervical diskectomy and fusion
    (ACDF)
  a. cervical fascia
  a. cervical fusion (ACF)
  a. cervical plate (ACP)
  a. cervical spine surgery

a. cervical surgery vocal cord
  damage
a. cervicothoracic junction surgery
a. collateral ligament
a. column disruption
a. column fracture
a. column osteosynthesis
a. compartment
a. compartment syndrome (ACS)
a. construct
a. cord compression
a. cord impingement
a. corpectomy
a. correction
a. cortex penetration
a. cruciate
a. cruciate deficit knee
a. cruciate instability with pivot
  shift
a. cruciate ligament (ACL)
a. cruciate ligament of knee
a. distraction instrumentation
a. drainage
a. drawer sign
a. drawer stress radiograph
a. drawer test (ADT)
a. epineurotomy
a. extensile approach
a. fiber-region
a. forceps
a. glenoid labrum
a. glide
a. heel
a. hip dislocation
a. hip release
a. horn
a. horn cell
a. horn meniscal tear
a. humeral line
a. iliofemoral technique
a. impingement syndrome
a. inferior iliac spine (AIIS)
a. innominate
a. innominate rotation
a. instability
a. internal fixation
a. internal fixation device
a. interosseous nerve syndrome
a. jugular vein
a. Kostuik-Harrington distraction
  system
a. kyphosis
a. labrum periosteum shoulder
  arthroscopic lesion (ALPSA)
a. ligament of head of fibula
a. locking plate system (ALPS)
a. longitudinal ligament (ALL)
a. long toe flexor

a. lower cervical spine surgery
a. lumbar interbody fusion
a. lumbar vertebral interbody fusion
a. margin
a. meniscofemoral ligament
a. metallic fixation
a. myocutaneous flap
a. neutralization
a. oblique ligament (AOL)
a. oblique meniscal tear
a. occipitocervical arthrodesis
a. occipitocervical spine
a. pelvic tilt
a. plate fixation
a. plate system (APS)
a. portal
a. and posterior (AP)
a. and posterior fusion
a. pronator teres
a. quadriceps musculocutaneous flap technique
a. quadrilateral triplane frame
a. radial collateral artery
a. recurrent tibial artery
a. retroperitoneal decompression
a. retroperitoneal flank approach
a. rotary drawer test
a. sacrococcygeal ligament
a. sacroiliac joint plate
a. sacroiliac ligament
a. scalene muscle
a. screw fixation
a. serratus muscle
a. shear
a. short-segment stabilization
a. shoulder dislocation
a. shoulder release
a. sliding tibial graft
a. slot graft arthrodesis
a. soft tissue impingement
a. spinal artery
a. spinal fixation
a. spinal fusion
a. spinal plating
a. spurring
a. stabilization procedure
a. sternoclavicular joint
a. sternomastoid approach
a. superior iliac spine (ASIS)
a. surgical exposure
a. talofibular ligament (ATFL)

a. talofibular ligament rupture
a. talus shift
a. tarsal tunnel syndrome
a. thoracic nerve
a. tibial artery
tibialis a.
a. tibial muscle
a. tibial sign
a. tibial syndrome
a. tibial tendon
a. tibiofibular ligament
a. tibiotalar ligament
a. transfer
a. translation
a. transthoracic approach
a. triangle
a. upper spine
a. Zielke instrumentation
anteriora
ligamenta sacroiliaca a.
anterior-inferior
a.-i. capsular ligament dysfunction
a.-i. dislocation
a.-i. movement
anterior-posterior
a.-p. compression (APC)
a.-p. fusion with SSI
a.-p. glide
a.-p. listhesis
a.-p. movement
anterius
ligamentum capitis fibulae a.
ligamentum longitudinale a.
ligamentum meniscofemorale a.
ligamentum sacrococcygeum a.
ligamentum talofibulare a.
ligamentum tibiofibulare a.
anterocentral portal
anterodistal
anteroinferior
a. portal
a. spondylolisthesis
anterolateral
a. approach
a. capsule
a. compression fracture
a. decompression
a. dislocation
a. drainage
a. femorotibial ligament tenodesis
a. portal
a. raphe

NOTES

anterolateral *(continued)*
    a. release
    a. rotary instability (ALRI)
    a. rotary knee instability
    a. sclerosis (ALS)
    a. ventricular opening (ALVO)
anterolateral-anteromedial rotary instability
anterolisthesis
anteromedial
    a. bundle
    a. capsule
    a. drainage
    a. incision
    a. portal
    a. retropharyngeal approach
    a. rotary instability
    a. tubercle transfer
anteromedial-posteromedial rotary instability
anteroposterior (AP)
    a. compression (APC)
    a. stress test
    a. sway
    a. talocalcaneal angle (APTC)
    a. talocalcaneal divergence
    a. tilt
    a. translation
anteroposterior/lateral sway
anteroproximal
anterosuperior (AS)
    a. external ilium movement (ASEx)
    a. iliac spine (ASIS)
    a. iliac spine graft
    a. ilium major
    a. internal ilium movement (ASIn)
antetorsion
    a. angle
    femoral a.
anteversion
    angle of a.
    a. determination
    femoral a.
    Magilligan technique for measuring a.
    neutral a.
    a. syndrome
anthropometric
    a. measuring tape
    a. method
    a. total hip (ATH)
anthropometry
antibacterial pillow
antibiosis
antibiotic
    a. bead pouch
    postoperative a.
    preoperative a.

    prophylactic a.
    a. and saline solution
antibiotic-impregnated
    a.-i. bead
    a.-i. polymethyl methacrylate (PMMA)
antibody
    AE1, AE3 a.
    antihistocompatibility a.
    antinuclear a. (ANA)
anticavitation drill
anticentromere
anticholinergic effect
anticipating financial compensation (AFC)
anticoagulant
    lupus a.
    a. therapy
anticoagulation
    prophylactic a.
anticonvulsant therapy
antidecubitus
    a. mattress
    a. pad
antidepressant
    tricyclic a.
antidromic stimulation
antiembolic
    a. position
    a. stockings
antifungal (AF)
    Absorbine Jr. A.
    Breezee Mist A.
antigen
    antiproliferating cell nuclear a.
    carcinoembryonic a. (CEA)
    epithelial membrane a. (EEMA)
    a.-extracted allogeneic (AAA)
    a.-extracted allogeneic bone (AAA bone)
    HLA-B27 blood a.
    human leukocyte a. (HLA)
    human lymphocyte a. (HLA)
    transplantation a.
antiglide plate
antigravity (AG)
antihistocompatibility antibody
antihypouricemic
antiinflammatory medication
antimalarial
antimicrobial benzalkonium chloride
antimigration system (AMS)
antinociceptive effect
antinuclear
    a. antibody (ANA)
    a. antibody test
antiosteoclastic agent
antiparkinsonism

antiplatelet drug
antiproliferating cell nuclear antigen
antipyretic agent
antiretroviral
antirotation
>   a. cable (ARC)
>   a. device

antiseptic
>   ACU-dyne a.
>   colored a.

Antishear gel sheet
antishock garment
Anti-Shox
>   A.-S. foot cushion
>   A.-S. heel cup
>   A.-S. orthosis
>   A.-S. orthotic

antistreptolysin-O titer (ASOT)
antitension line
antithrombin III
antithrombotic therapy
antithrust seat
antitipper wheelchair
antitoxin
antituberculosis drug
antivibration glove
Anturane
anular (*var. of* annular)
anulus (*var. of* annulus)
anvil
>   Bunnell a.
>   a. sign
>   a. test

Anxanil
any-angle splint
AO
>   ankle orthosis
>   Arbeitsgemeinschaft für
>   osteosynthesefragen
>   atlantooccipital
>   AO blade plate
>   AO brace
>   AO cancellous screw
>   AO classification
>   AO classification of ankle fracture
>   AO compression
>   AO compression apparatus
>   AO condylar blade plate
>   AO contoured T plate
>   AO contouring apparatus

>   AO cortex screw
>   AO-Denis-Weber classification of
>   ankle fracture
>   AO drill bit
>   AO dynamic compression plate
>   AO dynamic compression plate
>   construct
>   AO external fixation
>   AO femoral distractor
>   AO fixateur interne
>   AO fixateur interne instrumentation
>   AO group
>   AO group shoulder arthrodesis
>   AO guidepin
>   AO hook plate
>   AO internal fixator
>   AO lag screw
>   AO minifragment set
>   AO notched instrumentation
>   AO plate bender
>   AO procedure
>   AO pseudoisochromatic color plate
>   test
>   AO reconstruction plate
>   AO reduction forceps
>   AO semitubular plate
>   AO slotted medullary nail
>   AO small fragment plate
>   AO spinal internal fixation
>   AO spongiosa screw
>   AO spoon plate
>   AO-stopped drill guide
>   AO tap
>   AO technique
>   AO tension band

AOA
>   AOA cervical immobilization brace
>   AOA halo cervical traction

AO-ASIF, AO/ASIF
>   AO-ASIF compression plate
>   AO-ASIF compression technique
>   AO-ASIF fixateur interne
>   AO-ASIF orthopaedic implant
>   AO-ASIF screw

AOFAS
>   American Orthopaedic Foot and Ankle
>   Society

AOL
>   anterior oblique ligament

NOTES

AOPA
American Orthotic and Prosthetic
Association
aorta, pl. aortae
aortic stenosis (AS)
AP
action potential
anterior and posterior
anteroposterior
AP fusion
AP translatory motion
Apacet
APB
all-purpose boot
APC
anterior-posterior compression
anteroposterior compression
A-P cutter
APD
automated percutaneous diskectomy
ape hand
apelike hand
Apert
A. disease
A. syndrome
aperture
apex, pl. apices
A. ambulator
A. ambulator shoe
a. dorsal angulation
A. Energetics
a. of head of patella
A. insole
A. pin
A. Universal Drive and Irrigation
System
a. vertebra
Apfelbaum mirror
aphalangia
congenital a.
apical
a. corn
a. dental ligament
a. distraction
a. lordotic view
a. segment
a. vertebra
apices (*pl. of* apex)
APL
αa₂-plasmin inhibitor
APLD
automated percutaneous lumbar
diskectomy
Apley
A. compression test
A. distraction test
A. exam
A. grinding test

A. scratch test
A. sign
A. traction
apodia
Apofix cervical instrumentation
Apollo
A. hot/cold Pak
A. TM electric flexion table
A. total knee system
aponeurosis
adductor a.
digital a.
meniscal a.
palmar a.
plantar a.
quadriceps a.
a. of tendon
aponeurotic
a. band
a. fibroma
a. lengthening
a. tendon
a. triangle
a. troika
aponeurotomy
apophyseal
a. fracture
a. joint
apophysis, pl. apophyses
iliac a.
medial epicondylar a.
slipped vertebral a.
spinal process a.
vertebral ring a.
apophysitis
calcaneal a.
iliac a.
apoplexy
delayed a.
posttraumatic a.
APOPPS
adjustable postoperative protective
prosthetic socket
apparatus
Ace Unifix fixation a.
adjustable aiming a.
Anderson fixation a.
Anderson leg lengthening a.
AO compression a.
AO contouring a.
Axer compression a.
Bassett electrical stimulation a.
Bovie electrocautery a.
Buck convoluted traction a.
Calandruccio compression a.
Calandruccio triangular
compression a.
Cameron fracture a.

Charnley centering a.
compression a.
coracoclavicular fixation a.
coring a.
CPM a.
DeWald spinal a.
Deyerle fixation a.
driver tunnel locator a.
electrocautery a.
electronic bone stimulation a.
external skeletal fixation a.
fixating a.
four-bar external fixation a.
Fox internal fixation a.
Georgiade visor halo fixation a.
Giliberty a.
halo vest a.
Hamilton a.
Hare a.
Hoffmann-Vidal external fixation a.
Ilizarov a.
internal fixation a.
isokinetic joint a.
Kinetron muscle strengthening a.
Kronner external fixation a.
Küntscher traction a.
leg-holding a.
McLaughlin osteosynthesis a.
Mueller compression a.
nail plate a.
Nauth traction a.
Neufeld a.
optoelectric measuring a.
optoelectric signal detection a.
Orthofix a.
Parham-Martin fracture a.
Philips Angiodiagnostics 96 a.
Quengel a.
Rancho anklet foot control a.
Redi-Trac traction a.
Rezaian external fixation a.
rod-mounted targeting a.
Roger Anderson external fixation a.
snap-fit a.
Southwick pin-holding a.
Sutter-CPM knee a.
Telectronics electrical stimulation a.
Traumafix a.
triplanar protractor a.
Ultrafix a.
Vidal-Adrey modified Hoffman
  external fixation device a.

Volkov-Oganesian external
  fixation a.
Volkov-Oganesian-Povarov hinged
  distraction a.
Wagner external fixation a.
Wagner leg-lengthening a.
Wagner-Schanz screw a.
Zickel medullary a.
Zickel supracondylar fixation a.
Zimmer electrical stimulation a.

appearance
crabmeat-like a.
horseshoe a.
spongy a.

appendage clamp
appendiceal retractor
appendicular
Applause Super-Hemi wheelchair
appliance (*See* device, orthosis)
DeWald spinal a.
Jobst a.

application
cast a.
cold a.
diversified-type force a.
force a.
frame a.
Harrington rod instrumentation
  force a.
heat a.
ice a.
Isola spinal implant system a.
Kumar a.
paraspinal rod a.
traction a.
a. of traction device
transverse fixator a.

applicator
HEX heat a.
infrared a.

applied
a. kinesiology (AK)
a. load

applier
bayonet clip a.
bulldog clamp a.
clip a.
Ligaclip a.
Mayfield miniature clip a.
Mayfield temporary aneurysm
  clip a.
mini a.

NOTES

applier *(continued)*
    surgical staple a.
    vari-angle clip a.
apponensplasty
    ring sublimis a.
apposing articular surface
apposition
    axonal a.
    bayonet a.
    bone-to-bone a.
    facet a.
apprehension
    a. shoulder
    a. sign
    a. test
apprentice kyphosis
approach
    Abbott-Carpenter posterior a.
    Abbott knee a.
    acetabular extensile a.
    anterior acromioplasty a.
    anterior axillary a.
    anterior extensile a.
    anterior retroperitoneal flank a.
    anterior sternomastoid a.
    anterior transthoracic a.
    anterolateral a.
    anteromedial retropharyngeal a.
    axillary a.
    Bailey-Badgley anterior cervical a.
    Banks-Laufman a.
    Bennett posterior shoulder a.
    Berger-Bookwalter posterior a.
    bilateral ilioinguinal a.
    bilateral sacroiliac a.
    Bosworth a.
    Boyd a.
    Boyd-Sisk a.
    Brackett-Osgood knee a.
    Brackett-Osgood posterior a.
    Brodsky-Tullos-Gartsman a.
    Broomhead medial a.
    Brown knee a.
    Brown lateral a.
    Bruner a.
    Bruser knee a.
    Bruser lateral a.
    Bryan-Morrey elbow a.
    Bryan-Morrey extensive posterior a.
    Callahan a.
    Campbell elbow a.
    Campbell posterior shoulder a.
    Campbell posterolateral a.
    Carnesale acetabular extensile a.
    Carnesale hip a.
    Cave hip a.
    Cave knee a.
    cervical a.
    Cloward cervical disk a.
    Codman saber-cut shoulder a.
    Colonna-Ralston ankle a.
    Colonna-Ralston medial a.
    combined anterior and posterior a.
    combined low-cervical and
      transthoracic a.
    Coonse-Adams knee a.
    costotransversectomy a.
    Cubbins shoulder a.
    curved a.
    Darrach-McLaughlin a.
    deltoid-splitting shoulder a.
    deltopectoral a.
    Dickinson a.
    distal interphalangeal joint a.
    dorsal finger a.
    dorsal midline a.
    dorsalward a.
    dorsolateral a.
    dorsomedial a.
    dorsoplantar a.
    dorsoradial a.
    dorsorostral a.
    dorsoulnar a.
    Duran a.
    DuVries a.
    extended iliofemoral a.
    extensile a.
    extrabursal a.
    extraperitoneal a.
    extrapharyngeal a.
    Fahey a.
    Fernandez extensile anterior a.
    Fowler-Philip a.
    Gatellier-Chastang ankle a.
    Gatellier-Chastang posterolateral a.
    Gibson a.
    Gordon a.
    Guleke-Stookey a.
    Hardinge femoral a.
    Hardinge lateral a.
    Harmon cervical a.
    Harmon modified posterolateral a.
    Harmon posterolateral a.
    Harmon shoulder a.
    Harris anterolateral a.
    Harris lateral a.
    Hay lateral a.
    Henderson posterolateral a.
    Henderson posteromedial a.
    Henry anterior strap a.
    Henry anterolateral a.
    Henry extensile a.
    Henry posterior interosseous
      nerve a.
    Henry radial a.
    Hirschhorn compression a.

Hoffmann a.
Hoppenfeld-Deboer a.
Howorth a.
iliofemoral a.
ilioinguinal acetabular a.
inguinal a.
intraforaminal a.
ipsilateral a.
keyhole a.
Kikuchi-MacNap-Moreau a.
Kocher curved L a.
Kocher-Gibson posterolateral a.
Kocher-Langenbeck a.
Kocher lateral J a.
Koenig-Schaefer medial a.
lateral deltoid splitting a.
lateral Gatellier-Chastung a.
lateral J a.
lateral Kocher a.
lateral Ollier a.
lateral parapatellar a.
Lazepen-Gamidov anteromedial a.
Leslie-Ryan anterior axillary a.
Letournel-Judet a.
long deltopectoral a.
low cervical a.
Ludloff medial a.
Mayo a.
McAfee a.
McConnell extensile a.
McConnell median and ulnar
   nerve a.
McFarland-Osborne lateral a.
McLaughlin a.
McWhorter posterior shoulder a.
Mears-Rubash a.
medial parapatellar capsular a.
midlateral a.
midline medial a.
Minkoff-Jaffe-Menendez posterior a.
Mize-Bucholz-Grogen a.
Molesworth-Campbell elbow a.
Moore posterior a.
Moore-Southern a.
neurodevelopmental a.
Ollier arthrodesis a.
Ollier lateral a.
oropharyngeal a.
Osborne posterior a.
palmar a.
paramedian a.
pararectus a.

paraspinal a.
patella turndown a.
Perry extensile anterior a.
Pfannenstiel transverse a.
plantar a.
Pogrund lateral a.
posterior costotransversectomy a.
posterior inverted U a.
posterior midline a.
posterior occipitocervical a.
posterior transolecranon a.
posterolateral a.
posteromedial a.
proprioceptive neuromuscular
   facilitation a.
proximal interphalangeal joint a.
proximal metatarsal a.
pulp a.
Putti posterior a.
Reinert acetabular extensile a.
retroperitoneal a.
retropharyngeal a.
Roberts a.
Roos a.
Rowe posterior shoulder a.
saber-cut a.
sacral a.
screw-plate a.
Senegas hip a.
sensorimotor stimulation a.
Smith-Petersen a.
Smith-Petersen-Cave-Van Gorder
   anterolateral a.
Smith-Robinson cervical disk a.
Somerville anterior a.
Southwick-Robinson anterior
   cervical a.
Spetzler anterior transoral a.
split-heel a.
split patellar a.
stabilization a.
sternum-splitting a.
subclavicular a.
supraclavicular a.
surgical a.
Swedish a.
Thompson anterolateral a.
Thompson anteromedial a.
Thompson posterior radial a.
thoracic a.
thoracoabdominal a.
thoracolumbar retroperitoneal a.

NOTES

approach *(continued)*
    thoracotomy a.
    thumb metacarpophalangeal joint a.
    transacromial a.
    transaxillary a.
    transbrachioradialis a.
    transcalcaneal a.
    transclavicular a.
    transfibular a.
    transolecranon a.
    transoral a.
    transpedicular a.
    transperitoneal a.
    transsternal a.
    transthoracic a.
    transtrochanteric a.
    transverse a.
    triradiate acetabular extensile a.
    triradiate transtrochanteric a.
    unilateral sacroiliac a.
    volar finger a.
    volar midline a.
    volar radial a.
    volar ulnar a.
    volarward a.
    Wadsworth elbow a.
    Wadsworth posterolateral a.
    Wagner a.
    Wagoner posterior a.
    Watson-Jones anterior a.
    Watson-Jones lateral a.
    Wiltberger anterior cervical a.
    Wiltse a.
    Wiltse-Spencer paraspinal a.
    Yee posterior shoulder a.
    zigzag a.
    Z-plasty a.
approximation
approximator
    Acland clamp a.
    Acland double-clamp a.
    Bruni-Wayne clamp a.
    Bunke-Schulz clamp a.
    clamp a.
    double-clamp a.
    Henderson clamp a.
    hook a.
    Ikuta clamp a.
    Iwashi clamp a.
    Kleinert-Kutz clamp a.
    Lalonde tendon a.
    Lemmon sternal a.
    rib a.
    sternal a.
    Van Beek nerve a.
APR
    anatomic porous replacement
    APR acetabular prosthesis

    APR cement fixation
    APR cement fixation adhesive
    APR femoral prosthesis
    APR hip stem
    APR I femoral stem
    APR II hip system
    APR II prosthesis
    APR total hip system
apraxia
apraxic gait
Aprema III device
APRL
    Army Prosthetics Research Laboratory
    APRL hand prosthesis
    APRL prosthetic hook
apron
    quadriceps a.
APS
    air plasma spray
    anterior plate system
    APS hydroxyapatite
APTA
    American Physical Therapy Association
APTC
    anteroposterior talocalcaneal angle
APTT
    activated partial thromboplastin time test
Aqua
    A. PT water massage
    A. Spray
Aqua-Cel heating pad system
Aquachloral Supprettes
Aquaciser
    A. hydrodynamic measurement
    system
    A. pool
    A. 100R underwater treadmill
    system
    A. underwater treadmill
aquadynamic
Aquaflex gel pad
AquaGaiter treadmill
AquaMED
    A. dry hydrotherapy
    A. dry hydrotherapy equipment
AquaMotion pool
**Aquanex hydrodynamic measurement
system**
Aquaphor gauze dressing
Aquaplast
    A. splint
    A. splinting material
AquaSens fluid monitoring system
AquaShield
    A. orthopaedic cast cover
    A. reusable cast cover
Aquasonic Transmission Gel
Aquatech cast pad

A

aquatherapy
Aquatherm bed pad
aquatic
    a. cardiac evaluation and testing (ACET)
    a. rehabilitation
    a. stabilization program
Aqua-Trainer
Aquatrek device
Aquatrend water workout station
Aqua/Whirl bath
AquaWrap coding compression wrap
ARA
    Action Research Arm
    American Rheumatism Association
    ARA Test
ara-a
    adenine arabinoside
arabinoside
    adenine a. (ara-a)
arachidonate metabolism
arachidonic
arachnodactyly
arachnoid
arachnoiditis
arachnoid-shape Beaver blade
Arafiles
    A. elbow arthrodesis
    A. elbow prosthesis
Aralen Phosphate
Aran-Duchenne amyotrophy
Arava
Arbeitsgemeinschaft
    A. für osteosynthesefragen (AO)
    A. für osteosynthesefragen procedure
ARC
    antirotation cable
arc
    flexion-extension a.
    a. of motion
    painful a.
    reflex a.
    shoulder ROM a.
arcade
    a. of Frohse
    a. of Struthers
    superficialis a.
arch
    a. angle
    a. binder
    a. cookie

coracoacromial a.
    a. cushion
    a. fracture
    a. of Frohse
    Hapad metatarsal a.
    Hapad scaphoid a.
    Hillock a.
    a. index
    keystone of the calcar a.
    Langer a.
    longitudinal a.
    palmar a.
    a. peak area
    plantar a.
    posterior a.
    Roman a.
    superficial palmar a.
    a. support
    a.-up test
archer's shoulder
Archimedean drill
architectural alternation of bone
architecture
    bony a.
arch-lok
    Swede-O A.-l.
"arch and slouch" position
arch support
    plantar a. s.
    Plastizote a. s.
    Whitman a. s.
Archxerciser
ArCom processed polyethylene
Arctic Blaze hot/cold pack
arcuate
    a. complex
    a. foramen
    a. ligament
    a. movement
    a. osteotomy
    a. popliteal ligament
arcuatum
    ligamentum popliteum a.
arcus
    a. atlantis
    a. palmaris profundus
    a. palmaris superficialis
    a. parietooccipitalis
    a. pedis transversalis
    a. plantaris
    a. plantaris profundus
    a. pubicus

NOTES

arcus *(continued)*
    a. vertebrae
    a. vertebralis
    a. volaris profundus
    a. volaris superficialis
ardeparin sodium
ARDS
    adult respiratory distress syndrome
area
    arch peak a.
    dorsolumbar a.
    odontoid-axial a.
    performance a.
    pressure-sensitive a.
    puboischial a.
    a. scar
    trapezial a.
Aredia
Argesic-SA
Arglaes film dressing
ARGO
    Adjustable Advanced Reciprocating Gait
    Orthosis
Ariel computerized exercise system
Aristocort Forte
Arizona
    A. Health Science Center (AHSC)
    A. Health Science Center-Volz
    elbow prosthesis
    A. Health Sciences Center-Volz
    hinge
    A. leg support
arm
    abductor lever a.
    Action Research A. (ARA)
    articulating a.
    a. cuff
    a. cylinder cast
    a. elevator sling
    fail a.
    a. flap
    a. fossa test
    grenade-thrower's a.
    a. heel-strike synchrony
    a. holder
    lever a.
    Leyal a.
    linebacker's a.
    moment a.
    MonitorMate monitor a.
    outrigger a.
    Popeye a.
    a. positioner
    a. skate
    a. swathe
    tackler's a.
    Utah artificial a.

    wringer a.
    Yasargil Leyla retractor a.
armboard
    Flexisplint flexed a.
Armed Forces Institute of Pathology
Armistead
    A. technique
    A. ulnar lengthening
    A. ulnar lengthening operation
Armstrong
    A. acromionectomy
    A. plate
Army
    A. bone gouge
    A.-Navy retractor
    A. osteotome
    A. Prosthetics Research Laboratory
    (APRL)
Arnold-Chiari
    A.-C. malformation
    A.-C. syndrome
Arnold lumbar brace
AROM
    active range of motion
aromatherapy
Aron Alpha adhesive
Aronson-Prager technique
arrest
    epiphyseal a.
    greater trochanteric apophyseal a.
    growth a.
arrow
    Biofix a.
    Bionics a.
    A. pin clasp
Arrowsmith-Clerf pin-closing forceps
arsenical keratosis
ART
    active-release technique
art
    adjustive a.
ArtAssist arterial assist device
artefacta
    dermatitis a.
arterial
    a. aneurysm
    a. flap
    a. gas embolism
    a. graft
    a. occlusion sign
    a. oxygen saturation
    a. ring
    a. spasm
    a. trauma
arteria radicularis magna
arteriogram

arteriography
    a. block
    femoral a.
arteriosclerosis (AS)
    a. obliterans
arteriotomy
    ankle-level a.
arteriovenous
    a. fistula (AVF)
    a. malformation (AVM)
arteritis
    Takayasu a.
artery
    Adamkiewicz a.
    anomalous fibular nutrient a.
    anterior radial collateral a.
    anterior recurrent tibial a.
    anterior spinal a.
    anterior tibial a.
    ascending cervical a.
    axillary a.
    brachial a.
    carotid a.
    cervical a.
    circumflex iliac a.
    circumflex scapular a.
    collateral a.
    common carotid a.
    common iliac a.
    deep circumflex iliac a.
    digital a.
    dorsal digital a. (DDA)
    dorsalis pedis a.
    dorsal metatarsal a.
    end a.
    epiphyseal a.
    facial a.
    femoral circumflex a.
    first dorsal metatarsal a. (FDMA)
    first plantar metatarsal a. (FPMA)
    genicular a.
    geniculate a.
    gluteal a.
    hypogastric a.
    iliac a.
    iliofemoral flap a.
    iliolumbar a.
    inferior thyroid a.
    intercostal a.
    internal carotid a.
    internal iliac a.
    lingual a.

    medial geniculate a.
    metaphyseal a.
    metatarsal a.
    middle sacral a.
    nutrient a.
    obturator a.
    paramalleolar a.
    peroneal a.
    persistent sciatic a.
    plantar a.
    plantar digital a. (PDA)
    popliteal a.
    posterior radial collateral a.
    posterior tibial a.
    pudendal a.
    radial a.
    radicular a.
    rectal a.
    retinacular a.
    sacral a.
    segmental a.
    spinal a.
    subclavian a.
    superficial circumflex iliac a.
    superficial femoral a. (SFA)
    superficial temporal a.
    superior laryngeal a.
    superior thyroid a.
    supraclavicular fossa a.
    tarsal sinus a.
    thoracoacromial a.
    thrombosis radial a.
    tibial a.
    ulnar a.
    vertebral a.
    volar digital a.
Artha-G
arthralgia
    migratory a.
    subtalar a.
    temporomandibular joint a.
arthrectomy
arthrempyesis
Arthrex
    A. arthroscopy instrument
    A. sheathed interference screw
    A. zebra pin
arthrifluent abscess
arthritic
    a. shoe
    a. talonavicular change

NOTES

arthritide
arthritis, pl. **arthritides**
   acute hematogenous a.
   acute spinal a.
   allergenic a.
   Bekhterev a.
   Brucella a.
   calcaneocuboid joint a.
   Charcot a.
   crystal-induced a.
   degenerative a.
   enteropathic a.
   erosive a.
   A. Foundation Pain Reliever
   Fries score for rheumatoid a.
   fungal a.
   gonococcal septic a.
   gouty a.
   A. Helplessness Index (AHI)
   hemophiliac a.
   hypotrophic a.
   A. Impact Measurement Scale
    (AIMS)
   infectious a.
   juvenile rheumatoid a. (JRA)
   Marie-Strümpell a.
   migratory a.
   mutilans rheumatoid a.
   mycobacterial a.
   New York diagnostic criteria for
    rheumatoid a.
   oligoarticular a.
   Outerbridge staging of
    degenerative a.
   pantalocrural a.
   patellofemoral a.
   pauciarticular a.
   pisotriquetral a.
   polyarticular a.
   postinfectious a.
   postmenopausal a.
   psoriatic a.
   pyogenic a.
   radiocarpal a.
   rheumatoid a. (RA)
   Rome criteria for rheumatoid a.
   Salmonella a.
   septic a.
   seronegative a.
   seropositive a.
   silicone a.
   a. sock
   spinal a.
   staphylococcal a.
   Steinbrocker classification of
    rheumatoid a.
   suppurative a.
   tibiotalar a.

   Tom Smith a.
   traumatic a.
   tuberculous a.
   viral-associated a.
arthrocace
Arthrocare wand
arthrocele
arthrocentesis
arthrochalasis
arthrochondritis
arthroclasia
arthrodesed digit
arthrodesis
   Abbott-Fischer-Lucas hip a.
   Abbott-Lucas a.
   Adams transmalleolar a.
   Adkins technique spinal a.
   Albee hip a.
   ankle a.
   anterior occipitocervical a.
   anterior slot graft a.
   AO group shoulder a.
   Arafiles elbow a.
   atlantoaxial a.
   Baciu-Filibiu dowel ankle a.
   Baciu-Filibiu transmalleolar a.
   Badgley a.
   Barrasso-Wile-Gage a.
   Barr-Record ankle a.
   Batchelor-Brown extraarticular
    subtalar a.
   beak modification with triple a.
   Benyi modification of Lambrinudi
    triple a.
   bimalleolar approach to ankle a.
   Blair ankle a.
   Blair anterior a.
   Blair-Morris-Dunn-Hand ankle a.
   Blair tibiotalar a.
   Bosworth femoroischial a.
   Brett a.
   Brewster triple a.
   Brittain ischiofemoral a.
   Brockman-Nissen a.
   Brooks atlantoaxial a.
   calcaneocuboid a.
   calcaneocuboid distraction a.
    (CCDA)
   calcaneopelvic a.
   calcaneotibial a.
   Campbell-Akbarnia a.
   Campbell posterior a.
   Campbell-Rinehard-Kalenak
    anterior a.
   Carceau-Brahms ankle a.
   Carroll a.
   cervical a.
   Chandler a.

Chapchal knee a.
Charcot hip a.
Charnley ankle a.
Charnley compression a.
Charnley-Houston a.
Charnley-Houston shoulder a.
Chuinard-Peterson ankle a.
Chuinard-Peterson anterior a.
closing wedge a.
Cloward cervical a.
combined resection arthroplasty and a.
Compere-Thompson a.
compression a.
cone a.
coracoclavicular a.
cuneiform joint a.
Davis a.
Dennyson-Fulford subtalar a.
distal fibulotalar a.
distraction bone block a.
distraction/compression bone graft a.
dowel a.
Dunn-Brittain triple a.
Dunn triple a.
Elmslie triple a.
Enneking knee a.
excisional a.
extension injury posterior atlantoaxial a.
extraarticular a.
failed triple a.
fibulotalar a.
first cuneiform joint a.
first cuneiform-navicular joint a.
first metatarsal-first cuneiform a.
flexion injury posterior atlantoaxial a.
Gallie ankle a.
Gallie atlantoaxial a.
Gant hip a.
Garceau-Brahms a.
Ghormley a.
Gill a.
Gill-Stein a.
glenohumeral a.
Glissane a.
Goldner spinal a.
Graham ankle a.
Grice extraarticular subtalar a.

Grice-Green extraarticular subtalar a.
Guttmann subtalar a.
Haddad-Riordan a.
hallux interphalangeal joint a.
hallux rigidus a.
Harris-Beath a.
Heiple a.
Henderson a.
Hibbs a.
hindfoot a.
Hoke triple a.
Horwitz-Adams a.
Horwitz ankle a.
Horwitz transmalleolar a.
Ilizarov ankle a.
interbody a.
intercarpal a.
intertransverse process a.
intraarticular a.
Johannson-Barrington a.
John C. Wilson a.
joint a.
Kapandji-Sauvé a.
Key intraarticular knee a.
Kickaldy-Willis a.
knee a.
Kostuik-Alexander a.
Lambrinudi a.
lesser tarsal a.
Lionberger-Bishop-Tullos anterior a.
Lipscomb metatarsophaleangeal a.
Lipscomb modified McKeever a.
Lisfranc a.
Lucas-Murray knee a.
lunotriquetral a.
Mann-Coughlin a.
Mann modified McKeever a.
Mann-Thompson-Coughlin a.
Marcus-Balourdas-Heiple transmalleolar a.
McKeever metatarsophalangeal a.
metatarsocuneiform a.
metatarsophalangeal joint a.
midcarpal a.
Millender-Nalebuff wrist a.
Moberg a.
modified Boyd ankle a.
Morris-Hand-Dunn anterior a.
Mueller a.
Nalebuff a.
Naughton-Dunn triple a.

NOTES

arthrodesis *(continued)*
  naviculocuneiform joint a.
  occipitocervical a.
  panastragaloid a.
  pantalar a.
  paraarticular a.
  Pontenza a.
  posterior atlantoaxial a.
  Potter a.
  Pridie ankle a.
  a. for primary degenerative
    osteoarthritis
  Pritchett-Mallin-Matthews a.
  Putti knee a.
  radiocarpal a.
  resection a.
  Richards a.
  Richardson subtalar a.
  Robinson-Riley cervical a.
  Robinson-Smith spinal a.
  Robinson spinal a.
  Ryerson triple a.
  scaphocapitolunate a. (SCL)
  scaphotrapeziotrapezoid a.
  scapulothoracic a.
  Schneider hip a.
  Scranton transmalleolar a.
  a. screw
  Seoffert triple a.
  shoulder a.
  Shriver-Johnson interphalangeal a.
  Siffert-Forster-Nachamie a.
  Simmons spinal a.
  in situ a.
  sliding a.
  Smith-Robinson interbody a.
  Soren a.
  Spier elbow a.
  spinal a.
  Staples elbow a.
  Stark a.
  Steindler elbow a.
  Stewart-Harley transmalleolar
    ankle a.
  stone a.
  subtalar a.
  talar triple a.
  talonavicular a.
  tarsal a.
  tarsometatarsal joint a.
  tarsometatarsal truncated-wedge a.
  thoracoscapular a.
  tibia-hindfoot osteomusculocutaneous
    rotationplasty with
    calcaneopelvic a.
  tibiocalcaneal a.
  tibiotalar a.
  tibiotalocalcaneal a.
  transfibular a.
  transmalleolar ankle a.
  triple a.
  triquetrum-lunate a.
  triscaphe a.
  Trumble a.
  truncated tarsometatarsal wedge a.
  truncated-wedge a.
  Uematsu shoulder a.
  ulnocarpal a.
  Watson-Jones a.
  Whitecloud-LaRocca cervical a.
  White posterior a.
  Wilson cone a.
  Wilson-Johansson-Barrington cone a.
arthrodiastasis
arthrodynia
arthrodysplasia
arthroempyesis
arthroendoscopy
arthroereisis
  peg-in-hole a.
  subtalar a.
arthrofibrosis
Arthrofile orthopaedic rasp
Arthro-Flo
  A.-F. arthroscopic irrigation system
  A.-F. irrigator
arthrogenic gait
arthrogram
  nuclear a.
**arthrographic capsular distension and
  rupture technique**
arthrography
  Broström-Gordon a.
  contrast a.
  coronal computed tomographic a.
    (CCTA)
  double-contrast a.
  magnetic resonance a.
arthrogryposis
  a. multiplex congenita
  myopathic a.
  neurogenic a.
arthrogrypotic clubfoot
arthroidal protractor
arthrokatadysis
arthrokinematic
arthrokleisis
arthrolith
arthrology
Arthro-Lok system of Beaver blade
arthrolysis
arthromeningitis
arthrometer
  Acufex knee laxity a.
  Genucom a.
  KT1000 knee ligament a.

KT2000 knee ligament a.
KT1000/s surgical a.
Medmetric knee ligament a.
Medmetric KT-1000 knee laxity a.
Robinson a.
stress-testing a.
Stryker a.
a. testing
arthrometric knee laxity measurement
arthroncus
arthroneuralgia
arthronosos
arthroonychodysplasia syndrome
Arthropan
arthropathic
arthropathology
arthropathy
Charcot a.
crystal-related a.
cuff-tear a.
inflammatory a.
Jaccoud a.
joint a.
neuropathic a. (NA)
pyrophosphate a.
sacroiliac joint a.
seronegative a.
SLE a.
arthrophyte
arthroplasty
ablative a.
abrasion a.
acetabular cup a.
acromioclavicular a.
Albright-Chase a.
ankle a.
Ashworth hand a.
Ashworth implant a.
Aufranc cup a.
Aufranc-Turner a.
Austin Moore a.
autogenous interpositional
shoulder a.
Bechtol a.
bipolar hip a.
Bowers radial a.
Brain a.
Bryan a.
Campbell interpositional a.
Campbell resection a.
capitellocondylar total elbow a.
capsular interposition a.

carpometacarpal a.
Carroll a.
Carroll and Taber a.
Castle-Schneider resection
interposition a.
a. cement
cemented total hip a.
cementless total hip a.
Charnley low-friction a.
Charnley total hip a.
Clayton forefoot a.
Clayton resection a.
Colonna trochanteric a.
condylar implant a.
constrained ankle a.
constrained shoulder a.
convex condylar-implant a.
Coonrad-Morrey total elbow a.
Coonrad total elbow a.
Cracchiolo forefoot a.
Cracchiolo-Sculco implant a.
Crawford-Adams acetabular cup a.
Cubbins a.
cuff-tear a.
cup a.
Dewar-Barrington a.
distraction a.
duToit-Roux a.
DuVries a.
Eaton implant a.
Eaton volar plate a.
Eden-Hybbinette a.
elbow a.
ELP stem for hip a.
Ewald capitellocondylar total
elbow a.
Ewald elbow a.
Ewald-Walker kinematic knee a.
Ewald-Walker knee a.
excision a.
extensor brevis a.
failed implant a.
fascial a.
finger joint a.
forefoot a.
four-in-one a.
Ganley modification of Keller a.
Girdlestone resection a.
Global total shoulder a.
a. gouge
Gristina-Webb total shoulder a.
Gunston a.

NOTES

arthroplasty *(continued)*
Gustilo-Kyle cementless total hip a.
Harrington total hip a.
Head hip a.
Helal flap a.
hemijoint a.
hemiresection interposition a.
hip a.
Hungerford-Krackow-Kenna knee a.
ICLH double cup a.
implant a.
Inglis triaxial total elbow a.
Insall-Burstein-Freeman knee a.
interpositional elbow a.
interpositional shoulder a.
interpositional toe a.
Irvine ankle a.
Johnson resection a.
Jones resection a.
Kates forefoot a.
Keller-Lelièvre a.
Keller-Mann resection a.
Keller resection a.
knee a.
Kocher-McFarland hip a.
Koenig metatarsophalangeal joint a.
Koenig MPJ implant and a.
Kutes a.
Larmon forefoot a.
laser image custom a. (LICA)
Mann-DuVries a.
Mann resection a.
Mark II Sorrells hip a.
Matchett-Brown hip a.
Mayo ankle a.
Mayo resection a.
Mayo total elbow a.
McAtee-Tharias-Blazina a.
McKee-Farrar total hip a.
Memford-Gurd a.
metacarpophalangeal joint a.
Meuli a.
Millender a.
Miller-Galante knee a.
modified Keller resection a.
modified mold and surface
  replacement a.
mold acetabular a.
monospherical shoulder a.
monospherical total shoulder a.
Morrey-Bryan total elbow a.
Mould a.
Mueller hip a.
Mumford-Gurd a.
NEB a.
Neer unconstrained shoulder a.
New England Baptist hip a.
Niebauer trapeziometacarpal a.

noncemented total hip a.
Post total shoulder a.
Press-Fit condylar knee a.
primary a.
A. Products Consultants foot and
  legholder
prosthetic a.
Putti-Platt a.
Regnauld modification of Keller a.
resection a.
revision hip a.
rotator cuff-tear a.
Sauvé-Kapandji a.
Schlein elbow a.
semiconstrained total elbow a.
shoulder a.
Silastic lunate a.
silicone implant a.
silicone rubber a.
silicone wrist a.
Smith-Petersen cup a.
Speed a.
Stanmore shoulder a.
Steffee thumb a.
surface replacement hip a.
Swanson Convex condylar a.
Swanson interpositional wrist a.
Swanson metatarsophalangeal
  joint a.
Swanson PIP joint a.
Swanson radial head implant a.
Swanson silicone wrist a.
tendon interposition a.
total ankle a.
total articular replacement a.
  (TARA)
total articular resurfacing a.
  (TARA)
total elbow a.
total hip a. (THA)
total knee a. (TKA)
total patellofemoral joint a.
total shoulder a.
total wrist a.
triaxial total elbow a.
Tupper a.
UCLA anatomic shoulder a.
ulnar hemiresection interposition a.
unconstrained shoulder a.
unicompartmental knee a. (UKA)
Vainio a.
Valenti a.
Vitallium cup a.
volar plate a.
Volz total wrist a.
Wilson-McKeever a.
arthropneumotography

Arthropor
- A. acetabular cup
- A. cup pad
- A. cup prosthesis
- A. II acetabular prosthesis
- A. II porous socket
- A. oblong cup for acetabular defect

ArthroProbe
- A. arthroscopic laser
- Contact A.
- A. laser system

arthropyosis

arthrorheumatism

arthroscope
- angled a.
- Baxter angled a.
- Dyonics a.
- Eagle straight-ahead a.
- fiberoptic a.
- O'Connor operating a.
- Panoview a.
- Sapphire View a.
- a. sheath
- Storz oblique a.
- Stryker viewing a.
- triangulation technique for a.
- Wolf a.

arthroscopic
- a. abrasion chondroplasty
- a. acromioplasty
- a. augmentation
- a. cannula
- a. debridement
- a. entry portal
- a. examination
- a. grabber
- a. knife
- a. laser instrument
- a. laser surgery
- a. legholder
- a. meniscectomy
- a. microdiskectomy (AMD)
- a. osteotome
- a. probe
- a. punch
- a. scissors
- a. screw fixation
- a. shaver
- a. shaving
- a. sheath
- a. shield

- a. synovectomy
- a. syovector

arthroscopically assisted anterior cruciate ligament reconstruction

arthroscopy
- Allen shoulder a.
- a. basket forceps
- diagnostic a.
- diagnostic and operative a. (DOA)
- Gilquist a.
- a. grasping forceps
- Hawkeye suture needle for a.
- laser a.
- lateral hip a.
- midcarpal a.
- operative a.
- radiocarpal a.
- Ringer a.
- second-look a.

arthroscopy-assisted patellar tendon substitution

Arthro-sew

arthrosis
- crystal-induced a.
- degenerative a.
- Eaton CMC a. (stages I–IV)
- primary cystic a.
- subtalar a.
- trapezial a.
- uncovertebral a.

Arthrosol dressing

arthrosynovitis

Arthrotek
- A. calibrated cylinder
- A. Ellipticut hand instrumentation
- A. femoral aimer
- A. IES 1000
- A. tibial fixation device

arthrotome

arthrotomy
- Magnuson-Stack shoulder a.
- medial parapatellar a.
- operative a.
- parapatellar a.
- subtalar a.

arthroxesis

articular
- a. blockage
- a. capsule
- a. cartilage
- a. cartilage lesion
- a. cortex

NOTES

articular *(continued)*
  a. defect
  a. disk
  a. facet
  a. facet angle
  a. fragment
  a. insert
  a. instability
  a. labrum
  a.-ligamentous system
  a. mass separation
  a. mass separation fracture
  a. motion device (AMD)
  a. nerve
  a. pillar
  a. pillar fracture
  a. process
  a. strain
  a. structure
  a. surface
articulated
  a. AFO
  a. chin implant
  a. external fixator
  a. tension device
articulating
  a. arm
  a. bone end
articulatio humeri
articulation
  acromioclavicular a.
  atlantoaxial a.
  calcaneocuboid a.
  carpometacarpal a.
  carporadial a.
  Chopart a.
  collateral ligament of
    interphalangeal a.'s
  collateral ligament of MCP a.'s
  collateral ligament of MTP a.'s
  condylar a.
  coracoclavicular a.
  costovertebral a.
  coxofemoral a.
  DIP a.
  a. disturbance
  Goldman-Fristoe test of a.
  humeroradial a.
  humeroulnar a.
  intercarpal a.
  intermetacarpal a.
  interphalangeal a.
  Lisfranc joint a.
  metacarpophalangeal a.
  metatarsocuneiform a.
  occipitocervical a.
  palmar ligaments of
    interphalangeal a.'s

  patellofemoral a.
  PIP a.
  plane-type acromioclavicular a.
  plantar ligaments of
    interphalangeal a.'s
  plantar ligaments of MTP a.'s
  proximal radioulnar a.
  radiocapitellar a.
  radiocarpal a.
  radiohumeral a.
  radioscaphoid a.
  radioulnar a.
  scapuloclavicular a.
  subtalar a.
  talocalcaneonavicular ligament a.
  tarsometatarsal a.
  tibiofemoral a.
  tibiofibular a.
  ulnolunate a.
  ulnotriquetrum a.
  Vermont spinal fixator a.
articulatory procedure
Articulose-50 Injection
artifact
  electric a.
  friction a.
  movement a.
  a. on x-ray
  shock a.
  stimulus a.
artifactual
artificial
  a. fat pad
  a. joint implant
  a. ligament
  a. limb
  a. vertebral body
Artisan cement system
Arts
  Very Special A. (VSA)
ARUM Colles fixation pin
AS
  anterosuperior
  aortic stenosis
  arteriosclerosis
  AS ilium
  AS subluxation
ASA
  acetylsalicylic acid
  Lortab ASA
A.S.A.
ascending cervical artery
Asch
  A. forceps
  A. splint
ascites
  chylous a.
Ascriptin

ASE
    axilla, shoulder, elbow
    ASE bandage
aseptic
    a. fashion
    a. felon
    a. loosening
    a. necrosis
ASES
    American shoulder and elbow system
ASEx
    anterosuperior external ilium movement
    ASEx ilium
    ASEx subluxation
Asher physical build assessment technique
Ashhurst
    A. fracture classification system
    A. leg splint
    A. sign
Ashhurst-Bromer ankle fracture classification
Ashworth
    A. hand arthroplasty
    A. implant arthroplasty
    A. scale
    A. score of muscle spasticity
ASI
    acromial spur index
Asics shoe
ASICT
    amplitude-summation interferential current therapy
ASIF
    Association for the Study of Internal Fixation
    ASIF broad dynamic compression bone plate
    ASIF cancellous screw
    ASIF chisel
    ASIF cortical screw
    ASIF malleolar screw
    ASIF right-angle blade plate
    ASIF screw fixation technique
    ASIF screw pin
    ASIF system
    ASIF T-plate
    ASIF twist drill
ASIn
    anterosuperior internal ilium movement
    ASIn ilium
    ASIn subluxation

ASIS
    anterior superior iliac spine
    anterosuperior iliac spine
Asissto-Seat
    Maddapult A.-S.
Aslan endoscopic scissors
Asnis
    A. cannulated cancellous screw
    A. 2 guided-screw system
    A. pin
    A. pinning
    A. technique
ASOT
    antistreptolysin-O titer
ASP clip staple
aspect
    dorsal a.
    laminar cortex posterior a.
    medial a.
    posterolateral a.
    volar a.
Aspen
    A. cervical collar
    A. electrocautery
Aspercin Extra
aspergillosis infection
Aspergillus
    A. fumigatus
    A. niger
Aspergum
aspirated fat
aspiration
    anterior a.
    bone marrow a.
    joint a.
    lateral a.
    medial a.
    a. needle biopsy
aspirator
    Cavitron ultrasonic surgical a.
    Sonocut ultrasonic a.
aspirin
    Bayer Buffered A.
    carisoprodol and a.
    a. and codeine
    Extra Strength Bayer Enteric 500 A.
    A. Free Anacin Maximum Strength
    hydrocodone and a.
    methocarbamol and a.
    oxycodone and a.
    propoxyphene and a.

NOTES

45

aspirin *(continued)*
    Regular Strength Bayer Enteric
      500 A.
    Saint Joseph Adult Chewable A.
    St Joseph Adult Chewable A.
Asprimox
assay
    AlamarBlue osteoblast
      proliferation a.
    cefazolin a.
    chemiluminescent microtiter protein
      kinase activity a.
    deoxypyridinoline crosslinks
      urine a.
    enzyme-linked immunosorbent a.
      (ELISA)
    microtiter protein kinase a.
    osteoblast proliferation
      fluorometric a.
    Pyrilinks-D urine a.
    radioisotope clearance a.
assembly
    foot-ankle a.
    Massie nail a.
    multiple hook a.
    nail a.
    nail-screw sideplate a.
    proximal drill-guide a.
assessment
    Activity Loss A. (ALA)
    BFM arm impairment a.
    Brief Test of Head Injury A.
    ergonomic a.
    functional capacity a.
    Moire topographic scoliosis a.
    motor function a.
    Musculoskeletal Function A. (MFA)
    neurologic a.
    RIPA-2 A.
    RIPA-G A.
    Ross Information Processing A.
    Scales of Cognitive Ability for
      Traumatic Brain Injury A.
    SCATBI A.
    Tinetti gait a.
    vascular a.
    visual a.
    vocational a.
ASSI
    Accurate Surgical and Scientific
      Instruments Corporation
    ASSI coagulator
    ASSI wire-pass drill
assimilation
    atlantooccipital a.
ASSIST
    Thera-Band A.

assist
    Elite posterior spring a.
    knee extension a.
assistance
    ambulate with a.
Assistant
    A. Free calibrated femoral tibial
      spreader
    A. Free foot/ankle support
    A. Free long prong collateral
      ligament retractor
    A. Free self-retaining hip surgery
      retractor system
    A. Free Shubbs short prong
      collateral ligament retractor
    A. Free Stulberg leg positioner
    A. Free wide PCL retractor
assisted ambulation
assistive
    a. device
    a. technology device (ATD)
associated myofascial trigger point
Association
    American Nursing Home A.
    American Orthotic and
      Prosthetic A. (AOPA)
    American Physical Therapy A.
      (APTA)
    American Rheumatism A. (ARA)
    Canadian Physiotherapy A.
    A. of Chiropractic Colleges (ACC)
    Chiropractic Rehabilitation A.
      (CRA)
    Japanese Orthopaedic A. (JOA)
    A. Research Circulation Osseous
      classification system
    A. for the Study of Internal
      Fixation (ASIF)
astasia
astasia-abasia gait
astereognosis
asterixis
asthenia
asthenic
ASTM
    American Society for Testing and
      Materials
    ASTM augmented soft tissue
      mobilization
    ASTM designation of Biophase
Aston
    A. cartilage reduction
    A. patterning
astragalus
    aviator's a.
Astralac needle
Astramorph PF Injection

asymmetric
- a. incurvatum reflex
- a. skin fold
- a. subtalar joint development
- a. tonic neck reflex (ATNR)
- a. wear

asymmetrical growth
asymmetrically
asymmetry
- interinnominate a.

asyndesis
asyndetic communication
asynergia
asynergic
AT
- Achilles tendon
- activity training
- anaerobic threshold

Atarax
Atasoy
- A. triangular advancement flap
- A.-type flap for nail injury repair
- A. volar V-Y flap
- A. V-Y advancement
- A. V-Y technique

Atasoy-Kleinert flap
atavicus
- metatarsus primus a.

ataxia
- Bruns a.
- equilibratory a.
- Friedreich a.
- hereditary spinocerebellar a.
- locomotor a.
- spinocerebellar a.

ataxia-telangiectasia
ataxic cerebral palsy
A-T Bar
ATD
- assistive technology device

atelectasis
- plate-like a.
- pulmonary a.

Aten olecranon screw
ATFL
- anterior talofibular ligament

ATH
- anthropometric total hip

atherosclerosis
atherostenosis
athetoid cerebral palsy
athetotic

athlete's foot
athletic
- a. injury
- a. trainer

Ativan
Atkin epiphyseal fracture
Atkinson endoprosthesis
Atlanta
- A. brace orthosis
- A. hip brace

atlantal
- a. transverse ligament

Atlanta-Scottish
- A.-S. Rite abduction orthosis
- A.-S. Rite brace

Atlantic
- A. overlap brace
- A. rim brace

atlantis
- arcus a.
- A. cervical plate system
- ligamentum cruciforme a.
- ligamentum transversum a.

atlantoaxial
- a. alignment
- a. arthrodesis
- a. articulation
- a. dislocation (AAD)
- a. fracture-dislocation
- a. fusion
- a. impaction
- a. instability
- a. joint
- a. lesion
- a. ligament
- a. luxation
- a. rotary displacement
- a. rotatory fixation (AARF)
- a. rotatory subluxation
- a. stabilization
- a. subluxation (AAS)

atlantodens interval (ADI)
atlantodental
- a. interspace
- a. interval (ADI)

atlantooccipital (AO)
- a. anterior membrane
- a. assimilation
- a. disability
- a. fusion
- a. joint
- a. joint dislocation

NOTES

atlantooccipital *(continued)*
    a. junction
    a. ligament
    a. subluxation
atlantoodontoid
    a. interspace
    a. joint
atlas (C1)
    A. adjustable stand
    A. cable system
    cruciform ligament of a.
    a. fracture
    Jefferson fracture of a.
    a. laterality
    A. modular humeral prosthesis
    A. orthogonal percussion instrument
    transverse ligament of a.
atlas-axis
    a.-a. complex
    a.-a. movement
atlas-dens interval
ATM
    Awareness Through Movement
ATNR
    asymmetric tonic neck reflex
ATON
    adductor tenotomy and obturator
      neurectomy
atonia
atony
atopic dermatitis
ATO walker
ATR
    Achilles tendon rupture
    ATR brace
atracurium besylate
Atra-Grip clamp
atraumatic
    a., multidirectional, bilateral
      instability (AMBRI)
    a. multidirectional instability
    a. necrosis
    a. needle
atretic
atrophic
    a. fracture
    a. neuroarthropathy
    a. nonunion
atrophied
atrophy
    cortical a.
    disuse a.
    Duchenne muscular a.
    fat pad a.
    infantile spinal muscular a.
    muscular a.
    quadriceps a.
    scapular peroneal a.

    spinal muscular a. (SMA)
    Sudeck a.
    thenar a.
A/T/S Topical
attachment
    Accuvac smoke evacuation a.
    capsular a.
    femoral a.
    fibrous a.
    ligamentous a.
    muscular a.
    osseous a.
    Pearson splint a.
    PRAFO a.
    PRAFO KAFO a. (PKA)
    splint a.
    tendinous a.
    tendon-to-bone a.
    Thomas splint with Pearson a.
    a. versatility
attack
    adversive a.
Attenborough total knee prosthesis
attenuate
attenuation of tendon
Atton disease
attritional perforation
attrition of tendon
ATV
    all-terrain vehicle
    ATV accident
atypical dislocation
auditory
    a. defensiveness
    a. evoked potential (AEP)
Aufranc
    A. awl
    A. cobra retractor
    A. concentric hip mold
    A. cup arthroplasty
    A. gouge
    A. modification of Smith-Petersen
      cup
    A. osteotome
    A. periosteal elevator
    A. reamer
Aufranc-Cobra hip prosthesis
Aufranc-Turner
    A.-T. acetabular cup
    A.-T. arthroplasty
    A.-T. cemented hip prosthesis
    A.-T. femoral component
    A.-T. hip cup
    A.-T. hip prosthesis
    A.-T. stem
Aufricht glabellar rasp
auger

augmentation
>arthroscopic a.
>extraarticular a.
>hamstring ligament a.
>iliotibial band graft a.
>Leach-Schepsis-Paul a.
>slotted acetabular a.
>synthetic a.

Augustine boat nail
auranofin
aureus
>*Staphylococcus a.*

Aurolate
aurothioglucose
aurothiomalate
Aussies-Isseis unstable scoliosis
Austin
>A. bunionectomy
>A. chevron osteotomy fixation
>A. Medical Equipment (AME)
>A. Moore arthroplasty
>A. Moore chisel
>A. Moore extractor
>A. Moore femoral head prosthesis
>A. Moore hemiarthroplasty
>A. Moore hip prosthesis
>A. Moore hook
>A. Moore impactor
>A. Moore pin
>A. Moore rasp
>A. Moore reamer
>A. osteotomy

autoamputation
autochthonous graft
autoclavable
autoclave
autocompression plate
Autoflex II, III CPM unit
autofusion
autogéné
>Soudre a.

Autogenesis automator for Ilizarov screw
autogenic
autogenous
>a. bone graft
>a. fat
>a. fibular graft
>a. iliac bone
>a. interpositional shoulder arthroplasty

>a. patellar-ligament graft
>a. semitendinosus-gracilis graft

Auto Glide walker accessory
autograft
>bone-patellar tendon-bone a.
>a. bridge
>free revascularized a.
>patellar bone-tendon-bone a.
>Russell fibular head a.

autoimmunization
>surgical a.

Auto-Implant procedure
autologous
>a. blood
>a. blood transfusion
>a. cultured chondrocyte
>a. reverse graft
>a. reverse graft to ankle
>a. traction

automated
>a. percutaneous diskectomy (APD)
>a. percutaneous lumbar diskectomy (APLD)
>a. shaver

automatic
>a. screwdriver
>a. staple

Automator
>A. device

autonomic nervous system (ANS)
autonomous zone
Autophor
>A. ceramic total hip prosthesis
>A. femoral prosthesis

auto-reinforced polyglycolide rod
autosomal
autosuggestion
autotome drill
autotraction
autotransfusion suction
autotransfusion system
>Solcotrans a. s.

Autovac autotransfusion canister
Auvard clamp
A-V
>A-V Impulse system
>A-V Impulse System foot pump DVT prophylaxis device
>A-V Impulse System foot wrap DVT prophylaxis device

avascular
>a. fragment

NOTES

avascular *(continued)*
    a. microsis
    a. necrosis (AVN)
    a. necrosis of the femoral head
      (AVNFH)
    a. nonunion
    a. sequestrum
average evoked response
Averett hip prosthesis
Averill total hip replacement
AVF
    arteriovenous fistula
aviator's astragalus
Avila technique
avium
    Mycobacterium a.
avium-intracellulare
    Mycobacterium a.-i.
AVM
    arteriovenous malformation
AVN
    avascular necrosis
AVNFH
    avascular necrosis of the femoral head
avulse
avulsed ligament
avulsion
    bony a.
    a. chip fracture
    coracoid tip a.
    digitorum brevis a.
    a. fibular collateral ligament
    a. fragment
    a. injury
    isolated a.
    labral a.
    ligament a.
    nail a.
    a. of nail plate
    a. stress fracture
    syndesmotic a.
    a. technique
    tibial tubercle a.
    tubercle a.
awareness
    body a.
    kinesthetic a.
    sensory a.
    A. Through Movement (ATM)
awl
    angled a.
    Aufranc a.
    bone a.
    Carter Rowe a.
    curved a.
    DePuy a.
    Ender a.
    Ferran a.

    Küntscher a.
    Mark II Kodros radiolucent a.
    pointed a.
    reaming a.
    rectangular a.
    Rush pin reamer a.
    square-shaped a.
    Stedman a.
    Swanson scaphoid a.
    T-handled a.
    Zelicof orthopaedic a.
    Zuelzer a.
Axel wire twister
Axer
    A. compression apparatus
    A. compression device
    A. lateral opening wedge
      osteotomy
    A. varus derotational osteotomy
Axer-Clark procedure
axes (*pl. of* axis)
axial
    a. calcaneal projection
    a. calcaneus view
    a. compression
    a. compression injury
    a. compression load
    a. compression principle
    a. compression screw
    a. compression test
    a. fixation
    a. gripping strength
    a. instability
    a. loading
    a. loading injury
    a. loading of spine
    a. load test
    a. manual traction test
    a. multiplanar gradient refocused
      image
    a. multiplanar gradient refocused
      magnetic resonance image
    a. musculature
    a. neuritis
    a. pattern flap
    a. pin technique
    a. plane
    a. plane angular deformity
      biomechanics
    a. resistance exerciser
    a. rotation
    a. sesamoid projection
    a. sesamoid view
    a. spinal system
    a. stiffness
    a. traction
axilla, pl. **axillae**

A

a., shoulder, elbow (ASE)
a., shoulder, elbow bandage
axillary
  a. approach
  a. artery
  a. block
  a. contracture
  a. crutch
  a. flap
  a. nerve
  a. nerve injury
  a. vein
  a. view
Axiom modular knee system
axis, pl. **axes**
  anatomic a.
  bimalleolar-foot a.
  distal reference a. (DRA)
  femoral shaft a.
  A. fixation system
  flexion a.
  flexion-extension a.
  foot-thigh a.
  a. guide
  hypothalamic-pituitary-adrenal a.
  hypothalamoneurohypophyseal a.
    (HNA)
  interepicondylar a.
  leg a.
  ligamentum apicis dentis a.
  long a.
  longitudinal a.
  mechanical a.
  metatarsal a.
  proximal reference a. (PFA)

a. of rib motion
rotation a.
single a.
spinal a.
subtalar a.
a. traction
transcondylar a. (TCA)
transepicondylar a.
transmalleolar a. (TMA)
transverse a.
vertical a.
weightbearing a.
X a.
Y a.
Z a.
axle lock and bumper
axon
  a. degeneration
  a. reflex
  a. response
  a. sprout
  a. wave
axonal apposition
axonotmesis
axoplasmic
  a. flow
  a. transport
Ayers needle holder
Ayres tactile discrimination
Ayurveda
ayurvedic herbs
azathioprine
Azdone
azotemic osteodystrophy
aztreonam

NOTES

Baastrupi syndrome
Babcock forceps
Babinski
  B. hammer
  B. reflex
  B. sign
  B. test
Babinski-Fröhlich syndrome
baby
  b. Kocher clamp
  b. Lane forceps
  b. Satinsky clamp
bacampicillin
BacFix System
Baciguent Topical
bacitracin
  b., neomycin, and polymyxin B
  b., neomycin, polymyxin B, and
    hydrocortisone
  b., neomycin, polymyxin B, and
    lidocaine
  b. solution
Baciu-Filibiu
  B.-F. dowel ankle arthrodesis
  B.-F. transmalleolar arthrodesis
back
  b. brace
  B. Bubble gravity traction unit
  B. Bull lumbar support cushion
  B. Bull lumbar support system
  b. creaking
  b. crease
  b. exercise
  b. pain
  b. range of motion (BROM)
  b. range-of-motion device
  b. range-of-motion instrument
  rigid round b.
  B. Specialist electric table
  B. Specialist manual table
  b. strain
  b. support
backache
Backbar device
backboard
backcutting osteotome
BackCycler continuous passive motion
  device
Back-Ease aromatherapy hot/cold pack
backfire fracture
backfiring
Backhaus
  B. towel clamp
  B. towel forceps
Backhaus-Jones towel clamp

Backhaus-Kocher towel clamp
Back-Huggar
  Bodyline B.-H.
  B.-H. lumbar support
  B.-H. lumbar support cushion
Backjoy seat
back-knee deformity
Backnobber II massage tool
backout
  screw b.
backpack
  b. palsy
  b. paralysis
Back-Quell
"Back Shu" paraspinal point
Backstroke
  The B.
BackThing lumbar support
BackTracker
backward bending
backward-cutting knife
baclofen
Bacon
  B. bone rongeur
  B. rasp
bacteria
  aerobic b.
  airborne b.
  anaerobic b.
bacterial
  b. culture
  b. flora
Bacteroides
Bactocill
BactoShield Topical
Bac-Track
Bactroban
badger leg
Badgley
  B. arthrodesis
  B. combination procedure
  B. iliac wing resection
  B. laminectomy retractor
  B. plate
  B. resection of iliac wing
  B. technique
Bado classification
BAEP
  brainstem auditory evoked potential
BAER
  brainstem auditory evoked response
Baer
  B. bone-cutting forceps
  B. bone rongeur
  B. rib shears

bag
  B. Bath
  Infusible pressure infusion b.
  Versi-Splint carry b.
Bagby angled compression plate
bag-of-bones technique
Bahler hinge
Bahnson appendage clamp
Bailey
  B. bur
  B. conductor
  B. drill
  B. duckbill clamp
  B. rib contractor
  B. rib spreader
  B. saw guide
  B. wire saw
Bailey-Badgley
  B.-B. anterior cervical approach
  B.-B. cervical spine fusion
  B.-B. technique
Bailey-Cowley clamp
Bailey-Dubow
  B.-D. nail
  B.-D. osteotomy
  B.-D. rod
  B.-D. technique
Bailey-Gibbon rib contractor
Bailey-Gigli saw guide
Bailey-Morse clamp
bail-lock
  b.-l. brace
  b.-l. knee joint
  b.-l. knee joint orthosis
baja
  patella b.
BAK cage
Baker
  B. cyst
  B. lateral semitendinosus transfer
  B. patellar advancement operation
  B. technique
  B. trabecular traction
  B. translocation operation
Baker-Hill osteotomy
baker's leg
baking tin
Balacescu closing wedge osteotomy
Balacescu-Golden technique
balance
  b. beam scale
  b. board
  b. bridge
  dynamic b.
  electrolyte b.
  fluid b.
  B. Master
  b. pad

  b. padding orthosis
  postural b.
balanced
  b. hemivertebra
  b. skeletal traction
  b. splint
Baldan fracture splint
Balfour
  B. clamp
  B. self-retaining retractor
Balkan
  B. femoral splint
  B. fracture frame
ball
  b. bearing
  Body B.
  b. bur
  cold-weld femoral b.
  b. extractor
  Finger Fitness Spring B.
  b. of the foot
  Gertie b.
  Gripp squeeze b.
  b. guidepin
  gym b.
  Gymnastik b.
  Gymnic b.
  hand exercise b.
  HeavyMed b.
  Jurgan pin b.
  Ledraplastic exercise b.
  b.-peen splint
  PhysioGymnic exercise b.
  Physio-Roll VisuaLiser exercise b.
  b.-point guidepin
  b. reamer
  Silastic b.
  Slo-Mo b.
  squeeze b.
  Swiss b.
  Thera-Band exercise b.
  Theragym b.
  therapy b.
  b.-tipped Küntscher guide
  b.-valve tumor
  vestibular b.
ball-and-socket
  b.-a.-s. ankle prosthesis
  b.-a.-s. joint
  b.-a.-s. trochanteric osteotomy
Ballantine
  B. clamp
  B. hemilaminectomy retractor
Ballenger
  B. periosteotome
  B. swivel knife
Ballenger-Hajek chisel
Ballert Buildup foot wedge

ballistic
 b. information
 b. injury
balloon cell nevus
ballottable
ballotte
ballottement
 b. of patella
 b. test
ballpit
 multisensory b.
ball-tip
 b.-t. guidepin
 b.-t. spike
balmoral laced shoe
balneotherapy
Baló sclerosis
balsa wood filler block
Baltimore
 B. Therapeutic Equipment (BTE)
 B. Therapeutic Equipment Work
 Simulator
Bamberger-Marie disease
bamboo spine
Bamby clamp
banana
 b. Beaver blade
 b. finger extension splint
 b. knife
Bancap HC
band
 air b.
 AO tension b.
 aponeurotic b.
 big b.
 calf b.
 Can-Do Exercise B.
 congenital fibrous b.
 conjoined lateral b.
 exercise b.
 fascial b.
 fibrous b.
 Fit-Lastic therapy b.
 GelBand arm b.
 iliopatellar b.
 iliotibial b. (ITB)
 Jobst air b.
 lateral b.
 M b.
 palpable b.
 Parham b.
 Parham-Martin b.

 Partridge v.
 patellar b.
 pelvic b.
 pretendinous b.
 REP Bands exercise b.
 rigid metal pelvic b.
 sagittal b.
 scar b.
 Simonart b.
 taut b.
 tension b.
 True Blue exercise b.
 Xercise b.
 Z b.
bandage
 Ace adherent b.
 ankle traction b.
 ASE b.
 axilla, shoulder, elbow b.
 Barton b.
 capeline b.
 Champ elastic b.
 Comperm tubular elastic b.
 compression b.
 Conco elastic b.
 cotton elastic b.
 cravat b.
 Desault wrist b.
 Dressinet netting b.
 E Cotton b.
 Elastic Foam b.
 Elastomull elastic gauze b.
 Elastoplast b.
 Esmarch b.
 Fabco gauze b.
 fiberglass b.
 figure-of-eight b.
 Flex-Foam b.
 flexible b.
 Flexilite conforming elastic b.
 Flex-Master b.
 Fractura Flex b.
 Gibney b.
 Gibson b.
 gum rubber Martin b.
 Hamilton b.
 Helenca b.
 Heliodorus b.
 Hippocrates b.
 Hueter b.
 Hydron Burn B.
 immobilizing b.

B

NOTES

bandage *(continued)*
    Kerlix b.
    Kling elastic b.
    Martin sheet rubber b.
    Medi-Band b.
    MPM b.
    Nu Gauze b.
    Orthoflex elastic plaster b.
    Ortho-Trac adhesive skin
      traction b.
    Ortho-Vent b.
    Pavlik b.
    plaster-of-Paris b.
    polyurethane b.
    PRN b.
    Redigrip pressure b.
    replantation b.
    restrictive b.
    Ribble b.
    Richet b.
    Sayre b.
    scultetus b.
    Shur-Band self-closure elastic b.
    Silesian b.
    sling-and-swathe b.
    starch b.
    stockinette b.
    Thera-Boot b.
    Tricodur compression support b.
    Tricodur Epi compression b.
    Tricodur Omos compression b.
    Tricodur Talus compression b.
    Tru-Support EW b.
    Tru-Support SA b.
    TubeGauz b.
    Tubigrip b.
    Velpeau b.
    Webril b.
Bandi
    B. procedure
    B. technique
Band-It tennis elbow strap
band-like
    b.-l. adhesion
    b.-l. pain
bandy leg
Bane
    B. bone rongeur
    B. rongeur forceps
Bane-Hartmann bone rongeur
banjo
    b. cast
    b. splint
    b. traction
bank
    bone b.
    shoulder dislocation bone b.
    staple capsulorraphy bone b.

Bankart
    B. fracture
    B. operation
    B. procedure
    B. reconstruction
    B. shoulder dislocation
    B. shoulder lesion
    B. shoulder prosthesis
    B. shoulder repair
    B. shoulder repair set
Bankart-Putti-Platt operation
Banks
    American Association of Tissue B.
    (AATB)
    B. bone graft
Banks-Laufman
    B.-L. approach
    B.-L. incision
    B.-L. technique
Bannon-Klein implant
Banophen Oral
Bantam wire-cutting scissors
bantenadesis
BAP
    Behavioral Assessment of Pain
BAPS
    Biomechanical Ankle Platform System
    BAPS Ankle System
    BAPS board
bar
    b.-and-shoe orthosis
    A-T B.
    Bill b.
    b. bolt fixation
    bony b.
    broomstick b.
    calcaneonavicular b.
    cross b.
    Denis Browne b.
    derotator b.
    b. drill
    Fillauer b.
    Gerster traction b.
    grab b.
    intramedullary b.
    Leyla b.
    b.-like ventral defect on
      myelography
    Livingston intramedullary b.
    longitudinal spinal b.
    lumbrical b.
    metatarsal flatfoot b.
    MT b.
    opponens b.
    patellar b.
    posterior thigh b.
    b. resection
    rocker b.

B

screw alignment b.
b. section
spacer b.
spondylitic b.
spondylotic b.
stabilizing b.
stall b.
Stephen spreader b.
Thera-P exercise b.
Thornton b.
b.-to-bar clamp
Tommy trapeze b.
unsegmented vertebral b.
valgus b.
Zielke derotator b.
Bárány-Nylen maneuver
barbed
b. broach
b. staple
barber chair position
barbotage
Barbour
B. cervical fixation
B. technique
Bard clamp
Bardeleben
B. bone-holding forceps
B. rasp
Bard-Parker
B.-P. blade
B.-P. handle
B.-P. knife
B.-P. scalpel
Bareskin knee positioner
bark
prickly ash b.
barked injury
Barkow ligament
Barlow
B. cruciform infant splint
B. maneuver
B. provocative test
B. sign
Barnhart repair
barognosis
Baron suction tube
barotrauma
Barouk
B. button space for hallux valgus deformity
B. cannulated bone screw

B. microscrew with shortening osteotomy
B. microstaple
B. spacer
Barr
B. anterior transfer
B. bolt
B. bolt nail
B. hook
B. open reduction and internal fixation
B. pin
B. tendon transfer operation
B. tibial fracture fixation
Barraquer needle holder
Barrasso-Wile-Gage arthrodesis
barrel
b. bur
b. bur design
b. crawl
b. guide
b. plate
sideplate b.
barreled sideplate
Barre-Lieou syndrome
barrier
anatomic b.
elastic b.
B. lower extremity sheet
motion b.
pathologic b.
physiologic b.
side-bending b.
Barr-Record ankle arthrodesis
Barsky
B. cleft closure
B. macrodactyly reduction
B. procedure
B. technique
Barthel
B. ADL index
Bartlett
B. nail fold
B. nail fold excision
B. procedure
Barton
B. bandage
B. fracture
B. sling
B. tongs
B. traction handle

NOTES

Barton-Cone
- B.-C. tongs
- B.-C. tong traction

Bart-Phumphery syndrome

basal
- b. block cervical saddle
- b. joint
- b. neck
- b. neck fracture
- b. osteotomy

base
- Dycal b.
- b. of fingernail
- metacarpal b.
- b.-of-the-neck osteotomy
- plantar lateral b.
- Profix nonporous tibial b.
- b. of support
- b. wedge osteotomy
- b. wedge osteotomy/bunionectomy

baseball
- b. finger
- b. finger fracture
- b. finger splint
- b. pitcher's elbow
- b. shoulder

baseline
- b. capacity evaluation
- B. dynamometer
- b. view

basement membrane

basic
- #405 Econo 90 B.
- B. I, II cranial adjusting procedure
- b. multicellular remodeling unit
- B. Sequences ColorCards
- b. technique

basilar
- b. artery migraine
- b. crescentic osteotomy
- b. femoral neck fracture
- b. impression
- b. invagination
- b. metatarsal osteotomy

Basile hip screw

basioccipital

basket
- Acufex meniscal b.
- b. forceps
- b. rongeur
- rotary b.
- Schutte shovelnose b.
- b. stockinette
- walker b.

basketball foot

Basmajian technique

basocervical fracture

Bassett
- B. electrical stimulation apparatus
- B. electrical stimulation device
- B. electrical stimulation system
- B. sign

Basswood splint

Batchelor
- B. plaster
- B. plate

Batchelor-Brown extraarticular subtalar arthrodesis

Batch-Spittler-McFaddin
- B.-S.-M. knee disarticulation
- B.-S.-M. technique

Bateman
- B. femoral neck prosthesis
- B. finger prosthesis
- B. hemiarthroplasty
- B. modification of Mayer transfer operation
- B. shoulder operation
- B. UPF II bipolar knee system
- B. UPF II bipolar prosthesis
- B. UPF II shoulder prosthesis

bath
- Aqua/Whirl b.
- Bag B.
- contrast b. (CB)
- Dickson Paraffin b.
- galvanic b.
- hot water b.
- paraffin b. (PB)
- ThermaSplint heating b.
- whirlpool b. (WPB)

bathing and dressing ability

Bathlifter
- Leo B.

batrachian
- b. gait
- b. posture

Batson
- veins of B.

battered child syndrome

battery-driven hand drill

battery-pack Osteo-Stim bone stimulator

battery-powered instrument

batting
- Dacron b.

battledore incision

Battle sign

Batzdorf
- B. cervical wire passer
- B. cervical wire twister

Bauerfeind
- B. Achillotrain
- B. ankle brace
- B. comprifix knee brace

B. Malleolic Ankle Orthosis
B. SofSpot Heel Cup
Bauer-Jackson classification
Bauer-Tondra-Trusler
B.-T.-T. operation
B.-T.-T. technique
Baumann angle
Baumgard-Schwartz tennis elbow technique
Baumrucker clamp irrigator
Bavarian splint
Baxter
B. angled arthroscope
B. nerve release
B. personal Von-Loc ice pack
Baxter-D'Astous procedure
Bayer
B. Buffered Aspirin
B. Low Adult Strength
B. Select Pain Relief Formula
Baylor
B. adjustable cross splint
B. metatarsal splint
Bayne classification of radial agenesis
Bayne-Klug centralization
bayonet
b. apposition
b. clip applier
b. dislocation
b. fracture position
b. knife
b. leg
b. nonunion
b. osteotome
b.-point wire
b. position of fracture
b. rongeur
b. saw
b. sign
b. spacer
Bazooka support surface
BBC
biceps, brachialis, coracobrachialis
BBC muscles
BB to MM
belly button to medial malleolus
BB to MM examination
B. burgdorferi **titer for Lyme disease**
BDD
blistering distal dactylitis

BDH
biologically designed hip
BDH prosthesis
BE
below-elbow
beach chair position
bead
aminoglycoside-impregnated methyl methacrylate b.
antibiotic-impregnated b.
gentamicin b.
metallic b.
methyl methacrylate b.
b. pouch
Septobal b.
targeting b.
beaded
b. guidewire
b. hip pin
b.-pin wrench
b. reamer guidepin
beak
b. fingernail
b. fracture
b. ligament
metacarpal b.
b. modification with triple arthrodesis
b. nail
talar b.
beaked cervicomedullary junction
beaking
b. of head of talus
talar b.
beaklike osteophyte formation
Beall-Webel-Bailey technique
Beals test
beam
load b.
primary x-ray b.
beanbag
bearing
ball b.
pretibial b. (PTB)
radial b.
b.-seating forceps
Steinmann pin with ball b.
ulnar b.
bear's paw hand
Beasley-Babcock forceps
Beath
B. bone intramedullary peg

B

NOTES

Beath *(continued)*
    B. needle
    B. pin
    B. view
Beatson combined ankle angle
Beaty lateral release
Beaufort seating orthosis
Beau lines
Beaver
    B. blade handle
    B. cataract knife
    B. keratome blade
    B. saw
Beaver-DeBakey
    B.-D. blade
    B.-D. knife
Bebax
    B. Bootie
    B. orthosis
    B. shoe
    B. shoe for forefoot deformity
becaplermin
Bechterew
    B. disease
    B. test
Bechtol
    B. acetabular component
    B. arthroplasty
    B. hip prosthesis
    B. screw
    B. system prosthesis
Beck Depression Inventory
Beckenbaugh
    B. correction
    B. technique
Becker
    B. brace
    B. hand prosthesis
    B. 655 motion control limiter
    B. muscular dystrophy (BMD)
    B. orthopaedic spinal system
      (BOSS)
    B. orthopaedic spinal system
      orthotic device
    B. orthopedic thermoformable ankle
      system
    B. screwdriver
    B. technique
    B. tendon repair
    B. variant of Duchenne dystrophy
Beckman retractor
Beck-Steffee total ankle prosthesis
Beclard amputation
Becton
    B. open reduction
    B. technique

bed
    American Seating Access-O-
      Matic b.
    BioDyne b.
    bone graft b.
    Borg-Warner orthopaedic b.
    Burke Bariatric b.
    Cardiopulmonary Paragon 8500 b.
    Carrom orthopaedic b.
    Chick-Foster orthopedic b.
    CircOlectric b.
    Clinitron air b.
    b. cradle
    DMI orthopaedic b.
    Flexicair b.
    FluidAir b.
    Foster b.
    Gatch b.
    gatched b.
    Goodman orthopaedic b.
    Hausted orthopaedic b.
    high-air-loss b.
    high muscular resistance b.
    Hill-Rom orthopaedic b.
    hi-lo rehab b.
    Hollywood b.
    Inland Super Multi-Hite
      orthopaedic b.
    Inter-Royal frame orthopaedic b.
    Joerns orthopaedic b.
    Keane Mobility b.
    KinAir b.
    Lapidus b.
    low-air-loss b.
    Magnum 800 b.
    Medicus b.
    Mega-Air b.
    Mega Tilt and Turn b.
    nail b.
    obese b.
    orthopaedic b.
    Plastizote foot b.
    Pulmonair 40 b.
    b. rest
    Restcue b.
    ROHO b.
    Roto-Rest b.
    Simmons Multi-Matic
      orthopaedic b.
    Simmons Vari-Hite orthopaedic b.
    Skytron b.
    SMI 3000, 5000 b.
    Smith-Davis Converta-Hite
      orthopaedic b.
    Spa B.
    Stryker b.
    Superior Sleeprite Hi-Lo
      orthopaedic b.

Swinger car b.
Thera Pulse b.
Tilt and Turn Paragon b.
b.-to-chair transfer
Ultra-Flex orthopaedic b.
bedbound patient
Bednar tumor
bedroom fracture
Beebe wire-cutting scissors
Beery Test for Visual-Motor Integration
Beeson cast spreader
bee venom therapy
Beevor sign
behavior
compensatory b.
occupational b.
behavioral
B. Assessment of Pain (BAP)
B. Assessment of Pain
Questionnaire
b. mapping
Behcet syndrome
Behr syndrome
Bekhterev
B. arthritis
B. test
Bekhterev-Mendel reflex
Belcher clamp
Belix Oral
bell
Hydro-Tone B.
B. palsy
b. rasp
B. suture
B. table
B. Tawse procedure
belladonna
b. and opium
tincture of b.
Bell-Dally cervical dislocation
**Bellemore-Barrett closing wedge
osteotomy**
**Bellemore-Barrett-Middleton-Scougall-
Whiteway technique**
Bellergal-S
Bell-Tawse open reduction technique
Bellucci alligator scissors
belly
b. button to medial malleolus (BB
to MM)
b. button to medial malleolus
examination

muscle b.
b.-press test
Belos compression pin
below-elbow (BE)
b.-e. amputation
below-knee (BK)
b.-k. amputation (BKA)
b.-k. amputation using long
posterior flap
b.-k. prosthesis
b.-k. walking cast
belt
Carabelt therapeutic b.
gait b.
Meek pelvic traction b.
MicroTeq portable b.
Posey b.
PowerBelt lower back and
abdominal support b.
Reed cast b.
rib b.
sacroiliac b.
seat b.
Serola sacroiliac b.
SI b.
Silesian b.
Soma sacroiliac stabilization b.
Spine Power pelvic stabilizer b.
Sports Plus II back b.
TES b.
Tri-Flex auxiliary suspension b.
waist suspension b.
Zim-Zip rib b.
Benadryl Oral
Ben-Allergin-50 Injection
Bence Jones protein
bench
b. examination
Invacare vinyl transfer b.
Paramount 3-Way Press B.
pelvic b.
b. test
Winco Adjusting B.
bend
B.-A-Boot foot splint
deep knee b. (DKB)
sitting side b.
standing side b.
bender
AO plate b.
Bunnell knuckle b.
DePuy rod b.

NOTES

bender *(continued)*
    French rod b.
    Luque rod b.
    plate b.
    rod b.
    Rush b.
Benders
    Knuckle B.
bending
    backward b.
    cantilever b.
    forward b.
    lateral b.
    left side b.
    b. load
    right side b.
    rod b.
    side b.
    b. strength
    b. stress
    b. toward the side of injury
Bendixen-Kirschner traction
B-endorphin
benediction posture
BeneFin clinical shark cartilage
Benefoot & Birkenstock orthotic sandal
BeneJoint
Benemid
benign
    b. chondroblastoma
    b. congenital myopathy
    b. fasciculation
    b. tumor
Benink tarsal index
Bennet
    B. basic hand dislocation
    B. bone elevator
Bennett
    B. comminuted fracture
    B. dislocation
    B. elevator
    B. fracture-dislocation
    B. fracture of thumb
    B. lesion
    B. nail biopsy
    B. posterior shoulder approach
    B. quadriceps plastic operation
    B. quadriceps plastic procedure
    B. retractor
bent-knee cast
bent nail
Benyi modification of Lambrinudi triple arthrodesis
benzalkonium chloride
benzedrine
benzodiazepine
benzoic acid and salicylic acid

benzoin
    b. adherent tape
    tincture of b.
benztropine mesylate
BeOK hand exercise putty
Berens
    B. muscle clamp
    B. muscle clamp forceps
Berg balance test
Berger
    B. capsulodesis
    B. disease
    B. interscapular amputation
Berger-Bookwalter posterior approach
Bergman mallet
Bergstrom needle
Berke clamp
Berliner percussion hammer
Berman-Gartland
    B.-G. metatarsal osteotomy
    B.-G. procedure
Berman-Moorhead metal locator
Bermuda spica cast
Berndt-Hardy classification of transchondral fracture
Berndt hip ruler
Bernhard clamp
Berstein cast table
Bertin hip retractor
besylate
    atracurium b.
beta
    b. adrenergic
    b. blocker medication
    B. Pile II, III splint strap
    transforming growth factor b.
Betadine
    B. dressing
    B. First Aid Antibiotics + Moisturizer
    B. paint
    B. scrub
    B. scrub solution
    B. soak
    B.-soaked pledget
    B. soap
betamethasone
    b. and clotrimazole
    b. dipropionate
    b. sodium phosphate
Betasept
Bethesda bone
Bethune
    B. clamp
    B. periosteal elevator
Bethune-Coryllos rib shears
Beurrier connector
bevel

beveled
beveling
bevel-point Rush pin
Bevin-Aurglass technique
Bevin shoe
Bexophene
Beyer rongeur
Beyer-Stille bone rongeur
BFM
    Brunnstrom-Fugl-Meyer
    BFM arm impairment assessment
BFO
    BFO Kit
    BFO Orthosis
B.H. Moore procedure
BIA
    bioelectrical impedance analysis
Bi-Angular shoulder prosthesis
BIAS
    B. prosthesis
    B. rasp
    B. total hip system
bias-cut
    b.-c. stockinette
    b.-c. tape
BICAP cautery
bicentric prosthesis
biceps
    b., brachialis, coracobrachialis
    (BBC)
    b. brachialis muscle transfer
    b. brachialis tendon
    b. brachii muscle
    b. brachii tendon
    b. femoris
    b. femoris muscle
    b. femoris tendon
    b. groove
    b. interval lesion (BIL)
    b. jerk (BJ)
    b. jerk reflex test
    long head of b.
    b. reflex
    short head of b.
    b. tendinitis
bicepsplasty
bichloracetic acid
Bicillin C-R 900/300 Injection
bicipital
    b. groove
    b. rib
    b. syndrome

    b. tendinitis
    b. tendon
    b. tenosynovitis
    b. tuberosity
    b. tuberosity view
Bickel
    B. intramedullary nail
    B. intramedullary rod
    B. legholder
Bickel-Moe procedure
bicompartmental
    b. implant
    b. knee implant prosthesis
    b. soft-tissue sarcoma
bicondylar
    b. ankle prosthesis
    b. graft
    b. knee prosthesis
    b. tibial plateau
    b. T-shaped fracture
    b. Y-shaped fracture
Bicon-Plus Cup
Bicoral implant
bicorrectional Austin osteotomy
bicortical
    b. iliac bone
    b. iliac bone graft
    b. ilial strip graft
    b. screw
    b. screw fixation
bicycle, bike
    air b.
    Air-Dyne b.
    b. brace
    b. exerciser
    FES exercise b.
    b. injury
    Monark b.
    Schwinn Air-Dyne b.
    b. spoke fracture
BID
    bilateral interfacetal dislocation
Bielschowsky-Jansky disease
Bier
    B. amputation
    B. block
    B. block anesthesia
bifid
    b. condyle
    b. graft
    b. thumb
    b. thumb deformity

B

NOTES

bifida
    spina b.
bifilar needle recording electrode
biflanged drill
biframed distraction technique
bifrontal incision
bifurcated
    b. bladeplate
    b. vein graft (autologous pedal)
      for vascular reconstruction
bifurcate ligament
bifurcation osteotomy
bifurcatum
    ligamentum b.
big band
Bigelo calvarium clamp
Bigelow maneuver
biglycan
bike (*var. of* bicycle)
bikini skin incision
BIL
    biceps interval lesion
bilateral
    b. acute radicular syndrome
    b. amputation
    b. chronic radicular syndrome
    b. frame
    b. hemiplegia
    b. heterotopic ossification
    b. ilioinguinal approach
    b. interfacetal dislocation (BID)
    b. lateral fusion
    b. sacroiliac approach
    b. variable screw placement system
    b. V-Y Kutler flap
bilaterally
Bilhaut-Cloquet procedure
Bill bar
Billington yoke
biloba
    ginkgo b.
bilobed
    b. digital neurovascular island flap
    b. skin flap
Bilos
    B. pin
    B. pin extractor
bimalleolar
    b. angle
    b. ankle fracture
    b. approach to ankle arthrodesis
    b.-foot axis
Bi-Metric
    B.-M. hip prosthesis
    B.-M. Interlok femoral prosthesis
    B.-M. porous primary femoral
      prosthesis

    B.-M. tapered reamer with
      Zimmer-Hudson shank
Bindegewebsmassage
binder
    abdominal b.
    arch b.
    Helenca b.
    sacroiliac b.
    scultetus b.
binding
    biologic b.
binocular loupe
Bio-Absorbable interference screw
Bio-Boot
Biobrane
    B. adhesive
    B. glove
bioceramic implant material
Bio-Chromatic hand prosthesis
Bioclad with pegs reinforced acetabular
    prosthesis
Bioclusive select transparent film
    dressing
biocompartmental replacement of knee
biocompatibility
    implant b.
biocompatible
BioCompression Pneumatic Sleeve
bioconcave vertebra
Biocoral
biocorrosion
biodegradable
    b. plate
    b. surgical tack
Biodel implant
Biodex
    B. isokinetic dynamometer
    B. isokinetic testing machine
    B. Multi-Joint System 3 MVP
    B. test
Biodine
Biodynamic Molding System
BioDyne bed
bioelectric
    b. phenomenon
    b. potential
bioelectrical
    b. impedance
    b. impedance analysis (BIA)
    b. repair of delayed union or
     nonunion
bio-energy imbalance syndrome (BIS)
biofeedback
    b.-assisted method
    B. 5DX
BioFit Press-Fit acetabular prosthesis
Biofix
    B. absorbable fixation

B

B. absorbable fixation system
B. arrow
B. arrow gun
B. biodegradable implant
B. system pin

BIOflex

B. Magnet Back Support

Bioflex

B. magnetic brace
B. orthotic

Bio Flote air flotation system
Biofoot orthotic
Biofreeze

B. Roll-On
B. topical analgesic gel
B. with Ilex

Bio-Gel decubitus pillow
Bioglass prosthesis
Bio-Groove

B.-G. acetabular prosthesis
B.-G. Macrobond HA femoral
prosthesis

biokinetic remediation
Biokinetics pedobarograph
BioKnit garment electrode
biologic

b. binding
b. dressing
b. fixation

biologically

b. designed hip (BDH)
b. quiet interference screw

Biolox

B. ceramic ball head for hip
replacement
B. ceramic coating

biomagnet
biomaterial
biomechanical

b. analysis
B. Ankle Platform System (BAPS)
b. evaluation of foot function
during stance phase of gait
b. factor
b. frame of reference
b. principle
b. testing

biomechanics

axial plane angular deformity b.
bone b.
distraction instrumentation b.
Dwyer instrumentation b.

impact b.
b. of lifting
posterior fixation system b.
propulsion b.
soft tissue b.
walking b.

BioMed TENS unit
Biomet

B. acetabular cup
B. AGC knee prosthesis
B. button
B. cement-removal hand chisel
B. custom implant
B. fracture brace
B. hip prosthesis
B. MARS acetabular component
B. revision acetabular component
B. revision hip stem
B. revision knee system
B. shoulder component
B. total toe prosthesis
B. Ultra-Drive cement remover
B. Ultra-Drive ultrasonic revision
system

biometal
Biometric prosthesis
Bio-Modular total shoulder system
Bio-Moore endoprosthesis
Bionics arrow
Bionix self-reinforced PLLA smart
screw
Bio-Oss synthetic bone
Biophase

ASTM designation of B.
B. implant metal
B. implant metal prosthesis

biophysics

chiropractic b. (CBP)

bioplastic
BioPolyMeric graft
bioprosthesis

bovine collagen b.

biopsy (Bx)

aspiration needle b.
Bennett nail b.
bone marrow b.
channel-and-core b.
closed core needle b.
cone bone b.
Dunn b.
excisional b.
forage core b.

NOTES

biopsy *(continued)*
    b. forceps
    Fosnaugh nail b.
    freehand CT-guided b.
    incisional b.
    lumbar spine b.
    Michele vertebral b.
    needle b.
    open b.
    punch b.
    Scher nail b.
    shave b.
    spinal infection b.
    synovial b.
    thoracic spine b.
    trephine needle b.
    ultrasound-guided echo b.
    ultrasound-guided stereotactic b.
    Valls-Ottolenghim-Schajowicz
      needle b.
    Zaias nail b.
bioresorbable
    b. drug delivery system
    b. pin
BioRoc anchor
Bio-R-Sorb resorbable poly-L-lactic acid ministaple
BioSkin support
BioSphere
    B. suture anchor
    B. suture anchor implant
Biostop G cement restrictor
Biotens neurostimulator
Biotex
    B. implant metal
    B. implant metal prosthesis
Biothesiometer ROC
Biothotic
    B. foot orthosis
    B. orthotic
    B. orthotic mold
Biotone Polar lotion
BIOWARE software for Biodex isokinetic exercise system
Bio-Wick sock
BioZone nutrition system
Biozyme-C
bipartite
    b. fracture
    b. patella
    b. scaphoid
    b. tibial sesamoid
bipedal walking
bipedicle dorsal flap
biphasic
    b. action potential
    b. endplate activity
    b. (low-volt) waveform

bipivotal hinge knee brace
biplanar
    b. fixator
    b. radiography
biplane
    b. angiogram
    b. roentgenogram
    b. trochanteric osteotomy
biplaning of osteotomy
bipolar
    b. acetabular cup
    b. cauterization
    b. cautery
    b. coagulator
    b. femoral component
    b. femoral head prosthesis
    b. forceps
    b. hip arthroplasty
    b. hip arthroplasty component
    b. hip replacement prosthesis
    b. IF waveform
    b. needle recording electrode
    b. prosthetic cup
    b. release
    b. stimulating electrode
    b. vertebral traction
Bircher
    B. bone-holding clamp
    B. cartilage clamp
    B. meniscotome
    B. meniscus knife
Bircher-Ganske cartilage forceps
Bircher-Weber technique
birdcage splint
birefringent
    b. lipid crystals in tendinitis
    b. particle
Birkenstock Blue Footbed arch support
birth
    b. fracture
    b. injury
    b. trauma
BIS
    bio-energy imbalance syndrome
bisector line
Bishop
    B. bone clamp
    B. chisel
    B. classification
    B. gouge
    B. saw
Bishop-Black tendon tucker
Bishop-DeWitt tendon tucker
Bishop-Peter tendon tucker
bit
    AO drill b.
    cannulated drill b.
    drill b.

B

b. drill
femoral drill b.
Gore b.
Howmedica Microfixation System
  drill b.
Leibinger Micro System drill b.
Luhr Microfixation System drill b.
Storz Microsystems drill b.
Synthes Microsystem drill b.

bite
biter
  Stille bone b.
  suction b.
bivalved cylinder cast
bizarre
  b. high-frequency discharge
  b. repetitive discharge
  b. repetitive potential
BJ
  biceps jerk
Björk
  B. prosthesis
  B. rib drill
BK
  below-knee
  BK mole syndrome
  BK prosthesis
BKA
  below-knee amputation
black
  b. cohosh
  b.-dot heel
  b. heel syndrome
  B. Max mid size knee component
  B. peroneal tendon sheath injection
  B. rasp
  B. repair
  B. technique
Black-Broström staple technique
Blackburn
  B. technique
  B. traction
Blackburn-Peel
  B.-P. measurement
  B.-P. ratio
bladder
  b. ileus
  b. injury
blade
  arachnoid-shape Beaver b.
  Arthro-Lok system of Beaver b.
  banana Beaver b.

Bard-Parker b.
Beaver-DeBakey b.
Beaver keratome b.
Caspar b.
cast b.
cataract knife Beaver b.
Curdy b.
curved meniscotome b.
discission knife Beaver b.
Dynagrip handle of b.
Dyonics arthroscopic b.
Field b.
Gigli saw b.
Hebra b.
Hibbs b.
hook b.
Incisor arthroscopic b.
K b.
keratome Beaver b.
knife b.
Merlin arthroscopy b.
mini-meniscus b.
3 M Maxi Driver b.
MVR b.
notchplasty b.
Paufique b.
b. plate
b. plate driver
b. plate fixation
b.-point retractor
PowerCut drill b.
resector b.
retrograde Beaver b.
retrograde meniscal b.
rosette Beaver b.
sickle-shape Beaver b.
side-cutting b.
Smillie-Beaver b.
b.-spike retractor
Superblade b.
Swann-Morton surgical b.
Synovator arthroscopic b.
synovectomy b.
Taylor spinal retractor b.
Temperlite saw b.
Tiger b.
tri-radial resector b.
Zimmer-Gigli saw b.
bladeplate
  bifurcated b.
  fixed-angle AO b.

NOTES

Blair
- B. ankle arthrodesis
- B. ankle fusion
- B. anterior arthrodesis
- B. chisel
- B. elevator
- B. knife
- B. saw guide
- B. talar body fusion blade plate
- B. technique
- B. tibiotalar arthrodesis
- B. tibiotalar arthrodesis blade plate

Blair-Brown skin graft
Blair-Morris-Dunn-Hand ankle
  arthrodesis
Blair-Omer rerouting
Blajwas-Schwartz-Marcinko irrigation
  drainage system
Blalock clamp
blanch
Blanchard
- B. traction device
- B. traction device blade plate

blank
- Aliplast b.
- implant b.
- Nickelplast b.
- Plastazote b.

blanket
- EBI Temptek b.
- Hollister Hot/Ice knee b.
- Hot/Ice System III knee b.
- Rowe b.

Blastomyces dermatitidis
blastomycosis
- North American b.

blastomycotic osteomyelitis
Blatt
- B. capsulodesis
- B. procedure

Blatt-Ashworth procedure
Blauth knee prosthesis
Blazina prosthesis
bleb capsulodesis
Bleck
- B. iliopsoas recession
- B. metatarsus adductus classification
- B. method
- B. recession technique

Bledsoe
- B. cast brace
- B. knee brace
- B. leg brace

bleeders
- buzz b.

bleeding
- b. bone
- b. point

blind
- b. anchorage hole
- b. medullary nail
- b. medullary nailing

blink
- b. reflex
- b. response

Bliskunov implantable femoral distractor
blister
- b. of bone
- B. Film dressing
- fracture b.

blistering distal dactylitis (BDD)
Blis-To-Sol
Blix contractile force curve
bloc
- en b.

Blocadren
Bloch equation
block
- ankle b.
- anodal b.
- arteriography b.
- axillary b.
- balsa wood filler b.
- Bier b.
- bony b.
- brachial plexus b.
- Campbell posterior bone b.
- conduction b.
- condyle b.
- cutting b.
- 4-in-1 cutting b.
- depolarization b.
- differential spinal b.
- digital nerve b.
- facet joint b.
- femoral nerve b.
- field b.
- filler b.
- forefoot b.
- four-in-one b.
- ganglion b.
- Gill posterior bone b.
- graduated-height b.
- hand b.
- Hara infiltration b.
- Howard bone b.
- Inclan posterior bone b.
- interscalene b.
- Kohs b.
- Mayo nerve b.
- median nerve b.
- metacarpal b.
- Mikhail bone b.
- motor point b.
- musculocutaneous nerve b.
- nerve root b.

neurolytic b.
b. osteotomy
pelvic b.
peripheral nerve b.
plexus b.
posterior bone b.
push-up b.
recurrent median nerve b.
regional b.
scalene b.
sciatic leg b.
S-cutting b.
sphenopalatine ganglion b.
spinal cord b.
Steinberg infiltration b.
stellate sympathetic ganglion b.
Styrofoam filler b.
subarachnoid b.
sympathetic b.
b. test
tibial cutting b.
two-point nerve b.
ulnar nerve b.
blockage
articular b.
blocker
H2 b.
hook b.
blocker's exostosis
Block-Sulzberger syndrome
blood
autologous b.
b.-borne infection
b. cast
b. cell
b. culture
b. flow
b. glucose
b. loss
b. loss anemia
b. pressure
b. pressure monitor (BPM)
b. pressure monitoring
b. supply
b. transfusion
b. vessel tumor
b. volume pulse (BVP)
bloodless field
bloody effusion
Bloom-Raney
B.-R. modification

B.-R. modification of Smith-
Robinson technique
Bloom splint
Blount
B. anvil retractor
B. blade plate
B. bone spreader
B. brace
B. disease
B. displacement osteotomy
B. epiphysiodesis
B. fracture staple
B. knee retractor
B. knife
B. laminar spreader
B. osteotome
B. splint
B. stapling
B. technique for osteoclasis
B. tracing technique
Blount-Schmidt Milwaukee brace
blow-in fracture
blow-out fracture
B&L pinch gauge
blucher
b. laced shoe
b. opening
blue
B. Brand Therapy Putty
B. Line orthotic
methylene b.
b. nevus
b. rubber bleb nevus syndrome
Selsun B.
b. toe syndrome
Blumensaat line
Blumenthal bone rongeur
Blumer shelf
Blundell-Jones
B.-J. hip osteotomy
B.-J. technique
blunt
b. arthroscopic cannula
b. caliper
b. dissection
b. forceps
b. hook dissector
b. nose hemostat
b. stylet
b. tapered T-handled reamer
b. trocar

NOTES

blunt-tip
    b.-t. iris scissors
    b.-t. probe
BMC
    bone mineral content
BMD
    Becker muscular dystrophy
    bone mineral density
BME
    brief maximal effort
BMI
    body mass index
BMP
    bone marrow pressure
    BMP cabling and plating system
board
    American B. of Physical Therapy
      Specialists (ABPTS)
    balance b.
    BAPS b.
    Euroglide MKII slide b.
    Flexisplint flexed arm b.
    grid maze b.
    Hadfield hand b.
    hand b.
    J b.
    manipulation b.
    memory b.
    powder b.
    quad b.
    Rock ankle exercise b.
    rocker b.
    Rock & Roller exercise b.
    spinal b.
    b. splint
    Spri Xercise b.
    Steffensmeier b.
    string drawing b.
    Tegtmeier hand b.
    Visual Neglect B.
    wobble b.
    Yucca b.
boat nail
Bobechko
    B. sliding barrel hook
    B. spreader
Bobrath technique
Bock knee prosthesis
Bodenstab tourniquet
BODI
    BODI Dynamic Orthosis
    BODI knee extension orthosis
Bodnar retractor
body, pl. **bodies**
    alignment of vertebral bodies
    B. Armor walker cast
    artificial vertebral b.
    b. awareness

    B. Ball
    cartilaginous loose b.
    b. cast
    b.-exhaust suit
    fibrous loose b.
    foreign b. (FB)
    B. Gard neoprene support
    intraarticular loose b.
    b. jacket
    Kelvin b.
    b. logic rehabilitation system
    loose b.
    b. mass index (BMI)
    B. Master
    B. Masters MD 510 hi-lo pulley
      system
    Maxwell b.
    b. mechanics
    B. Mechanics Evaluation Checklist
    newtonian b.
    B. Oscillation Integrates
      Neuromuscular Gain (BOING)
    b. oscillation neuromuscular gain
      (BOING)
    osteocartilaginous loose b.
    B. Pedistal
    pedunculated loose b.
    B. Response system
    rice b.
    rigid b.
    b. side integration
    b. sway
    talar b.
    b. temperature
    Verocay b.
    vertebral b.
BodyBilt chair
BodyIce
    B. cold pack
    B. wrap
Bodyline
    B. Back-Huggar
    Satalite cushion by B.
"Bodyline sleeper" mattress overlay
Bodynapper Comfort Pillow
body-powered prosthetic device
Body-Solid exercise equipment
bodywork
Boeck sarcoid
Boehler (*var. of* Böhler)
bogginess
boggy
    b. consistency
    b. swelling
    b. synovitis
Bograb Universal offset ossicular
    prosthesis

Böhler, Boehler
- B. brace
- B. calcaneal angle
- B. calcaneal view
- B. cast breaker
- B. clamp
- B. extension bow
- B. fracture frame
- B. guideline
- B. lumbosacral angle
- B. lumbosacral view
- B. pin
- B. reducing frame
- B. skintight cast
- B. stirrup
- B. tongs
- B. tong traction
- B. wire splint

Böhler-Braun
- B.-B. frame
- B.-B. leg sling
- B.-B. splint

Böhler-Knowles hip pin

Böhler-Steinmann
- B.-S. pin
- B.-S. pin holder

Bohlman
- B. anterior cervical vertebrectomy
- B. cervical fusion technique
- B. pin
- B. triple-wire fusion
- B. triple-wire technique

Boies forceps

BOING

Body Oscillation Integrates Neuromuscular Gain

body oscillation neuromuscular gain

Boitzy open reduction

Boldrey brace

Bolero lift bath trolley

Bolin wedge filter system

Bollinger knee brace

Boloxie OT Prehension Game

bolster
- abduction b.
- cotton b.
- knee b.
- roll control b.
- rubber b.
- Telfa b.
- tie-over b.

bolt
- Alvar condylar b.
- Barr b.
- cannulated b.
- connecting b.
- b. cutter
- DePuy b.
- Fenton tibial b.
- fixation b.
- b. fixation
- Harris b.
- Herzenberg b.
- hexhead b.
- Holt b.
- Hubbard b.
- Hubbard-Nylok b.
- Moreira b.
- No-Lok b.
- Norman tibial b.
- Recon proximal drill guide b.
- Richmond b.
- solid hex b.
- tibial b.
- transfixion b.
- trochanteric b.
- Webb-Andreesen condylar b.
- Webb stove b.
- Wilson b.
- wire fixation b.
- Zimmer tibial b.

Boltzmann distribution

bolus

bombardment by nociceptor

Bombelli-Mathys-Morscher hip prosthesis

Bombelli-Morscher femoral component

Bond arm splint

Bondek suture

bonding

Poly-Lock b.

bone
- AAA b.
  - antigen-extracted allogeneic bone
- b. abscess
- b. absorption
- accessory b.
- b. age
- b. age according to Greulich and Pyle
- b. allograft
- allograft iliac b.
- antigen-extracted allogeneic b.
  - (AAA bone)

NOTES

bone *(continued)*
    architectural alternation of b.
    b. autogenous graft
    autogenous iliac b.
    b. awl
    b. bank
    Bethesda b.
    bicortical iliac b.
    b. biomechanics
    Bio-Oss synthetic b.
    b. biopsy needle
    b.-biting forceps
    bleeding b.
    blister of b.
    b. block procedure
    bone-patellar ligament-b. (BPB)
    bone-patellar tendon-b. (BPB)
    Bonfiglio b.
    b. borer
    b. bowing
    b.-breaking forceps
    bridging b.
    brittle b.
    b. bruise
    b. bur
    cadaver b.
    calcaneocuboid b.
    Calcitite b.
    b. callus
    cancellous versus cortical b.
    candle wax appearance of b.
    capitate b.
    carpal b.
    b. cement
    b.-cement interface
    chalky b.
    b. chip
    b. chip graft
    coalition of b.
    collar b.
    compact b.
    cortical versus cancellous b.
    corticocancellous b.
    b. crisis
    cuboid b.
    cuneiform b.
    b. curette
    b.-cutting forceps
    b. cyst excision
    b. cyst fracture probability
    b. cyst treatment
    b. debris
    b. defect
    demineralized b.
    b. densitometry
    b. deposition
    detritus b.
    b. development

    dimple the b.
    b. dissection
    b. dollop
    b. dowel
    b. drill set
    Durapatite b.
    eburnated b.
    ectopic b.
    enchondroma of b.
    b. end
    endochondral b.
    eosinophilic granuloma of b.
    b. extension clamp
    b. extractor
    b. femoral plug
    b. file
    b. flap fixation plate
    flat b.
    b.-forming tumor
    b. fragment
    fragmental b.
    freeze-dried b.
    freshening of b.
    fusiform periosteal new b.
    b. gouge
    b. graft bed
    b. graft collapse
    b. graft decompression
    B. Grafter instrument
    b. graft extrusion
    b. graft incorporation
    b. graft placement
    b. graft repair
    b. graft shoe horn
    b.-grasping forceps
    greater multangular b.
    b. growth
    b. growth stimulator
    hamate b.
    b. hand drill
    b. healing
    heterotopic b.
    b. holder
    b. hole punch
    b. hook
    hook of hamate b.
    hydroxyapatite b.
    hyoid b.
    b. impactor
    b. implant
    b.-implant interface
    b. implant material
    b. infarct
    b. infarction
    infected b.
    b. infection
    b. ingrowth
    b.-ingrowth fixation

innominate b.
Interpore b.
b. interstices
b. island
b. isograft
ivory b.
Kiel b.
lamellar b.
lamellated b.
laminar b.
b. lavage
lesser multangular b.
b. liner
long b.
long axis of b.
b. loss
lunate b.
lunocapitate b.
luxated b.
lyophilization of b.
b. mallet
marble b.
b. marrow
b. marrow aspiration
b. marrow biopsy
b. marrow graft
b. marrow pressure (BMP)
b. meal
medial metacarpal b.
b. metabolic unit
metacarpal b.
metatarsal b.
b. mill
b. mineral content (BMC)
b. mineral density (BMD)
morcellized b.
b. morphogenic protein
navicular b.
b. necrosis
b.-nibbling rongeur
Nicoll b.
nonlamellated b.
omovertebral b.
b.-on-bone
ossifying fibroma of long b.
osteonal lamellar b.
osteopenic b.
osteoporotic b.
os trapezium b.
os trapezoideum b.
b. overgrowth
pagetoid b.

particles of b.
b. paste
b. peg
b. peg epiphysiodesis
b. pegging
b. peg graft
b.-peg interface
perilesional b.
petrous temporal b.
Pirie b.
pisiform b.
b. plate selection
b. plug cutter
b. plug setter
porotic b.
primitive b.
b. production
b. prosthesis
b. punch forceps
b. punch rongeur
raw b.
b. reamer
b. remodeling
b. remodeling unit
b. resection
b. resorption
b. resurfacing
rider's b.
rudimentary b.
b. saw
b. scan
scaphoid b.
b. scintigraphy
b. screw
b. screw depth gauge
b.-screw interface strength
b. screw ruler gauge
b. screw targeter
semilunar b.
sesamoid b.
b. setting
short b.
b. skid
sliver of b.
b. slurry
b. spacer
spike of b.
split thickness cranial b.
b.-splitting forceps
spongy b.
b. spreader
b. spur

B

NOTES

bone *(continued)*
    b. stock
    subchondral b.
    subcoracoid b.
    subperiosteal new b.
    b. substance
    supernumerary b.
    supracollicular spike of cortical b.
    synthetic b.
    talonavicular b.
    b. tamp
    tarsal b.
    b. technique
    trabecular b.
    b. transfer
    b. trephine
    triangular wrist b.
    triquetrum b.
    b. trough
    b. tumor
    tumor-bearing b.
    b. union
    vascular bundle implantation
      into b.
    b. wax
    b. wax gelatin sponge
    b. wedge
    wormian b.
    woven b.
bone-holding
    b.-h. clamp
    b.-h. forceps
    b.-h. instrumentation
bonelet
Boneloc cement
bonemeal tablet
bone-patellar
    b.-p. ligament-bone (BPB)
    b.-p. tendon-bone (BPB)
    b.-p. tendon-bone autograft
    b.-p. tendon-bone preparation
BoneSource hydroxyapatite cement
bone-tendon-bone
    b.-t.-b. allograft
    b.-t.-b. graft
bone-to-bone
    b.-t.-b. apposition
    b.-t.-b. graft
Bonferroni correction
Bonfiglio
    B. bone
    B. bone replacement material
    B. graft
    B. modification
    B. modification of Phemister
      technique
Bonfiglio-Bardenstein technique
Bonner position

bonnet
    gluteal b.
Bonney clamp
Bonney-Kessel dorsiflexionary tilt-up
    osteotomy
Bonola technique
bony
    b. abnormality
    b. absorption
    b. ankylosis
    b. architecture
    b. avulsion
    b. bar
    b. block
    b. bridge
    b. bridge resection
    b. deformity
    b. demineralization
    b. distal end
    b. dysplasia
    b. eburnation
    b. element destruction
    b. encroachment
    b. erosion
    b. excrescence
    b. exostosis
    b. fragment
    b. interface
    b. island
    b. landmark
    b. lesion
    b. mass
    b. metastasis
    b. necrosis and destruction
    b. osteophyte
    b. overgrowth
    b. procedure
    b. prominence
    b. purchase
    b. skeleton
    b. slurry leakage
    b. spurring
    b. tenderness
    b. union
Boo-Boo Pacs
boot
    all-purpose b. (APB)
    Ambulator Chukka B.
    b. brace
    Bunny b.
    cast b.
    Chukka b.
    compression b.
    Cryo/Cuff b.
    derotation b.
    external sequential pneumatic
      compression b.
    fracture b.

gelatin compression b.
Gibney b.
Heelift suspension b.
L'Nard b.
Markell brace b.
Moon b.
pneumatic compression b.
Primer modified Unna b.
RIK FootHugger fluid heel b.
rocker b.
sequential pneumatic compression b.
SlimLine cast b.
Spenco b.
b.-top fracture
Unna paste b.
Venodyne b.
weight b.
Wilke b.
b. wrap

Booth test
Bootie
　　Bebax B.
Boplant Surgibone
Bora
　　B. centralization
　　B. operation
　　B. technique
borazone blade cutting machine
Borchardt olive-shaped bur
Borchgrevin traction
Borden-Spencer-Herman osteotomy
border
　　cryptotic medial b.
　　lateral acromial b.
　　medial b.
　　b. ray
　　b. ray amputation
　　scapulovertebral b.
　　superior b.
　　vertebral b.
bore needle
borer
　　bone b.
　　cork b.
Borge clamp
Borggreve
　　B. limb rotation
　　B. method
Borggreve-Hall technique
Borg-Warner orthopaedic bed
Bornholm disease
Boropak astringent solution

Borrelia burgdorferi
Bose
　　B. nail fold excision
　　B. procedure
BOSS
　　Becker orthopaedic spinal system
boss
　　carpometacarpal b.
bosselated
bosselation
bossing
　　frontal b.
Bostick staple
Boston
　　B. bivalve cast
　　B. brace thoracolumbosacral orthosis
　　B. Classification System
　　B. elbow system
　　B. LINAC
　　B. overlap brace
　　B. post-op hip orthosis
　　B. scoliosis brace
　　B. soft body jacket
　　B. thoracic brace
B&O Supprettes
Boswellin
Bosworth
　　B. approach
　　B. bone peg insertion
　　B. coracoclavicular screw
　　B. crown drill
　　B. femoroischial arthrodesis
　　B. femoroischial transplant
　　B. femoroischial transplantation
　　B. fracture
　　B. lumbar spinal fusion
　　B. screwdriver
　　B. shelf operation
　　B. shelf procedure
　　B. spine plate
　　B. splint
　　B. technique
　　B. tendo calcaneus repair
both-bone fracture
both-column fracture
botryoid sarcoma
bottle sign
bottom
　　hoof b.
　　Patten b.
　　weaver's b.

NOTES

B

Bottoms-Up posture system
botulinum toxin A (BtA)
Bouchard node
bouche de tapir
bouge needle
bounce home test
bouncing
 ligamentous b.
Bourneville disease
boutonnière
 b. deformity
 b. hand dislocation
 b. splint
Bovie
 B. cauterization
 B. cautery
 B. coagulating unit
 B. electrocautery apparatus
 B. electrocautery device
 B. knife
 underwater B.
bovine
 b. collagen
 b. collagen bioprosthesis
 b. collagen graft
 b. collagen implant
 b. collagen material prosthesis
bovis
 Mycobacterium b.
bow
 aiming b.
 B. & Arrow cannulated drill guide
 Böhler extension b.
 cupid's b.
 extension b.
 Framer finger extension b.
 Kirschner wire b.
 b. leg
 maximum radial b.
 posterior b.
 Schwarz finger extension b.
 b.-tie sign
 traction b.
Bowden cable suspension system
bowel training
Bowen
 B. chisel
 B. disease
 B. osteotome
 B. periosteal elevator
 B. suture drill
Bowen-Grover meniscotome
Bowers
 B. radial arthroplasty
 B. technique
bowing
 bone b.
 congenital posteromedial b.

 b. deformity
 b. fracture
 tibial b.
Bowlby arm splint
bowl curette
bowleg
 b. brace
 b. deformity
bowler's thumb
Bowman angle
bowstring
 b. sign
 b. tear
 b. test
box
 BTE Bolt B.
 b. chisel
 b. curette
 b.-end wrench
 high-toe b.
 ligamentous b.
 b. osteotome
 sit-and-reach b.
 toe b.
boxer's
 b. elbow
 b. fracture
 b. punch
boxwood mallet
Boyd
 B. ankle amputation
 B. approach
 B. classification
 B. dual-onlay bone graft
 B. hip disarticulation
 B. perforator
 B. podiatry chair
 B. type II fracture
Boyd-Anderson
 B.-A. biceps tendon repair
 B.-A. technique
Boyd-Bosworth procedure
Boyd-Griffin trochanteric fracture
 classification
Boyd-Ingram-Bourkhard treatment
Boyd-McLeod
 B.-M. procedure
 B.-M. tennis elbow technique
Boyd-Sisk
 B.-S. approach
 B.-S. posterior capsulorrhaphy
 B.-S. procedure
Boyer degenerative joint disease
 grading system
Boyes
 B. brachioradialis transfer technique
 B. muscle clamp
 B. transfer

Boyes-Goodfellow hook
Boyle-Davis retractor
Boyle-Thompson tendon transfer
Boytchev procedure
Bozzini light conductor
BPB
    bone-patellar ligament-bone
    bone-patellar tendon-bone
        BPB autologous graft
BPM
    blood pressure monitor
        Laserflo BPM
BPTB graft
BPTI
    brachial plexus traction injury
BR
    breathing reserve
brace
    Abbott b.
    abduction b.
    accommodative b.
    AFO pediatric b.
    Aircast Air-Stirrup b.
    Aircast ankle b.
    Aircast fracture b.
    Aircast leg b.
    Aircast pneumatic b.
    Aircast Swivel-Strap b.
    Aircast walking b.
    AirGEL ankle b.
    Air-Stirrup ankle b.
    Air-Stirrup ankle training b.
    Ank-L-Aid b.
    ankle ligament protector b.
    AO b.
    AOA cervical immobilization b.
    Arnold lumbar b.
    Atlanta hip b.
    Atlanta-Scottish Rite b.
    Atlantic overlap b.
    Atlantic rim b.
    ATR b.
    back b.
    bail-lock b.
    Bauerfeind ankle b.
    Bauerfeind comprifix knee b.
    Becker b.
    bicycle b.
    Bioflex magnetic b.
    Biomet fracture b.
    bipivotal hinge knee b.
    Bledsoe cast b.

Bledsoe knee b.
Bledsoe leg b.
Blount b.
Blount-Schmidt Milwaukee b.
Böhler b.
Boldrey b.
Bollinger knee b.
boot b.
Boston overlap b.
Boston scoliosis b.
Boston thoracic b.
bowleg b.
Buck knee b.
cable-twister b.
cage-back b.
caliper b.
Callender derotational b.
Camp b.
Cam Walker leg b.
Can Am b.
canvas b.
Capener b.
Carpal Lock wrist b.
carpenter's b.
CASH b.
Castaway leg b.
Castiglia ankle b.
Centec Propoint knee b.
cervical collar b.
chairback b.
Charleston nighttime bending b.
Charleston scoliosis b.
Charnley b.
CHH cervical b.
Chopart b.
Cincinnati ACL b.
clamshell b.
CM-Band 505N b.
CM-Band silicone rubber b.
Cole hyperextension b.
collar b.
contraflexion b.
controlled-motion b.
Cook walking b.
Count'R-Force arch b.
cowhorn b.
CRM rehab b.
CRS b.
CTEV b.
CTI b.
Cunningham b.
cutout patellar b.

B

NOTES

brace *(continued)*
DACO b.
DarcoGel ankle b.
Dennyson cervical b.
DePuy fracture b.
derotation b.
3D fracture walker b.
dial-lock b.
DonJoy ALP b.
DonJoy four-point Super Sport knee b.
DonJoy Gold Point knee b.
dorsiflexion stop b.
double Becker ankle b.
double-upright short leg b.
drop-foot b.
drop-lock knee b.
Duncan shoulder b.
dynamic abduction b.
Easy Lok ankle b.
Easy-On elbow b.
Eclipse Gel ankle b.
Edge knee b.
elastic-hinge knee b.
Elite knee b.
English b.
Equalizer cast b.
Exotec b.
figure-of-eight b.
Fisher b.
Flex Foam b.
flexor-hinge hand-splint b.
FLOAM ankle stirrup b.
Florida back b.
Florida cervical b.
Florida contraflexion b.
Florida extension b.
Florida hyperextension b.
Florida J-24, J-35, J-45, J-55 b.
Florida post-fusion b.
Florida spinal b.
foot-ankle b.
footdrop b.
Forrester cervical collar b.
four-point cervical b.
four-poster cervical b.
b.-free ambulation
Friedman b.
functional fracture b.
Futuro wrist b.
Galveston metacarpal b.
Generation II knee b.
Genutrain knee b.
GII Unloader ADJ knee b.
Gillette b.
GLS b.
GoldPoint b.
Goldthwait b.

Guilford cervical b.
halo b.
hand b.
head b.
Hennessy knee b.
Hessing b.
high-Knight b.
Hilgenreiner b.
hinged b.
Hi-Top foot/ankle b.
Hoke lumbar b.
Hudson-Jones knee-cage b.
Hudson TLSO b.
hyperextension b.
Ilfeld b.
InCare b.
Industrial Work b.
internal tibial torsion b.
I-Plus humeral b.
ischial weightbearing leg b.
Jewett-Benjamin cervical b.
Jewett contraflexion b.
Jewett hyperextension b.
Jewett post-fusion b.
J-59 Florida b.
Jones b.
J-55 postfusion b.
Kallassy b.
King cervical b.
Kleinert postoperative traction b.
Klengall b.
Klenzak spring b.
Kling cervical b.
knee b.
49er knee b.
knee cage b.
knee MD b.
Knight back b.
Knight-Taylor thoracic b.
knock-knee b.
Korn Cage knee b.
KSO b.
Küntscher-Hudson b.
Kydex b.
kyphosis b.
lace-on b.
lacing ankle b.
leaf-spring b.
LeCocq b.
leg b.
Lenox Hill derotational knee b.
Lenox Hill Spectralite knee b.
Lerman hinge b.
Lofstrand b.
long arm b.
long leg hinged b.
Lorenz b.

Lovitt-Uhler modification of Jewett post-fusion b.
LSU reciprocation-gait orthosis b.
lumbar b.
Lyman-Smith toe drop b.
MacAusland lumbar b.
McClintoch b.
McCollough internal tibial torsion b.
McDavid knee b.
McKee b.
McLight PCL b.
MD b.
Medical Design b.
Medipedic Multicentric knee b.
Metcalf spring drop b.
Miami fracture b.
Miami TLSO scoliosis b.
Milwaukee scoliosis b.
MKS II knee b.
Monarch knee b.
Moon Boot b.
Mooney b.
MTA b.
Mueller Ultralite b.
Multi-Lock knee b.
Murphy b.
Nakamura b.
neoprene hinged-knee b.
neoprene Osgood-Schlatter knee b.
neoprene wrist b.
New England scoliosis b.
Newington b.
Nextep knee b.
night b.
nonweightbearing b.
Northville b.
OA knee b.
Omni knee b.
Opiela b.
Oppenheim b.
Orbital shoulder stabilizer b.
Orthomedics b.
Ortho-Mold spinal b.
Orthoplast fracture b.
OS-5/Plus 2 knee b.
OsteoArthritic knee b.
Palumbo dynamic patellar b.
Palumbo knee b.
Palumbo stabilizing b.
pantaloon b.
patellar tendon-bearing b.

Patten-Bottom-Perthes b.
P.C. Williams b.
pediatric PRAFO b.
performer ultralight knee b.
Perlstein b.
PFT traction b.
Phelps b.
Philadelphia Plastizote cervical b.
piano-wire dorsiflexion b.
Pneu Knee b.
4-post cervical b.
Power Play knee b.
PPG-AFO b.
PPG-TLSO b.
Pro-8 ankle b.
PTB b.
PTS knee b.
Push medical b.
Quadrant advanced shoulder b.
QualCare knee b.
Raney flexion jacket b.
range of motion b.
ratchet-type b.
reamer b.
rigid postoperative b.
Rolyan tibial fracture b.
ROM knee b.
Saltiel b.
Sarmiento fracture b.
SAS II b.
SAWA shoulder b.
Schanz collar b.
scoliosis b.
Scottish Rite b.
Seton hip b.
short arm b.
short leg caliper b.
short leg double-upright b.
short leg walking b.
shoulder subluxation inhibitor b.
six-point knee b.
Smedberg b.
snap-lock b.
SOMI b.
Spinal Technology bivalve TLSO b.
Sports B.
Sports-Caster I, II knee b.
SSI b.
Stille b.
Stimprene electrotherapy b.
stirrup b.

NOTES

B

brace *(continued)*
    straight walker b.
    Strap Lok ankle b.
    Stromgren ankle b.
    Sully shoulder stabilizer b.
    Swede-O ankle b.
    Swede-O-Universal b.
    Swivel-Strap ankle b.
    Taylor back b.
    Taylor-Knight b.
    Taylor spine b.
    telescoping b.
    Teufel cervical b.
    Teurlings wrist b.
    The Richie b.
    Thermoskin b.
    Thomas cervical collar b.
    Thomas walking b.
    thoracolumbar standing orthosis b.
    TLSO b.
    toe-drop b.
    Tomasini b.
    Toronto b.
    Townsend b.
    Tracker knee b.
    Tri-angle shoulder abduction b.
    Trinkle b.
    turnbuckle ankle b.
    turnbuckle knee b.
    two-poster b.
    b.-type reamer
    UBC b.
    UCLA functional long leg b.
    Ultrabrace b.
    underarm b.
    unilateral calcaneal b. (UCB)
    University of British Columbia b.
    Unloader Adj. knee b.
    Varney acromioclavicular b.
    Verlow b.
    Victorian b.
    von Lackum transection shift
     jacket b.
    walking b.
    Warm Springs b.
    Watco b.
    weightbearing b.
    Wheaton b.
    Wilke boot b.
    Williams b.
    Wilmington scoliosis b.
    Wright Universal b.
    Yale b.
    Zimmer reamer b.
    Zinco CAM walker b.
brace/corset
    Hoke lumbar b.

bracelet
    Q-Ray b.
    b. test
braceRAP
brachial
    b. artery
    b. artery aneurysm
    b. artery injury
    b. plexus
    b. plexus block
    b. plexus injury
    b. plexus palsy
    b. plexus paralysis
    b. plexus repair
    b. plexus tendon
    b. plexus tension test
    b. plexus traction injury (BPTI)
brachialgia
brachialis
    b. muscle
    b. tendon
brachiocephalic vein
brachioradialis
    b. flap
    b. muscle
    b. tendon
    b. transfer
    b. transfer for wrist extension
brachium
brachymetatarsia
bracing
    cast b.
    fracture b.
    postoperative b.
bracket
    longitudinal epiphyseal b.
bracketed splint
Brackett-Osgood
    B.-O. knee approach
    B.-O. posterior approach
Brackett-Osgood-Putti-Abbott
    B.-O.-P.-A. operation
    B.-O.-P.-A. technique
Brackett osteotomy
Bradford
    B. fracture frame
    B. frame
    B. fusion
Brady
    B. balanced-suspension splint
    B. leg splint
Brady-Jewett technique
bradykinin
bradymetatarsalgia
Bragard
    B. reinforcement
    B. sign
    B. test

Bragg-peak photon-beam therapy
Brahms
    B. foot operation
    B. procedure
braid
    carbon fiber lamination b. (CFLB)
braided suture
Brailsford disease
brain
    B. arthroplasty
    b. damage
    b. injury
    B. reflex
    b. stem
brainstem
    b. auditory evoked potential
    (BAEP)
    b. auditory evoked response
    (BAER)
brake lever extension
Braly-Bishop-Tullos decompression
branch
    distal communicating b. (DCB)
    dorsal ulnar cutaneous b.
    interosseous b.
    motor b.
    posterior interosseous b.
    proper digital nerve b.
    proximal communicating b. (PCB)
    superior laryngeal nerve external b.
Brand
    B. tendon-holding forceps
    B. tendon passer
    B. tendon-passing forceps
    B. tendon stripper
    B. tendon transfer technique
Branhamella catarrhalis
Brannock
    B. Device shoe sizer
    B. foot measuring device
Brannon-Wickström technique
Brant aluminum splint
Brantigan-Voshell procedure
brassiere
    Jobst b.
Brattström condylar height ratio
Braun
    B. frame
    B. procedure
    B. shoulder tenotomy
    B. skin graft
Braun-Yasargil right-angle clip

break
    b. point
    b. test
breakage
    pedicle screw b.
    screw b.
    tack b.
breakaway
    b. lap cushion
    b. pin
    b. weakness
breakdancer's thumb
breakdown
    skin b.
breastbone
breaststroker's knee
Breast Vest EXU-DRY one-piece wound dressing
breathing reserve (BR)
Breck
    B. pin
    B. pin cutter
Breezee Mist Antifungal
bregmatomastoid suture
Bremer
    B. halo cervical traction
    B. halo system
Breslow classification of melanoma
Brett arthrodesis
Brett-Campbell tibial osteotomy
Breuerton x-ray view of hand
breve
    vinculum b.
brevis
    coxa b.
    extensor carpi radialis b. (ECRB)
    extensor digitorum b. (EDB)
    extensor pollicis b. (EPB)
    flexor digiti quinti b. (FDQB)
    flexor digitorum b. (FDB)
    flexor hallucis b. (FHB)
    flexor pollicis b. (FPB)
    peroneus b. (PB)
    radialis b.
    b. release
Brewster triple arthrodesis
Brickner position
bridge
    autograft b.
    balance b.
    bony b.
    b. graft

NOTES

bridge *(continued)*
    B. hip system
    iliac crest b.
    b. of meniscus
    osseous b.
    b. plate
    b. plate fixation
    tendon-bone b.
bridging
    b. bone
    b. callus
    b. of defect
    heterotrophic ossification b.
    myocardial b.
    b. osteophyte
bridle
    b. posterior tibial tendon transfer operation
    B. procedure
brief
    b. maximal effort (BME)
    b., small, abundant, polyphasic potential (BSAPP)
    b., small, abundant potential (BSAP)
    B. Test of Head Injury (BTHI)
    B. Test of Head Injury Assessment
Brigham prosthesis
Brighton electrical stimulation system
brim
    pelvic b.
    proximal medical b.
    quadrilateral b.
brisement
    b. therapy
Bristow
    B. operation
    B. periosteal elevator
    B. procedure
    B. rasp
Bristow-Helfet procedure
Bristow-May procedure
British test
Brittain
    B. chisel
    B. ischiofemoral arthrodesis
brittle bone
brittleness
broach
    barbed b.
    cemented b.
    cementless b.
    Charnley femoral b.
    drilling b.
    ELP b.
    b. extractor
    femoral prosthesis b.

    Harris b.
    Koenig metatarsal b.
    Mittlemeir b.
    orthopaedic b.
    root canal b.
    smooth b.
    square-hole b.
    Swanson metatarsal b.
    Zimmer femoral canal b.
broad
    b. AO dynamic compression plate
    b.-based gait
    b. thumb-big toe syndrome
Broadbent-Woolf four-limb Z-plasty
Broberg-Morrey
    B.-M. elbow function scale
    B.-M. fracture
Brockman
    B. foot operation
    B. incision
    B. procedure
Brockman-Nissen arthrodesis
Brodén
    B. stress examination
    B. stress radiography
Broden view
Brodie
    B. disease
    B. metaphyseal abscess
Brodsky-Tullos-Gartsman approach
BROM
    back range of motion
bromfenac sodium
bromhidrosis, bromidrosis
    plantar b.
Brooke Army Hospital splint
Brooker
    B. classification of heterotopic ossification I–IV
    B. double-locking unreamed tibial nail
    B. femoral nail
    B. frame
    B. heterotopic bone formation classification
    B. wire
Brooker-Jones tendon transfer
Brooker-Wills nail
Brooks
    B. atlantoaxial arthrodesis
    B. cervical fusion
    B. cervical fusion operation
    B. technique
    B.-type fusion
Brooks-Gallie
    B.-G. cervical fusion
    B.-G. cervical operation

Brooks-Jenkins
  B.-J. atlantoaxial fusion
  B.-J. atlantoaxial fusion technique
  B.-J. cervical fusion
  B.-J. cervical operation
Brooks-Jones tendon transfer
Brooks-Seddon
  B.-S. pectoralis major tendon
    transfer
  B.-S. tendon transfer
  B.-S. transfer technique
Broomhead
  B. medial approach
broomstick
  b. bar
  b. cast
  b. curl-up
Brophy periosteal elevator
Broström
  B. injection technique
  B. procedure
Broström-Gordon arthrography
Broström-Gould ankle instability
  operation
Broughton-Olney-Menelaus tibial
  diaphyseal shortening
brown
  B. dermatome
  b. fat tumor
  B. fibular transfer
  B. knee approach
  B. knee joint reconstruction
  B. lateral approach
  B. periosteotome
  B. rasp
  B. technique
  B. tissue forceps
  b. tumor of hyperparathyroidism
Brown-Adson forceps
Brown-Cushing forceps
Browne splint
Brown-Mueller T-fastener set
Brown-Séquard
  B.-S. lesion
  B.-S. syndrome
Brucella
  B. agglutination test
  B. arthritis
  B. osteomyelitis
brucellosis
  spinal b.

Bruce protocol
Brudzinski
  B. sign
  B. test
Bruening chisel
Bruening-Citelli rongeur
Bruger
  cul-de-sac of B.
Bruininks-Oseretsky Test of Motor
  Proficiency
bruisability
bruise
  bone b.
Brun bone curette
Bruner
  B. approach
  B. incision
Brunhilde strain
Bruni-Wayne clamp approximator
Brunner
  B. modified incision
  B. palmar incision
  B. rib shears
Brunn plaster shears
Brunnstrom-Fugl-Meyer (BFM)
Bruns
  B. ataxia
Brunswick-Mack rotating drill
Bruser
  B. knee approach
  B. lateral approach
  B. skin incision
  B. technique
brush
  Cohort bone b.
  Plak-Vac oral suction b.
  b. test
bruxism
Bryan
  B. arthroplasty
  B. procedure
  B. total knee implant prosthesis
Bryan-Morrey
  B.-M. elbow approach
  B.-M. extensive posterior approach
  B.-M. technique
Bryant
  B. sign
  B. traction
BSAP
  brief, small, abundant potential

NOTES

BSAPP
brief, small, abundant, polyphasic potential

BtA
botulinum toxin A

BTE
Baltimore Therapeutic Equipment
BTE Assembly Tree
BTE Bolt Box
BTE Dyamic Pedobarograph
BTE dynamic lift
BTE Work Simulator

BTHI
Brief Test of Head Injury

BTM hip system

buccal

buccinator
b. muscle
b. myomucosal flap

Buchanan disease

Buch-Gramcko gouge

Buchholz
B. acetabular cup
B. prosthesis

Buck
B. bone curette
B. cement restrictor inserter
B. convoluted traction apparatus
B. convoluted traction device
B. extension splint
B. fascia
B. femoral cement restrictor inserter
B. knee brace
B. method
B. neurological hammer
B. periosteal elevator
B. plug
B. traction
B. traction splint

bucket
Denis Browne b.
kick b.
Lenox b.

bucket-handle
b.-h. fracture
b.-h. plica
b.-h. rib
b.-h. rib motion
b.-h. rim motion
b.-h. tear
b.-h. tear of meniscus

Buck-Gramcko
B.-G. pollicization
B.-G. technique

buckle
b. fracture
wire-fixation b.

Buckley chisel

Bucky
B. diaphragm
B. x-ray tray

bud
limb b.

buddy
b. splint
b. strap
b. taping

Budin
B. hammertoe splint
B. toe splint

Budin-Chandler
B.-C. anteversion determination
B.-C. method

Buerger-Allen exercise

Buerger disease

buffalo hump

Bufferin

Buffex

Buffinol Extra

Buford complex

Bugg-Boyd technique

buggy
cruiser b.
Maclaren mobile b.

Buhl spirometer

Builder Grip hand exerciser

buildup (noun)

build up (verb)

bulb
b. dynamometer
irrigation b.
b. neuroma
b. suture
b. and thumb screw valve

bulbar abnormality

bulbocavernosus reflex

bulge
disk b.

bulging disk

bulk graft

bulky
b. hand dressing

bulla, pl. **bullae**

bulldog
b. clamp
b. clamp applier
b. clamp-applying forceps

bullet driver

bullosa
epidermolysis b.

bullous

Bullseye femoral guide

bump
hip b.
inion b.

pump b.
runner's b.
bumper
axle lock and b.
b. cast
dorsiflexion b.
flexion b.
b. fracture
b. wedge
Buncke
B. technique
B. transfer
bundle
anteromedial b.
b. dressing
b. function
intermediate b.
medial neurovascular b.
b.-nailing method
neurovascular b.
posterolateral b.
superior gluteal neurovascular b.
Bunge amputation
bunion
b. deformity
b. dissector
dorsal b.
Estersohn osteotomy for tailor's b.
b. formation
juvenile b.
b. shield
tailor's b.
bunionectomy
Akin b.
Austin b.
chevron b.
DuVries-Mann modified b.
Hauser b.
Joplin b.
Kelikian modified Z b.
Keller b.
Kreuscher b.
Lapidus b.
Mayo b.
McBride b.
Mitchell b.
modified Mau b.
modified McBride b.
osteotomy b.
Reverdin b.
Reverdin-Laird b.
Reverdin-McBride b.

Silver b.
Stone b.
tailor's b.
tricorrectional b.
Wilson b.
Wu b.
bunionette excision
bunionette-hallux valgus-splayfoot complex
bunion-hallux valgus complex
bunk bed fracture
Bunker footpiece
Bunke-Schulz clamp approximator
Bunnell
B. active hand and finger splint
B. anvil
B. atraumatic technique
B. bone drill
B. crisscross suture
B. digital exertion measurer
B. dissecting probe
B. dressing
B. figure-eight suture
B. finger extension splint
B. finger loop
B. forwarding probe
B. gutter splint
B. hand drill
B. knuckle bender
B. knuckle-bender splint
B. modification of Steindler flexorplasty
B. opponensplasty
B. outrigger splint
B. posterior tibial tendon transfer
B. posterior tibial tendon transfer operation
B. pullout wire
B. reverse knuckle bender splint
B. safety-pin splint
B. solution
B. stitch
B. tendon needle
B. tendon passer
B. tendon repair
B. tendon stripper
B. tendon suturing technique
B. tendon transfer technique
B. test
B. wire pull-out suture
B. zigzag fashion
Bunnell-Littler test

NOTES

B

Bunnell-Williams procedure
Bunny
    B. boot
    B. Boot foot splint
buoyancy
bupivacaine
Buprenex
buprenorphine
bur, burr
    Adson b.
    Albee olive-shaped b.
    Bailey b.
    ball b.
    barrel b.
    bone b.
    Borchardt olive-shaped b.
    Burwell b.
    Caparosa b.
    carbide b.
    coarse carbide cone b.
    coarse-olive b.
    cone b.
    conical b.
    crosscut b.
    Cushing b.
    cutting b.
    decortication b.
    dental b.
    D'Errico enlarging drill b.
    D'Errico perforating drill b.
    diamond b.
    3-in-1 diamond b.
    b.-down technique
    Doyen cylindrical b.
    Doyen spherical b.
    b. drill
    Dyonics arthroplasty b.
    enlarging b.
    fine-olive b.
    finish b.
    flame-tip b.
    Hall b.
    high-speed b.
    high-torque b.
    b. hole
    Hudson brace with b.
    large-nail spicule b.
    long coarse b.
    long-stemmed powered b.
    McKenzie enlarging b.
    medium carbide cone b.
    medium fine b.
    Midas Rex b.
    MTM 2 b.
    new happy b.
    old smoothie b.
    orthopaedic b.

    Ossotome b.
    paronychia b.
    pear b.
    perforating b.
    pilot b.
    power b.
    right-ankle b.
    Rosen b.
    Rotablator rotating b.
    rotary b.
    round b.
    Shannon b.
    short coarse b.
    short fine b.
    small nail spicule b.
    smoothie junior b.
    spherical b.
    Stille b.
    Zimmer rotary b.
Burch-Greenwood tendon tucker
Burford-Finochietto rib spreader
Burford rib spreader
burgdorferi
    Borrelia b.
Burgess
    B. below-knee amputation
    B. technique
buried K-wire fixation in digital fusion
Burke Bariatric bed
Burkhalter
    B. modification of Stiles-Bunnell
      technique
    B. transfer technique
Burkhalter-Reyes method phalangeal
    fracture
burn
    B. bench test
    b. boutonnière deformity
    chemical b.
    circumferential chemical b.
    b. contracture
    electrical b.
    irrigation b.
    mafenide acetate for b.
    plaster cast application b.
    b. syndactyly
Burnham
    B. finger splint
    B. thumb splint
burning
    b. feet
    b. pain
burning-feet syndrome
Burns
    B. disease
    B. plate
Burns-Haney incision

Burow
    B. skin flap technique
    B. triangle
burr (*var. of* bur)
Burroughs solution
Burrows technique
bursa, pl. **bursae**
    adventitious b.
    deltoid b.
    intermetatarsophalangeal b.
    ischiogluteal b.
    Luschka b.
    olecranon b.
    pisiform b.
    prepatellar b.
    radial b.
    retrocalcaneal b.
    subacromial b.
    subdeltoid b.
    trochanteric b.
    ulnar b.
    Voshell b.
bursal
    b. cyst
    b. debridement
    b. flap
    b. fluid
    b. inflammation
    b. projection
    b. sac
    b. tissue
bursitis
    anserine b.
    chronic retrocalcaneal b.
    cubital b.
    iliopsoas b.
    infracalcaneal b.
    infrapatellar b.
    intermetatarsophalangeal b.
    ischiogluteal b.
    medial gastrocnemius b.
    olecranon b.
    patellar b.
    pigmented villonodular b.
    postcalcaneal b.
    prepatellar b.
    pyogenic b.
    retrocalcaneal b.
    semimembranosus b.
    septic b.
    subdeltoid b.
    subgluteal b.

    subscapularis b.
    tarsal navicular b.
    Tornwaldt b.
    trochanteric b.
    tuberculous trochanteric b.
bursocentesis
bursography
    Mikasa subacromial b.
    subacromial b.
bursolith
bursopathy
bursotomy
burst
    b. fracture
    b. injury
    b.-type laceration
bursting dislocation
Burton-Pelligrini excising trapezium
Burton sign
Burwell bur
Burwell-Charnley
    B.-C. classification of fracture
        reduction
    B.-C. fracture reduction
        classification
**Burwell-Scott modification of Watson-
    Jones incision**
Busenkell posterior hip retractor
bushing
    guide b.
    Uniflex drill b.
butabarbital sodium
Butalan
butalbital
    b. compound and codeine
Butazolidin
butenafine
Buticaps
Butisol Sodium
Butler
    B. fifth toe operation
    B. procedure to correct overlapping
        toes
butorphanol
butterfly
    B. cushion
    B. cushion with strap
    b. fracture
    b. fracture fragment
    b. vertebra
**butterfly-shaped monoblock vertebral
    plate**

NOTES

buttocks
    heart-shaped b.
    b. pad
button
    b. abscess
    Biomet b.
    Charnley suture b.
    Drummond b.
    Endo b.
    Hewson ligament b.
    b. hook
    ligament b.
    padded b.
    patellar b.
    polyethylene b.
    pull-out b.
    Silastic b.
    B. Spacer
    b. suture
    b. toe amputation
    Wisconsin b.
buttonhole
    b. deformity

    b. fracture
    b. rupture
buttress
    OMNI pretibial b.
    b. pie plate
    b. thread screw
    b.-type plate
buttressed hook
buttressing in internal fixation
"buttress" pad
buzz bleeders
BVP
    blood volume pulse
Bx
    biopsy
Byars mandibular prosthesis
bypass
    dorsal pedal b.
    extended tibial in situ b.
    femorodistal b.
    b. graft angiography
    popliteus b.
    b. surgery

C

C angle
C clamp
C knife
C Stance ankle
C washer

C1

atlas

C-2

C-2 hip system
C-2 OsteoCap hip prosthesis

C1–C3 cruciate pulley
CA-5000 drill-guide isometer
CA-6000 spine motion analyzer
cabinet

grid c.

cable

antirotation c. (ARC)
chrome-cobalt c.
Dall-Miles c.
Dwyer scoliosis c.
fiberoptic c.
Gallie fusion-using c.
c.-hook compression instrumentation
interspinous c.
liquid c.
Oklahoma City c. (OKC)
scoliosis correction with Dwyer c.
Songer c.
c. suspension system
c. tensioner
titanium c.
twister c.
c.-twister brace
c.-twister orthosis

Cabot

C. leg splint
C. posterior splint

Cacchione syndrome
CAD

computer-assisted design
CAD femoral stem prosthesis

cadaver

c. bone
c. bone graft

cadaveric knee
CAD/CAM

computer-assisted design-controlled
alignment method
CAD/CAM prosthesis

cadence of gait
Cadenza

C. girdle
C. panty

café au lait spot

caffeine

acetaminophen, aspirin, and c.
orphenadrine, aspirin, and c.

Caffey

C. disease
C. hyperostosis

Caffinière, de La Caffinière

C. trapeziometacarpal prosthesis

cage

c.-back brace
BAK c.
carbon-fiber-composite c.
carbon-fiber-reinforced c.
fusion c.
lumbar intersomatic fusion
expandable c. (LIFEC)
Moss c.
protrusio c.
Pyramesh c.
rib c.
SL c.
stereolithography c.
Swedish knee c.
threaded fusion c.

CAH

Camber axis hinge

Cairns hemostatic forceps
caisson worker's disease
Calan
Calandriello

C. hip reduction
C. procedure

Calandruccio

C. cemented hip prosthesis
C. clamp
C. compression apparatus
C. fixation
C. fixation device
C. impaction screw-plate
C. side plate
C. triangular compression apparatus

calcaneal

c. apophysitis
c. avulsion fracture
c. displaced fracture
c. fat pad
c. fracture reduction
c. gait
c. inclination angle
c. L osteotomy
c. malunion
c. pin
c. resection
c. spur
c. spur cookie orthosis

calcaneal *(continued)*
  c. spur pad in shoe
  c. spur syndrome
  c. tendon
  c. tenodesis
  c. valgus
  c. varus
  c. Y plate
calcaneal-second metatarsal angle
  inclination angle
calcanectomy
calcanei (*pl. of* calcaneus)
calcaneocavovarus deformity
calcaneocavus
  c. deformity
  c. feet
  c. foot
  talipes c.
calcaneoclavicular ligament
calcaneocuboid (CC)
  c. arthrodesis
  c. articulation
  c. bone
  c. distraction arthrodesis (CCDA)
  c. joint
  c. joint arthritis
  c. ligament
  c. subluxation
calcaneocuboideum
  ligamentum c.
calcaneofibulare
  ligamentum c.
calcaneofibular ligament (CFL)
calcaneonavicular
  c. bar
  c. bar resection
  c. bar section
  c. coalition
  c. joint
  c. ligament
  c. ligament-tibialis posterior tendon
    advancement
calcaneonaviculare
  ligamentum c.
calcaneopelvic arthrodesis
calcaneoplantar angle
calcaneotibial
  c. angle
  c. arthrodesis
  c. fusion
  c. ligament
calcaneotibiale
  ligamentum c.
calcaneovalgus
  c. deformity
  c. flatfoot

  c. foot
  talipes c.
calcaneus, pl. **calcanei**
  accessory ossification center of c.
  displaced intraarticular c.
  distal c.
  c. gait
  c. secondarius
  talipes c.
  tendo c.
  White-Kraynick tendo c.
calcar
  c. collar
  c. femorale
  c. femorale development
  pivot of c.
  c. pivot
  c. planer
  c. reamer
  c. replacement
  c. replacement femoral prosthesis
  c. replacement stem
  c. trimmer with Zimmer-Hudson
    shank
Cal Carb-HD
Calcichew
Calciday-667
calcifediol
Calciferol
  C. Injection
  C. Oral
calcificans
  chondrodystrophia c.
calcification
  flocculent foci of c.
  heterotopic c.
  juvenile intervertebral disk c.
    (JIDC)
  paraarticular c.
calcific tendinitis
calcified osteoid
calcify
calcifying aponeurotic fibroma
Calcijex
Calcimar Injection
Calci-Mix
calcinosis
  c. circumscripta
  c., Raynaud, esophageal,
    sclerodactyly, telangiectasia
    (CREST)
  tumoral c.
calciphylaxis
calcis
  os c.
Calcitite
  C. bone

C. graft
C. graft material
calcitonin
salmon c.
calcitonin-salmon
calcitriol
calcium
c. alginate dressing
c. aluminate
c. carbonate
c. deposit
c. glubionate
c. hydroxyapatite
c. lactate
c. phosphate
c. phosphate ceramic
c. phosphate, dibasic
c. pyrophosphate dihydrate deposition (CPPD)
c. pyrophosphate dihydrate deposition disease
serum c.
Calderol
Caldesene Topical
Caldwell-Coleman
C.-C. flatfoot operation
C.-C. flatfoot technique
Caldwell-Durham
C.-D. tendon operation
C.-D. tendon transfer
Caldwell hanging cast
calf
c. band
c. circumference
c. hypertension
c. shell
c. squeeze test
calibrated
c. clubfoot splint
c. guidepin
c. guide wire
c. pin
c. pin guide
c. probe
calibration curve
calibrator
screw depth c.
caliper
blunt c.
c. brace
Harpenden c.
Lafayette skinfold c.

Lange skinfold c.
Mitutoyo digital c.
pluri-cal c.
c. rib movement
skinfold c.
skinfold c.
Thomas walking c.
Townley femur c.
Vernier c.
weight-relieving c.
Callahan
C. approach
C. extension of cervical injury
C. fusion technique
Callander amputation
Callaway test
Calleja exercise
Callender
C. derotational brace
C. technique hip prosthesis
callosal lesion
callosity
callotasis distraction
callous
c. bone union
callus
bone c.
bridging c.
elephant-foot c.
florid c.
c. formation
fracture c.
horse's foot c.
irritation c.
c. massage
pinch c.
shearing c.
c. weld
Calnan-Nicolle
C.-N. finger implant
C.-N. finger prosthesis
calor
Cal-Plus
Caltagirone chisel
Caltrate
C. 600
C. Jr.
Calvé-Perthes disease
CAM
complimentary alternative medicine
controlled ankle motion
CAM Walker

C

NOTES

Cam
- C. Lock knee joint
- C. walker
- C. Walker leg brace

Cama Arthritis Pain Reliever
Camber axis hinge (CAH)
camelback sign
camera
- DyoCam 550 arthroscopic video c.
- DyoCam arthroscopic view c.
- gamma c.
- Saticon tube c.
- Sony CCD/RGB DXC-151 color video c.
- Stryker c.
- Vidicon vacuum chamber pickup tube for video c.

Cameron
- C. femoral component removal
- C. fracture apparatus
- C. fracture device

Cameron-Haight periosteal elevator
Camino catheter technique
Camitz
- C. technique
- C. tendon transfer

camouflage prosthesis
Camp
- C. brace
- C. corset

Campbell
- C. ankle procedure
- C. cannulated screw
- C. elbow approach
- C. gouge
- C. interpositional arthroplasty
- C. nerve root retractor
- C. onlay bone graft
- C. osteotome
- C. periosteal elevator
- C. posterior arthrodesis
- C. posterior bone block
- C. posterior shoulder approach
- C. posterolateral approach
- C. reamer
- C. resection arthroplasty
- C. rongeur
- C. screw fixation
- C. technique
- C. tibial osteotomy
- C. traction splint
- C. transfer
- C. triceps reflection

Campbell-Akbarnia
- C.-A. arthrodesis
- C.-A. procedure

Campbell-Goldthwait procedure

Campbell-Rinehard-Kalenak anterior arthrodesis
Camper
- C. chiasma
- C. fascia

Campho-Phenique
camphor and phenol
camptocormia
camptodactyly
CamStar
- C. exercise machine
- C. power leg press

Canadian
- C. crutch
- C. hip disarticulation prosthesis
- C. Knee Orthosis
- C. Physiotherapy Association

Canakis beaded hip pin
canal
- Alcock c.
- cartilage c.
- cortical bone primary c.
- femoral c.
- c. finder
- Guyon c.
- haversian c.
- humeral c.
- Hunter c.
- hydrops c.
- c. innominate osteotomy
- intramedullary c.
- medullary c.
- Richet tibio-astragalocalcaneal c.
- spinal c.
- talar c.
- tarsal c.
- Volkmann c.

Canale
- C. osteotomy
- C. technique

Canale-Kelly
- C.-K. talar neck fracture
- C.-K. talar neck fracture classification
- C.-K. view

canaliculus, pl. canaliculi
Can Am brace
Canavan leukodystrophy
Canavan-van Bogaert-Bertrand disease
cancellectomy
cancellous
- c. bone screw
- c. chip
- c. chip bone graft
- c. and cortical bone graft
- c. insert
- c. insert graft
- c. morselized bone graft

c. pin
c. surface
c. versus cortical bone
Candida
candle wax appearance of bone
Can-Do Exercise Band
cane
Double Duty c.
MAFO c.
offset c.
quad c.
quadrapod c.
single-point c.
small-base quad c.
TheraCane c.
tripod c.
canister
Autovac autotransfusion c.
Cannon Law of Denervation Supersensitivity
cannula
Acufex double-lumen arthroscopic c.
arthroscopic c.
blunt arthroscopic c.
Concept c.
Dyonics c.
Eriksson muscle biopsy c.
inflow c.
large-bore inflow c.
McCain TMJ c.
microirrigating c.
outflow c.
self-sealing c.
suprapatellar c.
c. system
Teflon c.
zone-specific c.
cannulated
c. bolt
c. cortical step drill
c. drill bit
c. drill point
c. expulsion piston
c. guided hip screw system
c. Henderson reamer
c. hip screw
c. nail
C. Plus screw system
c. reaming technique
c. wrench

cannulation
unilateral pedicle c.
canted finger hook
Cantelli sign
cantilever bending
canvas brace
cap
acetabular c.
c.-and-anchor plate
Carnation corn c.'s
cartilaginous c.
Cloward drill guard c.
Compoz Gel C.'s
digit c.
Feverall Sprinkle C.'s
flexor c.
nerve c.
plaster toe c.
plastic end c.'s
Silipos mesh c.
c. splint
Zang metatarsal c.
Zimmer tibial nail c.
capacitive sensor
capacity
forced vital c. (FVC)
Caparosa
C. bur
C. wire crimper
CAPE
continuous anatomical passive exerciser
capeline bandage
Capello
C. slim-line abduction pillow
C. technique
C. total hip replacement
Capener
C. brace
C. coil splint
C. finger splint
C. lateral rhachotomy
capillary
c. filling time
c. hemangioma
c. ischemia
c. refill
c. refill time
CAPIS
CAPIS bone plate system
CAPIS screw
CAPIS screw assortment tray
CAPIS screwdriver

NOTES

capital
C. and Codeine
c. epiphyseal angle
c. epiphysis (CE)
c. femoral epiphysis
c. fragment
c. ligament
capitate
c. bone
c.-hamate joint
capitate-lunate
c.-l. instability
c.-l. joint
capitellar fracture
capitellocondylar
c. total elbow arthroplasty
c. unconstrained elbow prosthesis
capitellum
Hahn-Steinthal fracture of c.
Kocher-Lorenz fracture of c.
capitolunate angle
capitular epiphysis
capitulum
c. radiale humeri fracture
Caplets
Miles Nervine C.
Capner
C. gouge
C. splint
Caprolactam suture
capsaicin
capsaicoid topical cream
Capsin
capsular
c. adhesion
c. attachment
c. flap
c. imbrication
c. imbrication procedure
c. incision
c. interposition arthroplasty
c. layer
c. length insufficiency
c. ligament
c. plication
c. reefing
c. release
c. shift procedure
c. strap
c. support tissue
capsular-ligamentous tension
capsular-shift reconstruction
capsulatum
Histoplasma c.
capsule
anterior c.
anterolateral c.
anteromedial c.

articular c.
dorsal c.
elbow c.
facet c.
fibrous c.
Gerota c.
joint c.
Kadian C.
medial c.
meniscofemoral c.
meniscotibial c.
metatarsophalangeal joint c.
midlateral c.
midmedial c.
plantar c.
posterior c.
posterolateral c.
posteromedial c.
suprasellar c.
talanavicular c.
trapeziometacarpal c.
capsulectomy
capsulitis
adhesive c.
glenohumeral adhesive c.
capsulodesis
Berger c.
Blatt c.
bleb c.
dorsal c.
Zancolli flexion c.
capsulolabral complex
capsuloligamentous
c. complex
c. mechanism
c. system
c. tissue
capsuloperiosteal envelope
capsuloplasty
Zancolli c.
capsulorrhaphy
Boyd-Sisk posterior c.
duToit-Roux staple c.
medial c.
pants-over-vest c.
posterior c.
Rockwood posterior c.
Roux-duToit staple c.
c. staple
staple c.
Tibone posterior c.
capsulotomy
Curtis PIP joint c.
dorsal transverse c.
dorsolateral and medial c.
L-shaped c.
medial V-Y c.
posterior c.

stereotaxic anterior c.
subtalar c.
talonavicular c.
transmetatarsal c.
transverse c.
T-shaped c.
Capzasin-P
CAQ
Clinical Analysis Questionnaire
Carabelt
C. lower back support
C. therapeutic belt
Cara Klenz cleansing agent
carbamate
chlorphenesis c.
carbamazepine
Carbapenem
carbenicillin
Carb-HD
Cal C.-H.
carbide bur
carbidopa-levodopa
Carbocaine
CarboFlex odor-control dressing
carbohydrate
c. analysis
c. oxidation
carbol-fuchsin solution
carbon
C. Copy II Foot prosthesis
C. Copy II light foot
C. Copy II Light prosthesis
c. dioxide laser
c. fiber
c. fiber fixator
c. fiber graft
c. fiber half ring
c. fiber lamination braid (CFLB)
c. fiber-reinforced plate
c. fiber-reinforced polyethylene
c. implant
C. Monotube long bone fracture
external fixation system
pyrolytic c.
c. steel drill point
carbonate
calcium c.
carbon-fiber-composite cage
carbon-fiber-reinforced cage
carbon-tungsten rasp

Carboplast
C. II sheeting
C. II sheet orthotic material
Carborundum grinding wheel
Carceau-Brahms ankle arthrodesis
carcinoembryonic antigen (CEA)
Carcon stent
card
memory exercise c.
pace c.
pattern matching c.
Similarity Discrimination C.
Size Discrimination C.
Cardan screwdriver
cardinal axes (X,Y,Z)
cardiogenic shock
Cardiopulmonary Paragon 8500 bed
cardiovascular disease
Cardona keratoprosthesis prosthesis
care
corrective spinal c.
Miami Acute C. (MAC)
palliative c.
postoperative wound c.
Caregiver Strain Index (CSI)
Carex ambulatory aid
CARF
Commission on Accreditation of
Rehabilitation Facilities
carisoprodol
c. and aspirin
c., aspirin, and codeine
Carl P. Jones traction splint
C-arm
C.-a. fluoroscope
C.-a. fluoroscopy
C.-a. fluoroscopy unit
Carmody perforator drill
Carnation corn caps
Carnesale
C. acetabular extensile approach
C. hip approach
C. technique
Carnesale-Stewart-Barnes
C.-S.-B. classification of hip
dislocation
C.-S.-B. hip dislocation
classification
Carolon AFO sock
carotid
c. artery
c. artery compression

NOTES

C

carotid *(continued)*
    c. content
    c. sheath
    c. vein
carpal
    c. bone
    c. bone fracture ankylosis
    c. bone stress fracture
    C. Care Exerciser
    C. Care rehabilitative program
    c. compression test
    c. instability
    c. ligament
    C. Lock wrist brace
    C. Lock wrist splint
    c. lunate implant prosthesis
    c. navicular fracture
    c. pedal spasm
    c. row
    c. scaphoid
    c. scaphoid bone fracture
    c. scaphoid implant prosthesis
    c. scaphoid screw
    c. synovectomy
    c. tunnel
    c. tunnel release (CTR)
    c. tunnel surgery relief kit
    c. tunnel syndrome (CTS)
    c. tunnel view
carpal-intercarpal joint
carpal-metacarpal (CMC)
carpectomy
    distal row c.
    Omer-Capen c.
    proximal row c.
carpenter's brace
Carpenter syndrome
carpi
    os triangulare c.
    c. radialis brevis tendon
    c. radialis longus tendon
carpometacarpal (CMC)
    c. arthroplasty
    c. articulation
    c. boss
    c. fracture-dislocation
    c. joint
    c. joint dislocation
    c. joint fracture
    c. joint radiography
carpophalangeal joint
carporadial articulation
carposcope
carprofen
carpus
    complex instability of c. (CIC)
Carrell
    C. fibular substitution

    C. fibular substitution technique
    C. resection
Carrell-Girard screw
Carrie car seat
carrier
    Cave-Rowe ligature c.
    clamp c.
    double-headed stereotactic c.
    Finochietto clamp c.
    ligature c.
    Yasargil ligature c.
Carrington Dermal wound gel
Carroll
    C. arthrodesis
    C. arthroplasty
    C. bone-holding forceps
    C. dressing forceps
    C. hand retractor
    C. skin hook
    C. and Taber arthroplasty
    C. tendon-pulling forceps
    C. tissue forceps
Carroll-Bennett retractor
Carroll-Bunnell drill
Carroll-Legg
    C.-L. osteotome
    C.-L. periosteal elevator
Carroll-Smith-Petersen osteotome
Carrom orthopaedic bed
Carr-Purcell-Meiboom-Gill sequence
Carr-Purcell sequence
carrying
    c. angle
    c. angle of forearm
Carstan reverse wedge osteotomy
cart
    Harloff c.
Cartam-Treander reverse wedge
  osteotomy
Carter
    C. elevation pillow
    C. immobilization cushion
    C. Rowe awl
    C. splint
Carter-Rowe view
Carticel
cartilage
    c. ablation
    c. abrader
    articular c.
    BeneFin clinical shark c.
    c. canal
    c. cell
    c. clamp
    costal c.
    cryopreserved c.
    eburnation of c.
    c. elastic pullover kneecap splint

c. forceps
free flap of c.
glenoid c.
c. graft
c.-hair hypoplasia
c. healing
hyaline c.
c. hypertrophy
c. implant
McMurray maneuver for torn
  knee c.
patellofemoral groove c.
physeal c.
quadrangular c.
c. scissors
shelling off of c.
thyroid c.
triradial c.
triradiate c.

cartilaginous
c. anlage
c. cap
c. cap of phalangeal head
c. coalition
c. degeneration
c. growth plate
c. hamartoma
c. hypertrophy
c. lesion
c. loose body
c. metaplasia
c. spur
c. tissue
c. tumor

cartwheel fracture
Cartwright implant
cascade
C. Up and About system
Cascading Tower Technology
Casey pelvic clamp
CASH
cruciform anterior spinal hyperextension
CASH brace
CASH orthosis
CASP
contoured anterior spinal plate
Caspar
C. anterior instrumentation
C. blade
C. retractor
Caspari
C. arthroscopic portal

C. repair
C. shuttle
C. suture punch
Casselberry suture punch
cast
above-elbow c.
accessory navicular c.
airplane c.
c. application
arm cylinder c.
banjo c.
below-knee walking c.
bent-knee c.
Bermuda spica c.
bivalved cylinder c.
c. blade
blood c.
body c.
Body Armor walker c.
Böhler skintight c.
c. boot
Boston bivalve c.
c. bracing
broomstick c.
bumper c.
Caldwell hanging c.
circular c.
Comfort C.
corrective c.
Cotrel scoliosis c.
cottonloader position c.
c. cover
C. Cozy toe covering
c. cushion
Cutter c.
c. cutter
cylinder walking c.
Dehne c.
double hip spica c.
EDF scoliosis c.
elbow c.
Equilizer short leg walking c.
extension body c.
fiberglass c.
figure-of-eight c.
flexion body c.
Fractura Flex c.
Frejka c.
full thumb spica c.
gaiter c.
C. Gard cast protector
gauntlet c.

C

NOTES

cast *(continued)*
    Gelocast c.
    groin-to-ankle c.
    gutter c.
    Gypsona c.
    halo c.
    handshake c.
    hanging arm c.
    Hexcelite c.
    hinged cylinder c.
    hip spica c.
    hyperextension c.
    c. immobilization
    inhibitive c.
    intermediate c.
    "intern's triangle" in hip spica c.
    Kite clubfoot c.
    Kite metatarsal c.
    c. knife
    leg walking c.
    light c.
    c. liner
    localizer c.
    long arm c. (LAC)
    long arm finger c.
    long bent-knee leg c.
    long leg c. (LLC)
    long leg walking c. (LLWC)
    long leg weightbearing c.
      (LLWBC)
    Lorenz c.
    Lovell clubfoot c.
    MaxCast c.
    medial malleolus c.
    3M fiberglass c.
    Minerva c.
    modified Cotrel c.
    Moe modified Cotrel c.
    Mooney c.
    Neufeld c.
    nonwalking c.
    O'Donoghue cotton c.
    one-and-one-half spica c.
    one-half spica c.
    onlay bone graft c.
    Orfizip knee c.
    Orthoplast slipper c.
    outrigger c.
    c. padding
    pantaloon spica c.
    pantaloon walking c.
    patellar dislocation c.
    patellar tendon weightbearing c.
    petaling the c.
    Petrie spica c.
    plaster c.
    plaster-of-Paris c.
    plastic c.

polyurethane c.
pontoon spica c.
PTB c.
quadriceps femoris muscle c.
Quengel c.
removable c.
c. removal
rigid below-the-knee c.
Risser localizer scoliosis c.
Risser turnbuckle c.
Sarmiento short leg patellar
  tendon-bearing c.
Sbarbaro spica c.
Schmeisser spica c.
scoliosis c.
semirigid fiberglass c. (SRF)
serial wedge c.
c. shoe
short arm c. (SAC)
short arm fiberglass c.
short arm gauntlet c.
short arm navicular c. (SANC)
short leg c. (SLC)
short leg plaster c.
short leg walking c. (SLWC)
short walking c. (SLWC)
shoulder spica c.
single-leg spica c.
skin-tight c.
slipper-type c.
c. sock
spica c.
sugar-tong c.
c. syndrome
c. table
c. tape
three-finger spica c.
three-point pressure c.
thumb spica c.
toe spica c.
toe-to-groin c.
toe-to-midthigh c.
tone-inhibiting leg c.
total contact c. (TCC)
traction c.
turnbuckle c.
underarm c.
univalve c.
Unna boot c.
Velpeau c.
c. walker
walking boot c.
warm-and-form c.
c. wedge
wedging c.
well-leg c.
c. window
windowed c.

c. with dorsal toe plate extension
c. with volar toe plate extension
zipper c.
castaway
    C. ankle walker
    C. leg brace
    C. leg walker
    US manufacturing air c.
castbelt
    Posey below-the-knee c.
cast breaker
    Böhler c. b.
    Wolfe-Böhler c. b.
Castech extremity support
Castellani paint
Castiglia ankle brace
casting
    intermittent c.
    negative c.
    postoperative c.
    serial c.
    total contact c. (TCC)
Castle procedure
Castle-Schneider resection interposition arthroplasty
Castroviejo
    C. bladebreaker knife
    C. needle holder
    C. trephine
cast spreader
    Beeson c. s.
    Hoffer-Daimler c. s.
CAT
    computerized axial tomography
Cataflam Oral
Catagni criteria
Catapres
cataract knife Beaver blade
catarrhalis
    Branhamella c.
cat-back
    rachitic c.-b.
CAT-CAM
    contoured adduction trochanteric-controlled alignment method
catch and clunk test
catching sensation
catch-up clunk
Categories
    Functional Ambulation C. (FAC)
category
    Westin-Turco c.

Cateye Ergociser
Cathcart Orthocentric hip prosthesis
cathepsin
catheter
    Abramson c.
    c. entrapment
    Foley c.
    c. kinking
    Mentor Self-Cath soft c.
    tracer c.
    wicking c.
cathode
Catlin amputating knife
Caton method
Cat's Paw Exerciser
Catterall classification
cauda
    c. equina
    c. equina compression
    c. equina syndrome
caudad anterior mold
caudal
    c. lamina resection
    c. retinaculum
    c. spinal agenesis
    c. translation
caudally
caudocephalad
caudocranial
causalgia
causalgic pain
cauterization
    bipolar c.
    Bovie c.
    phenol c.
    unipolar c.
cautery
    Aesculap bipolar c.
    BICAP c.
    bipolar c.
    Bovie c.
    Concept hand-held c.
    intraarticular c.
    Mira c.
    monopolar c.
    slow c.
    unipolar c.
cava
    inferior vena c.
    superior vena c.
    vena c.

C

NOTES

Cavanaugh-Rogers
    C.-R. classification of footprints
    C.-R. footprint classification
Cave
    C. hip approach
    C. knee approach
cavern chordoma
cavernous
    c. hemangioma
    c. lymphangioma
Cave-Rowe
    C.-R. ligature carrier
    C.-R. shoulder dislocation operation
    C.-R. shoulder dislocation technique
Cavin osteotome
cavitary
    c. deficiency
    glenoid c.
cavitation
    joint c.
    manual c.
Cavitron ultrasonic surgical aspirator
cavity
    absorption c.
    cotyloid c.
    glenoid c.
    joint c.
    marrow c.
    Meckel c.
    saclike c.
    synovial c.
cavo abducto varus deformity
cavocalcaneovalgus deformity
cavoequinovarus
cavovalgus
    pes c.
    talipes c.
cavovarus
    c. deformity
    c. foot
    pes c.
    talipes c.
cavus
    combined c.
    c. deformity
    c. foot
    C. foot support
    metatarsus c.
    pes c.
CAWO
    closing abductory-wedge osteotomy
CB
    contrast bath
C-bar orthosis
CBP
    chiropractic biophysics
    CBP technique

CBTP
    Cognitive Behavior Therapy Package
CBWO
    closed base wedge osteotomy
CC
    calcaneocuboid
    chief complaint
    coracoclavicular
    Adalat CC
    CC joint
    CC Rider closed-chain rehabilitation
      system
CCD
    central collodiaphyseal angle
    central collodiaphysial
    CCD angle
CCDA
    calcaneocuboid distraction arthrodesis
CCPQ
    Children's Comprehensive Pain
    Questionnaire
CCS
    chronic compartment syndrome
CCTA
    coronal computed tomographic
    arthrography
C-D
    C-D hook
    C-D instrumentation
    C-D instrumentation device
    C-D instrumentation fixation
      strength
    C-D instrumentation rigidity
    C-D rod insertion
    C-D screw modification
CDH
    congenital dislocation of hip
    congenital dysplasia of hip
    CDH cup inserter
    CDH Precoat Plus hip prosthesis
CE
    capital epiphysis
    CE angle
CEA
    carcinoembryonic antigen
Cebotome drill
Cedell-Magnusson
    C.-M. arthritis classification
    C.-M. classification of arthritis on
      x-ray
CEEG
    computerized electroencephalography
Cefadyl
cefamandole
cefazolin
    c. assay
    c. clearance
    c. sodium

Cefizox
cefmetazole
Cefobid
cefonicid
cefoperazone
Cefotan
cefotaxime
cefotetan
cefoxitin
ceftazidime
Ceftin Oral
ceftizoxime
ceftriaxone
cefuroxime
Celebrex
celecoxib
Celestone Soluspan
cell
- anterior horn c.
- blood c.
- cartilage c.
- chondrosarcoma c.
- c. cushion
- endothelial c.
- c.-mediated immunity
- Merkel c.
- mesenchymal c.
- multipotential c.
- myxomatous c.
- osteoclastic giant c.
- osteogenic c.
- osteoprogenitor c.
- packed red c.
- Schwann c.
- senescent c.
- specialized c.
- spindle c.
- squamous c.
- c. therapy

cellular
- c. periosteal osteocartilaginous mass
- c. schwannoma

cellulitis
- aerobic c.
- anaerobic c.

celluloid implant material
CEM
- central extensor mechanism

cement
- acrylic bone c.
- arthroplasty c.
- bone c.

- c.-bone interface
- Boneloc c.
- BoneSource hydroxyapatite c.
- c. centralizer
- centrifugation of c.
- CMW bone c.
- c. compactor
- c. disease
- doughy c.
- Duall #88 c.
- C. Eater
- C. Eater drill
- Howmedica c.
- Implast bone c.
- c. injection gun
- c. interface
- Ketac c.
- key the c.
- c. line
- low viscosity bone c.
- c. mantle
- c. mantle grade classification
- master c.
- methyl methacrylate c.
- Norian SRS c.
- Orthocomp c.
- orthopaedic c.
- Orthoset c.
- Osteobond copolymer bone c.
- Palacos radiopaque bone c.
- c. patty
- c. plug
- PMMA bone c.
- polymerization of bone c.
- polymerized c.
- polymethyl methacrylate bone c.
- pressurization of c.
- Pronto c.
- prosthetic antibiotic-loaded acrylic c. (PROSTALAC)
- Protoplast c.
- Refobacin Palacos c.
- c. removal
- c.-removal hand chisel
- c. restrictor
- c. restrictor inserter
- Simplex P bone c.
- c. spacer inserter
- c. spatula
- Sulfix-6 c.
- Surgical Simplex P bone c.
- Surgical Simplex P radiopaque c.

NOTES

C

101

cement *(continued)*
    c. syringe
    c. technique
    Zimmer bone c.
    Zimmer low-viscosity c.
cemental fracture
cemented
    c. broach
    c. component
    c. total hip arthroplasty
cementless
    c. broach
    c. disease
    c. femoral component
    c. technique
    c. total hip arthroplasty
cementome
    Anspach c.
cementophyte
cementum fracture
Centec Propoint knee brace
center
    c. of axial rotation
    c.-edge angle
    c.-edge angle of Wiberg
    c. of gravity (COG)
    c. of mass
    Midwest Regional Spinal Cord
      Injury C.
    ossification c.
centering
    c. drill
    c. hole
central
    c. canal stenosis
    c. collodiaphyseal angle (CCD)
    c. collodiaphysial (CCD)
    c. column
    c. cord
    c. cord syndrome
    c. core disease
    c. deficiency
    c. disk protrusion
    c. dislocation
    c. electromyography
    c. extensor mechanism (CEM)
    c. fiber-region
    c. fracture
    c. heel pad syndrome
    c. herniation
    c. horn
    c. nervous system (CNS)
    c. physiolysis
    c. polydactyly
    c. posterior-anterior pressure
    c. ray
    c. ray amputation
    c. segment

    c. slip
    c. slip sparing technique
    c. spine spondylosis
    c. transpatellar tendon portal
    c. venous pressure monitoring
Centralign precoat hip prosthesis
centralization
    Bayne-Klug c.
    Bora c.
      Manske-McCarroll-Swanson c.
    c. of radius operation
    tendon c.
centralizer
    cement c.
    PMMA c.
centralizing rod
centrifugation of cement
centrifuged methyl methacrylate
centrocentral coaptation
centrode
centromedullary
    c. nail
    c. nailing
centronuclear myopathy
cephalad
    c. anterior mold
    c. translation
cephalexin
cephalic
    c. angulation
    c. vein
cephalocaudal
cephalomedullary nail fracture
cephaloscapular projection
cephalosporin
cephalothin
cephapirin
cephazolin
cephradine
Ceptaz
ceramic
    c. acetabular cup
    calcium phosphate c.
    c. implant
    c. ossicular prosthesis
    resorbable c.
    c. vertebral spacer
ceramide trihexosidase deficiency
Ceramion prosthesis
**Ceraver Osteal knee replacement
system**
cerclage
    Dall-Miles cable c.
    Howmedica c.
    c. wire
    c. wire fixation
    c. wire inserter
    c. wire twister

cerebellar retractor
cerebellopontine angle tumor
cerebellum
cerebral
    c. palsy (CP)
    c. palsy pathologic fracture
cerebral palsy (CP)
    ataxic c. p.
    athetoid c. p.
    dyskinetic c. p.
    flaccid c. p.
    spastic c. p.
cerebroside reticulocytosis
cerebrospinal fluid (CSF)
cerebrovascular accident (CVA)
Ceres Secret aloe vera gel
Certification
    American Board of C. (ABC)
certified
    c. orthotist (CO)
    c. pedorthist (CPed)
    c. prosthetist (CP)
    c. prosthetist/orthotist (CPO)
Cerva Crane halter
cervical
    c. acceleration/deceleration syndrome
    c. AOA halo traction
    c. approach
    c. artery
    c. arthrodesis
    c. chair
    c. collar
    c. collar brace
    c. compaction test
    c. corpectomy
    c. Derifield procedure
    electromyocardiography
    c. disk
    c. disk disease
    c. diskectomy
    c. disk excision
    c. diskography
    c. disk surgery
    c. dorsal glide
    c. dorsal outlet syndrome
    c. drill
    c. extension strength
    c. fascia
    c. fracture tongs
    c. general rotation
    c. halter traction
    c. hypolordosis

c. interbody fusion
c. joint
c. laminectomy punch
c. lordosis
c. mallet
c. manual traction
c. microtrauma
c. midline disk herniation
c. mover ligament
c. nerve root encroachment
c. nerve root injection
c. nerve root injury
c. oblique facet wiring
c. orthosis (CO)
c. plate
c. plexus
c. punch forceps
c. radiculitis
c. radiculopathy
c. range-of-motion device
c. range-of-motion instrument (CROM)
c. rib
c. roll
c. rongeur
c. root
c. rotation in extension
c. saddle
c. screw insertion technique
c. sidegliding test
c. sleep pillow
c. specific rotation in flexion
c. spinal cord
c. spinal injury
c. spine (C-spine)
c. spine decompression
c. spine internal fixation
c. spine kyphotic deformity
c. spine laminectomy
c. spine posterior fusion
c. spine posterior ligament disruption
c. spine rheumatoid disease
c. spine screw-plate fixation
c. spine stabilization
c. spine trauma
c. spondylolysis
c. spondylotic myelopathy
c. spondylotic myelopathy fusion technique
c. spondylotic myelopathy vertebrectomy

NOTES

cervical *(continued)*
    c. stairstep
    c. support
    c. sympathectomy
    c. sympathetic chain location
    c. synostosis
    c. tension myositis (CTM)
    c. triangle
    c. trochanteric fracture
cervical/lumbar hammer
cervicocranial
cervicoencephalic syndrome
cervicogenic
    c. headache
    c. syndrome
cervicooccipital fusion
cervicothoracic
    c. curve
    c. jacket
    c. junction
    c. junction stabilization
    c. junction surgery
    c. orthosis
    c. pedicle anatomy
    c. pedicle angle
    c. transition
cervicothoracolumbosacral orthosis (CTLSO)
cervicotrochanteric
    c. displaced fracture
Cervitrak device
CES
    cranial electrical stimulation
Cetaphil
CFL
    calcaneofibular ligament
CFLB
    carbon fiber lamination braid
C-Flex supine cervical traction
CFS
    contoured femoral stem
        CFS hip prosthesis
CH
    coracohumeral
        CH ligament
Chaddock
    C. sign
    C. test
Chadwick-Bentley classification
CHAG
    coralline hydroxyapatite Goniopora
        CHAG bone graft substitute
        material
chain
    closed c.
    closed kinetic c. (CKC)
    kinetic c.
    open kinetic c.

    paravertebral sympathetic c.
    pelvic kinematic c.
    sympathetic c.
chair
    BodyBilt c.
    Boyd podiatry c.
    cervical c.
    dynamic integrated stabilization c. (DISC)
    ergonomic c.
    EZ Rider support c.
    Gardner c.
    Hogg c.
    Invacare padded shower c.
    Kaleidoscope c.
    Orthokinetics travel c.
    Pogon c.
    Portal Pro 2 treatment c.
    sit/stand c.
    STC 900-series travel c.
    Vess c.
chairback
    c. brace
    c. orthosis
Chalet frame
chalky bone
chamber
    monoplace hyperbaric c.
    multiplace hyperbaric c.
    Portable Topical Hyperbaric
        Oxygen Extremity C.
    Pudenz flushing c.
Chamberlain line
Chambers
    C. osteotomy
    C. procedure
chamfer
    c. cut
    c. cut jig
    c. reamer
chamfered cylinder acetabular component
chamomile
Champ
    C. elastic bandage
    C. Insulated Propac II
Champion
    C. Power Sox
    C. Trauma Score (CTS)
Championnière bone drill
Chance
    C. fracture thoracolumbar spine
    C. vertebral fracture
Chandler
    C. arthrodesis
    C. bone elevator
    C. felt collar splint
    C. hip fusion

C. knee retractor
C. patellar advancement
C. procedure
C. spinal perforating forceps
C. tendon transfer
C. unreamed interlocking tibial nail

change
age-associated degenerative c.
arthritic talonavicular c.'s
Charcot c.
degenerative arthritic c.
diurnal c.
Iowa degenerative c.
kinematic gait pattern c.
neuromuscular gait pattern c.
sarcomatous c.
trophic c.

Chang-Miltner incision
channel
c.-and-core biopsy
interosseous anastomosing c.
tibial c.

Chapchal knee arthrodesis
Chaput
C. fracture
C. tubercle

characteristic
receiver operating c. (ROC)

Charcot
C. arthritis
C. arthropathy
C. change
C. deformity
C. disruption
C. foot
C. hip arthrodesis
C. joint
C. joint disease
C. restraint orthotic walker
(CROW)
C. spine

Charcot-Bouchard intracerebral aneurysm
Charcot-Marie-Tooth (CMT)
C.-M.-T. disease

Charest head frame
Charleston
C. nighttime bending brace
C. scoliosis brace

charley horse
Charlie Chaplin type of gait

Charnley
C. acetabular cup
C. acetabular cup prosthesis
C. ankle arthrodesis
C. arthrodesis clamp
C. bone clamp
C. bone curette
C. brace
C. brace handle
C. cemented prosthesis
C. centering apparatus
C. centering drill
C. classification of function
C. compression
C. compression arthrodesis
C. compression clamp
C. compression-type knee fusion
C. deepening reamer
C. device
C. expanding reamer
C. external fixation clamp
C. femoral broach
C. femoral condyle drill
C. femoral condyle radius gauge
C. femoral inlay aligner
C. femoral inlay guillotine
C. femoral prosthesis neck punch
C. femoral prosthesis pusher
C. flat-back femoral component
C. foam suture pad
C. functional classification
C. hip score
C. horizontal retractor
C. implant
C. incision
C. initial incision retractor
C. laminar flow room
C. low-friction arthroplasty
C. low-friction hip prosthesis
C. narrow-stem component
C. offset-bore cup
C. pain and function grading scale
C. pilot drill
C. pin
C. pin clamp
C. pin retractor
C. rasp
C. self-retaining retractor
C. socket gauge
C. standard-stem component
C. starting drill
C. suction drain

C

NOTES

Charnley *(continued)*
    C. suture button
    C. taper reamer
    C. template
    C. tibial onlay jig
    C. total hip arthroplasty
    C. total hip prosthesis
    C. total hip replacement
    C. total hip system
    C. towel
    C. trochanter holder
    C. trochanter reamer
    C. wire-holding forceps
    C. wire passer
Charnley-Hastings prosthesis
Charnley-Houston
    C.-H. arthrodesis
    C.-H. shoulder arthrodesis
Charnley-Maerle D'Aubigné disability grading system
Charnley-Mueller hip prosthesis
Charriere bone saw
chart
    Reality Orientation C.
    sclerotome pain c.
Chatfield-Girdlestone splint
chattering
Chatzidakis hinged Vitallium implant prosthesis
chauffeur's fracture
Chaves muscle transfer
Chaves-Rapp
    C.-R. muscle transfer
    C.-R. muscle transfer technique
    C.-R. paralysis
check
    Derifield pelvic leg c.
Checkerboard wheelchair cushion
checklist
    Body Mechanics Evaluation C.
    Low Back Pain Symptom C.
    McGill pain c.
checkrein
    c. deformity
    c. ligament
    c. procedure
check-socket
Chédiak-Higashi syndrome
cheese-grater hemispherical reamer
cheilectomy
    dorsal c.
    Garceau c.
    Mann-Coughlin-DuVries c.
    Sage-Clark c.
cheilotomy
cheiralgia paresthetica
cheirarthritis
cheiroarthropathy

cheirobrachialgia
cheiromegaly
cheiroplasty
cheiropodalgia
chelation therapy
chelonei
    Mycobacterium c.
chemical
    c. burn
    c. matrixectomy
    c. sympathectomy
chemiluminescent microtiter protein kinase activity assay
chemonucleolysis
    chymopapain c.
    double-needle c.
chemotactic factor
chemotherapy
    adjuvant c.
    neoadjuvant c.
Cherf
    C. cast stand
    C. legholder
Cherry
    C. drill
    C. osteotome
    C. screw extractor
    C. tongs
    C. tong traction
Cherry-Austin drill
chest
    c.-band transmitter
    c. roll
    c. tube
chevron
    c. bunionectomy
    c. fusion
    c. hallux valgus correction
    c. incision
    c. laceration
    c. osteotomy
    c. osteotomy with rigid screw fixation
    c. procedure
    c. technique
chevron-Akin double osteotomy
Cheyne periosteal elevator
CHH cervical brace
chi
    t'ai c.
Chi'Am International
Chiari
    C. innominate osteotomy
    C. technique
Chiari-Foix-Nicolesco syndrome
Chiari-Salter-Steel pelvic osteotomy
chiasma
    Camper c.

Chiba spinal system
Chick
    C. CLT operating frame
    C. fracture table
    C. nail
Chick-Foster orthopedic bed
Chick-Langren orthopaedic table
chief complaint (CC)
Chiene test
chilblain, chilblains
child
    battered c. syndrome
children
    C.'s Advil Oral Suspension
    C.'s Comprehensive Pain
      Questionnaire (CCPQ)
    C.'s Dynafed Jr.
    C.'s Hospital hand drill
    C.'s Hospital screwdriver
    C.'s Motrin Oral Suspension
    C.'s Silapap
    Total Knee for c.
Childress
    C. ankle fixation technique
    C. duck waddle test
Chinese
    C. fingertrap
    C. fingertrap suture
    C. flap
    C. red line sign
chin-occiput piece
chin-to-chest test
ChinUpps cervicofacial support
chip
    bone c.
    cancellous c.
    c. fracture
    c. graft
Chippaux-Smirak arch index
Chiro-Klenx tea
chiropractic
    c. adjustment
    c. analysis
    c. biophysics (CBP)
    c. lesion
    c. manipulative reflex technique
      (CMRT)
    C. Rehabilitation Association (CRA)
    C. Strength Flexall 454
    c. treatment of fracture
Chiroslide
    C. Jamar Hand Dynamometer

Chirotech x-ray system
chisel
    Adson laminectomy c.
    Alexander c.
    ASIF c.
    Austin Moore c.
    Ballenger-Hajek c.
    Biomet cement-removal hand c.
    Bishop c.
    Blair c.
    Bowen c.
    box c.
    Brittain c.
    Bruening c.
    Buckley c.
    Caltagirone c.
    cement-removal hand c.
    Cinelli-McIndoe c.
    Cloward c.
    cold c.
    Converse c.
    Cottle c.
    Dautrey c.
    D'Errico lamina c.
    c.-edge elevator
    Fomon c.
    c. fracture
    Freer c.
    gold-paneled c.
    Hajek c.
    Harmon c.
    Hibbs c.
    Kerrison c.
    Lambert-Lowman c.
    Lexer c.
    Lowman c.
    Lowman-Hoglund c.
    Lucas c.
    Magnum c.
    Martin cartilage c.
    Metzenbaum c.
    Meyerding c.
    Miles bone c.
    Moore prosthesis-mortising c.
    Oratek c.
    orthopaedic c.
    Partsch c.
    Passow c.
    Pick c.
    Puka c.
    Schwartze c.
    seating c.

NOTES

C

chisel *(continued)*
    Sheehan c.
    Simmons c.
    Smillie cartilage c.
    Smillie meniscectomy c.
    square-hollow c.
    Stille bone c.
    swan-neck c.
    Trautmann c.
    U.S. Army bone c.
    West bone c.
    White c.
chi-square test
chloral hydrate
chlorambucil
chloramphenicol osteomyelitis
chlordiazepoxide
chlorhexidine gluconate
chloride
    antimicrobial benzalkonium c.
    benzalkonium c.
    ethyl c.
    polyvinyl c. (PVC)
chloroprocaine
chloroquine phosphate
chlorotrianisene
chlorphenesin
chlorphenesis carbamate
chlorpromazine
chlorprothixene
chlorzoxazone
Cho
    C. anterior cruciate ligament
      reconstruction
    C. tendon technique
cholesterol
Cholestin
choline
    c. magnesium trisalicylate
    c. salicylate
cholinergic vagal function
chondral fragment
chondralgia
chondrectomy
chondrification
chondritis
chondroblast
chondroblastoma
    benign c.
chondrocalcinosis
chondroclast
chondrocyte
    autologous cultured c.
    hypertrophic c.
chondrodiastasis
chondrodysplasia

chondrodystrophia
    c. calcificans
    c. fetalis
chondrodystrophy
chondroepiphysis
chondroepiphysitis
chondrofibroma
chondroid syringoma
chondroitin
chondroitin/glucosamine sulfate complex
chondrolipoma
chondrolysis
chondroma
    extraskeletal c.
    juxtacortical c.
    periosteal c.
chondromalacia
    Outerbridge scale for joint or
      articular surface damage in c.
    c. patellae
chondromalacic
chondromatosis
    Henderson-Jones c.
    synovial c.
chondrometaplasia
chondromyofibroma
chondromyxofibroma
chondromyxoid fibroma
chondromyxoma
chondromyxosarcoma
chondronecrosis
chondroosseous
    c. growth
    c. spur
chondroosteodystrophy
chondropathology
chondrophyte
chondroplastic
    c. dwarfism
    c. myotonia
chondroplasty
    abrasion c.
    arthroscopic abrasion c.
    c. knife
chondroporosis
chondroprotective agent
chondrosarcoma
    c. cell
    clear cell c.
    dedifferentiated c.
    differentiated c.
    extraskeletal c.
    mesenchymal c.
    myxoid c.
    parosteal c.
    periosteal c.
chondrosarcomatosis
chondrosis

chondrosteoma
chondrosternoplasty
chondrotomy
Chooz
chop amputation
Chopart
  C. ankle dislocation
  C. articulation
  C. brace
  C. hindfoot amputation
  C. midtarsal joint
  C. osseous joint injury
  C. partial foot prosthesis
Cho-Pat
  C.-P. Achilles tendon strap
  C.-P. elbow strap
  C.-P. knee strap
choppy sea sign
chordoblastoma
chordocarcinoma
chordoma
  cavern c.
  sacrococcygeal c.
chordosarcoma
chordotomy
chorea
  Huntington c.
choreatic gait
choreiform
Chow technique
Choyce MK II keratoprosthesis
  prosthesis
CHPS
  chronic heel pain syndrome
Chrisman-Snook
  C.-S. ankle technique
  C.-S. procedure
  C.-S. reconstruction
  C.-S. reconstruction of ankle
    ligament
Christensen interlocking nail
Christiani maneuver
Christiansen hip prosthesis
Christmas
  C. hemophiliac disease
  C. tree adapter
  C. tree reamer
chromatolysis
chrome
  cobalt c.
  c.-cobalt cable
chromium-cobalt-alloy implant

chromium-cobalt mesh
chromium implant
chromomycosis
chronaxie, chronaxy
chrondroblastoma
chronic
  c. compartment syndrome (CCS)
  c. functional instability
  c. heel pain syndrome (CHPS)
  c. intractable benign pain syndrome
    (CIBPS)
  c. low back pain (CLBP)
  c. musculoskeletal pain syndrome
    (CMPS)
  c. pyogenic osteomyelitis
  c. recurrent ankle joint dislocation
  c. recurrent dislocation of the
    ankle joint
  c. retrocalcaneal bursitis
  c. tophaceous disease
  c. tophaceous gout
CHSD
  congenital hyperphosphatasemic skeletal
    dysplasia
chuck
  c. adapter
  c. drill
  gold-handled c.
  hand c.
  Jacobs c.
  pin c.
  Steinmann pin with pin c.
  T-handle Zimmer c.
  three-jaw c.
Chuinard autogenous bone graft
Chuinard-Peterson
  C.-P. ankle arthrodesis
  C.-P. ankle fusion
  C.-P. anterior arthrodesis
Chukka boot
Chvostek sign
Chvostek-Weiss sign
chyloretroperitoneum
chylothorax
chylous
  c. ascites
  c. leakage
Chymar
  Alpha C.
Chymodiactin
chymopapain
  c. blocking agent

NOTES

C

chymopapain *(continued)*
    c. chemonucleolysis
    c. injection
chymotrypsin
    alpha c.
CI
    confidence interval
Cibacalcin Injection
CIBPS
    chronic intractable benign pain syndrome
CIC
    complex instability of carpus
Cica Care wound dressing
cicatrix, pl. **cicatrices**
cicatrization
Cicherelli bone rongeur
ciclopirox
Cida-foam
Cida-Gel powder
Cida-soak
Cida-spray
Cierny-Mader technique
ciguatera
cilastatin
    imipenem and c.
cimetidine
cinch
    joint c.
Cincinnati
    C. ACL brace
    C. incision
    C. Knee Rating System
    C. knee scoring questionnaire
    C. technique
cinearthrography
    triple-injection c.
Cinelli-McIndoe chisel
Cinelli osteotome
cine-magnetic resonance imaging (cine-MRI)
cine-MRI
    cine-magnetic resonance imaging
cineradiography
cine view
cingulate gyrus activity
cingulotomy, cingulumotomy
Cinti knee rating scale
Cintor knee prosthesis
Cipro
    C. Injection
    C. Oral
ciprofloxacin
CircOlectric
    C. bed
    C. frame
CircPlus bandage/wrap system
Circul'Air shoe process system

circular
    c. cast
    c. external fixator
    c. laminar hook with offset top
    c. open amputation
    c. saw
    c. supracondylar amputation
    c. wire
    c. wire fixator
circulation
    collateral c.
    femoral c.
    perichondral c.
circulation, muscle sensation (CMS)
Circulator boot system
circulatory embarrassment
circulus articuli vasculosis
circumduction maneuver
circumductor table
circumference
    calf c.
    pelvic c.
circumferential
    c. chemical burn
    c. dressing
    c. fracture
    c. grommet
    c. ligamentous sleeve
    c. release of clubfoot
    c. wire
    c. wire-loop fixation
    c. wiring
circumflex
    c. iliac artery
    c. scapular artery
circumscribed
circumscribing incision
circumscripta
    calcinosis c.
    Dubreuilh melanosis c.
Cirrus
    C. composite prosthetic foot
    C. foot prosthesis
    C. foot prosthetic
cirsoid angioma
cisplatin
Citanest
    C. Forte
    C. Plain
Citelli
    C. angle
    C. punch forceps
citrate
    orphenadrine c.
    sufentanil c.
CIVRA
    continuous intravenous regional anesthesia

CKC
  closed kinetic chain
CKS
  Continuum knee system
  CKS implant
  CKS knee system
Claforan
Claiborne external fixator
clamp
  Acland c.
  Adair breast c.
  Aesculap c.
  Allen-Kocher c.
  Allis c.
  angled DeBakey c.
  Ann Arbor double towel c.
  appendage c.
  c. approximator
  Atra-Grip c.
  Auvard c.
  baby Kocher c.
  baby Satinsky c.
  Backhaus-Jones towel c.
  Backhaus-Kocher towel c.
  Backhaus towel c.
  Bahnson appendage c.
  Bailey-Cowley c.
  Bailey duckbill c.
  Bailey-Morse c.
  Balfour c.
  Ballantine c.
  Bamby c.
  Bard c.
  bar-to-bar c.
  Belcher c.
  Berens muscle c.
  Berke c.
  Bernhard c.
  Bethune c.
  Bigelo calvarium c.
  Bircher bone-holding c.
  Bircher cartilage c.
  Bishop bone c.
  Blalock c.
  Böhler c.
  bone extension c.
  bone-holding c.
  Bonney c.
  Borge c.
  Boyes muscle c.
  bulldog c.
  C c.

  Calandruccio c.
  c. carrier
  cartilage c.
  Casey pelvic c.
  Charnley arthrodesis c.
  Charnley bone c.
  Charnley compression c.
  Charnley external fixation c.
  Charnley pin c.
  Clevis c.
  Cooley graft c.
  Cooley iliac c.
  Cooley multipurpose angled c.
  Cooley multipurpose curved c.
  Davidson muscle c.
  Demel wire c.
  Demos tibial artery c.
  Diethrich bulldog c.
  disposable muscle biopsy c.
  dissecting c.
  distraction c.
  Doctor Collins fracture c.
  Edna towel c.
  exclusion c.
  extension bone c.
  femoral c.
  Ferguson bone c.
  c. fixator
  c. forceps
  Frahur cartilage c.
  Frazier-Adson osteoplastic flap c.
  Frazier-Sachs c.
  Freeman c.
  Friedrich c.
  Friedrich-Petz c.
  full-curved c.
  Gerster bone c.
  Goodwin bone c.
  Greenberg c.
  Halifax interlaminar c.
  Harrington hook c.
  hemostatic thoracic c.
  Hex-Fix Universal swivel c.
  Hoen c.
  Hoffmann ligament c.
  c. holder
  Hugh Young pedicle c.
  iliac c.
  c. insert
  interlaminar c.
  Jackson bone c.
  Jackson bone-extension c.

C

NOTES

clamp *(continued)*

Jackson bone-holding c.
Jacobson bulldog c.
Jameson muscle c.
Jarit anterior resection c.
Jarit cartilage c.
Jarit meniscal c.
Jarit small bone-holding c.
Johns Hopkins bulldog c.
Jones thoracic c.
Jones towel c.
Kantrowitz thoracic c.
Kelly c.
Kern bone-holding c.
Kocher c.
Lahey c.
Lalonde bone c.
Lambert-Lowman bone c.
Lambotte bone-holding c.
Lamis patellar c.
Lane bone-holding c.
Lewin bone-holding c.
ligament c.
lobster-type c.
Locke bone c.
locking c.
Lowman bone-holding c.
Lowman-Gerster bone c.
Lowman-Hoglund c.
Lulu c.
Malis hinge c.
Martin cartilage c.
Martin meniscal c.
Martin muscular c.
Masterson curved c.
Masterson pelvic c.
Masterson straight c.
Mastin muscular c.
Matthew cross-leg c.
Mayo c.
meniscal c.
metal c.
microvascular c.
miniature multipurpose c.
mini-Ullrich bone c.
Mitchel-Adam multipurpose c.
Mixter ligature-carrier c.
Mixter right-angle c.
mosquito c.
Moynihan towel c.
multipurpose angled c.
multipurpose curved c.
muscle biopsy c.
muscular c.
Naraghi-DeCoster reduction c.
osteoplastic flap c.
padded c.
Parham-Martin bone-holding c.

patellar cement c.
patellar reduction c.
Pean c.
pedicle c.
pelvic C-c.
Pemberton spur-crushing c.
phalangeal c.
pin-to-bar c.
point-of-reduction c.
Price muscular biopsy c.
ratchet c.
Rayport muscular biopsy c.
reamer c.
Richards bone c.
rod c.
rubber-shod c.
Rumel myocardial c.
Rumel rubber c.
Rumel thoracic c.
Rush bone c.
Seidel bone-holding c.
self-retaining c.
Semb bone-holding c.
Slocum meniscal c.
Smith bone c.
Southwick c.
speed-lock c.
spur-crushing c.
stainless steel c.
Steinhauser bone c.
Steri-Clamp c.
Surgi-Med c.
towel c.
trochanter-holding c.
Ulrich bone-holding c.
Universal wire c.
Verbrugge bone c.
vessel c.
VSF c.
Walton meniscal c.
Wells pedicle c.
Wester meniscal c.
West Shur cartilage c.
wire-tightening c.
Wylie lumbar bulldog c.
X c.
Zimmer cartilage c.

clamping mechanism
clamp-on
clamshell

c. brace
c. prosthesis

Clancy

C. cruciate ligament reconstruction
C. lateral compartment
C. ligament technique
C. patellar tendon graft

Clancy-Andrews reconstruction

Clanton-DeLee algorithm
Clark
C. classification of melanoma
C. pectoralis major transfer
C. sign
C. transfer technique
Clarke arch angle
Clark-Southwick-Odgen modification
Clarus SpineScope
clasp
Arrow pin c.
EPI Sport epicondylitis c.
clasped
c. thumb
c. thumb deformity
class
Aitken hip c.
classification
AAOS acetabular abnormalities c.
acromioclavicular injury c.
Aitken epiphyseal fracture c.
Allman acromioclavicular injury c.
Anderson-D'Alonzo odontoid
fracture c.
Anderson modification of Berndt-
Harty c.
Anderson tibial pseudarthrosis c.
AO c.
Ashhurst-Bromer ankle fracture c.
Bado c.
Bauer-Jackson c.
Berndt-Harty c. of transchondral
fracture
Bishop c.
Bleck metatarsus adductus c.
Boyd c.
Boyd-Griffin trochanteric fracture c.
Brooker heterotopic bone
formation c.
Burwell-Charnley fracture
reduction c.
Canale-Kelly talar neck fracture c.
Carnesale-Stewart-Barnes hip
dislocation c.
Catterall c.
Cavanaugh-Rogers footprint c.
Cedell-Magnusson arthritis c.
cement mantle grade c.
Chadwick-Bentley c.
Charnley functional c.
Clatter c.
Codman c.

Colonna hip fracture c.
Colton c.
Copeland-Kavat metatarsophalangeal
dislocation c.
CP Sports Balance C.
Crowe congenital hip dysplasia c.
D'Antonio acetabular c.
Darrow pain c.
Daseler-Anson plantaris muscle
anatomy c.
Delbert hip fracture c.
DeLee c.
Denis Browne sacral fracture c.
Denis Browne spinal fracture c.
Dias-Tachdijian physeal injury c.
Dickhaut-DeLee discoid meniscus c.
Dorr bone c.
Dyck-Lambert c.
Eckert-Davis c.
Ellis c.
Enna c.
Enneking c.
Epstein hip dislocation c.
Epstein-Thomas c.
Essex-Lopresti calcaneal fracture c.
Estok and Harris c.
Evans intertrochanteric fracture c.
Ficat and Arlet c.
Ficat femoral head osteonecrosis c.
Ficat stage of avascular necrosis c.
Fielding femoral fracture c.
Fielding-Magliato subtrochanteric
fracture c.
Flatt c.
fracture c.
Fränkel neurologic deficit c.
Franz-O'Rahilly c.
Freeman calcaneal fracture c.
Fries score for rheumatoid
arthritis c.
Frykman distal radius fracture c.
Garden femoral neck fracture c.
Gartland humeral supracondylar
fracture c.
Gartland Universal radial
fracture c.
Grantham femur fracture c.
Greenfield spinocerebellar ataxia c.
Gumley seat beat injury c.
Gustilo-Anderson open fracture c.
Gustilo puncture wound c.

C

NOTES

classification *(continued)*
Hahn-Steinthal capitellum
fracture c.
Hannover c.
Hansen fracture c.
Hardcastle c.
Hardy-Clapham sesamoid c.
Hawkins talar fracture c.
Henderson c.
Herbert-Fisher fracture system c.
Herbert scaphoid bone fracture c.
Herring lateral pillar c.
Hoaglund-States c.
Hohl-Luck tibial plateau fracture c.
Hohl-Moore c.
Hohl tibial condylar fracture c.
Holdsworth spinal fracture c.
Hughston c.
Ideberg glenoid fracture c.
Ingram-Bachynski hip fracture c.
Insall patellar injury c.
Jahss ankle dislocation c.
Jahss metatarsophalangeal joint
dislocation c.
Jeffery radial fracture c.
Johner-Wruhs tibial fracture c.
Johnson-Boseker scale c.
Johnson-Jahss posterior tibial
tendon tear c.
Jones-Barnes-Lloyd-Roberts c.
Jones congenital tibial deficiency c.
Jones diaphyseal fracture c.
Kalamchi c.
Kelikian nail deformity c.
Kellam-Waddel c.
Key-Conwell pelvic fracture c.
Kilfoyle humeral medial condylar
fracture c.
Kocher c.
Kostuik-Errico spinal stability c.
Kyle-Gustilo c.
Kyle-Gustilo-Premer c.
LaGrange humeral supracondylar
fracture c.
Langenskiöld c. (stage I–VI)
Lauge-Hansen ankle fracture c.
Letournel-Judet acetabular
fracture c.
Leung thumb loss c.
Lindell c.
Lloyd-Roberts-Catteral-Salamon c.
Macewen c.
MacNichol-Voutsinas c.
Mason radial head fracture c.
Mast-Spieghel-Pappas c.
Mathews olecranon fracture c.
Mayo carpal instability c.
McDermott radiological c.

McLain-Weinstein spinal tumor c.
Melone distal radius fracture c.
Meyers-McKeever tibial fracture c.
Milch condylar fracture c.
Milch elbow fracture c.
Minaar coalition c.
Moore tibial plateau fracture c.
MRC muscle function c.
Mueller femoral supracondylar
fracture c.
Mueller tibial fracture c.
Neer femur fracture c.
Neer-Horowitz c.
Neer humerus fracture c.
Neer shoulder fracture c.
Neviaser frozen shoulder c.
Newman radial neck and head
fracture c.
Nicoll c.
Nurick spondylosis c.
O'Brien radial fracture c.
Oden peroneal tendon
subluxation c.
Ogden epiphyseal fracture c.
Ogden knee dislocation c.
O'Rahilly limb deficiency c.
ordinal c.
Orthopaedic Trauma Association c.
Outerbridge c.
Ovadia-Beals tibial plafond
fracture c.
Paley c.
Palmer triangular fibrocartilage
complex lesion c.
Papavasiliou olecranon fracture c.
Pauwels femoral neck fracture c.
Pennal c.
Pipkin posterior hip dislocation c.
Pipkin subclassification of Epstein-
Thomas c.
Poland epiphyseal fracture c.
Prosthetic Problem Inventory
Scale c.
Quénu-Küss tarsometatarsal
injury c.
Quinby pelvic fracture c.
Ranawat c.
Ratliff avascular necrosis c.
Riordan club hand c.
Riseborough-Radin intercondylar
fracture c.
Rockwood c.
Rowe calcaneal fracture c.
Rowe-Lowell hip dislocation c.
Ruedi-Allgower c.
Russe c.
Russell-Taylor c.
Rüter c.

Sage-Salvatore c.
Saha shoulder muscle c.
Sakellarides calcaneal fracture c.
Salter epiphyseal fracture c.
Salter-Harris c.
Salter-Harris-Rang epiphyseal
  fracture c.
Sanders CT C.
scalar c.
Schatzker tibial plateau fracture c.
Seddon c.
Seinsheimer femoral fracture c.
Severin c.
Shelton femoral fracture c.
Singh osteoporosis c.
Sorbie calcaneal fracture c.
Speed radial head fracture c.
Steinbrocker rheumatoid arthritis c.
Steinert epiphyseal fracture c.
Steward-Milford fracture c.
Sunderland c. of nerve injury
Swanson c.
Tachdjian c.
Thomas c.
Thompson-Epstein c.
Three Color Concept of wound c.
Tile c.
Torg c.
Torode-Zieg c.
Toronto pelvic fracture c.
Tronzo fracture c.
Tscherne c.
Tscherne-Gotzen tibial fracture c.
Universal distal radius fracture c.
Venn-Watson c.
Vostal radial fracture c.
Wagner c.
Warren-Marshall c.
Wassel thumb duplication c.
Watanabe discoid meniscus c.
Watson-Jones spinal fracture c.
Watson-Jones tibial fracture c.
Weber c.
Weber-Danis ankle injury c.
Weiland c.
Weissman c.
Wiberg patellar c.
Wiley-Galey c.
Wilkins radial fracture c.
Winquist femoral shaft fracture c.
Winquist-Hansen femoral fracture c.
Young pelvic fracture c.

Zickel c.
Zlotsky-Ballard acromioclavicular
  injury c.
Clatter classification
claudication
  neurogenic c. (NC)
clavicectomy
clavicle
  c. excision
  floating c.
  intraarticular c.
  c. pin
  weightlifter's c.
clavicular
  c. birth fracture
  c. cross splint
  c. epiphysis
  c. fracture aneurysm
  c. notch
claviculectomy
clavipectoral
  c. fascia
  c. triangle
clavulanate
clavus foot
claw
  c. finger
  c.-type basic frame
clawfoot
  c. contracture
  c. deformity
  c. foot
clawhand deformity
clawtoe deformity
clay shoveler's fracture
Clayton
  C. forefoot arthroplasty
  C. greenstick splint
  C. osteotome
  C. procedure
  C. procedure with panmetatarsal
    head resection
  C. resection arthroplasty
Clayton-Fowler technique
CLBP
  chronic low back pain
cleaner
  Orthozime instrument c.
cleanser
  ClinsWound wound c.
  MPM antimicrobial wound c.

NOTES

cleanser *(continued)*
    Restore AF antimicrobial skin c.
    SeptiCare antimicrobial wound c.
Cleanwheel
    C. disposable neurological pinwheel
    C. presterilized disposable device
clear
    c. cell chondrosarcoma
    c. cell sarcoma
clearance
    cefazolin c.
    radioactive xenon c.
cleavage
    c. fracture
    horizontal c.
    c. lesion
    c. line
    c. tear
Cleeman sign
cleft
    c. closure
    c. foot
    gluteal c.
    Hahn c.
    c. hand
    intergluteal c.
    interinnominoabdominal c.
    retropharyngeal fascial c.
    c. spinous process
    venous c.
    c. vertebra
clefthand deformity
clefting of meniscus
clefts of Hahn
cleidocranial
    c. dysostosis
    c. dysplasia
Cleland
    C. ligament
    C. ligament in the hand
clenched-fist syndrome
Cleocin
    C. HCl
    C. Pediatric
    C. Phosphate
Cleveland
    C. bone-cutting forceps
    C. bone rongeur
Cleveland-Bosworth-Thompson technique
Clevis clamp
CLI
    critical limb ischemia
click
    hip c.
    Mulder c.
    Ortolani c.
    c. sign

clicker
    compression c.
Climara Transdermal
climber
    Fitstep II stair c.
    Sprint C.
clindamycin
clinical
    C. Analysis Questionnaire (CAQ)
    c. conservatism
    c. diagnosis
    c. examination
    c. trial
Clinisert mattress
Clinitron air bed
clinodactyly
Clinoril
ClinsWound wound cleanser
clioquinol
clip
    c. applier
    c.-applying forceps
    c.-bending forceps
    Braun-Yasargil right-angle c.
    c.-cutting forceps
    c.-introducing forceps
    Khodadad c.
    Michel c.
    palmar c.
    towel c.
clivus
cloacae
    Enterobacter c.
clock
    shoulder c.
clockwise
clog
    Hollander c.
    Markell Mobility Health C.'s
    wooden postoperative c.'s
clomipramine
Clomycin
clonazepam
clonus
    ankle c.
    drawn ankle c.
    patellar c.
    persistent c.
    sustained ankle c.
    three-beat c.
    unsustained c.
Clorpactin WCS-90
close
    c. encounter nut
    c. wedge osteotomy/bunionectomy
closed
    c. amputation
    c. base wedge osteotomy (CBWO)

c. chain
c.-chain exercise
c. core needle biopsy
c. Cotrel-Dubousset hook
c. drainage system
c. femoral diaphyseal shortening
c.-flap amputation
c. intramedullary nailing with reaming
c. intramedullary osteotomy
c. irrigation
c. kinetic chain (CKC)
c. kinetic chain progressive-resistance exercise
c. Küntscher nail
c. Küntscher nailing
c. manipulative maneuver
c. medullary nailing
c. pinning
c. pseudarthrosis
c.-reak fracture
c. reduction (CR)
c. soft tissue injury
c. transverse process TSRH hook
c. treatment
c.-wedge osteotomy
c. wound

closing
c. abductory-wedge osteotomy (CAWO)
c. base wedge
c. base-wedge osteotomy
voluntary c. (VC)
c. wedge arthrodesis
c. wedge greenstick dorsal proximal metatarsal osteotomy
c. wedge manipulation and reapplication of plaster

clostridial
c. infection
c. myonecrosis
c. myositis

Clostridium perfringens
closure
Barsky cleft c.
cleft c.
delayed c.
epiphyseal c.
myofascial c.
physeal c.
premature c.
primary c.

secondary c.
skin c.
Sureclosure c.
visual c.
wound c.

clot
exogenous fibrin c.
fibrin c.

cloth
AliMold stretch c.

clothespin spinal fusion graft
clotrimazole
betamethasone and c.

clotting disorder
Cloutier unconstrained knee prosthesis
cloven-hoof fracture of finger
cloverleaf
c. condylar plate fixation
c. counterbore
c. Küntscher nail
c. met foot pad
c. pattern
c. pin
c. pin extractor
c. plate

Cloward
C. anterior spinal fusion
C. back fusion
C. blade retractor
C. bone graft impactor
C. cervical arthrodesis
C. cervical disk approach
C. cervical drill
C. cervical drill guard
C. cervical drill tip
C. chisel
C. depth gauge
C. dowel cutter
C. drill guard cap
C. drill guide
C. drill shaft
C. fusion diskectomy
C. fusion diskography
C. hammer
C. osteophyte elevator
C. periosteal elevator
C. rongeur
C. spinal fusion osteotome
C. spreader
C. surgical saddle
C. technique

Cloward-Cone curette

C

NOTES

cloxacillin
CLS hip system
clubbed
   c. nail
   c. toe
clubbing
   c. of finger
   c. of toe
clubfoot
   acquired c.
   arthrogrypotic c.
   circumferential release of c.
   c. deformity
   c. release
   resistant c.
   c. splint
clubhand
   radial c.
   ulnar c.
clumsy gait
clunk
   catch-up c.
   c. test
Clyburn
   C. Colles fracture fixator
   C. external fixator
CM
   combined mechanical
CMAP
   compound muscle action potential
   compound muscle-motor action potential
CM-Band
   CM-B. 505N brace
   CM-B. silicone rubber brace
CMC
   carpal-metacarpal
   carpometacarpal
   CMC fusion
   CMC joint
   CMC splint
CME-MRI
   contrast medium-enhanced magnetic
     resonance imaging
CMO hydrocollator
CMPS
   chronic musculoskeletal pain syndrome
CMRT
   chiropractic manipulative reflex
     technique
CMS
   circulation, muscle sensation
CMT
   Charcot-Marie-Tooth
   CMT disease
CMW
   C. bone cement
   C. cement gun

CNS
   central nervous system
CO
   certified orthotist
   cervical orthosis
coach's finger
coagulase
   c. negative
   c. positive
coagulated plasma
coagulating forceps
coagulation
   c. disorder
   disseminated intravascular c. (DIC)
   c. factor
coagulator
   ASSI c.
   bipolar c.
   Concept bipolar c.
   Malis CMC-II bipolar c.
   Polar-Mate c.
coalescence
coalition
   c. of bone
   calcaneonavicular c.
   cartilaginous c.
   complete c.
   congenital complete subtalar c.
   fibrous talocalcaneal c.
   incomplete c.
   lunate-triquetral c.
   Minaar classification of c.
   osseous c.
   talocalcaneal c.
   tarsal c.
   c. view
coapt
coaptating
coaptation
   centrocentral c.
   c. plate
coapted
coarse
   c. carbide cone bur
   c.-olive bur
coated implant
coating
   aluminum oxide ceramic c.
   Biolox ceramic c.
   cobalt-chrome powder c.
   Porocoat porous c.
   porous c.
   sintering of cobalt-chrome
     powder c.
coaxial needle electrode
Coballoy
   C. implant metal

C. implant metal prosthesis
C. twist drill

cobalt
c.-based alloy
c. chrome
c. implant

cobalt-chrome
c.-c. powder coating
c.-c. power sintering

cobalt-chromium
c.-c. alloy
c.-c. head
c.-c. implant
ion-bombarded c.-c.
smooth c.-c.

cobalt-chromium-alloy prosthesis
cobalt-chromium-molybdenum (Co-Cr-Mo)
cobalt-chromium-tungsten-nickel (Co-Cr-W-Ni)

Coban
C. elastic dressing
C. elastic wrap

Cobb
C. attachment for Albee-Compere fracture table
C. curette
C. gauge
C. lumbar angle
C. measurement of scoliosis
C. method
C. method for measuring scoliosis
C. osteotome
C. periosteal elevator
C. scoliosis angle
C. scoliosis measuring technique
C. spinal gouge
C. syndrome
technique of C.

cobra
c.-design femoral component
c.-head plate
c. retractor

Coccidioides immitis
coccidioidin skin test
coccidioidomycosis
c. infection

coccygeal spine
coccygodynia
coccygotomy
coccyx
c. fracture

posterior surgical exposure of sacrum and c.

cocked-half flap
Cocke maxillectomy
cocking injury
Cocklin toe operation
cock-robin head tilt
cock-up
c.-u. arm splint
c.-u. deformity
c.-u. hand splint
c.-u. splint orthosis
c.-u. toe
c.-u. wrist support

co-contraction exercise
Co-Cr-Mo
cobalt-chromium-molybdenum
Co-Cr-Mo alloy implant metal
Co-Cr-Mo alloy prosthesis
Co-Cr-Mo pin

Co-Cr-W-Ni
cobalt-chromium-tungsten-nickel
Co-Cr-W-Ni alloy implant metal
Co-Cr-W-Ni alloy prosthesis

codeine
acetaminophen and c.
aspirin and c.
butalbital compound and c.
Capital and C.
carisoprodol, aspirin, and c.
Empirin With C.
Fiorinal with C.
Phenaphen With C.
Tylenol With C.

codfish
c. deformity
c. vertebra

Codivilla
C. bone graft
C. tendon lengthening
C. tendon lengthening technique

Codman
C. ACP system
C. angle
C. anterior cervical plate system
C. anterior cervical plating system
C. classification
C. exercise
C. saber-cut shoulder approach
C. sign
C. Ti-frame posterior fixation system

C

NOTES

119

Codman *(continued)*
C. triangle
C. tumor
C. wire-passing drill
Codoxy
coefficient
c. of friction
interclass correlation c. (ICC)
c. of variation (CV)
Coe-pak
C.-p. paste
C.-p. paste adhesive
Cofield
C. shoulder prosthesis
C. technique
C. total shoulder system
CoFilm dressing
Coflex wrap
COG
center of gravity
Cogent
C. light
C. LightWear headlight
C. XL illuminator
Co-Gesic
cognition
Cognitive
C. Behavior Therapy Package (CBTP)
C. Error Questionnaire
C. Strategies Questionnaire
cogwheel
c. gait
c. rigidity
c. sign
Cohen
C. periosteal elevator
C. rongeur
cohesion
glenohumeral joint c.
COH hip abduction splint
cohort
C. anterior plate system
C. bone brush
C. bone screw
C. spinal impactor
c. study
C. Ti-spacer
cohosh
black c.
COI
combination of isotonics
coilette
FLX flexible treatment c.
coin
fracture en c.
Coker-Arnold collar

ColBenemid
colchicine and probenecid
Colclough laminectomy rongeur
cold
c. application
c. chisel
c.-curing polymer
c. injury
c. intolerance
c.-mold prosthesis
c. pad
c. phase as in bone scanning
c. pressor test
c. rolled rod
c. therapy
c. weld
Coldflo cold therapy and sequential compression
Coldhot pack
coldPaq
cold-weld
c.-w. femoral ball
c.-w. femoral prosthesis
Cole
C. fracture frame
C. hyperextension brace
C. hyperextension frame
C. osteotomy
C. osteotomy for midfoot deformity
C. procedure
C. technique
C. tendon fixation
Coleman
C. flatfoot technique
C. lateral block test
C. plasty
coli
Escherichia c.
colinear alignment
colistin
collagen
bovine c.
c. fiber
microcrystalline c.
c. scaffold
c. vascular disease
collagenase
collagenous schwannoma
collagraft
C. bone graft matrix
collapse
bone graft c.
foot c.
hindfoot-midfoot c.
neuropathic c.
scapholunate advanced c. (SLAC)
vertebral c.

collapsible
- c. internal fixation device
- c. pin

collapsing pes valgo planus

collar
- c.-and-cuff sling
- Aspen cervical c.
- c. bone
- c. brace
- calcar c.
- c.-calcar support femoral prosthesis
- cervical c.
- Coker-Arnold c.
- Colpack c.
- c. and cuff
- Exo-Static cervical c.
- Forrester-Brown c.
- hard c.
- Headmaster c.
- implant c.
- Lewin c.
- MAC cervical c.
- Marlin cervical c.
- Mayo-Thomas c.
- Miami J cervical c.
- myocervical c.
- Nec Loc cervical c.
- periosteal bone c.
- Philadelphia cervical c.
- plastic c.
- Plastizote cervical c.
- Pneu-trac cervical c.
- 2+2 Rehab C.
- Schanz c.
- serpentine foam c.
- soft c.
- Thomas c.

collared
- c. femoral head
- c. Press-Fit femoral stem implantation

collarless
- c. polished taper (CPT)
- c. stem

collat
- collateral

collateral (collat)
- c. artery
- c. circulation
- c. fibular ligament
- c. ligament instability

- c. ligament of interphalangeal articulations
- c. ligament of MCP articulations
- c. ligament of MTP articulations
- c. ligament rupture
- c. radial ligament
- c. tibial ligament
- c. ulnar ligament

collectomy
- shortening c.

College
- American C. of Occupational and Environmental Medicine (ACOEM)
- Association of Chiropractic C.'s (ACC)
- C. Park TruStep foot
- C. Park TruStep foot prosthesis

Colles
- C. fascia
- C. fracture
- C. splint

Collet
- C. screwdriver adapter
- tibial C.

colli
- fibromatosis c.
- pterygium c.

collicular fracture

Collier sign

collimation

Collimator
- Multileaf C.
- C. plugging pattern

Collin amputating knife

Collins
- C. dynamometer
- C. rib shears

Collis
- C. broken femoral stem technique
- C. retractor
- C. TDR instrument

Collis-Dubrul femoral stem removal

Collison
- C. body drill
- C. cannulated hand drill
- C. plate
- C. screw
- C. screwdriver
- C. tap drill

Collis-Taylor retractor

collodiaphysial
- central c. (CCD)

C

NOTES

collodion dressing
colloid
    c. cyst
    c. solution
colocutaneous fistula
Colonna
    C. hip fracture classification
    C. shelf operation
    C. trochanteric arthroplasty
Colonna-Ralston
    C.-R. ankle approach
    C.-R. incision
    C.-R. medial approach
color
    c.-coded therapy putty
    c. of digit
    c. Doppler echography
    c. duplex imaging
Colorado Cycle
ColorCards
    Adjective C.
    Basic Sequences C.
    Everyday Objects C.
    Preposition C.
    Verb C.
    What's Wrong C.
colored antiseptic
Colpack collar
Colpacs pack
Coltart
    C. calcaneotibial fusion
    C. fracture technique
Colton classification
Columbus
    C. McKinnon assist for lifting or
      transfer
    C. McKinnon Hugger device
column
    central c.
    contrast c.
    radial c.
    spinal c.
    ulnar c.
    vertebral c.
comb
    toe c.
Combat Task Test
CombiDERM nonadhesive absorbent
dressing
Combi Multi-Traction System
combination
    film-screen c.
    Futureplex Flower Essence C.'s
    Isola spinal implant system plate-
      rod c.
    c. of isotonics (COI)
    c. of isotonics technique

combined
    c. anterior and posterior approach
    c. cavus
    c. cavus deformity
    c. curve
    c. fixation device
    c. flexion-distraction injury and
      burst fracture
    c.-flexion phenomenon
    c. instability
    c. low-cervical and transthoracic
      approach
    c. mechanical (CM)
    c. nerve palsy
    penicillin g benzathine and
      procaine c.
    c. radial-ulnar-humeral fracture
    c. resection arthroplasty and
      arthrodesis
    c. scintigraphy
Comfeel Ulcus dressing
Comforfoam splint
comfort
    C. Cast
    c. level
    C. Take-Along wheelchair cushion
    C. wrist immobilizer
comforter
    Thermo hand c.
    Thermo knee c.
Comf-Orthotic
    C.-O. 3/4 length insole
    C.-O. sports replacement insole
Comfortseat
    Flo-Fit C.
Comfy
    C. Elbow Orthosis
    C. elbow splint
    C. Knee Orthosis
    C. walker
comitans, pl. comitantes
    vena c.
comitantes
    venae c.
Command
    C. hip instrumentation system
    C. instrument system surgical
      instrument
commemorative sign
comminuted
    c. intraarticular fracture
Commission on Accreditation of
Rehabilitation Facilities (CARF)
commissural myelorrhaphy
Committee
    Fitness Safety Standards C.
    International Knee
      Documentation C. (IKDC)

Policy and Review C. for Human
Research
common
c. carotid artery
c. dural sac
c. extensor tendon
c. iliac artery
c. iliac vein
c. peroneal nerve
c. peroneal nerve syndrome
communicans
Gray ramus c.
communicating hydrosyringomyelia
communication
asyndetic c.
communis
extensor digitorum c. (EDC)
flexor digitorum c. (FDC)
ligamentum caudale integumenti c.
Comolli sign
compact bone
compaction
vertical sacral c.
compactor
acetabular cement c.
cement c.
comparative radiographic examination
comparison
pairwise c.
compartment
anterior c.
Clancy lateral c.
deep posterior c.
c. fasciotomy
interosseous c.
lateral c.
medial c.
Mueller lateral c.
osseofascial c.
osteofascial c.
patellofemoral c.
posterior c.
posterolateral c.
posteromedial c.
superficial posterior c.
c. syndrome
compartmental
C. II knee prosthesis
c. pressure
Compass
C. hinge
C. stereotactic system

Compazine
Compeed protective dressing
compensable accident
compensated talipes equinus
compensating filter
compensation
anticipating financial c. (AFC)
c. reaction
Workers' C.
compensatory
c. basilar osteotomy
c. behavior
c. curve
c. deformity
c. hypermobility
c. movement
c. scoliosis
c. structural subluxation
c. wedge
Compere
C. lengthening
C. osteotome
C. threaded pin
C. wire
Compere-Thompson arthrodesis
Comperm tubular elastic bandage
complaint
chief c. (CC)
complement
complete
c. amputation
c. coalition
c. common peroneal nerve lesion
c. dislocation
c. fracture
c. subtalar release (CSR)
c. syndactyly
complex
c. acetabular reconstruction
ankle joint c. (AJC)
arcuate c.
atlas-axis c.
Buford c.
bunionette-hallux valgus-splayfoot c.
bunion-hallux valgus c.
capsulolabral c.
capsuloligamentous c.
chondroitin/glucosamine sulfate c.
Edinger-Westphal c.
epiphyseal c.
fabellofibular c.
fibrocartilage c.

C

NOTES

complex *(continued)*
>forearm c.
>c. fracture
>gastrocnemius-soleus c.
>gastroc-soleus c.
>Ghon-Sachs c.
>hallux valgus-metatarsus primus
> varus c.
>hindfoot joint c.
>c. instability of carpus (CIC)
>knee c.
>lateral quadruple c.
>ligament-bone c.
>ligamentous c.
>Lisfranc joint c.
>lumbopelvic c.
>medial quadruple c.
>c. meniscal tear
>c. motor unit action potential
>plantar capsuloligamentous c.
>postural c.
>quadruple c.
>c. repetitive discharge
>semimembranosus c.
>shoulder c.
>soleus c.
>spinal cord-meningeal c.
>c. syndactyly
>talocalcaneonavicular c.
>talonavicular-cuneiform c.
>three-joint c.
>trialkylphosphine gold c.
>triangular fibrocartilage c. (TFC,
> TFCC)
>vertebral subluxation c. (VSC)
>zygomatic-malar c. (ZMC)

compliance

complicated complex syndactyly

complication
>intraoperative c.
>neurologic c.
>neurovascular c.
>postoperative c.
>pulmonary c.
>urologic c.

complimentary alternative medicine (CAM)

component
>acetabular c.
>AML trial hip c.
>Amstutz femoral c.
>anatomically graduated c. (AGC)
>Aufranc-Turner femoral c.
>Bechtol acetabular c.
>Biomet MARS acetabular c.
>Biomet revision acetabular c.
>Biomet shoulder c.
>bipolar femoral c.

>bipolar hip arthroplasty c.
>Black Max mid size knee c.
>Bombelli-Morscher femoral c.
>cemented c.
>cementless femoral c.
>chamfered cylinder acetabular c.
>Charnley flat-back femoral c.
>Charnley narrow-stem c.
>Charnley standard-stem c.
>cobra-design femoral c.
>Definition PM femoral implant c.
>DePuy trispiked acetabular c.
>dorsi stop c.
>Duramer polyethylene c.
>femoral c.
>c. of gait
>glenoid c.
>Gustilo-Kyle femoral c.
>Harris-Galante hip replacement
> acetabular c.
>Harris-Galante I porous-coated
> acetabular c.
>Healey revision acetabular c.
>humeral c.
>hybrid fixation of hip
> replacement c.
>Infinity femoral c.
>keel of glenoid c.
>kinesiopathologic c.
>large-head humeral c.
>Lubinus acetabular c.
>MARS revision acetabular c.
>Meridian ST femoral implant c.
>metal-backed acetabular c.
>Metasul hip joint c.
>modular large-head c.
>monoblock femoral c.
>Morse taper lock of modular hip
> implant c.
>Neer II humeral c.
>neuromuscular c.
>NexGen c.
>Ogee acetabular c.
>Osteolock acetabular c.
>Osteolock HA femoral c.
>Osteonics Omnifit-HA c.
>performance c.
>polyethylene liner implant c.
>porous cementless c.
>porous-coated c.
>posterior c.
>postural c.
>Press-Fit femoral c.
>Profix porous femoral c.
>prosthesis c.
>Reliance CM femoral implant c.
>roof-reinforcement ring hip
> arthroplasty c.

sensory c.
Smith & Nephew reflection
  acetabular cup implant c.
Springlite G foot c.
Springlite II foot c.
structural c.
c. subsidence
sympathetic c.
Taperloc femoral c.
Tharies femoral resurfacing c.
Tharies hip c.
Ti-Bac acetabular c.
tibial c.
c. trial
trial femoral c.
Tri-Con c.
Tricon-M c.
uncemented femoral c.
Universal radial c.
V40 femoral head implant c.
Vitalock cluster acetabular c.
Vitalock solid-back acetabular c.
Zimmer NexGen LPS knee
  femoral c.

composite
c. defect
E-A-R specialty c.
c. fracture
c. free tissue transfer
c. groin fascial free flap
c. material
c. rib graft
c. skin graft
c. spring elastic splint

compound
dihydrocodeine c.
c. mixed nerve action potential
c. motor nerve action potential
c. muscle action potential (CMAP)
c. muscle-motor action potential
  (CMAP)
c. nevus
OCT c.
Pediplast moldable footcare c.
pentazocine c.
c. sensory nerve action potential
c. shattered elbow
Soma C.
Talwin C.

Compoz
C. Gel Caps
C. Nighttime Sleep Aid

compressed nitrogen
compressible
compression
anterior cord c.
anterior-posterior c. (APC)
anteroposterior c. (APC)
AO c.
c. apparatus
c. arthrodesis
axial c.
c. bandage
c. boot
carotid artery c.
cauda equina c.
Charnley c.
c. clicker
Coldflo cold therapy and
  sequential c.
cord c.
disk c.
c. dressing
duodenal c.
dynamic c. (DC)
elastic c.
c. extension
c. flexion
c. glove
c. Harrington instrumentation
Harrington rod instrumentation c.
c. hip screw
c. hook
c. inserter-extractor
c. instrumentation posterior
  construct
interfragmental c.
interfragmentary c.
intermittent impulse c.
ischemic c.
c. lag screw
lateral c. (LC)
c. load
c. loading
median nerve c.
c.-molded prosthesis
c. molding
napkin ring c.
nerve root c.
neuraxial c.
c. overload
c. pattern
c. plate
c. plate fixation

NOTES

C

compression *(continued)*
    pneumatic pedal c.
    c. rod
    c. rod treatment
    c. screw-plate device
    c. sideplate
    c. sleeve shin splint
    spinal cord c.
    c. spring
    static c.
    c. strain
    c. technique
    c. test
    c. testing
    c. ultrasonography
    c. ultrasound
    c. U-rod instrumentation
    vasopneumatic intermittent c.
    venous c.
    vertebral c.
    vertical c.
    c. wire
    c. wiring

compression-plus-torque theory of cervical injury

compressive
    c. centripetal wrapping
    c. dressing
    c. flexion injury
    c. hyperextension injury
    c. neuropathy
    c. rod

compressor
    Adair screw c.
    screw c.

Comprifix
    C. active ankle support
    C. ankle splint

Compton clavicle pin

Compudriver digital torque-meter

computed tomography (CT)

computer-assisted
    c.-a. design (CAD)
    c.-a. design/computer assisted
      manufacturing prosthesis
    c.-a. design-controlled alignment
      method (CAD/CAM)

computerized
    c. axial tomography (CAT)
    c. electroencephalography (CEEG)
    c. isokinetic dynamometer
    c. musculoskeletal analysis
    c. patient record (CPR)

ComputeRow
    Universal C.

Conaxial ankle prosthesis

concave
    c. articular surface
    c. loading socket
    c. rod
    c.-surface reamer

concavity
    flexural c.
    glenoid c.

concealed straight leg raising test

concentrate
    platelet c.

concentration
    minimal bactericidal c.
    minimal inhibitory c.
    motion c.
    serum bactericidal c.
    serum urate c.

concentric
    c. contraction
    c. function
    c. lamella
    c. loading
    c. needle electrode
    c. reduction
    c. work

concept
    C. arthroscopy power system
    C. beach chair shoulder positioning
      system
    C. bipolar coagulator
    C. cannula
    Eftekhar c.
    C. hand-held cautery
    C. II rowing ergometer
    "one wound-one scar" c.
    C. Precise ACL guide system
    C. rotator cuff repair system
    C. self-compressing cannulated
      screw system
    C. Sterling arthroscopy blade
      system
    three-column c.
    C. two-pin passer

conceptual ability

Concise
    C. cementing sculp
    C. side plate

Conco elastic bandage

concomitant

concretion

concurrent force system

concussion

condensing osteitis

condition
    degenerative spine c.
    dysvascular c.
    sterile c.
    tumorous c.

conditioned stimulus (CS)

conditioner
Shuttle cardiomuscular c.
conditioning
c. stimulus
work c.
conductance
conduction
c. block
c. distance
c. time
c. velocity (CV)
c. velocity test
volume c.
conductive Hydrogel wound dressing
conductor
Bailey c.
Bozzini light c.
light c.
condylar
c. angle
c. articulation
c. femoral fracture
c. implant
c. implant arthroplasty
c. plate
c. screw fixation
condyle
bifid c.
c. block
femoral c.
flare of the c.
humeral c.
lateral femoral c.
lateral tibial c.
medial femoral c.
medial humerus c.
medial/lateral femoral c.
occipital c.
odontoid c.
tibial c.
volar c.
condylectomy
DuVries phalangeal c.
DuVries plantar c.
phalangeal c.
plantar c.
condylocephalic
Ender nail c.
c. nail
c. nailing
condylopatellar sulcus
condylotomy

cone
c. arthrodesis
c. bone biopsy
c. bur
C. checkers game
hand c.
Posey Palm C.
C. ring curette
C. splint
stacking c.
C. suction biopsy curette
coned-down view
confidence interval (CI)
configuration
activity c.
Cotrel-Dubousset hook claw c.
Dudley J. Morton foot c.
triangular base transverse bar c.
confirmatory testing
confluent
Conform dressing
confrontational test
confusion test
congenita
amyoplasia c.
amyotonia c.
arthrogryposis multiplex c.
dyskeratosis c.
fragilitas ossium c.
luxatio coxae c.
myotonia c.
paramyotonia c.
congenital
c. above-elbow amputation
c. annular band
c. anomaly
c. aphalangia
c. atlantoaxial instability
c. band syndrome
c. below-elbow amputation
c. clasped thumb
c. complete subtalar coalition
c. convex pes plano valgus
c. dislocation of hip (CDH)
c. disorder disease
c. dysplasia of hip (CDH)
c. dystrophy
c. fibrous band
c. fracture
c. general fibromatosis
c. hemivertebra
c. hip dislocation

C

NOTES

congenital *(continued)*
   c. hip dysplasia
   c. hip subluxation
   c. hyperphosphatasemic skeletal dysplasia (CHSD)
   c. hypotonia
   c. intercalary limb absence
   c. kyphosis (type I, II)
   c. laxity of ligament
   c. limb deficiency
   c. metatarsus adductus
   c. myotonia
   c. osseous
   c. posteromedial bowing
   c. predisposition
   c. radioulnar synostosis
   c. ring
   c. ring syndrome
   c. scapular elevation
   c. scoliosis
   c. spondylolisthesis
   c. talipes equinovarus
   c. terminal limb absence
   c. tibial pseudarthrosis
   c. torticollis
   c. trigger digit
   c. trigger finger
   c. ulnar drift
   c. vertical talus (CVT)
   c. vertical talus foot deformity
   c. wryneck
congestion
   flap c.
   intraosseous vascular c.
congestive heart failure
congruence
   c. angle
   patellofemoral c.
congruency
   joint c.
congruent metatarsophalangeal joint
congruity
   joint c.
congruous
conical
   c. bur
   c. obturator
   c. reamer
conjoined
   c. lateral band
   c. tendon
conjugated
   estrogens, c.
Conley pin
connecting
   c. bolt
   c. plate

connection
   Martin-Gruber c.
   Riche-Cannieu c.
connective
   c. tissue
   c. tissue disease
   c. tissue massage (CTM)
   c. tissue plasticity
connector
   adjustable pedicle c.
   Beurrier c.
   domino spinal instrumentation c.
   dual (bypass) c.
   intrinsic transverse c.
   longitudinal member to anchor c.
   longitudinal member to longitudinal member c.
   pedicle c.
   tandem c.
   transverse c.
Connolly
   C. procedure
   C. technique
conoid
   c. ligament
   c. tubercle
conoideum
   ligamentum c.
Conrad-Bugg
   C.-B. trapping
   C.-B. trapping of soft tissue in ankle fracture
Conray contrast media
consecutive dislocation
consensual light reflex
conservatism
   clinical c.
conservative
   c. management
   c. therapy
consistency
   boggy c.
   doughy c.
consolidated graft
consolidation
   delayed c.
   fracture line c.
   premature c.
constancy
   form c.
constant
   c. direct current stimulator
   c.-friction knee
   c. massive motion
   C. and Murley shoulder scoring system
   c.-touch perception

ConstaVac
    C. autoreinfusion system
    C. drainage
constellation of clinical findings
constrained
    c. ankle arthroplasty
    c. condylar knee
    c. hinged knee prosthesis
    c. nonhinged knee prosthesis
    c. shoulder arthroplasty
constriction
    c. band syndrome
    hourglass c.
    c. ring
construct
    anterior c.
    AO dynamic compression plate c.
    compression instrumentation
      posterior c.
    disease c.
    double-rod c.
    Edwards modular system bridging
      sleeve c.
    Edwards modular system
      compression c.
    Edwards modular system
      distraction-lordosis c.
    Edwards modular system
      kyphoreduction c.
    Edwards modular system
      neutralization c.
    Edwards modular system rod
      sleeve c.
    Edwards modular system
      scoliosis c.
    Edwards modular system
      spondylo c.
    Edwards modular system standard
      sleeve c.
    hook-to-screw L4-S1 compression c.
    iliosacral and iliac fixation c.
    pedicle screw c.
    c. pedicle screw-laminar claw c.
    posterior c.
    rod-hook c.
    screw-to-screw compression c.
    segmental compression c.
    single-rod c.
    spondylo c.
    triplane c.
    TSRH double-rod c.
    upper cervical spine anterior c.

    upper cervical spine posterior c.
    Wiltse system double-rod c.
    Wiltse system H c.
    Wiltse system single-rod c.
Constructa-Foam
constructional ability
contact
    C. ArthroProbe
    c. force
    c. healing
    c. laser delivery system
    c. manipulation
    manual c.
    c. point
    c. shield
    C. SPH cups system
    standing knee bend PSIS-sacrum c.
container
    Quickbox c.
content
    bone mineral c. (BMC)
    carotid c.
    hydrolyze disc c.
context
    performance c.
contiguous
    c. articular surface
    c. vertebral structure
continuity
continuous
    c. anatomical passive exerciser
      (CAPE)
    c. cryotherapy
    c. intravenous regional anesthesia
      (CIVRA)
    c. passive motion (CPM)
    c. passive motion machine
    c. wave arthroscopy pump
Continuum
    C. knee system (CKS)
    C. knee system implant (CKS
      implant)
contour
    C. DF-80 total hip operation
    double hump c.
    C. internal prosthesis
    patellar c.
    polyethylene proximal brims in
      quadrilateral c.
    spinal c.
    Wiberg type II patellar c.

C

NOTES

contoured
    c. adduction trochanteric-controlled alignment method (CAT-CAM)
    c. anterior spinal plate (CASP)
    c. anterior spinal plate drill guide
    c. anterior spinal plate technique
    c. felt padding
    c. femoral stem (CFS, CSF)
    c. T-plate plate
    c. washer
contouring
contract
    Contract Relax Agonist C. (CRAC)
    c.-relax technique
contractility
    muscle c.
contraction
    active c.
    concentric c.
    direct c.
    eccentric c.
    extrafusal fiber c.
    c. fasciculation
    isometric c.
    isotonic c.
    lengthening c.
    maintained c.
    maximal voluntary c. (MVC)
    muscular c.
    reflex muscular c.
    repeated quick stretch superimposed upon an existing c. (RQS-SEC)
    shortening c.
    tetanic c.
    c. tremor
    c. type
    volitional c.
contractor
    Bailey-Gibbon rib c.
    Bailey rib c.
    Lemmon rib c.
    rib c.
    Sellors rib c.
contracture
    abduction c.
    acute ischemic c.
    adduction c.
    axillary c.
    burn c.
    clawfoot c.
    digital c.
    Dupuytren c.
    equinus c.
    established c.
    c. exercise
    extension c.
    external rotation c.
    fixed flexion c. (FFC)

    flexion c.
    flexion, abduction, external rotation c.
    forearm c.
    gastroc-soleus c.
    hip flexor c.
    intrinsic c.
    ischemic c.
    lumbrical intrinsic c.
    muscle c.
    opposition c.
    paralytic c.
    pelvic flexion c. (PFC)
    postpoliomyelitic c.
    pronation c.
    quadriceps c.
    rectus femoris c.
    retropatellar fat pad c.
    rotational c.
    Skoog procedure for release of Dupuytren c.
    soft tissue c.
    spastic intrinsic c.
    supination c.
    valgus c.
    varus c.
    Volkmann ischemic c.
    web c.
contraflexion brace
contraindication
contralateral
    c. hypoplastic/agenetic pedicle
    c. pain
    c. sign
    c. spondylolysis
    c. straight leg raising
    c. straight leg raising test
contrast
    c. agent
    air c.
    c. arthrography
    c. bath (CB)
    c. column
    c. media
    c. medium-enhanced magnetic resonance imaging (CME-MRI)
contrecoup
    fracture by c.
    c. fracture
    c. injury
control
    3D positional c.
    Dupaco knee c.
    exsanguination tourniquet c.
    habitual c.
    hip joint aspiration under fluoroscopic c.
    image c.

maximum c. (MC)
monitored anesthesia c.
motion c.
postural c.
pronation c.
PSC pronation/spring c.
swing-phase c.
tourniquet c.
trunk c.
verticality c.
voluntary c. (VC)
controlled
c. ankle motion (CAM)
c. ankle walker
c. comminuted fracture
c.-motion brace
c. rotational osteotomy
controller
shoulder c.
C. Shoulder Orthosis
contusion
hip c.
pulmonary c.
rib c.
conus medullaris syndrome
ConvaDERM Plus dressing
Conve back support
conventional
c. osteosarcoma
c. silicone elastomer (CSE)
c. technique
c. tomography
Conventry proximal tibial osteotomy
convergence
angle of c.
c. facilitation
c. projection
Converse
C. chisel
C. periosteal elevator
C. splint
conversion
Tilt-In-Space wheelchair c.
Convery polyarticular disability index
convex
c. condylar-implant arthroplasty
c. fusion
c. pes valgus
c. rod
convexity
distal ulnar c.
left lumbar c.

c. of the spine
ulnar c.
convulsion
Conyers technique
Cook-Gordon mechanism
cookie
arch c.
c. cutter
Gelfoam c.
met c.
metatarsal c.
navicular shoe c.
scaphoid shoe c.
shoe c.
Cook walking brace
cool
c. pack
c. pack cryotherapy
Cool-Aid continuous controlled cold
therapy
coolant
Cooley
C. graft clamp
C. iliac clamp
C. multipurpose angled clamp
C. multipurpose curved clamp
C. rib retractor
C. rib shears
Cooley-Baumgarten wire twister
cooling machine
CoolSorb absorbent cold transfer
dressing
Coombs bone biopsy system
Coonrad
C. hinged prosthesis
C. semiconstrained elbow prosthesis
C. total elbow arthroplasty
Coonrad-Morrey
C.-M. elbow prosthesis
C.-M. total elbow arthroplasty
Coonse-Adams
C.-A. knee approach
C.-A. quadricepsplasty
C.-A. technique
Coopercare Lastrap support wrap
Coopernail sign
Cooper reduction
Coopervision irrigation/aspiration
handpiece
Coordinate
C. complete revision knee system
coordinated mobility

NOTES

coordinate system (X,Y,Z)
coordination
    muscular c.
Copeland-Howard
    C.-H. scapulothoracic fusion
    C.-H. shoulder operation
Copeland-Kavat
    C.-K. classification of
      metatarsophalangeal dislocation
    C.-K. metatarsophalangeal
      dislocation classification
copolymer
    c. ankle-foot orthosis
    c. orthotic material
copper
    c. deficiency syndrome
    c. wire effect
copropraxia
coracoacromial
    c. arch
    c. ligament
    c. ligament transfer
    c. process
coracoacromiale
    ligamentum c.
coracobrachialis
    biceps, brachialis, c. (BBC)
coracoclavicular (CC)
    c. arthrodesis
    c. articulation
    c. distance
    c. fixation apparatus
    c. joint
    c. ligament
    c. screw fixation
    c. suture fixation
    c. technique
coracoclaviculare
    ligamentum c.
coracohumeral (CH)
    c. ligament
coracohumerale
    ligamentum c.
coracoid
    c. fracture
    c. impingement syndrome
    c. notch
    c. process
    c. tip avulsion
Coraderm dressing
Corail
    C. HA-coated stem
    C. HA-coated stem hip implant
    C. hip system
coralline
    c. hydroxyapatite
    c. hydroxyapatite Goniopora
      (CHAG)

Corb bone biopsy instrument
Corbett bone rongeur
cord
    central c.
    cervical spinal c.
    c. compression
    digital c.
    heel c.
    lateral c.
    natatory c.
    c. portion
    pretendinous c.
    retrovascular c.
    space available for the c. (SAC)
    spinal c.
    spiral c.
    Sport C.
    tenodesis of the heel c.
    tethered spinal c.
    c.-traction syndrome
    vocal c.
Cordis implantable drug reservoir
  device
cordlike structure
Cordon-Colles fracture splint
cordotomy
core
    c. biopsy obturator
    c. decompression
    c. decompression of femoral head
    c. drilling procedure
    C. Hibak Rest
    C. Lobak Rest
    C. Max-Relax Cushion
    C. Sitback Rest
    C. Slimrest
    c. suture
Corfit System 7000 Series Lumbosacral
  Support
coring
    c. apparatus
    c. device
cork
    c. borer
    sheet c.
corkscrew femoral head extractor
corn
    apical c.
    end c.
    hard c.
    interdigital c.
    Lister c.
    neurovascular c.
    plantar c.
    soft c.
    web c.
Cornelia de Lange syndrome

corner
> c. fracture
> 4-c. midcarpal fusion
> posteromedial c.

corneum
> stratum c.

cornuate navicular

cornu cutaneum

coronal
> c. computed tomographic arthrography (CCTA)
> c. incision
> c. plane
> c. plane correction
> c. plane deformity
> c. plane deformity sagittal translation
> c. scalp incision
> c. split fracture
> c. tilting

coronary
> c. angiography
> c. artery disease
> c. ligament

coronoid
> c. line
> c. process
> c. process fracture

corpectomy
> anterior c.
> cervical c.
> c. model
> vertebral body c.

Corporation
> Accurate Surgical and Scientific Instruments C. (ASSI)

corporectomy amputation

corporotransverse
> c. inferior ligament
> c. superior ligament

cor pulmonale

corpuscle
> pacinian c.
> Vater-Pacini c.

correction
> anterior c.
> Beckenbaugh c.
> Bonferroni c.
> chevron hallux valgus c.
> coronal plane c.
> cubitus varus c.
> hallux varus c.

Johnson-Spiegl hallux varus c.
Kilsyn-Evans principle of frontal plane c.
King type IV curve posterior c.
kyphosis c.
mechanism of c.
neuromechanical c.
oligosegmental c.
phalangeal malunion c.
rotational c.
Ruiz-Mora c.
scoliosis c.
somatovisceral c.
Steel c.

corrective
> c. cast
> c. lengthening osteotomy
> c. orthosis
> c. spinal care

corrodens
> *Eikenella c.*

corrosion
> crevice c.
> fretting c.
> metal implant c.

corrugated reamer

corset
> Camp c.
> elastic ankle c.
> Hoke lumbar c.
> Kampe c.
> leather ankle c.
> lumbosacral c.
> soft c.
> c. suspension
> thigh c.

Cort
> S-T C.

Cortef

cortex, pl. **cortices**
> adrenal c.
> articular c.
> femoral c.
> lateral c.
> c. screw
> vertebral body anterior c.

cortical
> c. atrophy
> c. bone graft
> c. bone modeling
> c. bone primary canal
> c. bone remodeling

C

NOTES

cortical *(continued)*
    c. cancellous screw
    c. debridement
    c. defect
    c. desmoid
    c. desmoid tumor
    c. destruction
    c. fibrous dysplasia
    c. fracture
    c. fragment
    c. index
    c. lucency
    c. perforation
    c. pin
    c. plate
    c. step drill
    c. strut graft
    c. thickening
    c. versus cancellous bone
    c. window
    c. windowing
corticocancellous
    c. bone
    c. bone graft
    c. chip graft
corticosteroid
    depot c.
    c.-induced avascular necrosis
    c. injection
    postoperative c.
    c. therapy (CS)
corticotomy
    DeBastiani c.
    Ilizarov c.
    percutaneous c.
    c. of proximal tibia
corticotropin
cortisone
    c. acetate
    c. injection
Cortisporin
    C. Topical Cream
    C. Topical Ointment
Cortone Acetate
corundum ceramic implant material
Coryllos-Doyen periosteal elevator
Coryllos rasp
Corynebacterium
Cosmeceuticals
    Dead Sea C. (DSC)
Cosmegen
cosmesis
    foot c.
    poor c.
Cosmolon closure for splint
costal
    c. angle
    c. cartilage

    c. notch
    c. periosteotome
costectomy
Costen syndrome
costochondral
    c. joint
    c. junction of ribs
costochondritis
costoclavicular
    c. ligament
    c. maneuver
    c. space
    c. syndrome
    c. syndrome test
costoclaviculare
    ligamentum c.
costolumbar angle
costophrenic angle
costosternal angle
costotransversarium
    ligamentum c.
costotransverse
    c. joint
    c. ligament
costotransversectomy
    c. approach
    Seddon dorsal spine c.
    c. technique
costovertebral
    c. angle (CVA)
    c. angle tenderness
    c. articulation
    c. joint
cot
    finger c.
Coton test
Cotrel
    C. pedicle screw
    C. pedicle screw fixation strength
    C. pedicle screw rigidity
    C. scoliosis
    C. scoliosis cast
    C. traction
Cotrel-Dubousset
    C.-D. derotation operation
    C.-D. dynamic transverse traction device
    C.-D. hook claw configuration
    C.-D. hook-rod
    C.-D. pedicle screw instrumentation
    C.-D. pedicular instrumentation
    C.-D. rod
    C.-D. rod flexibility
    C.-D. spinal instrument
Cottle
    C. chisel
    C. mallet
    C. osteotome

C. rasp
C. saw
Cottle-MacKenty
    C.-M. elevator
    C.-M. rasp
cotton
    C. ankle fracture
    c. bolster
    c. cast padding
    c. dressing
    c. elastic bandage
    C. reduction of elbow dislocation
    c. roll
    c. sheet wadding
    c. suture
Cotton-Berg syndrome
cottonloader
    c. position
    c. position cast
cottonoid patty
Cottony
    C. Dacron
    C. Dacron suture
cotyloid
    c. cavity
    c. notch
cotyloplasty technique
Couch-Derosa-Throop transfer
couche spongoide
cough
    c. fracture
    c. test
Coulter counter
Coumadin
Council
    Medical Research C. (MRC)
count
    instrument, sponge, and needle c.
    lymphocyte c.
    platelet c.
    potassium-40 c.
    white blood cell c.
counter
    Coulter c.
    extended medial shoe c.
    Geiger c.
    heel c.
    c. nutation
    c. rotating saw
    C. Rotation System (CRS)
    c. sink
counterbalance

counterbore
    cloverleaf c.
counterclockwise
counterrotational splint
countersinking osteotomy
countersink screw head
countersunk
countertraction splint
Count'R-Force arch brace
coupled
    c. discharge
    c. motion
coupler
    Ferrier c.
Couvelaire incision
Coventry
    C. distal femoral osteotomy
    C. screw
    C. staple
    C. vagal osteotomy
    C. vagus osteotomy
cover
    Accu-Flo polyethylene bur hole c.
    Accu-Flo silicone rubber bur
      hold c.
    AliTane cushion c.
    AliTex cushion c.
    AquaShield orthopaedic cast c.
    AquaShield reusable cast c.
    cast c.
    Dryspell cast c.
    ShowerSafe waterproof cast and
      bandage c.
    SofStep wheelchair footplate c.
    Springlite polyolefin BK c.
    Springlite polyurethane AK, BK
      conical c.
coverage
    skin c.
covering
    Cast Cozy toe c.
    epineural c.
    fascial sheath c.
Coverlet
    C. adhesive
    C. adhesive surgical dressing
    C. Strips wound dressing
Cover-Roll
    C.-R. adhesive gauze dressing
    C.-R. gauze
Covertell composite secondary dressing
Cowden disease

C

NOTES

Cowen-Loftus toe-phalanx
  transplantation
cowhorn brace
Co-Wrap dressing
coxa
    c. adducta
    c. brevis
    c. magna
    c. plana
    c. saltans
    c. senilis
    c. valga
    c. vara
    c. vara deformity pelvic
      radiotherapy
    c. vara luxans
coxarthria
coxarthritis
coxarthropathy
coxarthrosis
Cox flexion-distraction technique
coxitis
coxofemoral
    c. articulation
    c. joint
Cozen-Brockway
    C.-B. technique
    C.-B. Z-plasty
Cozen test
CP
    cerebral palsy
    certified prosthetist
      CP Sports Balance Classification
CP2 inflatable cold pack
CPed
    certified pedorthist
CPM
    continuous passive motion
      AIM CPM
      CPM apparatus
      CPM device
      CPM machine
CPO
    certified prosthetist/orthotist
CPPD
    calcium pyrophosphate dihydrate
      deposition
CPR
    computerized patient record
cps, c/sec
    cycles per second
CPT
    collarless polished taper
      CPT hip system
CR
    closed reduction
CRA
    Chiropractic Rehabilitation Association

crab gait
crabmeat-like appearance
CRAC
    Contract Relax Agonist Contract
Cracchiolo
    C. forefoot arthroplasty
    C. procedure
Cracchiolo-Sculco
    C.-S. implant arthroplasty
    C.-S. implant operation
crack fracture
cracking
    c. of joint
    stress-corrosion c.
cradle
    c. arm sling
    bed c.
    Posey bed c.
Crafoord thoracic scissors
Craig
    C. abduction splint
    C. pin
    C. pin remover
    C. vertebral biopsy set
Craig-Scott orthosis
Cramer wire splint
cramp
    c. discharge
    muscular c.
Cram test
Crane
    C. mallet
    C. osteotome
    C. shoulder exercise
cranial
    c. bone graft
    c. electrical stimulation (CES)
    c. Jacobs hook
    c. nerve abnormality
    c. nerves II-XII intact
    c.-sacral respiratory mechanism
      (CRSM)
    c. tongs
craniocaudal glide
craniocervical plate
craniofacial
    c. angle
    c. dysjunction fracture
craniomandibular dysfunction
craniosacral
    c. therapy (CST)
    c. therapy technique
craniospinal trauma
craniotabes
craniovertebral
crank
    c. frame retractor

c. table
c. test
cravat bandage
Crawford
C. head frame
C. incision
C. low lithotomy crutch
C. small parts dexterity test
Crawford-Adams
C.-A. acetabular cup
C.-A. acetabular cup arthroplasty
Crawford-Marxen-Osterfeld technique
crawl
barrel c.
C-reactive protein
creaking
alar c.
back c.
distal medial c.
flexion c.
infragluteal c.
metatarsal-phalangeal c.
palmar c.
PIP flexion c.
popliteal flexion c.
skin c.
thenar c.
ulnar c.
wrist c.
cream (*See also* creme)
AliDeep massage c.
capsaicoid topical c.
Cortisporin Topical C.
Diapedic foot c.
DSC Foot C.
Free-Up massage c.
Lamisil C.
Lotrimin AF C.
Maximum Strength Desenex
  Antifungal C.
Neosporin C.
Noritate C.
Oxistat c.
terbinafine hydrochloride c.
Thera-Gesic c.
Ureacin-20 c.
Vita ADE c.
crease
alar c.
back c.
distal palmar c. (DPC)

flexor skin c.
infragluteal c.
metatarsal phalangeal c.
palmar c.
popliteal c.
skin c.
thenar palmar c. (TPC)
creatine:height index
creatine phosphokinase
creation
kyphosis c.
lordosis c.
Credo razor
creep
viscoelastic c.
web space c.
creeping substitution
Crego
C. elevator
C. femoral osteotomy
C. hip reduction
C. retractor
C. tendon transfer technique
Crego-McCarroll
C.-M. pin
C.-M. traction
cremasteric reflex
creme (*See also* cream)
Aloe Grande c.
Fungoid C.
Hydrisinol c.
Lactinol-E c.
Ureacin-20 c.
crepitans
peritendinitis c.
crepitation
patellofemoral c.
crepitus
crescent
C. memory pillow
c. pillow
c. sign
crescentic
c. base wedge osteotomy
c. base wedge
  osteotomy/bunionectomy
c. calcaneal osteotomy
c. rupture
c. saw
c. shelf osteotomy (CSO)
Crescent-Pillo pillow

C

NOTES

crescent-shaped
> c.-s. fibrocartilaginous disk
> c.-s. osteotomy

CREST
> calcinosis, Raynaud, esophageal,
>   sclerodactyly, telangiectasia
> CREST syndrome

crest
> iliac c.
> neural c.
> palpation of iliac c.
> c. sign
> c. sign side

cretinism

crevice corrosion

cricoid ring

cricopharyngeal sphincter muscle

cricothyroid membrane

Crile
> C. head traction
> C. hemostat

Crile-Wood needle holder

crimped Dacron prosthesis

crimper
> Caparosa wire c.
> pin c.
> Simmons c.
> washer c.
> wire c.

crisis, pl. crises
> bone c.

crista

criteria
> Catagni c.
> Harris c.
> Hodgkinson acetabular component
>   loosening c.
> Insall c.
> Mackinnon-Dellon c.
> New York diagnostic c.
> Rome c.
> Severin hip c.

Criticaid lotion

critical
> c. limb ischemia (CLI)
> c. load

CRM
> CRM cup
> CRM rehab brace
> CRM stem
> CRM system

CROM
> cervical range-of-motion instrument

Crosby reduction

cross
> c.-arm flap
> c. bar
> c.-finger flap

> c. friction
> c.-legged gait
> c. leg pain
> c.-linking
> c.-screw fixation
> c.-slot screwdriver
> c.-union

cross-bracing
> spinal rod c.-b.
> Wiltse system c.-b.

crosscut
> c. bur
> c. saw

crossed
> c. extensor reflex
> c. intrinsic transfer
> c. straight leg raising

crossed-leg straight leg raising

crosshead displacement

crossing
> nerve c.

cross-leg
> c.-l. flap
> c.-l. gait

crosslink
> Edwards modular system rod c.
> Galveston fixation with TSRH c.
> c. plate
> c. plate size
> TSRH c.

crossover
> c. second toe
> c. test

crossover-toe deformity

cross-table
> c.-t. lateral radiograph
> c.-t. view

crotch strap

crouch gait

Crouzon syndrome

CROW
> Charcot restraint orthotic walker

Crowe
> C. congenital hip dysplasia
>   classification
> C. congenital hip dysplasia
>   classification system
> C. congenital hip dysplasia (type
>   I–IV)
> C. pilot point
> C. pilot point on Steinmann pin
> C. subluxation
> C. tip pin

crown
> Adaptic c.
> c. and collar scissors
> c. drill

c. drill screw
Unitek steel c.
CRS
Counter Rotation System
CRS brace
CRS Tibial Torsion System
CRSM
cranial-sacral respiratory mechanism
cruciate
anterior c.
c. condylar knee system
c. fashion
c. head bone screw
c. ligament
c. ligament reconstruction
c. ligament rupture
c. ligaments of knee
c. paralysis
posterior c.
c. punch
c.-retaining prosthesis
c.-sacrificing prosthesis
cruciform
c. anterior spinal hyperextension
(CASH)
c. anterior spinal hyperextension
orthosis
c. head bone screw
c. ligament of atlas
c. screwdriver
c. tibial base plate
cruiser buggy
crural fascia
cruris
ligamentum cruciatum c.
ligamentum transversum c.
crush
c. fracture
c. injury
"crushed eggshell" fracture
crushing osteochondritis
crutch
c. ambulation
axillary c.
c. and belt femoral closed nail
c. and belt femoral closed nailing
Canadian c.
Crawford low lithotomy c.
EuroCuff forearm c.
Hardy aluminum c.
Lofstrand c.

c. walking
weightbearing c.
Crutchfield
C. bone drill
C. drill point
C. hand drill
C. pin
C. skeletal tong traction
Crutchfield-Raney
C.-R. drill
C.-R. tongs
cryoanalgesia
Cryo/Cuff
C. ankle dressing
C. boot
C. Knee Compression Dressing
System
Cryocup ice massager
cryoepiphysiodesis
percutaneous c.
cryohypophysectomy
cryoprecipitate
cryopreserved cartilage
cryosurgery
cryotherapy
continuous c.
cool pack c.
liquid nitrogen c.
verruca c.
cryptococcal infection
cryptococcosis
Cryptococcus neoformans
cryptotic
c. medial border
crystal
monosodium urate c.
C. polymer gel
c.-related arthropathy
uric acid c.
crystal-induced
c.-i. arthritis
c.-i. arthrosis
c.-i. synovitis
crystalloid
c. solution
CS
conditioned stimulus
corticosteroid therapy
CSC3 cervical support cushion
CSE
conventional silicone elastomer

C

NOTES

c/sec (*var. of* cps)
    cycles per second
CSF
    cerebrospinal fluid
    contoured femoral stem
        CSF prosthesis
C-shaped
        C.-s. foot
        C.-s. plate
CSI
    Caregiver Strain Index
CSO
    crescentic shelf osteotomy
C-spine
    cervical spine
CSR
    complete subtalar release
        McKay-Simons CSR
CST
    craniosacral therapy
CT
    computed tomography
        CT scan
CT1 suture
CTD
    cumulative trauma disorder
CTEV brace
CTI brace
CTLSO
    cervicothoracolumbosacral orthosis
        CTLSO orthosis
CTM
    cervical tension myositis
    connective tissue massage
CTR
    carpal tunnel release
CTS
    carpal tunnel syndrome
    Champion Trauma Score
        CTS gauge
        CTS Gripfit splint
Cubbins
        C. arthroplasty
        C. bone screwdriver
        C. incision
        C. open reduction
        C. screw
        C. shoulder approach
        C. shoulder dislocation technique
cube
    Temper Foam c.
cubital
        c. bursitis
        c. tunnel
        c. tunnel splint
        c. tunnel syndrome
cubiti (*pl. of* cubitus)
cubitocarpal

cubitoradial
cubitus, pl. cubiti
    patella cubiti
    c. pseudovarus
    c. recurvatum
    c. varus
    c. varus correction
cuboid
    c. bone
    c. fracture
    c. syndrome
cubonavicular joint
cucullaris muscle
cucumber heel
cuff
    Aircast Cryo C.
    arm c.
    collar and c.
    Cryo/C.
    c. of fascia
    hand c.
    joint distraction c.
    leather c.
    C. Link orthopaedic device
    musculotendinous c.
    pneumatic tourniquet c.
    push c.
    Push-Ease Quad C.
    c. resection
    rotator c. (RC)
    shoulder c.
    Steri-Cuff disposable tourniquet c.
    c. suspension
    c.-tear arthropathy
    c.-tear arthroplasty
    thigh c.
CUI
    CUI dorsal implant
    CUI malar implant
    CUI tendon prosthesis
cuing strategy
cul-de-sac of Bruger
Culler hook
Culley ulnar splint
culture
    bacterial c.
    blood c.
    urine c.
    wound c.
cumulative trauma disorder (CTD)
cuneatus
    fasciculus c.
cuneiform
    c. bone
    c.-first metatarsal exostosis
    c. fracture
    c. injury
    c. joint

c. joint arthrodesis
c. mortise
c. osteotomy

Cuniard and Campell technique
cuniculatum
epithelioma c.
Cunningham brace
cup
AccuPressure heel c.
acetabular c.
c.-and-ball osteotomy
Anti-Shox heel c.
c. arthroplasty
Arthropor acetabular c.
Aufranc modification of Smith-
Petersen c.
Aufranc-Turner acetabular c.
Aufranc-Turner hip c.
Bauerfeind SofSpot Heel C.
Bicon-Plus C.
Biomet acetabular c.
bipolar acetabular c.
bipolar prosthetic c.
Buchholz acetabular c.
c.-cement interface
ceramic acetabular c.
Charnley acetabular c.
Charnley offset-bore c.
c. and cone method
Crawford-Adams acetabular c.
CRM c.
custom-made acetabular c.
DePuy bipolar c.
Flo-Trol drinking c.
Gemini c.
Hallister heel c.
Harris-Galante acetabular c.
heel c.
c. holder
c. holder handle
Integrity acetabular c.
Interseal acetabular c.
Kennedy spillproof c.
Laing concentric hip c.
Lord c.
low-profile c.
Luck hip c.
McKee-Farrar acetabular c.
metal-backed acetabular c.
migration of acetabular c.
Mueller c.
NEB acetabular c.

oblong polyethylene acetabular c.
c.-on-cup arthroplasty of the hip
Opti-Fix II acetabular c.
Osteonics acetabular c.
plastic heel c.
Polysorb heel c.
c. positioner
Press-Fit c.
prosthesis c.
c. reamer
Reflection I, V, and FSO
acetabular c.
Restoration GAP acetabular c.
retroversion of acetabular c.
Riecken PQ premium heel c.
screw-in ceramic acetabular c.
Silipos silicone wonder c.
Smith-Petersen c.
Sorbuthane II heel c.
S-ROM Super C.
trial acetabular c.
Tuli gel-heel c.
Tuli heel c.
Wonder-Cup heel c.
Wonder-Spur heel c.
Wonderzorb heel c.
ZTT acetabular c.
ZTT I, II c.
cupid's bow
cupped
c. curette
c. grasping forceps
Cuprimine
Curdy blade
curettage
curette, curet
Acufex c.
angled Scoville c.
bone c.
bowl c.
box c.
Brun bone c.
Buck bone c.
Charnley bone c.
Cloward-Cone c.
Cobb c.
Cone ring c.
Cone suction biopsy c.
cupped c.
curved c.
Daubenspeck bone c.
Dawson-Yuhl-Cone c.

NOTES

curette *(continued)*

Epstein c.
Faulkner c.
fine c.
fine-angled c.
Gillquist suction c.
Halle bone c.
Hardy hypophysial c.
Hatfield bone c.
hex handle c.
Hibbs c.
hypophysial c.
Innomed bone c.
Jansen bone c.
Kerpel bone c.
Kerrison c.
Kevorkian c.
Lempert bone c.
long c.
Magnum c.
Malis c.
Martini bone c.
mastoid c.
McCain TMJ c.
McElroy c.
meniscal c.
Meyhoeffer bone c.
Microsect c.
Moe bone c.
orthopaedic c.
oval curved-cup c.
Piffard c.
Schede bone c.
Scoville c.
short c.
Spratt bone c.
Spratt mastoid c.
stout-neck c.
straight c.
T-handle c.
Volkmann bone c.
Walker ruptured disk c.
Whitney single-use plastic c.
Williger bone c.

curiosity reaction

curl

dynamic trunk c.
neutral wrist c.
reverse wrist c.
seated hamstring c.
trunk c.
wrist c.

curl-up

broomstick c.-u.

curly

c. toe
c. toe deformity

current

action c.
amplitude-summation interferential c.
cutting c.
direct c. (DC)
interferential c.
low-frequency alternating c. (LFAC)

Currey model

Curry

C. hip nail
C. walking splint

Curschmann-Steinert disease

Curtin

C. incision
C. plantar fibromatosis excision

Curtis

C. PIP joint capsulotomy
C. technique

Curtis-Fisher knee technique

curvature

dorsal kyphotic c.
humpbacked spinal c.
Pott spinal c.
radius of c.

curve

accommodation c.
Blix contractile force c.
calibration c.
cervicothoracic c.
combined c.
compensatory c.
displacement c.
double major spinal c.
double thoracic c.
flattening of normal lordotic c.
fractional c.
full c.
Hadley S-c.
King type thoracic and lumbar c.
  (type I–IV)
kyphotic c.
length-tension c.
load-deflection c.
load-deformation c.
load-displacement c.
lordotic c.
low single thoracic c.
lumbar lordotic c.
major c.
c. measurement
minor c.
nonstructural c.
normal lordotic c.
c. pattern
primary c.
c. progression
c. progression in scoliosis
right thoracic c.

off

C

rigid c.
scoliotic c.
severe rigid thoracic c.
specific c.
strain-stress c.
strength c.
strength-duration c.
stress-strain c.
structural c.
thoracic c.
thoracolumbar c.
torque c.

curved
c. approach
c. awl
c. basket forceps
c. bone rongeur
c. curette
c. gouge
c. incision
c. Küntscher nail system
c. Mayo scissors
c. meniscotome
c. meniscotome blade
c. osteotome
c. osteotomy
c. passer
c. periosteal elevator
c. retractor

curvilinear
c. chin implant
c. incision

CurvTek TSR bone drill

Cushing
C. bur
C. flat drill
C. perforator drill
C. retractor
C. rongeur
C. saw guide
C. syndrome

Cushing-Gigli saw guide

Cushing-Hopkins periosteal elevator

cushion
abduction c.
alarm c.
AliEdge edge rest c.
amputee c.
Anti-Shox foot c.
arch c.
Back Bull lumbar support c.
Back-Huggar lumbar support c.

breakaway lap c.
Butterfly c.
Carter immobilization c.
cast c.
cell c.
Checkerboard wheelchair c.
Comfort Take-Along wheelchair c.
Core Max-Relax C.
CSC3 cervical support c.
Disc-O-Sit Jr. c.
Dry Flotation wheelchair c.
Easebak lumbar support c.
Easy Up c.
enhancer c.
FB cast c.
FloFit c.
gel c.
Gel-Foam Ultra-Wedge c.
Geo-Matt contour c.
C. Grip Flatware
Healthier seating c.
heel c.
c. heel
Hudson Hydrofloat C.
hydro c.
hydrofloat c.
invalid c.
Isch-Dish Plus c.
J2 c.
Jay basic c.
Jay combi c.
Jay Rave c.
Jay Triad c.
Jay Xtreme c.
LapTop c.
latex c.
MaxiFloat wheelchair c.
Pediplast c.
PERI-COMFORT c.
pommel c.
Posture Curve lumbar c.
Posture Wedge seat c.
pressure-relief c.
Prop'r Toes hammer toe c.
Quadtro c.
ring c.
ROHO Pack-It c.
saddle c.
Sat-A-Lite contoured wedge seat c.
Shockmaster heel c.
c. shoe liner
Sit-Straight wheelchair c.

NOTES

143

cushion *(continued)*
    Skil-Care c.
    Sorbothane heel c.
    Temper Foam c.
    T-Foam c.
    T-Gel c.
    trilaminate c.
    Viscoheel K heel c.
    Viscoheel N c.
    Viscoheel SofSpot viscoelastic
      heel c.
    Viscolas heel c.
    Y B Sore c.
cushioned shoe insert
cushion-throat wire cutter
Custodis implant
custom
    c. implant
    c.-made acetabular cup
    c. prosthesis
    c. rasp
    c.-threaded prosthesis
cut
    chamfer c.
    freehand c.
    horizontal gantry c.
    notch c.
cutaneous
    c. axon reflex
    c. distribution
    c. flap
    c. graft
    c. horn
    c. mycosis
    c. nerve
cutaneum
    cornu c.
cuticle
Cutinova
    C. cavity dressing
    C. foam dressing
    C. thin dressing
cutout
    c. patellar brace
    c. table
cut-out shoe
cutter
    A-P c.
    bolt c.
    bone plug c.
    Breck pin c.
    cast c.
    C. cast
    Cloward dowel c.
    cookie c.
    cushion-throat wire c.
    diamond pin c.

    double-action c.
    end c.
    Hefty-bite pin c.
    Horsley bone c.
    Howmedica Microfixation Sytem
      plate c.
    C. implant
    Jarit pin c.
    Kalish Duredge wire c.
    Kirschner wire c.
    Kleinert-Kutz bone c.
    Leibinger Micro System plate c.
    Luhr Microfixation System plate c.
    Martin diamond wire c.
    Midas Rex AM1 bone c.
    milling c.
    motorized meniscal c.
    M-Pact cast c.
    multiaction pin c.
    multiple action c.
    pin c.
    plug c.
    Redi-Vac cast c.
    rib c.
    Rochester harvest bone c.
    Rochester recipient bone c.
    Roos rib c.
    side c.
    side-cut pin c.
    Sklar pin c.
    Spartan jaw wire c.
    Storz Microsystems plate c.
    Synthes Microsystem plate c.
    T-C pin c.
    toothed c.
    wire c.
    Wister wire/pin c.
cutting
    c. block
    c. bur
    c. current
    c. current knife
    c. forceps
    c. jig
    c. jig for chevron osteotomy
    c. needle
    c. shaver
CV
    coefficient of variation
    conduction velocity
CVA
    cerebrovascular accident
    costovertebral angle
    CVA Sling
CVT
    congenital vertical talus
C-wire inserter

cyanoacrylate
    c. adhesive
    c. glue
cyanosis
Cybex
    C. back rehabilitation equipment
    C. cycle ergometer
    C. device
    C. I, II+ exercise system
    C. II, II+ isokinetic exerciser
    C. II isokinetic dynamometer
    C. 340 isokinetic rehabilitation and
    testing system
    C. machine
    C. test
    C. tester
    C. testing
    C. Torso Rotation Testing and
    Rehabilitation Unit
    C. training system
    C. Trunk Extension Flexion unit
cycle
    Colorado C.
    Ergociser exercise c.
    c. ergometer
    Exer-Pedic c.
    gait c.
    Power Trainer c.
    recumbent c.
    Saratoga c.
    c. time
cycleciser
cycles per second (cps, c/sec)
cyclic loading
cyclobenzaprine HCl
cyclooxygenase product
cyclophosphamide
cyclops
    C. formation
    c. lesion
cyclosporin A
cyclosporine
cyclothymia
cyclothymic disorder
cylinder
    air c.
    Arthrotek calibrated c.
    Feldenkrais c.
    c. walking cast
cylindrical
    c. osteotomy
    c. sleeve

cyma line
cyproheptadine
Cyriax
    C. evaluation
    C. technique
cyst
    c. ablation
    acetabular c.
    acromioclavicular c.
    aneurysmal bone c. (ABC)
    Baker c.
    bursal c.
    colloid c.
    epidermal inclusion c.
    epidermoid c.
    expansile c.
    ganglion c.
    giant synovial c.
    inclusion c.
    c. index
    juxtaarticular bone c.
    lateral meniscal c.
    lipid inclusion c.
    meniscal c.
    mucous c.
    pilar c.
    pilonidal c.
    popliteal giant synovial c.
    postfracture c.
    rheumatoid c.
    sacral c.
    sebaceous c.
    subarticular c.
    subchondral bone c.
    synovial c.
    trichilemmal c.
    unicameral bone c.
cystic
    c. bone lesion
    c. defect
    c. disease
    c. hygroma
    c. tumor
cystica
    osteitis fibrosa c.
cystogram
cystography
cystometrogram
cytoarchitectonic abnormality
cytokine
cytotoxic drug

NOTES

Cytoxan · Cytoxan

Cytoxan
    C. Injection

C. Oral

3D
three-dimensional
3D fracture walker brace
3D plate
3D positional adjustability
3D positional control
D/3
distal third
DACO brace
Dacron
D. batting
Cottony D.
D. graft
D.-impregnated silicone rod
D. stent
D. suture
dactinomycin
dactylitis
blistering distal d. (BDD)
tuberculous d.
dactyly
DAF
dynamic axial fixator
DAI
diffuse axonal injury
Daily Adjusted Progressive Resistance Exercise (DAPRE)
Dakin
D. solution
D. tubing
Dalalone
D. D.P.
D. L.A.
Dale first rib rongeur
Dalgan
Dall-Miles
D.-M. cable
D.-M. cable cerclage
D.-M. cable/crimp cerclage system
D.-M. cable grip system
D.-M. cerclage wire
Dalmane
dalteparin
DALYs
Disability Adjusted Life Years
dam
dental d.
damage
anterior cervical surgery vocal
cord d.
brain d.
physeal d.
Damason-P
D'Ambrosia test

DANA
designed after natural anatomy
DANA shoulder prosthesis
danaparoid
danazol
dance
high-impact aerobic d. (HIAD)
low-impact aerobic d. (LIAD)
Saint Vitus d.
dancer pad
dancing
d. bear gait
d. bear syndrome
d. gait
Dandy maneuver
Dandy-Walker deformity
dangling foot
Daniel iliac bone graft
Danis-Weber
D.-W. classification of ankle injury
D.-W. fracture
Danniflex CPM exerciser
Danocrine
D'Antonio
D. acetabular classification
D. classification of acetabular
abnormalities
Dantrium
dantrolene
dantrone
DAPRE
Daily Adjusted Progressive Resistance
Exercise
DAPRE strength training
Darco
D. moldable insole
D. Podospray
D. shoe
D. toe alignment splint
D. Wedge shoe
DarcoGel ankle brace
Darier
D. disease
D. sign
Darrach
D. periosteal elevator
D. procedure
D. resection
D. retractor
Darrach-Hughston-Milch fracture
Darrach-McLaughlin
D.-M. approach
D.-M. shoulder technique
Darrow pain classification

D

Darvocet-N
   D.-N. 100
Darvon Compound-65 Pulvules
Darvon-N
Das
   D. Gupta procedure
   D. Gupta scapular excision
   D. Gupta scapulectomy
DASA
   distal articular set angle
Dasco
   D. Pro angle finder
   D. Pro angle finger
Daseler-Anson
   D.-A. classification of plantaris
     muscle anatomy
   D.-A. plantaris muscle anatomy
     classification
dashboard
   d. dislocation
   d. fracture
   d. injury
DataHand system
Daubenspeck
   D. bone curette
d'Aubigne
   d. femoral prosthesis
   d. femoral reconstruction
   d. hip status system
   d. patellar transplant
   d. resection reconstruction
Dautrey
   D. chisel
   D. osteotome
Davey-Rorabeck-Fowler decompression technique
David drainage
Davidson muscle clamp
Davidson-Sauerbruch-Doyen periosteal elevator
Davis
   D. arthrodesis
   D. drainage technique
   D. fusion
   D. metacarpal splint
   D. muscle-pedicle graft
   D. pin
   D. saw guide
   D. series
Dawbarn sign
DawSkin
   D. flexible protective skin system
   D. prosthetic
Dawson-Yuhl
   D.-Y. gouge
   D.-Y. impactor
   D.-Y. osteotome
   D.-Y. periosteal elevator

   D.-Y. rongeur forceps
   D.-Y. suction tube
Dawson-Yuhl-Cone curette
Dawson-Yuhl-Kerrison rongeur forceps
Dawson-Yuhl-Key elevator
Dawson-Yuhl-Leksell rongeur forceps
DAW Strap-Pad
Day
   D. fixation device
   D. fixation pin
   D. fixation staple
Daypro
DayTimer Carpal Tunnel Support
Daytona cervical orthosis
DBM
   demineralized bone matrix
DBS
   deep bonding system
   Denis Browne splint
DC
   direct current
   dynamic compression
DCB
   distal communicating branch
DCP
   dynamic compression plate
DCS
   dorsal column stimulator
   Dynamic condylar screw
     DCS pin
DDA
   dorsal digital artery
ddC
   dideoxycytidine
DDD
   degenerative disk disease
DDH
   developmental dislocated hip
   developmental dysplasia of the hip
     DDH orthosis
ddI
   dideoxyinosine
DDP
   dual drop pelvic
     DDP table
DDT
   DDT lock screw inserter
   DDT screw
de
   d. Barsy syndrome
   d. Kleyn position
   d. Kleyn test
   d. La Caffinière trapeziometacarpal
     prosthesis
   d. Lange syndrome
   d. Morgan spot
   d. Quervain tendinitis

dead
>d.-arm syndrome
>D. Sea Cosmeceuticals (DSC)
>d. space

deafferentation pain
Deane unconstrained knee prosthesis
Dean scissors
Deaver retractor
DeBakey prosthesis
DeBastiani
>D. corticotomy
>D. distractor
>D. external fixator
>D. femoral lengthening
>D. technique

Debeyre-Patte-Elmelik
>D.-P.-E. rotator cuff operation
>D.-P.-E. rotator cuff technique

debonding
debride
debridement
>Ahern trochanteric d.
>arthroscopic d.
>bursal d.
>cortical d.
>diagnostic arthroscopy and d.
>exploration and d.
>hemidiaphyseal d.
>irrigation and d. (I&D)
>Magnuson d.
>d. patella

debris
>bone d.
>fibrin d.
>d.-incited osteolysis
>joint d.
>metallic d.
>particulate d.
>polyethylene d.
>polymeric d.
>d.-retaining reamer
>wear d.

Debrisan
Debrunner kyphometer
debulk
debulking
>d. procedure
>Tsuge d.

deburring
Decadron-LA
Decadron Phosphate
Decaject

Decaject-LA
decalcification
decay
>free induction d. (FID)

deceleration
decerebrate posture
dechondrification
deciduous
Decker rongeur
deck plate
declination angle
decoder
>TeleCaption d.

decompression
>anterior retroperitoneal d.
>anterolateral d.
>bone graft d.
>Braly-Bishop-Tullos d.
>cervical spine d.
>core d.
>d. equipment
>extensive posterior d.
>d. of fasciotomy
>d. fasciotomy
>foot d.
>Getty d.
>d. laminectomy
>lateral d.
>leg d.
>lumbar spine d.
>Mubarak-Hargens d.
>nerve root d.
>posterior nerve d.
>posterolateral d.
>retroperitoneal d.
>d. rhachotomy
>sacral spine d.
>subacromial d.
>d. technique
>thoracic spine d.
>thoracolumbar spine d.
>timing of d.
>vertebral body d.

decompressive
>d. acromioplasty
>d. osteotomy

deconditioned syndrome
deconditioning syndrome
decorticate posture
decortication
>d. bur
>d. technique

D

NOTES

decorum
decremental response
decub
    decubitus position
Decubinex
    D. pad
    D. pad/protector
    D. protector
Decubitene oxygenated oil
decubitus
    d. position (decub)
    d. ulcer
decussation
dedifferentiated chondrosarcoma
Dee
    D. elbow hinge
    D. totally constrained elbow
      prosthesis
deep
    d. bonding system (DBS)
    d. circumflex iliac artery
    d. collateral ligament
    d. delayed infection
    d. fascia
    d. friction massage
    d. iliac dissection
    d. intracompartmental soft-tissue
      sarcoma
    d. kneading massage
    d. knee bend (DKB)
    d. peroneal nerve
    d. posterior compartment
    d. posterior sacrococcygeal ligament
    d. retractor
    d.-shelled acetabulum
    d. stroking and kneading massage
    d. tendon reflex (DTR)
    d. transverse carpal ligament
    d. transverse metacarpal ligament
    d. TV metatarsal ligament
    d. vein insufficiency (DVI)
    d. vein thrombosis (DVT)
    d. venous thrombosis (DVT)
    d. venous thrombosis prophylaxis
    d. wound infection
deepening reamer
deepithelialized rectus abdominis muscle
  (DRAM)
Deerfield test
defect
    Arthropor oblong cup for
      acetabular d.
    articular d.
    bone d.
    bridging of d.
    composite d.
    cortical d.
    cystic d.

    developmental d.
    diaphyseal d.
    fibrous cortical d.
    fusiform d.
    impression d.
    Klippel-Feil segmentation d.
    mapping the d.
    nonsubperiosteal cortical d.
    d. nonunion
    osseous d.
    osteoarticular d.
    osteochondral d.
    pars d.
    segmentation d.
    skeletal d.
    step d.
    subcortical d.
    subperiosteal cortical d.
    tibial d.
    triangular d.
    trochlear d.
    unremodeled d.
defensiveness
    auditory d.
    oral d.
    tactile d.
defervesce
defervescence
deficiency
    Aitken femoral d.
    American Academy of Orthopaedic
      Surgeons classification of
      acetabular d.
    cavitary d.
    central d.
    ceramide trihexosidase d.
    congenital limb d.
    factor VIII, IX d.
    focal d.
    Jones classification of congenital
      tibial d.
    Kalamchi-Dawe classification of
      congenital tibial d.
    long bone d.
    longitudinal d.
    magnesium d.
    O'Rahilly classification of limb d.
    proximal femoral focal d. (PFFD)
    radial d.
    segmental d.
    skeletal limb d.
    transverse d.
    vitamin C, D, K d.
deficient
    d. knee
    d. spinous process
deficit
    motor d.

neurologic d.
osteoporosis with vertebral collapse
  and neurologic d.
perceptual d.
proprioceptive d.
sensorimotor d.
sensory or motor d.
Definition PM femoral implant
  component
definitive
d. cerclage wire
d. stabilization
deformability
deformans
dystonia musculorum d.
osteitis d.
Page osteitis d.
deformation
elastic d.
plastic d.
stem d.
deformer
active d.
deformity
abduction d.
acetabular protrusio d.
adduction d.
adduction-internal rotation d.
adductovarus d.
adult-acquired flatfoot d.
d. analysis
angular d.
angulation d.
back-knee d.
Barouk button space for hallux
  valgus d.
Bebax shoe for forefoot d.
bifid thumb d.
bony d.
boutonnière d.
bowing d.
bowleg d.
bunion d.
burn boutonnière d.
buttonhole d.
calcaneocavovarus d.
calcaneocavus d.
calcaneovalgus d.
cavo abducto varus d.
cavocalcaneovalgus d.
cavovarus d.
cavus d.

cervical spine kyphotic d.
Charcot d.
checkrein d.
clasped thumb d.
clawfoot d.
clawhand d.
clawtoe d.
clefthand d.
clubfoot d.
cock-up d.
codfish d.
Cole osteotomy for midfoot d.
combined cavus d.
compensatory d.
congenital vertical talus foot d.
coronal plane d.
crossover-toe d.
curly toe d.
Dandy-Walker d.
digitus flexus d.
DISI d.
elevatus d.
equinocavovarus d.
equinovalgus d.
equinovarus hindfoot d.
equinus d.
eversion-external rotation d.
extension d.
femoral head d.
finger d.
fishtail d.
fixed d.
flat back d.
flatfoot d.
flexion-internal rotational d.
flexion valgus d.
forefoot abduction d.
garden spade d.
genu valgum d.
genu varum d.
gun stock d.
Haglund d.
hallux limitus d.
hallux valgus d.
hammer toe d.
hatchet-head d.
Hill-Sachs d.
hindfoot d.
hook-nail d.
hourglass d.
humpback d.
hyperextension d.

D

NOTES

deformity *(continued)*
    internal rotation d.
    intrinsic minus d.
    intrinsic plus d.
    joint d.
    Kelikian classification of nail d.
    Kirner d.
    knock-knee d.
    kyphotic d.
    lobster-claw d.
    lumbar spine kyphotic d.
    Madelung d.
    mallet finger d.
    mallet toe d.
    Michal d.
    multiplanar d.
    neuropathic midfoot d.
    oblique osteotomy for tibial d.
    one-plane d.
    pannus d.
    pencil and cup d.
    pes planovalgus d.
    pes planus d.
    pes valgoplanus d.
    planovalgus d.
    plantar flexion-inversion d.
    posttraumatic spinal d.
    procurvatum d.
    procurvature d.
    protrusio d.
    pseudoboutonnière d.
    pseudo-Hurler d.
    recurvatum angulation d.
    rockerbottom foot d.
    rotational d.
    round shoulder d.
    sabre shin d.
    sagittal d.
    shepherd's crook d.
    silver fork d.
    spastic thumb-in-palm d.
    spinal coronal plane d.
    spine d.
    splayfoot d.
    split-hand d.
    split-nail d.
    Sprengel d.
    S-shaped d.
    subcondylar d.
    supination d.
    swan-neck finger d.
    talipes cavus d.
    thoracic spine kyphotic d.
    thoracic spine scoliotic d.
    three-plane d.
    thumb d.
    thumb-in-palm d.
    triphalangeal thumb d.
    turned-up pulp d.
    two-plane d.
    ulnar deviation d.
    ulnar drift d.
    valgus d.
    varus hindfoot d.
    Velpeau d.
    volar angulation d.
    Volkmann clawhand d.
    windblown d.
    windswept d.
    wrist d.
    Zancolli procedure for clawhand d.
    zigzag compensatory d.
deformity/instability
    spinal d./i.
Defourmentel bone rongeur
Dega pelvic osteotomy
degeneration
    axon d.
    cartilaginous d.
    disk d.
    endoneurium d.
    immobilization d.
    joint d.
    Kirkaldy-Willis three phases of d.
    retrograde d.
    spinal d.
    spinocerebellar d.
    wallerian d.
    wear-and-tear d.
degenerative
    d. arthritic change
    d. arthritis
    d. arthrosis
    d. disk disease (DDD)
    d. disorder
    d. joint disease (DJD)
    d. lumbar scoliosis
    d. lumbar spine fusion
    d. meniscus
    d. osteoarthritis
    d. spine condition
    d. spondylolisthesis (type 3)
    d. spondylosis
    d. spondylosis decompression and fusion
    d. tear
degloving
    d. injury
    d. procedure
degradable polyglycolide rod
degradation
    proteoglycan d.
degrees
    d. of freedom (DOF)
    d.-of-freedom joint motion

d. of valgus angulation
d. of varus angulation
degree of separation
"deh chi" response
dehiscence
wound d.
Dehne cast
Déjérine sign
Déjérine-Sottas
D.-S. disease
D.-S. syndrome
Deknatel orthopedic autotransfusion system
delamination
DeLaura knee prosthesis
DeLaura-Verner knee prosthesis
delay
sensory d.
delayed
d. apoplexy
d. bone imaging
d. closure
d. consolidation
d. femoral osteotomy
d. fracture union
d. graft
d. onset
d.-onset muscle soreness (DOMS)
d. open reduction
d. primary repair
d. reflex
d. response
Delbert hip fracture classification
Delbet
D. splint
D. splint for heel fracture
DeLee classification
deliberate therapy
Delitala
D. T-nail nail
D. T-pin
Del-Mycin Topical
DeLorme exercise
Delrin-handle bone saw
Delrin joint
delta
d. femoral nail
d. frame
d. phalanx
d. receptor
D. Recon nail
D. Recon proximal drill guide

d. rod
d. tibial nail
D. walker
Delta-Cortef Oral
Deltafit Keel
Delta-Lite
D.-L. casting tape
D.-L. FlashCast
Delta-Rol cast padding
Deltasone
deltoid
d. bursa
d. fascia
d. flap
d. insertion over joint
d. ligament
d. ligament tear
d. muscle
d. origin
Deltoid-Aid arm support
deltoid-splitting
d.-s. incision
d.-s. shoulder approach
deltopectoral
d. approach
d. flap
d. groove
d. interval
deltotrapezius fascial ligament
deluxe
d. FIN pin
d. FIN pin inserter
demand
motion d.
specific adaptation to imposed d. (SAID)
demarcate
demarcation
line of d.
Demariniff protractor
DeMarneffe meniscotomy knife
DeMartel-Wolfson clamp holder
DeMayo suture passer
Demel wire clamp
dementia
Guam amyotrophic lateral sclerosis-parkinsonism d.
Demerol
Demianoff sign
demineralization
bony d.

D

NOTES

demineralized
    d. bone
    d. bone graft
    d. bone matrix (DBM)
Demos tibial artery clamp
Demser
DeMuth hip screw
demyelination
denatured alcohol
denervation
    d. disease
    d. potential
    d. supersensitivity
Denham
    D. external fixation
    D. external fixation device
    D. pin
Denis
    D. Browne bar
    D. Browne bar foot orthosis
    D. Browne bucket
    D. Browne clubfoot splint
    D. Browne hip splint
    D. Browne sacral fracture
      classification
    D. Browne spinal fracture
      classification
    D. Browne splint (DBS)
    D. Browne talipes hobble splint
    D. Browne three-column model
    D. Browne three-column spine
      theory
    D. Browne tray
    D. spinal fracture
Dennyson cervical brace
Dennyson-Fulford subtalar arthrodesis
DENS
    direct electrical nerve stimulation
dens
    d. anterior screw fixation
    d. fracture
    d. x-ray view
densitometry
    bone d.
    dual photon d. (DPD)
    photon d.
density
    bone mineral d. (BMD)
    fiber d.
    lumbosacral junction bone d.
dental
    d. bur
    d. dam
    d. drill
    d. freer
    d. mirror
    d. pick
dentate fracture

dentinogenesis imperfecta
denudation
denude
deodorant
    Deoshoes d.
Deon
    D. hip prosthesis
    D. stem
Deoshoes deodorant
deossification
deoxypyridinoline crosslinks urine assay
Depakote
DePalma
    D. hip prosthesis
    D. modified patellar technique
    D. staple
Depen
dependent edema
depGynogen Injection
depMedalone Injection
Depo-Estradiol Injection
Depogen Injection
Depoject Injection
depolarization block
depolarizing drug
depolymerization
    increased d.
    unbalanced d.
Depo-Medrol Injection
Depopred Injection
deposit
    calcium d.
    gouty tophaceous d.
    rotator cuff calcified d.
    tophaceous d.
deposition
    bone d.
    calcium pyrophosphate dihydrate d.
      (CPPD)
    pseudotumorous mucin d.
depot corticosteroid
depressed
    d. fracture
    d. reflex
depression
    d. fracture
    d. of fragment
    Hamilton Rating Scale for D.
    postactivation d.
depressor
depth
    d. caliper-meter stick method
    d.-check drill
    d. gauge
    wire penetration d.
DePuy
    D. acetabular liner
    D. acetabular lining

D. aeroplane splint
D. AML Porocoat stem prosthesis
D. any-angle splint
D. awl
D. bipolar cup
D. bolt
D. calcar grinder
D. coaptation splint
D. drill
D. femoral acetabular overlay guide
D. fracture brace
D. halter
D. hip prosthesis with Scuderi head
D. interference screw
D. open-spindle splint
D. open-thimble splint
D. orthopaedic implant
D. pin
D. plate
D. rainbow frame
D. rasp
D. reamer
D. reducing frame
D. rocking leg splint
D. rod bender
D. rolled Colles splint
D. screwdriver
D. support
D. trispiked acetabular component
DePuy-Pott splint
de Quervain
    d. Q. disease
    d. Q. fracture
    d. Q. injury
    d. Q. stenosing tenosynovitis
derangement
    internal d.
    structural d.
    vertebral d.
Derby nail
Dercum disease
Derifield pelvic leg check
derivatives
    undecylenic acid and d.
dermabrader
Dermacentor
    D. andersoni
    D. variabilis
Dermaflex Gel

Dermagran
    D. wound cleanser with zinc
    D. wound dressing
dermal
    d. fasciectomy
    d. fibromatosis
    d. graft
DermaTemp infrared thermographic sensor
dermatitidis
    Blastomyces d.
dermatitis
    d. artefacta
    atopic d.
    shoe d.
dermatoarthritis
dermatocele
dermatofibrosarcoma protuberans
dermatomal
    d. pain
    d. pattern
dermatome
    Brown d.
    d. mapping
    mechanical d.
    Padgett electric d.
    Reese d.
    Stryker d.
dermatomyositis
dermatosensory evoked potential
dermatosis
    juvenile plantar d.
Dermiflex dressing
dermodesis
    resection d.
dermographia
dermometer
dermomyotome
dermoplast-plastizote orthosis
Dero hole-in-one prosthetic sock
Derosa-Graziano step-cut osteotomy
derotate
derotation
    d. boot
    d. brace
    oblique osteotomy with d.
derotational
    d. osteotomy
    d. pin
derotator bar
DeRoyal/LMB finger splint

D

NOTES

D'Errico
- D. enlarging drill bur
- D. lamina chisel
- D. perforating drill
- D. perforating drill bur
- D. perforator drill
- D. retractor

Desault
- D. sign
- D. wrist bandage
- D. wrist dislocation

Deschamps needle

Descot fracture

Desenex
- Prescription Strength D.

design
- barrel bur d.
- computer-assisted d. (CAD)
- Harris d. (HD)
- hook hollow-ground connection d.
- hook V-groove connection d.
- mechanical plate d.
- metal-on-metal d.
- pedicle screw linkage d.
- prosthetic d.
- prototype d.
- screw d.
- spinal implant d.
- transpedicular fixation system d.
- V-groove hollow-ground connection d.

designed after natural anatomy (DANA)

DesignLine orthotic

desipramine

desirudin

Desk-rest arm support

desmalgia

desmectasis

desmitis

desmocytoma

desmoid
- cortical d.
- d. fibroma
- d. lesion
- periosteal d.
- d. tumor

desmoma

desmopathy

desmoplasia

desmoplastic fibroma

desmopressin

desmorrhexis

desmosis

desmotomy

Desormaux endoscope

Desoxyn

desoxyribonuclease
- fibrinolysin and d.

Destot sign

destruction
- bony element d.
- bony necrosis and d.
- cortical d.

destructive lesion

desyndactylization
- Weinstock d.

detector
- analogous signal d.
- Isometer bone graft placement site d.

determination
- anteversion d.
- Budin-Chandler anteversion d.
- fusion limit d.
- leg length d.
- skin blood flow d.
- transcutaneous oxygen tension d.
- Whitesides tissue pressure d.

detritus
- d. bone
- foci of hyaline cartilage d.

Deune knee prosthesis

development
- asymmetric subtalar joint d.
- bone d.
- calcar femorale d.
- General Education D. (GED)
- postural d.

developmental
- d. coxa vara
- d. defect
- d. dislocated hip (DDH)
- d. dislocated hip orthosis
- d. disorder disease
- d. dysplasia
- d. dysplasia of the hip (DDH)

Deverle fixation

deviation
- angular d.
- lateral d.
- radial d.
- rotary d.
- standard d.
- ulnar d.

Devic disease

device
- Ace Unifix fixation d.
- acrylic orthotic d.
- Acufex bioabsorbable fixation d.
- adjustable aiming d.
- adjustable 2-point caliper sensory assessment d.
- Agee 4-pin fixation d.
- Altona finger extension d.
- Anderson fixation d.
- Anderson leg lengthening d.

Antense anti-tension d.
anterior internal fixation d.
antirotation d.
application of traction d.
Aprema III d.
Aquatrek d.
ArtAssist arterial assist d.
Arthrotek tibial fixation d.
articular motion d. (AMD)
articulated tension d.
assistive d.
assistive technology d. (ATD)
Automator d.
A-V Impulse System foot pump
  DVT prophylaxis d.
A-V Impulse System foot wrap
  DVT prophylaxis d.
Axer compression d.
Backbar d.
BackCycler continuous passive
  motion d.
back range-of-motion d.
Bassett electrical stimulation d.
Becker orthopaedic spinal system
  orthotic d.
Blanchard traction d.
body-powered prosthetic d.
Bovie electrocautery d.
Brannock foot measuring d.
Buck convoluted traction d.
Calandruccio fixation d.
Cameron fracture d.
C-D instrumentation d.
cervical range-of-motion d.
Cervitrak d.
Charnley d.
Cleanwheel presterilized
  disposable d.
collapsible internal fixation d.
Columbus McKinnon Hugger d.
combined fixation d.
compression screw-plate d.
Cordis implantable drug
  reservoir d.
coring d.
Cotrel-Dubousset dynamic transverse
  traction d.
CPM d.
Cuff Link orthopaedic d.
Cybex d.
Day fixation d.
Denham external fixation d.

Deyerle fixation d.
Deyo d.
DIGIT-grip d.
Disk-Criminator nerve stimulation
  measuring d.
distal targeting d.
DressFlex orthotic d.
Dunn fracture d.
Dwyer d.
dynamic transverse traction d.
EBI d.
Edwards modular system sacral
  fixation d.
electrocardiographic recording d.
Electronics electrical stimulation d.
Evershears surgical instrument d.
EX-FI-RE external fixation d.
E-Z Flex jaw exercising d.
EZ-Trac orthopaedic suspension d.
FastOut d.
fixation d.
Fox internal fixation d.
fracture fixation d.
Fromm triangle orthopaedic d.
Georgiade fixation d.
Giliberty d.
Golgi d.
Graftmaster d.
Grip-Ease d.
halo-gravity traction d.
halo vest d.
Hare splint d.
Harrington-Kostuik distraction d.
Harrington rod instrumentation
  distraction outrigger d.
Harris-Aufranc d.
Heyer-Schulte antisiphon d.
Hoffmann fixation d.
Hoffmann-Vidal external fixation d.
Ikuta fixation d.
Ilizarov d.
Insta-Nerve d.
intraarticular cautery d.
Intracell mechanical muscle d.
Intracell myofascial trigger-point d.
isometric d.
JACE W550 CPM wrist d.
JAS elbow motion d.
Kaneda distraction d.
Kendrick extrication d. (KED)
Kennedy ligament augmenting d.
Kin-Con d.

D

NOTES

device *(continued)*

kinetic rehab d. (KRD)
Kirschner d.
Knott rod distraction d.
KRD L2000 rehab d.
Kronner external fixation d.
Kuhlman cervical traction d.
Küntscher traction d.
Legasus support CPM d.
leg-holding d.
Leinbach d.
ligament augmentation d. (LAD)
Lite-Gait partial weight-bearing gait
   therapy d.
Luque fixation d.
McAtee compression screw d.
McLaughlin osteosynthesis d.
MicroFET2 muscle testing d.
Mobilimb CPM d.
Mueller fixation d.
muscle and neurological stimulation
   electrotherapy d.
MyoTrac d.
MyoTrac 2, C d.
nail-bending d.
nail plate d.
Nauth traction d.
Necktrac traction d.
Neufeld d.
Neuro-Aide testing d.
newer-generation d.
notcher d.
Ogden Anchor soft tissue d.
Ommaya reservoir d.
Omni-Flexor d.
Oppociser exercise d.
Oratek d.
Original Jacknobber II muscle-
   massage d.
Orthofix external fixation d.
Ortholav irrigation and suction d.
orthotic d.
Oxford uncompartmental d.
Parham-Martin fracture d.
passive motion d.
passive positioning d.
peg board lateral positioning d.
Plastizote orthotic d.
PlexiPulse intermittent pneumatic
   compression d.
PLM d.
pneumatic external compression d.
Polar Care 500 cryotherapy d.
PPT orthotic d.
pronation spring-control d.
ProTrac measurement d.
pulsatile pneumatic plantar-
   compression d.

Quartzo d.
Quengel d.
Rancho ankle foot control d.
Redi-Trac traction d.
Reichert-Mundinger stereotactic d.
Rezaian external fixation d.
Rezaian interbody d.
Richards lag screw d.
RMC knee replacement d.
Rochester bone trephine d.
rod distraction d.
rod-mounted targeting d.
Roeder manipulative aptitude
   test d.
Roger Anderson compression d.
Roger Anderson external
   fixation d.
Roger Anderson stabilization d.
RollerBack self-massage d.
Rolz d.
rotation d.
SAFHS ultrasound d.
sequential compression d. (SCD)
Servox d.
shear-off d.
sliding fixation d.
sliding nail d.
Slot distraction d.
snap-fit d.
Sofamor spinal d.
SOLEutions custom orthotic d.
SOLEutions Prefab orthotic d.
Sorbothane orthotic d.
Southwick pin-holding d.
Spenco orthotic d.
SplintsRite stabilization d.
sports terminal d.
SporTX stimulation d.
StairClimber assist d.
Statak soft tissue attachment d.
Stellbrink fixation d.
Stone clamp-locking d.
Stress-Ray varus-valgus d.
STx lumbar traction d.
STx Saunders lumbar disc d.
Sukhtian-Hughes fixation d.
Suretac bioabsorbable shoulder
   fixation d.
Sutter-CPM knee d.
Tacticon peripheral neuropathy
   screening d.
Tekscan in-shoe monitoring d.
Telectronics electrical stimulation d.
Tenderlett d.
terminal d. (TD)
thermocouple skin temperature d.
The Rope stretching d.
The Rope stretch and traction d.

Thumper d.
transpedicularly implanted anterior
  spinal support d.
transverse loading d.
d. for transverse traction (DTT)
triangular compression d.
TriggerWheel d.
TSRH corkscrew d.
TSRH mini-corkscrew d.
Vidal-Adrey modified Hoffmann
  external fixation d.
visor halo fixation d.
Volkov-Oganesian elbow
  distraction d.
Volkov-Oganesian external
  fixation d.
voluntary closing terminal d.
voluntary opening terminal d.
Wagner external fixation d.
Wagner-Schanz screw d.
Wasserstein fixation d.
Wrist Pro wrist support d.
Xercise tube resistive d.
XTB knee extension d.
Zickel supracondylar d.
Zielke distraction d.
Zimmer electrical stimulation d.
Zipper anti-disconnect d.
devitalized
  d. bone graft
  d. tissue
DeWald
  D. spinal apparatus
  D. spinal appliance
Dewar
  D. posterior cervical fixation
    procedure
  D. posterior cervical fusion
  D. posterior cervical fusion
    technique
Dewar-Barrington
  D.-B. arthroplasty
  D.-B. clavicular dislocation
    technique
Dewar-Harris
  D.-H. paralysis
  D.-H. shoulder technique
dexamethasone
  neomycin and d.
DEXA scan
Dexasone L.A.
Dexone LA

Dexon suture
dextranomer
dextran prophylaxis
dextromethorphan
  acetaminophen and d.
dextropropoxyphene
dextrorotary scoliosis
dextrorotoscoliosis
dextroscoliosis scoliosis
dextrose
  d. solution
  tetracaine and d.
Deyerle
  D. drill
  D. femoral fracture technique
  D. fixation apparatus
  D. fixation device
  D. II pin
  D. plate
  D. sciatic tension test
  D. screw
Deyo device
dezocine
DF80 hip internal prosthesis
DFA
  hallux dorsiflexion angle
D-Foam
DHC Plus
DH pressure relief walker
DHS hip screw
DHT
Diab-A-Foot
  D.-A.-F. protection system
  D.-A.-F. rocker insole
Diab-A-Pad insole
Diab-A-Sheet
Diab-A-Sole insole
Diab-A-Thotics orthotic
diabetes mellitus
diabetic
  d. Charcot foot
  D. Diagnostic Insole
  D. D-Sole foot orthosis
  d. femoral mononeuropathy
  d. insole
  d. neurotrophic ulcer
  d. orthosis kit
  d. patient
  d. polyradiculopathy
  d. pressure relief shoe
  d. sock
diacondylar fracture

D

NOTES

diadochokinesia
diagnosis (dx)
    clinical d.
    differential d.
    palpatory d.
diagnostic
    d. arthroscopy
    d. arthroscopy and debridement
    d. arthroscopy, operative
      arthroscopy, and possible
      operative arthrotomy (AAA)
    d. imaging
    d. and operative arthroscopy
      (DOA)
    d. strategy
diagonal stretch
diagram
    free body d.
dial
    d.-lock brace
    d.-lock orthosis
    d. pelvic osteotomy
    d. periacetabular osteotomy
    d. test
diameter
    horizontal pedicle d.
    lumbar spine pedicle d.
    neck d.
    pedicle d.
    sagittal pedicle d.
    sagittal spinal canal d.
    thoracic spine pedicle d.
    transpedicular fixation effective
      pedicle d.
    transverse pedicle d.
    vertical pedicle d.
diametral
diametric pelvic fracture
diamond
    D. biomechanical table
    d. bur
    d. high-speed drill
    d.-inlay graft
    D. nail
    d. pin cutter
    d.-shaped medullary nail
Diamond-Gould
    D.-G. reduction syndactyly
    D.-G. syndactyly operation
diapedesis
Diapedic foot cream
diapering
    triple d.
diaphragm
    Bucky d.
    urogenital d.
diaphyseal
    d. aclasis

    d. defect
    d. dysplasia
    d.-epiphyseal fusion
    d. fracture
    d. osteotomy
    d. plating
    d. tuberculosis
diaphysectomy
diaphysis, pl. diaphyses
    femoral d.
diaplasis
diarthrodial joint
diarthrosis
Dias-Giegerich
    D.-G. fracture technique
    D.-G. open reduction
Dias-Tachdijian physeal injury
    classification
diastasis
    ankle mortise d.
    d. fibula
    pubic d.
    symphysis pubis d.
    tibiofibular d.
    transsyndesmotic bolt in
      tibiofibular d.
diastatic fracture
diastematomyelia
diastrophic
    d. dwarfism
    d. dysplasia
diathermy
    microwave d. (MWD)
    short-wave d. (SWD)
diathesis
    Dupuytren d.
Diaz disease
diazepam
dibasic
    calcium phosphate, d.
Dibenzyline
DIC
    disseminated intravascular coagulation
Dicarbosil
DiChiara hand try
dichlorodifluoromethane and
    trichloromonofluoromethane
dichlorotetrafluoroethane
    ethyl chloride and d.
Dick AO fixateur interne
Dickhaut-DeLee
    D.-D. classification of discoid
      meniscus
    D.-D. discoid meniscus
      classification
Dickinson
    D. approach
    D. calcaneal bursitis technique

Dickinson-Coutts-Woodward-Handler
  osteotomy
Dickson
    D. geometric osteotomy
    D. Paraffin bath
    D. paralysis
    D. transplant technique
Dickson-Diveley
    D.-D. foot operation
    D.-D. procedure
diclofenac sodium and misoprostol
dicloxacillin
dicondylar fracture
didanosine
dideoxycytidine (ddC)
dideoxyinosine (ddI)
Didiee view
Didronel
Diebold-Bejjani osteotomy
die punch fracture
diet
    Gerson d.
    low-purine d.
    tea-and-toast d.
    d. therapy
dietary modification
Diethrich bulldog clamp
diethylstilbestrol
difference
    KT side-to-side d.
differential
    d. diagnosis
    d. spinal block
    temperature d. (TD)
differentiated chondrosarcoma
differentiation failure
diffuse
    d. axonal injury (DAI)
    d. idiopathic sclerosing hyperostosis
    (DISH)
    d. idiopathic skeletal hyperostosis
    (DISH)
    d. idiopathic skeletal hyperostosis
    syndrome
    d. infantile fibromatosis
diffusion
diflunisal
digastric muscle
DiGeorge syndrome
Digi-Flex
    D.-F. exercise system

D.-F. finger exerciser
D.-F. hand exerciser
Digikit finger tourniquet
Digi Sleeve stockinette dressing
digit
    1st d.
      thumb
    2nd d.
      index finger
    3rd d.
      long finger
    accessory d.
    arthrodesed d.
    d. cap
    color of d.
    congenital trigger d.
    fifth d.
    first d.
    flail d.
    fourth d.
    infantile trigger d.
    multiple d.'s
    second d.
    d. splint
    supernumerary d.
    4th d.
      ring finger
    5th d.
      little finger
    third d.
    trigger d.
    d. tube
    d. wrap
Digit-Aide fifth toe splint
digital
    AHP d.
    d. amputation
    d. aponeurosis
    d. artery
    d. artery protection
    D. Biofeedback System
    d.-block anesthesia
    d. blood perfusion
    D. Care kit
    d. contracture
    d. cord
    d. edge-detection
    d. extensor mechanism
    d. extensor tendon
    d. flexor tendinitis
    d. flexor tendon
    d. flexor tendon sheath

D

NOTES

digital *(continued)*
  d. impaction
  d. nail
  d. nerve
  d. nerve block
  d. opposers
  d. pad
  d. palpation
  d. photoplethysmography
  d. plethysmography
  d. prosthesis
  d. response test
  d. shortening
  d. subtraction angiography (DSA)
  d. theca
  d. tourniquet
  d. vibrogram
DIGIT-grip device
digiti quinti proprius tendon
digitizer
  Amfit d.
  Metrecom d.
digitorum brevis avulsion
digitus
  d. abductus
  d. flexus deformity
Di Guglielmo disease
dihydrocodeine compound
dihydroergotamine
dihydroergotamine-heparin
dihydrostreptomycin
dihydrotachysterol
diisocyanate
  methylene bisphenyl d.
Dilantin
dilator
  Eder-Puestow metal olive d.
  lacrimal duct d.
  vessel d.
Dilaudid
  D.-5
  D.-HP
Dillwyn-Evans
  D.-E. osteotomy
  D.-E. resection
Dilocaine
dimelia
  ulnar d.
dimenhydrinate
dimension
  D. hip prosthesis
  D. hip system
  pedicle d.
Dimension-C femoral stem prosthesis
dimethyl sulfoxide (DMSO)
diminished sensation
Dimon-Hughston
  D.-H. fracture fixation

  D.-H. intertrochanteric osteotomy
  D.-H. technique
Dimon osteotomy
dimple
  d. the bone
  pilonidal d.
Dingman
  D. bone-holding forceps
  D. mouth gag
  D. osteotome
diode
  infrared light-emitting d.
Dioval Injection
DIP
  distal interphalangeal
  DIP articulation
  DIP fusion
  DIP joint
DiPalma shoe lift
diparesis
  spastic d.
diphasic
Diphenhist
diphenhydramine
  acetaminophen and d.
diphenylhydantoin
diphosphonate
  aminohydroxy propylidene d.
  technetium labeled methylene d.
  technetium-99 methylene d.
DIPJ
  distal interphalangeal joint
diplegia
  spastic d.
Diplococcus pneumoniae
diplomyelia
diploscope
dipropionate
  betamethasone d.
dipyridamole thallium imaging
direct
  d. contraction
  d. current (DC)
  d. electrical nerve stimulation
    (DENS)
  d. lateral portal
director
  grooved d.
disability
  D. Adjusted Life Years (DALYs)
  atlantooccipital d.
  permanent d.
Disalcid
disappearing bone disease
disarticular amputation
disarticulate
disarticulation
  Batch-Spittler-McFaddin knee d.

Boyd hip d.
elbow d. (ED)
joint d.
Lisfranc d.
Mazet d. of knee
metatarsophalangeal joint d.
sacroiliac d.
shoulder d. (SD)
wrist d. (WD)

DISC
dynamic integrated stabilization chair

disc (*var. of* disk)

discectomy (*var. of* diskectomy)

discerta
porokeratosis plantaris d.

discharge
bizarre high-frequency d.
bizarre repetitive d.
complex repetitive d.
coupled d.
cramp d.
double d.
d. frequency
grouped d.
multiple d.
myokymic d.
myotonic d.
neuromyotonic d.
paired d.
pseudomyotonic d.
repetitive d.
d. summary
triple d.
waning d.

disci (*pl. of* discus)

discission knife Beaver blade

discitis
juvenile d.

discogenic (*var. of* diskogenic)

discogram (*var. of* diskogram)

discography (*var. of* diskography)

discoid lateral meniscus

discoligamentous injury

discometry (*var. of* diskometry)

discontinuity
pelvic d.

discopathogenic

discopathy

Disc-O-Sit Jr. cushion

discotome
Pheasant d.

discrepancy
leg length d. (LLD)
limb length d.

discrete
d. activity
d. blood supply to a bone graft

discrimination
Ayres tactile d.
right-left d.
two-point d.
Weber static two-point d.

discus, pl. **disci**

disease
Albers-Schönberg d.
allograft coronary artery d.
Apert d.
Atton d.
Bamberger-Marie d.
B. burgdorferi titer for Lyme d.
Bechterew d.
Berger d.
Bielschowsky-Jansky d.
Blount d.
Bornholm d.
Bourneville d.
Bowen d.
Brailsford d.
Brodie d.
Buchanan d.
Buerger d.
Burns d.
Caffey d.
caisson worker's d.
calcium pyrophosphate dihydrate
deposition d.
Calvé-Perthes d.
Canavan-van Bogaert-Bertrand d.
cardiovascular d.
cement d.
cementless d.
central core d.
cervical disk d.
cervical spine rheumatoid d.
Charcot joint d.
Charcot-Marie-Tooth d.
Christmas hemophiliac d.
chronic tophaceous d.
CMT d.
collagen vascular d.
congenital disorder d.
connective tissue d.
d. construct

D

NOTES

disease *(continued)*
coronary artery d.
Cowden d.
Curschmann-Steinert d.
cystic d.
Darier d.
degenerative disk d. (DDD)
degenerative joint d. (DJD)
Déjérine-Sottas d.
denervation d.
de Quervain d.
Dercum d.
developmental disorder d.
Devic d.
Diaz d.
Di Guglielmo d.
disappearing bone d.
diver's d.
double Charcot d.
Duchenne d.
Duplay d.
Dupuytren d.
Ehrenfeld d.
Ellis-vanCreveld d.
embolic d.
end-organ d.
Engelmann d.
Erb-Goldflam d.
Erb-Landouzy d.
Erdheim-Chester d.
Erhenfeld d.
facet joint d. (FJD)
facioscapulohumeral muscle
  atrophy d.
Farber d.
Fazio-Londe d.
Felix d.
fibromuscular d.
Forestier d.
fracture d.
Freiberg d.
Freiberg-Kohler d.
Friedreich d.
Garré d.
Garrod d.
Gaucher d.
genetic d.
Gilbert d.
glenohumeral joint d.
Gorham d.
Haas d.
Hand-Schüller-Christian d.
Hansen d.
Hass d.
hereditary neuropathic d.
herniated disk d.
histiocytosis X group of d.'s
hydroxyapatite deposition d.

hypophosphatemic bone d.
inheritable d.
intrinsic vascular d.
ischemic d.
Iselin d.
Jaffe d.
Joseph d.
Kashin-Bek d.
Kawasaki d.
Kienböck d.
Kimura d.
Kinnier-Wilson d.
Köhler d.
König d.
Kugelberg-Welander d.
Kümmell d.
Landouzy-Dejerine d.
lederhosen d.
Legg-Calvé-Perthes d. (LCPD)
Legg-Perthes d.
Letterer-Siwe d.
Lewis upper limb cardiovascular d.
lipid storage d.
liver d.
Lou Gehrig d.
lower motor neuron d.
Lyme d.
Mafucci d.
Marie-Bamberger d.
Marie-Charcot-Tooth d.
Marie-Strümpell d.
marrow d.
Mauclaire d.
McArdle d.
metabolic bone d.
metastatic d.
milk-alkali d.
Milroy d.
mini-core d.
mitochondrial d.
Morquio d.
Morton d.
Munchmeyer d.
neoplastic disorder d.
neurogenic d.
neurologic d.
neuromuscular d.
neuronal degenerative d.
neuropathic hereditary d.
Niemann-Pick d.
oligoarticular d.
Ollier d.
Oppenheim d.
Osgood-Schlatter d.
osteoarthritis d.
Paget d.
Panner d.
Parkinson d.

Pelligrini-Stieda d.
peripheral arterial occlusive d.
  (PAOD)
peripheral vascular d. (PVD)
Perthes d.
Peyronie d.
phytanic acid storage d.
posttest likelihood of d.
Pott d.
Preiser d.
pretest likelihood of d.
Raynaud d.
Refsum d.
Reiter d.
rheumatoid d.
Rosai-Dorfman d.
Roussy-Levy d.
scapuloperoneal muscle atrophy d.
Scheuermann d.
Sever d.
severe degenerative disk d.
sickle-cell d.
Sinding-Larsen-Johansson d.
skeletal hypoplasia d.
Still d.
Sudeck d.
synovial d.
Taratynov d.
Thiemann d.
Thomsen d.
thoracolumbar degenerative d.
thromboembolic d. (TED)
traumatic disorder d.
upper motor neuron d.
Van Neck d.
venous thromboembolic d. (VTED)
von Recklinghausen d.
von Willebrand d.
Voorhoeve d.
Wartenberg d.
Werdnig-Hoffmann d.
Whipple d.
Wilson d.
Woringer-Kolopp d.

**disease-modifying antirheumatologic drug
  (DMARD)**
disengage
DISH
diffuse idiopathic sclerosing hyperostosis
diffuse idiopathic skeletal hyperostosis
  DISH syndrome

dish
scoop d.
DISI
distal intercalated segment instability
dorsal intercalary segment instability
dorsiflexed intercalated segment
  instability
  DISI collapse pattern
  DISI deformity
disk, disc
amphiarthrodial d.
articular d.
d. bulge
bulging d.
cervical d.
d. compression
crescent-shaped fibrocartilaginous d.
d. degeneration
d. diffusion method
d. diffusion test
d. excision
excision of intervertebral d.
extruded d.
d. extrusion
fibrocartilaginous d.
d. forceps
d. fragment
d. grabber
herniated cervical d.
herniated contained d.
herniated intervertebral d. (HID)
d. herniation
intervertebral d.
d. lesion
lumbar d.
massive herniated d.
ortho d.
d. plication
d. pressure
d. prolapse
protruding d.
d. protrusion
d. rongeur
sequestered d.
sequestrated d.
slipped d.
d. space
d. space saline acceptance test
swollen d.
vacuum d.
Diskard head halter

D

NOTES

Disk-Criminator

D.-C. nerve stimulation measuring device

D.-C. sensory testing

diskectomy, discectomy

automated percutaneous d. (APD)

automated percutaneous lumbar d. (APLD)

cervical d.

Cloward fusion d.

laminotomy and d. (LAM)

microlumbar d. (MLD)

microsurgery d.

microsurgical d. (MSD)

Nucleotome system for lumbar d.

partial d.

percutaneous lumbar d.

Robinson anterior cervical d.

Smith-Robinson anterior cervical d.

Williams d.

Wiltse d.

d. with Cloward fusion

diskogenic, discogenic

d. neck pain

diskogram, discogram

d. needle

diskography, discography

cervical d.

Cloward fusion d.

lumbar d.

microlumbar d.

Williams d.

diskometry, discometry

Disl

dislocation

dislocated

d. knee

d. patella

dislocation (Disl)

acromioclavicular joint d.

antenatal d.

anterior hip d.

anterior-inferior d.

anterior shoulder d.

anterolateral d.

atlantoaxial d. (AAD)

atlantooccipital joint d.

atypical d.

Bankart shoulder d.

bayonet d.

Bell-Dally cervical d.

Bennet basic hand d.

Bennett d.

bilateral interfacetal d. (BID)

boutonnière hand d.

bursting d.

Carnesale-Stewart-Barnes classification of hip d.

carpometacarpal joint d.

central d.

Chopart ankle d.

chronic recurrent ankle joint d.

complete d.

congenital hip d.

consecutive d.

d. contour abnormality

Copeland-Kavat classification of metatarsophalangeal d.

Cotton reduction of elbow d.

dashboard d.

Desault wrist d.

divergent elbow d.

dorsal perilunate d.

dorsal transscaphoid perilunar d.

elbow d.

facet d.

d. fracture

frank d.

gamekeeper's thumb d.

glenohumeral joint d.

habitual d.

Hill-Sachs shoulder d.

hip d.

incomplete d.

interphalangeal joint d.

intraarticular d.

isolated d.

Jahss classification of ankle d.

joint d.

Kienböck d.

knee d.

Lisfranc d.

lumbosacral d.

lunate d.

luxatio erecta shoulder d.

medial swivel d.

metacarpophalangeal d.

metatarsophalangeal joint d.

Meyn reduction of elbow d.

milkmaid's elbow d.

Monteggia d.

Nélaton ankle d.

occipitoatlantal d.

old, unreduced d.

Otto pelvis d.

Palmer transscaphoid perilunar d.

panclavicular d.

parachute jumper's d.

Pare reduction of elbow d.

partial d.

patellar intraarticular d.

pathologic d.

perilunar transscaphoid d.

perilunate carpal d.

peroneal d.

phalangeal d.

posterior hip d.
posterior shoulder d.
posteromedial d.
prenatal d.
primitive d.
proximal tibiofibular joint d.
radial head d.
recent d.
recurrent patellar d.
retrosternal d.
sacroiliac d.
shoulder d.
Smith d.
spontaneous hyperemic d.
sternoclavicular joint d.
subastragalar d.
subcoracoid shoulder d.
subglenoid shoulder d.
subspinous d.
subtalar d.
superior d.
swivel d.
talar d.
talonavicular d.
taratologic d.
tarsal d.
tarsometatarsal d.
temporomandibular joint d.
tibialis posterior d.
tibiofibular joint d.
transscaphoid perilunate d.
traumatic d.
triquetrolunate d.
unilateral interfacetal d.
unreduced d.
volar semilunar wrist d.

dislodgment
hook d.

DISMAL
dorsiflexed intercalated segment
instability

disodium
etidronate d.

disorder
adrenal d.
clotting d.
coagulation d.
cumulative trauma d. (CTD)
cyclothymic d.
degenerative d.
fluoroquinolone-associated Achilles
tendon d.

intervertebral disk d.
lumbar disk d.
motor d.
muscle d.
nail d.
narcissistic personality d.
neoplastic d.
neurogenic d.
nontotal-contact d.
parathyroid d.
patellofemoral d.
peripheral neurocompressive d.
posttraumatic stress d. (PTSD)
progressive neurologic d.
recurrent d.
repetitive trauma d. (RTD)
respiratory d.
rheumatoid d.
spastic d.
tendon d.
trophic joint d.

disorientation
hypnotic time d.

disparity
limb-length d.

dispenser
Jet Vac cement d.

dispersion
temporal d.

displaced
d. intraarticular calcaneus
d. intraarticular fracture

displacement
angular d.
atlantoaxial rotary d.
crosshead d.
d. curve
Ellis-Jones peroneal tendon d.
hypnotic d.
interregional d.
lateral rotary d.
left-right leg d.
load-to-grip d.
medial d.
oblique d.
d. osteotomy
peroneal tendon d.
rotary d.
significant d.
spondylolisthesis with significant d.
tendon d.

D

NOTES

displacement *(continued)*
    traumatic d.
    Y-axis translatory d.
disposable muscle biopsy clamp
Disposatrode disposable electrode
disproportion
    fiber-type d.
disrelationship
    persistent occiput/atlas d.
disruption
    anterior column d.
    cervical spine posterior ligament d.
    Charcot d.
    end-stage d.
    facet capsule d.
    joint d.
    lateral compartment d.
    ligamentous d.
    medial compartment d.
    pedicle cortex d.
dissecans
    osteochondritis d. (OCD)
    osteochondrosis d.
    patellar osteochondritis d.
    talar osteochondritis d.
dissecting
    d. clamp
    d. probe
    d. scissors
dissection
    blunt d.
    bone d.
    deep iliac d.
    extracapsular d.
    field of d.
    Pack-Ehrlich deep iliac d.
    sharp d.
    subligamentous d.
    subperiosteal d.
dissector
    Angell James d.
    blunt hook d.
    bunion d.
    Effler-Groves d.
    Freer d.
    grooved d.
    joker d.
    Kidner d.
    Kocher d.
    Lewin bunion d.
    Marino transsphenoidal d.
    McDonald d.
    Penfield 4 d.
    sesamoidectomy d.
    transphenoidal d.
    West hand d.
disseminata
    osteitis fibrosa d.

disseminated
    d. intravascular coagulation (DIC)
    d. pigmented villonodular synovitis
dissipate
dissociation
    hypnotic d.
    lunotriquetral d.
    d. movement
    radioulnar d.
    scapholunate d.
    scapulothoracic d.
distal
    d. Akin phalangeal osteotomy
    d. articular set angle (DASA)
    d. biceps brachii tendon rupture
    d. bone end
    d. calcaneus
    d. clavicular excision
    d. communicating branch (DCB)
    d. concave articular surface
    d. femoral cutting guide
    d. femoral epiphyseal fracture
    d. femur
    d. fibula
    d. fibulotalar arthrodesis
    d. first metatarsal osteotomy
    d. forearm
    d. fragment
    d. humeral epiphysis
    d. humeral fracture
    d. humerus
    d. intercalated segment instability (DISI)
    d. interlocking
    d. interphalangeal (DIP)
    d. interphalangeal joint (DIPJ)
    d. interphalangeal joint approach
    d. intrinsic release
    d. latency
    d. locking
    d. locking screw
    d. L osteotomy
    d. medial creaking
    d. metaphysis
    d. metatarsal articular angle
    d. neurolysis
    d. oblique sliding osteotomy
    d. palmar crease (DPC)
    d. phalanx (DP)
    d. phocomelia
    d. radial fracture
    d. radioulnar joint (DRUJ)
    d. radioulnar joint prosthesis
    d. radioulnar joint stabilization
    d. radius
    d. realignment
    d. reference axis (DRA)
    d. row carpectomy

d. segment weight
d. soft tissue release (DSTR)
d. targeting
d. targeting device
d. third (D/3, distal/3)
d. third of shaft
d. tibia
d. tibial epiphyseal injury
d. tibiofibular fusion
d. tibiofibular joint
d. transfer
d. tuft
d. ulna
d. ulnar convexity
d. Wagner femoral metaphyseal
  shortening

distal/3
distal third
distally
distalward
distance
conduction d.
coracoclavicular d.
focal film d. (FFD)
fulcrum d.
source image d. (SID)
tube-to-film d.
distension
distolateral
distoocclusal
distortion
multisegmental spinal d.
sacral base d.
structural intersegmental d.
distract
distraction
apical d.
d. arthroplasty
d. bone block arthrodesis
callotasis d.
d. clamp
fixed d.
flexion d.
d. force
d. of fracture
Guhl d.
halo-cast d.
halo-femoral d.
halo-pelvic d.
d. histogenesis
d. hook
d. injury

d. instrumentation
d. instrumentation biomechanics
joint d.
d. lengthening
longitudinal d.
manipulation with d.
Monticelli-Spinelli d.
physeal d.
d. pin
d. rod
d. screw
slow d.
spinal d.
d. technique
d. test
distraction/compression
d./c. bone graft arthrodesis
d./c. scoliosis treatment
distractive
d. extension
d. flexion
d. motion
distractor
Acufex ankle d.
Anderson d.
AO femoral d.
Bliskunov implantable femoral d.
DeBastiani d.
femoral d.
hook d.
Ilizarov d.
joint d.
Kessler metacarpal d.
Mark II distal femur d.
Monticelli-Spinelli d.
Mueller d.
Orthofix M-100 d.
d. pin
Pinto d.
Santa Casa d.
turnbuckle d.
Wagner d.
distribution
Boltzmann d.
cutaneous d.
stress d.
disturbance
articulation d.
disuse atrophy
diurnal
d. change
d. variation in straight leg raising

D

NOTES

divergence
>angle of d.
>anteroposterior talocalcaneal d.

divergent elbow dislocation
diver's disease
diversified
>D. chiropractic manipulative therapy
>d. manipulation
>d.-type force application

diversional activity
diverticulum
>Zenker d.

division
>Swafford-Lichtman d.

divisionary line
divot
Dix-Hallpike maneuver
DJD
>degenerative joint disease

DKB
>deep knee bend

DMA angle
DMARD
>disease-modifying antirheumatologic
>drug

D-Med Injection
DMI orthopaedic bed
DMSO
>dimethyl sulfoxide

DOA
>diagnostic and operative arthroscopy

Doane knee retractor
Doan's
>Extra Strength D.
>D., Original

dobutamine echocardiography
Doctor Collins fracture clamp
documentation
documented pseudarthrosis
Dodd perforator
DOF
>degrees of freedom

dog-ear repair
dogleg fracture
Dolacet
Dolene
dolens
>phlegmasia cerulea d.

dolichostenomelia
doll
>Lizzie d.
>D. trochanteric reattachment
>D. trochanteric reattachment
>technique

dollar
>d. sign
>d. sign side

dollop
>bone d.

Dolobid
Dolophine
Dolorac
dolorimeter
dolorosa
>adiposis d.
>hallux d.

dome
>d. fracture
>Maquet d.
>d. osteotomy
>d. plunger
>d.-shaped osteotomy
>shoulder d.
>talar d.
>weightbearing acetabular d.

dominance
>hand d.
>left-hand d.
>right-hand d.

dominant
>left-hand d.
>right-hand d.

domino spinal instrumentation connector
DOMS
>delayed-onset muscle soreness

Donaghy angled suture needle holder
Donati suture
DonJoy
>D. ALP brace
>D. four-point Super Sport knee
>brace
>D. Gold Point knee brace
>D. wrist splint

donning-doffing skill
donor
>d. site
>d. team

Dooley nail
DOOR syndrome
Doppler
>D. bidirectional test
>D. echocardiography
>D. measurement
>D. pulse evaluation
>D. scope
>D. study
>D. technique
>D. ultrasound flowmeter
>D. ultrasound segmental blood
>pressure testing

Doral
Dormarex 2 Oral
Dormin Oral

Dorrance
- D. hand prosthesis
- D. procedure

Dorr bone classification

dorsal
- d. aspect
- d. bunion
- d. calcaneonavicular ligament
- d. capsule
- d. capsulodesis
- d. carpometacarpal ligament
- d. cheilectomy
- d. closing wedge osteotomy
- d. columella implant
- d. column stimulator (DCS)
- d. column stimulator implant
- d. cross-finger flap
- d. cuboideonavicular ligament
- d. cuneocuboid ligament
- d. cuneonavicular ligament
- d. digital artery (DDA)
- d. drainage
- d. extension block splint
- d. finger approach
- d. glide
- d. hood
- d. intercalary segment instability (DISI)
- d. intercarpal ligament
- d. intercuneiform ligament
- d. interosseous muscle
- d. kyphotic curvature
- d. ligaments of tarsus
- d. linear incision
- d. lithotomy position
- d. longitudinal incision
- d. metacarpal ligament
- d. metatarsal artery
- d. metatarsal ligament
- d. midline approach
- d. neuroma
- d. pedal bypass
- d. perilunate dislocation
- d. point
- d. proximal metatarsal osteotomy
- d. radial slope
- d. radiocarpal ligament
- d. rami
- d. recumbent position
- d. reflex
- d. root entry zone (DREZ)
- d. root ganglion (DRG)
- d. root ganglionectomy
- d. scapular nerve
- d. skin
- d. spine (D-spine)
- d. subcutaneous nerve transposition
- d. synovectomy
- d. tarsometatarsal ligament
- d. tenosynovectomy
- d. translation
- d. transscaphoid perilunar dislocation
- d. transverse capsulotomy
- d. transverse incision
- d. ulnar cutaneous branch
- d. wing
- d. wing fracture
- d. wire-loop fixation
- d. wrist splint with outrigger

dorsale
- ligamentum calcaneonaviculare d.
- ligamentum cuboideonaviculare d.
- ligamentum cuneocuboideum d.
- ligamentum radiocarpale d.

dorsalia
- ligamenta carpometacarpalia d.
- ligamenta cuneonavicularia d.
- ligamenta intercuneiformia d.
- ligamenta metacarpalia d.
- ligamenta metatarsalia d.
- ligamenta tarsi d.
- ligamenta tarsometatarsalia d.

dorsalis
- d. pedis (DP)
- d. pedis artery
- d. pedis artery anatomy
- d. pedis flap
- d. pedis pulse
- tabes d.

dorsal-V osteotomy

dorsalward approach

Dorsey screw-holding screwdriver

dorsi
- elastofibroma d.
- d. jam syndrome
- latissimus d.
- d. stop component

dorsiflexed intercalated segment instability (DISI, DISMAL)

dorsiflexion
- d. bumper
- d.-eversion
- d. flexion

D

NOTES

dorsiflexion *(continued)*
    d. foot splint
    d.-plantar flexion position
    resisted d.
    d. stop brace
dorsiflexor gait
dorsiflexory wedge osteotomy
Dorsiwedge night splint
dorsolateral
    d. approach
    d. and medial capsulotomy
dorsolumbar area
dorsomedial
    d. approach
    d. incision
dorsoplantar
    d. approach
    d. projection
    d. talometatarsal angle
    d. talonavicular angle
    d. view
dorsoradial
    d. approach
    d. ligament (DRL)
dorsorostral approach
dorsoulnar approach
dorsum of hand
Dosepak
    Medrol D.
double
    d.-arc sign
    d. Becker ankle brace
    d. bent Hohmann acetabular
      retractor
    d. binocular operating microscope
    d. camelback sign
    d.-cannula system
    d. Charcot disease
    d.-clamp approximator
    d. Cobra plate
    d.-contrast arthrography
    d. contrast study
    d. crush syndrome
    d. discharge
    D. Duty cane
    D. Duty cane reacher
    d.-flexion knee motion
    d. flexion wave
    d. fracture
    d.-headed stereotactic carrier
    d. hemiplegia
    d. hip spica cast
    d.-hook Lovejoy retractor
    d.-H plate
    d. hump contour
    d. incision
    d.-incision fasciotomy
    d. inflow cannula system

    d.-leg stance phase of gait
    d.-L spinal rod
    d. major curve pattern
    d. major curve scoliosis
    d. major spinal curve
    d.-needle chemonucleolysis
    d.-occlusal splint
    d.-open hook
    d. osteotomy
    d.-pendulum action
    d. portal technique
    d. right-angle suture
    d.-ring frame
    d. simultaneous sensory stimulation
    d.-step gait
    d. support time
    d. thoracic curve
    d. thoracic curve scoliosis
    d.-threaded Herbert screw
    d.-thumb thrust
    d. tourniquet
    d. Zielke instrumentation
double-action
    d.-a. cutter
    d.-a. rongeur
double-ended
    d.-e. nail
    d.-e. right-angle retractor
double-looped
    d.-l. gracilis graft
    d.-l. semitendinous and gracilis
      hamstring graft knee
      reconstruction technique
double-rod
    d.-r. construct
    d.-r. technique
double-stem
    d.-s. implant
    d.-s. silicone lesser MP joint
doublet
double-tap gait
double-upright short leg brace
doughnut
    d. headrest
    d. ring
doughy
    d. cement
    d. consistency
Douglas skin graft
Dow
    D. Corning implant prosthesis
    D. Corning titanium hemi-implant
    D. Corning Wright finger joint
      prosthesis
dowager's hump
dowel
    d. arthrodesis
    bone d.

d. bone graft
d. graft technique
d. grip
d. spinal fusion
threaded cortical d.
doweled
doweling
d. spondylolisthesis
d. spondylolisthesis technique
down
d.-angle hook
D. epiphyseal knife
d. syndrome
downbiting rongeur
Downey
D. hemilaminectomy retractor
D. object recognition test
D. texture discrimination test
Downey-McGlamery procedure
downgoing toe
Downing
D. cartilage knife
D. staple
downsized circular laminar hook
doxepin
doxorubicin
Doyan periosteal elevator
Doyen
D. bone mallet
D. costal rasp
D. cylindrical bur
D. cylindrical drill
D. rib elevator
D. rib rasp
D. spherical bur
Dozier radiolucent Bennett retractor
DP
distal phalanx
dorsalis pedis
D.P.
Dalalone D.P.
DPA
dual-photon absorptiometry
DPC
distal palmar crease
DPD
dual photon densitometry
DPX
dual-photon absorptiometry
Dr
Dr Scholl's Athlete's Foot

Dr Scholl's Maximum Strength
Tritin
Dr.
Dr. Joseph's footbrush
Dr. Kho's CMC Support
DRA
distal reference axis
drafting
overlay d.
Dragstedt skin graft
drag-to gait
drain
Charnley suction d.
Hemovac Hydrocoat d.
Heyer-Schulte wound d.
Jackson-Pratt d.
Nélaton rubber tube d.
open fracture wound d.
Penrose d.
polyethylene d.
PVC d.
rubber d.
Shirley d.
Silastic d.
subcutaneous d.
Surgivac d.
Wound-Evac d.
drainage
anterior d.
anterolateral d.
anteromedial d.
ConstaVac d.
David d.
dorsal d.
elikian d.
ilium d.
incision and d. (I&D)
Klein d.
lateral d.
medial d.
Ober posterior d.
open d.
pelvic d.
posterior d.
posterolateral d.
posteromedial d.
suction d.
draining infected nonunion
DRAM
deepithelialized rectus abdominis muscle
DRAM flap
Dramamine

D

NOTES

drape
  fenestrated d.
  incise d.
  Loban adhesive d.
  3M skin d.
  NeuroDrape surgical d.
  OPMI microscopic d.
  Opraflex d.
  reprep and d.
draped out
drawer
  flexion-rotation-d. (FRD)
  d. sign
  d. test
drawing
  pain d.
  preoperative d.
drawn ankle clonus
Dream
  D. Pillow
  D. Ride car seat
Drennan
  D. metaphyseal-epiphyseal angle
  D. posterior transfer
DressFlex
  D. orthotic
  D. orthotic device
Dressinet netting bandage
dressing
  abdominal d.
  ACU-derm wound d.
  Adaptic d.
  Aeroplast d.
  Alginate d.
  Algisite Alginate wound d.
  Allevyn Island d.
  Allevyn wound d.
  Aquaphor gauze d.
  Arglaes film d.
  Arthrosol d.
  Betadine d.
  Bioclusive select transparent
    film d.
  biologic d.
  Blister Film d.
  Breast Vest EXU-DRY one-piece
    wound d.
  bulky hand d.
  bundle d.
  Bunnell d.
  calcium alginate d.
  CarboFlex odor-control d.
  Cica Care wound d.
  circumferential d.
  Coban elastic d.
  CoFilm d.
  collodion d.

CombiDERM nonadhesive
  absorbent d.
Comfeel Ulcus d.
Compeed protective d.
compression d.
compressive d.
conductive Hydrogel wound d.
Conform d.
ConvaDERM Plus d.
CoolSorb absorbent cold transfer d.
Coraderm d.
cotton d.
Coverlet adhesive surgical d.
Coverlet Strips wound d.
Cover-Roll adhesive gauze d.
Covertell composite secondary d.
Co-Wrap d.
Cryo/Cuff ankle d.
Cutinova cavity d.
Cutinova foam d.
Cutinova thin d.
Dermagran wound d.
Dermiflex d.
Digi Sleeve stockinette d.
dry d.
dry sterile d. (DSD)
DuoDerm d.
Eakin cohesive seal d.
Elastikon d.
Elastomull d.
Elastoplast d.
Ensure-It d.
Epigard d.
Esmarch d.
Exu-Dry wound d.
Fabco gauze d.
figure-of-eight d.
Flexderm wound d.
FLEXIGRID d.
Flexinet d.
fluff d.
Fuller shield d.
Furacin gauze d.
FyBron d.
gauze d.
Geliperm d.
Glasscock ear d.
Granuflex d.
Hydrocol d.
hydrocolloid occlusive d.
Hydrocol wound d.
Hydrogel wound d.
HypaFix wound d.
immediate postoperative
  prosthesis d.
Inerpan flexible burn d.
Intact d.
Intrasite d.

J&J Ulcer d.
Jones d.
Kaltostat d.
Kelikian foot d.
Kerlix d.
Kling adhesive d.
Koch-Mason d.
Kollagen d.
LYOfoam C d.
LYOfoam wound d.
Medi-Rip d.
Microfoam d.
Mills d.
modified Robert Jones d.
Mother Jones d.
neoprene d.
nonadherent gauze d.
N-Terface d.
Nu Gauze d.
occlusive d.
O'Donoghue d.
Omniderm d.
Opraflex d.
OpSite wound d.
Orthoflex d.
Orthoplast d.
OsmoCyte Island wound-care d.
Owen gauze d.
palm-to-axilla d.
Panogauze Hydrogel wound d.
patch d.
pledget d.
PolyMem wound-care d.
Polyskin d.
PolyWic d.
pressure d.
Primaderm d.
Primapore wound d.
ProCyte transparent d.
Profore wound d.
PVD d.
RepliCare wound d.
Reston d.
Restore CalciCare d.
rigid d.
Robert Jones d.
Schanz d.
Scherisorb d.
Setopress d.
SignaDRESS hydrocolloid d.
Silastic gel d.
silk mesh gauze d.

SkinTemp collagen skin d.
sling d.
Sof-Rol d.
soft bulky d.
Sof-Wick d.
Spenco Second Skin d.
stent d.
sterile dry d. (SDD)
d. stick
Stimson d.
SuperSkin thin film d.
Surgilast tubular elastic d.
Synthaderm d.
Tegaderm d.
Telfa gauze d.
THINSite d.
toe-to-groin modified Jones d.
Tricodur Epi compression d.
Tricodur Omos compression d.
Tricodur Talus compression d.
Tubex gauze d.
Tubigrip d.
Ultec thin d.
Uniflex d.
Velpeau d.
Vi-Drape d.
Vigilon d.
Webril d.
wet-to-dry d.
wide-mesh petroleum gauze d.
Xeroform gauze d.

Dreyer formula
Dreyfus
    D. prosthesis forceps
    D. prosthesis placement instrument
DREZ
    dorsal root entry zone
    DREZ lesion
    DREZ modification of Eriksson
      technique
DRG
    dorsal root ganglion
Driessen hinged plate
drift
    congenital ulnar d.
    osseous d.
    pronator d.
    radial d.
    ulnar d.
drill
    ACL d.
    Acra-Cut wire pass d.

D

NOTES

175

drill *(continued)*
Acufex d.
Adson-Rogers perforating d.
Adson spiral d.
Adson twist d.
Aesculap d.
agility d.
air d.
air-powered cutting d.
Albee d.
Amico d.
Anspach power d.
anticavitation d.
Archimedean d.
ASIF twist d.
ASSI wire-pass d.
autotome d.
Bailey d.
bar d.
battery-driven hand d.
biflanged d.
bit d.
d. bit
Björk rib d.
bone hand d.
Bosworth crown d.
Bowen suture d.
Brunswick-Mack rotating d.
Bunnell bone d.
Bunnell hand d.
bur d.
cannulated cortical step d.
Carmody perforator d.
Carroll-Bunnell d.
Cebotome d.
Cement Eater d.
centering d.
cervical d.
Championnière bone d.
Charnley centering d.
Charnley femoral condyle d.
Charnley pilot d.
Charnley starting d.
Cherry d.
Cherry-Austin d.
Children's Hospital hand d.
chuck d.
Cloward cervical d.
Coballoy twist d.
Codman wire-passing d.
Collison body d.
Collison cannulated hand d.
Collison tap d.
cortical step d.
crown d.
Crutchfield bone d.
Crutchfield hand d.
Crutchfield-Raney d.

CurvTek TSR bone d.
Cushing flat d.
Cushing perforator d.
dental d.
depth-check d.
DePuy d.
D'Errico perforating d.
D'Errico perforator d.
Deyerle d.
diamond high-speed d.
Doyen cylindrical d.
driver nail d.
Elan d.
Elan-E power d.
extractor nail d.
fingernail d.
Fisch d.
flat d.
Galt hand d.
Gates-Glidden d.
glenoid d.
Gray bone d.
d. guard
d. guide
d. guide forceps
Hall air d.
Hall-Dundar d.
Hall Micro-Aire d.
Hall power d.
Hall step-down d.
Hall Versipower d.
Hamby twist d.
hand d.
hand-operated d.
Harold Crowe d.
Harris-Smith anterior interbody d.
Hewson d.
high-speed twist d.
d. hole
hollow mill d.
Hudson bone d.
initiator d.
intramedullary d.
Jacobs chuck d.
d. jig
Jordan-Day d.
Kerr electro-torque d.
Kerr hand d.
Kirschner bone d.
Kirschner wire d.
Kodex d.
Küntscher d.
Lentulo spiral d.
Loth-Kirschner d.
Luck bone d.
Lusskin bone d.
Macewen d.
Magnuson twist d.

Mathews hand d.
Mathews load d.
McKenzie bone d.
McKenzie perforating twist d.
Michelson-Sequoia air d.
Micro-Aire d.
Midas Rex d.
mini-Stryker power d.
Minos air d.
Mira d.
Modny d.
Moore bone d.
nail d.
Neil-Moore perforator d.
Neurain d.
Neurairtome d.
nippers nail d.
Orthairtome II d.
orthopaedic surgical d.
orthopaedic Universal d.
Osseodent surgical d.
Osteone air d.
Patrick d.
Pease bone d.
pencil-tip d.
penetrating d.
Penn finger d.
perforating twist d.
perforator d.
pilot d.
d. pin
pistol-grip hand d.
d. point
Portmann d.
power d.
pronator d.
Ralks bone d.
Ralks fingernail d.
Raney bone d.
Raney perforator d.
retention d.
rib d.
Rica bone d.
Richards Lovejoy bone d.
Richards pistol-grip d.
Richmond subarachnoid twist d.
Richter bone d.
right-angle dental d.
scissors nail d.
Shea d.
Sherman-Stille d.
Sklar bone d.

d. sleeve
Smedberg hand d.
Smedberg twist d.
SMIC sternal d.
Smith d.
spiral d.
spiral or twist d.
Spirec d.
step d.
step-down d.
Stille bone d.
Stille hand d.
Stille-Sherman bone d.
Stiwer hand d.
Stryker d.
Surgairtome air d.
surgical-orthopaedic d.
suture hole d.
Synthes d.
tap d.
Thornwald antral d.
d.-tipped guidewire
Toti trephine d.
Treace stapes d.
trephine d.
Trinkle bone d.
Trinkle power d.
Trinkle Super-Cut twist d.
Trowbridge-Campau bone d.
Trowbridge triple-speed d.
twist d.
Ullrich drill-guard d.
Uniflex calibrated step d.
union broach retention d.
Universal two-speed hand d.
Vitallium d.
Warren-Mack rotating d.
wire d.
Wolferman d.
Wullstein d.
Xomed d.
Zimalate twist d.
Zimmer hand d.
Zimmer-Kirschner hand d.
Zimmer Universal d.
drill-guide
Acufex d.-g.
drilling
d. broach
d. jig
d. technique

D

NOTES

drill point
    cannulated d. p.
    carbon steel d. p.
D-ring strap
drip-tube feeding
Drisdol Oral
drive
    Jacobs chuck d.
    worm d.
drive-extractor
driver
    blade plate d.
    bullet d.
    Eby band d.
    femoral head d.
    Flatt d.
    graft d.
    Hall d.
    Harrington hook d.
    Jewett d.
    Ken d.
    Kirschner wire d.
    Küntscher nail d.
    K-wire d.
    Linvatec d.
    Lloyd nail d.
    Massie d.
    Maxi-Driver d.
    McNutt d.
    McReynolds d.
    Micro Series wire d.
    Milewski d.
    Moore d.
    Moore-Blount d.
    nail d.
    d. nail drill
    Neufeld d.
    Nystroem nail d.
    Nystroem-Stille d.
    Orthoairtome wire d.
    ParaMax angled d.
    polyethylene-faced d.
    prosthesis d.
    Pugh d.
    Put-In D.
    Rush d.
    Sage d.
    Schneider nail d.
    Sharbaro d.
    staple d.
    supine position d.
    surgical pin d.
    Sven-Johansson d.
    Teflon-coated d.
    tibial d.
    trial d.
    d. tunnel locator apparatus

    wire d.
    Zimmer Orthair ream d.
driver-bender-extractor
    Rush d.-b.-e.
driver-extractor
    Hansen-Street d.-e.
    Ken d.-e.
    McReynolds d.-e.
    Sage d.-e.
    Schneider d.-e.
    Zimmer d.-e.
drivethrough sign
DRL
    dorsoradial ligament
dromedary gait
droopy shoulder syndrome
drop
    foot d.
    wrist d.
    d. wrist splint
drop-arm
    d.-a. sign
    d.-a. test
drop-entry (closed body) hook
droperidol and fentanyl
drop-foot
    d.-f. brace
    d.-f. gait
    d.-f. redression stockings
    d.-f. splint
drop-lock
    d.-l. knee brace
    d.-l. ring
dropped foot
drug
    antiplatelet d.
    antituberculosis d.
    cytotoxic d.
    depolarizing d.
    disease-modifying
      antirheumatologic d. (DMARD)
    d.-induced myotonia
    plasmapheresis d.
    slow-acting antirheumatic d.
      (SAARD)
DRUJ
    distal radioulnar joint
    DRUJ instability
    DRUJ prosthesis
drummer-boy palsy
Drummond
    D. button
    D. hook
    D. hook holder
    D. spinal instrumentation
    D. spinous wiring technique
    D. wire
    D. wire technique

drunken sailor gait
dry
    d. dressing
    D. Flotation wheelchair cushion
    d. gangrene
    d. hydrotherapy
    d. infected nonunion
    d. sterile dressing (DSD)
Drysol
Dryspell cast cover
DS
    Tolectin D.
DSA
    digital subtraction angiography
DSC
    Dead Sea Cosmeceuticals
    DSC Foot Cream
    Parafon Forte DSC
DSD
    dry sterile dressing
DSIS orthotic
D-Soles
    D.-S. insole
    D.-S. orthotic
D-spine
    dorsal spine
DSTR
    distal soft tissue release
DTR
    deep tendon reflex
DTT
    device for transverse traction
    DTT implant
    DTT system
dual
    d. (bypass) connector
    d. compression scoliosis treatment
    d. drop pelvic (DDP)
    d.-energy x-ray absorptiometry (DXA)
    d.-lock total hip prosthesis
    d. nerve root suction retractor
    d.-onlay cortical bone graft
    d.-photon absorptiometry (DPA, DPX)
    d. photon densitometry (DPD)
    d. photon densitometry test
    d. photon densitometry test for osteoporosis
    d.-photon electrospinal orthosis
    d. plate

    D. Range Limiter System
    d. square-ended Harrington rod
Duall #88 cement
Dubreuilh
    D. melanosis circumscripta
    melanosis circumscripta preblastomatosis of D.
Duchenne
    D. disease
    D. muscular atrophy
    D. muscular dystrophy
duckbill rongeur
duck waddle
    d. w. gait
    d. w. test
duct
    thoracic d.
ductility
Dudley J. Morton foot configuration
Dugas test
dull aching pain
dumbbell
    d. tumor
    d. wagon
Dumon-Gilliard prosthesis introducer
Duncan
    D. loop
    D. prone rectus test
    D. shoulder brace
Duncan-Lovell modification
Dunlop-Shands view
Dunlop traction
Dunn
    D. biopsy
    D. fracture device
    D. hip operation
    D. multiple comparison test
    D. osteotomy
    D. technique
    D. triple arthrodesis
Dunn-Brittain
    D.-B. foot stabilization
    D.-B. foot stabilization technique
    D.-B. triple arthrodesis
Dunn-Hess trochanteric osteotomy
DuoCet
Duo-Cline Dual Support contoured bed wedge
Duocondylar knee prosthesis
duodenal compression
DuoDerm dressing
Duo-Drive screw

NOTES

Duofilm Solution
Duo-Lock hip prosthesis
Duo-Patellar knee prosthesis
Duopress
    D. guide
    D. plate
Dupaco
    D. knee control
    D. knee prosthesis
Duplay disease
duplex
    d. Doppler ultrasonography
    d. ultrasound
duplicate
    d. sternum
    d. thumb
duplication
    Marks-Bayne technique for
       thumb d.
    symmetric thumb d.
    thumb d.
    Wassel type IV thumb d.
duPont Bunion Rating Score
Dupont distal humeral plate system
Dupuytren
    D. contracture
    D. contracture release
    D. diathesis
    D. disease
    D. exostosis
    D. fasciitis
    D. fracture
    D. sign
    D. splint
dura
    d. mater
    d. mater graft
Duracon
    D. knee implant
    D. prosthesis
    D. total knee replacement system
Duract
Duragesic Transdermal
Dura-Kold reusable compression ice wrap
dural
    d. ectasia
    d. ligament
    d. repair
Duraleve custom molded foot orthotic
Durallium implant
Duraloc
    D. acetabular cup system
    D. acetabular liner
Duralone Injection
Duramer polyethylene component
Duramorph Injection
Duran approach

Duran-Houser
    D.-H. protocol
    D.-H. wrist splint
Durapatite
    D. bone
    D. bone replacement material
    D. implant
DuraPrep
Dura-Soft soft-compression reusable ice or heat wrap
Dura-Stick adhesive electrode
Duraval Hook & Loop strap material
Duray-Reed gouge
Durham
    D. flatfoot
    D. flatfoot operation
    D. plasty
Durkan
    D. carpal compression test
    D. CTS gauge
durometer
durum
    heloma d. (HD)
dust
    nail d.
Dutchman's roll
duToit-Roux
    d.-R. arthroplasty
    d.-R. staple capsulorrhaphy
duToit shoulder staple
Duverney fracture
DuVries
    D. approach
    D. arthroplasty
    D. deltoid ligament reconstruction
       technique
    D. hammertoe repair
    D. incision
    D. modified McBride hallux valgus
       operation
    D. phalangeal condylectomy
    D. plantar condylectomy
    D. procedure
    D. technique for overlapping toe
DuVries-Mann modified bunionectomy
DVI
    deep vein insufficiency
Dvorak test
DVT
    deep vein thrombosis
    deep venous thrombosis
    Flowtron DVT
    DVT prophylaxis
Dwar-Barrington resection
dwarfism
    achondroplastic d.
    chondroplastic d.
    diastrophic d.

Laron d.
Russell-Silver d.
Dwyer
D. calcaneal osteotomy
D. clawfoot operation
D. correction of scoliosis
D. device
D. incision
D. instrumentation biomechanics
D. procedure
D. scoliosis cable
D. spinal instrumentation
D. spinal mechanical stapler
D. spinal screw
D. tensioner
Dwyer-Hall plate
Dwyer-Wickham electrical stimulation system
dx
diagnosis
DXA
dual-energy x-ray absorptiometry
Dycal base
Dycem roll matting
Dycill
Dyck-Lambert classification
Dycor prosthetic foot
dye
methylene blue d.
d. punch injury
Dyke-Davidoff-Masson syndrome
DynaDisc exercise equipment
DYNAfabric material
Dynafed IB
DynaFix external fixation system
DynaFlex Gyro exerciser
Dyna-Flex multilayer compression system
DynaGraft implant
Dynagrip
D. blade handle
D. handle of blade
DynaHeat hot pack
Dyna-Hex Topical
Dyna knee splint
DynaLator ultrasound unit
Dyna-Lok
D.-L. pedicle screw system
D.-L. plate system
D.-L. plating system
dynametric testing

dynamic
d. abduction brace
d. alignment
d. axial fixator (DAF)
d. balance
d. compression (DC)
d. compression plate (DCP)
d. compression plate fixation
d. compression plate instrumentation
D. condylar screw (DCS)
d. condylar screw fixation
d. condylar screw tap
D. digit extensor tube
d. double tendon replacement
D. elbow orthosis
d. electromyography
d. fault
D. foot stabilizer
d. hallux varus
d. integrated stabilization chair (DISC)
d. joint force
D. knee orthosis
d. listing
d. listing nomenclature
d. locking nail
d. lumbar stabilization
d. magnetic resonance imaging
d. metatarsus adductus
d. movement
d. MRI
d. muscle transfer
d. repair
d. splint
d. splinting
d. stabilizing innersole system
d. stump exercise
d. traction method
d. transverse traction device
d. trunk curl
D. wrist orthosis
dynamization
dynamometer
Baseline d.
Biodex isokinetic d.
bulb d.
Chiroslide Jamar Hand D.
Collins d.
computerized isokinetic d.
Cybex II isokinetic d.
electromechanical d.
hand grip d.

NOTES

D

dynamometer *(continued)*
    handheld d. (HHD)
    Harpenden d.
    Isobex d.
    Jamar hydraulic hand d.
    KinCom electromechanical d.
    Lido isokinetic d.
    orthopaedic d.
    Smedley d.
    Spark handheld d.
dynamometry
    isokinetic d.
    tip-pinch d.
DynaPak electrode kit
Dynapen
Dynaphor iontophoresis
Dynaplex knee prosthesis
DynaPrene splinting thermoplastic
Dynatron
    D. 50, 125, 525 electrotherapy
    D. Mini 2000 electrotherapy
    D. 2000 muscle test
    D. TX 900 electrotherapy
    D. 150 ultrasound
DynaWraps
dyne
dynometer
dynorphin
DyoCam
    D. 550 arthroscopic video camera
    D. arthroscopic view camera
Dyonic arthroscopic instrument
Dyonics
    D. arthroplasty bur
    D. arthroscope
    D. arthroscopic blade
    D. cannula
    D. Golden Retriever magnet
    D. shaver
dysarthria
    lingual d.
    spinal d.
dysarthric lesion
dysarthrosis
    patellofemoral d.
dysautonomia
    familial d.
dysbaric
    d. osteonecrosis
    d. oxygen
dyschondroplasia
dyscollagenosis
dyscrasic fracture
dyscratic
dysdiadochokinesia
dysesthesia
dysfunction
    anterior-inferior capsular ligament d.

craniomandibular d.
extensor mechanism d.
facet joint d.
flexor hallucis longus d. (FHLD)
joint d.
kidney d.
mechanical d.
motor d.
neuroarticular d.
painful minor intervertebral d.
  (PMID)
patellofemoral d.
pilomotor d.
posttraumatic sacroiliac d.
segmental d.
somatic d.
dysgenesis
    alar d.
    epiphyseal d.
dyshidrosis, dyshydrosis
dyskeratosis congenita
dyskinesia
    positional d.
    poststatic d. (PSDK)
    retrolisthesis positional d.
dyskinetic cerebral palsy
dyskinsia
dysmetria
dysostosis
    cleidocranial d.
    Jansen metaphyseal d.
    Schmid metaphyseal d.
    Spahr metaphyseal d.
dysplasia
    acropectorovertebral d.
    bony d.
    cleidocranial d.
    congenital hip d.
    congenital hyperphosphatasemic
      skeletal d. (CHSD)
    cortical fibrous d.
    Crowe congenital hip d. (type
      I–IV)
    developmental d.
    diaphyseal d.
    diastrophic d.
    epiarticular osteochondromatous d.
    epiphyseal d.
    d. epiphysealis hemimelia
    femoral head d.
    fibrous d.
    d. of hip
    Holt-Oram atriodigital d.
    intracortical fibrous d.
    Meyer d.
    Mondini d.
    monostotic fibrous d.
    multiple epiphyseal d.

Namaqualand hip d.
oculoauriculovertebral d.
osteofibrous d.
patellofemoral d.
polyostotic fibrous d.
progressive diaphyseal d.
rhizomesomelic bone d.
Sponastrine d.
spondyloepiphyseal d.
Streeter d.
vertebral (defects), (imperforate)
  anus, tracheoesophageal (fistula),
  radial and renal (d.) (VATER)

dysplastic
d. acetabulum
d. fibula
d. nevus syndrome
d. spondylolisthesis

dysponetic
dysraphism
spinal d.

dystaxia
dystonia
focal d.
d. musculorum deformans

dystopia
shoulder d.

dystrophic
d. gait

d. nail
d. toenail

Dystrophile exercise unit
dystrophy
Becker muscular d. (BMD)
Becker variant of Duchenne d.
congenital d.
Duchenne muscular d.
Erb muscular d.
fascioscapulohumeral d.
Fröhlich adiposogenital d.
Gowers muscular d.
humeroperoneal muscular d.
juvenile muscular d.
Kiloh-Nevin ocular form of
  progressive muscular d.
limb-girdle d.
muscular d. (MD)
myotonic muscular d.
osseous d.
posttraumatic d.
progressive muscular d. (PMD)
reflex neurovascular d.
reflex sympathetic d. (RSD)
sex-linked muscular d.
sympathetic d.
sympathetic reflex d.

dysvascular condition

D

NOTES

EACS
exertional anterior compartment
syndrome
Eagle
E. straight-ahead arthroscope
E. syndrome
Eagle-Barrett syndrome
Eakin cohesive seal dressing
Earle sign
EARLY
ergonomic assessment of risk and
liability
Early Fit night splint
E-A-R specialty composite
earth electrode
EAS
endoskeletal alignment system
Easebak lumbar support cushion
Easprin
EAST
external rotation-abduction stress test
Easton cock-up splint
East-West retractor
Eastwood technique
Easy
E. Access foot splint
E. Lok ankle brace
E. Up cushion
Easy-On elbow brace
EasyStep pressure relief walker
eater
Anspach Cement E.
Cement E.
Zimmer Cibatome cement e.
Eaton
E. closed reduction
E. CMC arthrosis (stages I–IV)
E. implant arthroplasty
E. splint
E. trapezium finger joint
replacement prosthesis
E. volar plate arthroplasty
Eaton-Lambert syndrome
Eaton-Littler
E.-L. ligament reconstruction
E.-L. technique
Eaton-Malerich
E.-M. fracture-dislocation operation
E.-M. fracture-dislocation technique
E.-M. reduction
Eberle
E. contracture release
E. contracture release technique
EBI
electronic bone stimulation

EBI device
EBI external fixator
EBI Medical OsteoGen bone
growth stimulator
EBI Medical Systems bone healing
system
EBI Medical Systems Orthofix
fixation system
EBI Temptek blanket
EBIce
eburnate
eburnated bone
eburnation
bony e.
e. of cartilage
Eby band driver
eccentric
e. axis of ankle rotation
e. axis of rotation of the ankle
e. contraction
e. drill guide
e. dynamic compression plate
(EDCP)
e. exercise
e. function
e. loading
e. work
ecchondroma
ecchondrotome
ecchymosis
eccrine
e. poroma
e. sweat gland
ECG
electrocardiogram
echinococcosis
Echlin
E. duckbill rongeur
E. rongeur forceps
echo
e. time (TE)
e. train length (ETL)
echocardiography
dobutamine e.
Doppler e.
M-mode transesophageal e.
transesophageal e. (TEE)
transthoracic e. (TTE)
echography
color Doppler e.
Ecker-Lotke-Glazer
E.-L.-G. patellar tendon repair
E.-L.-G. tendon reconstruction
E.-L.-G. tendon reconstruction
technique

E

Eckert-Davis classification
Eclipse
    E. Gel ankle brace
    E. Gel elbow strap
    E. TENS unit
EC-Naprosyn
econazole
#405 Econo 90 Basic
Econo-Strap
Econo 90 traction unit
Ecotrin
    E. Low Adult Strength
E Cotton bandage
ECRB
    extensor carpi radialis brevis
        ECRB muscle
        ECRB tendon
ECRL
    extensor carpi radialis longus
        ECRL muscle
        ECRL tendon
ECT
    European compression technique
        ECT bone screw
        ECT internal fracture fixation
ectasia
    dural e.
ectomesomorphic physique
ectomorph
ectomorphic physique
ectopic
    e. bone
    e. ossification
ECTR
    endoscopic carpal tunnel release
ECTRA
    endoscopic carpal tunnel release
        ECTRA carpal tunnel instruments
        ECTRA system
Ectra
ECU
    European Chiropractic Union
    extensor carpi ulnaris
ED
    elbow disarticulation
EDB
    extensor digitorum brevis
        EDB muscle
        EDB tendon
EDC
    extensor digitorum communis
EDCP
    eccentric dynamic compression plate
edema
    dependent e.
    intracompartmental e.
    mushy e.
    nonpitting e.

    pitting e.
    posttraumatic e.
    pretibial e.
    pulmonary e.
    e. sock
    stump e.
edematous
Eden-Hybbinette
    E.-H. arthroplasty
    E.-H. procedure
Eden-Lange procedure
Eden test
Eder-Puestow metal olive dilator
EDF scoliosis cast
EDG
    electrodynogram
    EDG system
Edgarton-Grand thumb adduction
edge
    Acufex E.
    Factor Eleven: The E.
    E. knee brace
    patellar e.
edge-detection
    digital e.-d.
Edinger-Westphal complex
EDit
    electric differential therapy
EDL
    extensor digitorum longus
EDM
    extensor digiti minimi
Edna towel clamp
EDPCS
    exertional deep posterior compartment
      syndrome
EDQ
    extensor digiti quinti
EDS
    Ehlers-Danlos syndrome
education
    lifestyle e. (LSE)
Edwards
    E. D-L modular fixator
    E. hook
    E. instrumentation
    E. modular system
    E. modular system bridging sleeve
      construct
    E. modular system compression
      construct
    E. modular system construct
      selection
    E. modular system distraction-
      lordosis construct
    E. modular system dynamic
      loading

E. modular system kyphoreduction
construct

E. modular system load sharing

E. modular system neutralization
construct

E. modular system rod crosslink

E. modular system rod sleeve
construct

E. modular system sacral fixation
device

E. modular system scoliosis
construct

E. modular system spinal rod-
sleeve

E. modular system spinal/sacral
screw

E. modular system spondylo
construct

E. modular system standard sleeve
construct

E. modular system Universal rod

E. polyethylene sleeve

E. procedure

E. seamless prosthesis

E. syndrome

Edwards-Levine

E.-L. hook

E.-L. rod

E.-L. sleeve

Edwin Smith papyrus

EDX, EDx

electrodiagnosis

EEA

end-to-end anastomosis

EEA stapler

EEMA

epithelial membrane antigen

effect

anticholinergic e.

antinociceptive e.

copper wire e.

neurophysiologic e.

rake-handle e.

spindle e.

steal e.

Steindler e.

tenodesis e.

tethering e.

efferent nerve impulse

efficacy

Effler-Groves

E.-G. dissector

E.-G. hook

effleurage massage

effort

brief maximal e. (BME)

effusion

bloody e.

joint e.

pleural e.

Efodine

Eftekhar

E. broken femoral stem technique

E. concept

Eftekhar-Charnley hip prosthesis

Egawa sign

Eggers

E. bone plate

E. contact splint

E. neurectomy

E. screw

E. tendon transfer technique

E. tenodesis

E. transfer

Eggsercizer resistive hand exerciser

EHL

extensor hallucis longus

EHL tendon

Ehlers-Danlos syndrome (EDS)

Ehrenfeld disease

EI

external ilium

Eicher

E. femoral prosthesis

E. hip prosthesis

eicosanoid

eighty-nine-newton test

Eikenella corrodens

**Eilers-Armstrong unicompartmental knee
prosthesis**

EIP

extensor indicis proprius

EJ

elbow jerk

Ekbom restless leg syndrome

**El-Ahwany classification of humeral
supracondylar fracture**

Elan drill

Elan-E power drill

Elase-Chloromycetin

E.-C. ointment

E.-C. Topical

E

NOTES

Elase Topical
Elastafit tubing kit
ElastaTrac
    E. home lumbar traction system
    E. home lumbar traction unit
elastic
    e. ankle corset
    e. barrier
    e. compression
    e. deformation
    E. Foam bandage
    e.-hinge knee brace
    e. knee cage orthosis
    e. limit
    e. plaster-of-Paris
    e. property
    e. stable intramedullary nail (ESIN)
    e. stable intramedullary nailing
      (ESIN)
    e. stockings
    e. strain
    e. stretch
    e. traction
    e. twister orthosis
    e. zone
elasticity
    modulus of e.
Elastikon
    E. dressing
    E. tape
elastofibroma dorsi
Elasto-Gel
    E.-G. hot/cold wrap
    E.-G. shoulder therapy wrap
elastoidosis
Elasto-Link joint wrap
elastoma
elastomer
    conventional silicone e. (CSE)
    high performance silicone e.
    medical e. X7-2320
    polyolefin e.
    e. skin molding
    thermoplastic e. (TPE)
Elastomull
    E. dressing
    E. elastic gauze bandage
Elastoplast
    E. bandage
    E. dressing
elastosis
Elavil
elbow
    above e.
    e. arthroplasty
    axilla, shoulder, e. (ASE)
    baseball pitcher's e.
    boxer's e.

    e. capsule
    e. cast
    compound shattered e.
    e. disarticulation (ED)
    e. dislocation
    epicondylitis of the e.
    e. extension splint
    e. extensor tendon
    fat pad of e.
    e. flexion splint
    e. flexion test
    floating e.
    e. fracture
    Frohse arcade of the e.
    golfer's e.
    e. hinge
    e. injury
    javelin thrower's e.
    e. jerk (EJ)
    e. jerk reflex test
    e. magnet
    milkmaid's e.
    e. orthosis (EO)
    e. pad
    e. prosthesis
    pulled e.
    e. radiography
    e. reflex
    reverse tennis e.
    e. sleeve
    slipped e.
    e. stability
    supermarket e.
    temper tantrum e.
    tennis e.
    thrower's e.
    varus/valgus stress of the e.
    Wilson procedure for extraarticular
      fusion of e.
    wrestler's e.
elbow-wrist-hand orthosis (EWHO)
Elderberry Sambu Internal Cleansing
    Program
electric
    e. artifact
    e. cast saw
    e. differential therapy (EDit)
electrical
    e. bone-growth stimulator
    e. burn
    e. implant
    e. inactivity
    e. injury
    e. modality
    e. nerve stimulation
    e. potential
    e. silence
    e. stimulation therapy

e. stimulator waveform
e. surface stimulation
e. surface stimulation treatment for
  scoliosis
Electri-Cool
  E.-C. cold therapy system
  E.-C. continuous controlled cold
    therapy
electroacupuncture
Electro-Acuscope 85 stimulator
electrocardiogram (ECG)
electrocardiographic recording device
electrocardiography
electrocautery
  e. apparatus
  Aspen e.
electrocoagulated
electrocoagulation
electrode
  active e.
  bifilar needle recording e.
  BioKnit garment e.
  bipolar needle recording e.
  bipolar stimulating e.
  coaxial needle e.
  concentric needle e.
  Disposatrode disposable e.
  Dura-Stick adhesive e.
  earth e.
  Electro-Mesh e.
  Excel Plus e.
  exploring e.
  e. glove
  ground e.
  indifferent e.
  iontophoresis e.
  LSI Easy Stims self-adhesive e.
  LSI silver self-adhesive
    disposable e.
  macro-EMG needle e.
  microcurrent e.
  monopolar needle recording e.
  multilead e.
  needle e.
  Prizm Electro-Mesh Sock e.
  recording e.
  reference e.
  single fiber needle e.
  e. sock
  stigmatic e.
  stimulating e.

surface e.
Teq-Trode e.
Ultra Stim silver e.
unipolar needle e.
Versa-Stim self-adhering e.
electrodesiccated bleeding point
electrodiagnosis (EDX, EDx)
**Electro-Diagnostic Instruments Model
  720 Bilateral Tetrapolar**
electrodiagnostic medicine
electrodynogram (EDG)
electroencephalography
  computerized e. (CEEG)
electrogoniometer
  Ankle-Foot Elgon e.
  parallelogram e.
  six-degrees-of-freedom e.
electrokinetic potential
Electro-Link joint wrap
electrolyte
  e. balance
  e. replacement
electromagnet
  spring-mounted e.
electromechanical dynamometer
Electro-Mesh
  E.-M. electrode
  E.-M. sleeve
electromyocardiography
  cervical Derifield procedure   e.
electromyogram (EMG)
electromyography (EMG)
  central e.
  dynamic e.
  integrated e.
  single fiber e. (SFEMG)
  surface e. (sEMG)
electron beam therapy
electroneuromyography (ENMG)
electroneurophysiologic
electronic
  e. bone stimulation (EBI)
  e. bone stimulation apparatus
  e. goniometer
Electronics electrical stimulation device
electronystagmography (ENG)
**electrostimulation for nonunion of
  fracture**
electrosurgical
  e. generator

E

NOTES

electrosurgical *(continued)*
    e. instrument
    e. pencil
electrotherapeutic point stimulation (ETPS)
electrotherapy
    Dynatron 50, 125, 525 e.
    Dynatron Mini 2000 e.
    Dynatron TX 900 e.
    Mettler e.
    PET e.
    e. system (ES)
    ultrasound e.
Elekta stereotactic head frame
element
    neural e.
    posterior e.
elementary fracture
elephant-ear clavicular splint
elephant-foot
    e.-f. callus
    e.-f. fracture nonunion
elevated rim acetabular liner
elevation
    congenital scapular e.
    e. exercise
    e. of extremity
    protection, restricted activity, ice, compression, e. (PRICE)
    rest, ice, compression, e. (RICE)
    scapular e.
elevator
    Adson periosteal e.
    Alexander periosteal e.
    Aufranc periosteal e.
    Bennet bone e.
    Bennett e.
    Bethune periosteal e.
    Blair e.
    Bowen periosteal e.
    Bristow periosteal e.
    Brophy periosteal e.
    Buck periosteal e.
    Cameron-Haight periosteal e.
    Campbell periosteal e.
    Carroll-Legg periosteal e.
    Chandler bone e.
    Cheyne periosteal e.
    chisel-edge e.
    Cloward osteophyte e.
    Cloward periosteal e.
    Cobb periosteal e.
    Cohen periosteal e.
    Converse periosteal e.
    Coryllos-Doyen periosteal e.
    Cottle-MacKenty e.
    Crego e.
    curved periosteal e.

Cushing-Hopkins periosteal e.
Darrach periosteal e.
Davidson-Sauerbruch-Doyen periosteal e.
Dawson-Yuhl-Key e.
Dawson-Yuhl periosteal e.
Doyan periosteal e.
Doyen rib e.
Farabeuf periosteal e.
Fomon periosteal e.
fracture reducing e.
Freer periosteal e.
Freer septal e.
Gardner e.
Harrington spinal e.
Henahan e.
Herczel rib e.
Hibbs chisel e.
Hoen periosteal e.
Iowa University periosteal e.
Jannetta duckbill e.
joker periosteal e.
Joseph periosteal e.
J-periosteal e.
Kahre-Williger periosteal e.
Kennerdell-Maroon e.
Key periosteal e.
Kirmission periosteal e.
Kocher e.
Lambotte e.
lamina e.
Lane periosteal e.
Langenbeck periosteal e.
Lempert periosteal e.
Lewis periosteal e.
Locke e.
Love-Adson periosteal e.
lumbosacral fusion e.
Malis e.
Matson-Alexander rib e.
Matson periosteal e.
Matson rib e.
McClamary e.
McGlamry e.
Mead periosteal e.
Molt periosteal e.
Moore bone e.
nasal e.
orthopaedic shoulder e.
OSI extremity e.
osteophyte e.
Penfield periosteal e.
periosteal e.
Phemister e.
Presbyterian Hospital staphylorrhaphy e.
Ray-Parsons-Sunday staphylorrhaphy e.

Rhoton e.
rib e.
Roberts-Gill periosteal e.
Rochester lamina e.
Rochester spinal e.
Rolyan arm e.
Rosen e.
Sauerbruch rib e.
Sayre e.
Scott-McCracken periosteal e.
Sebileau periosteal e.
Sedillot periosteal e.
Sheffield hand e.
Sisson fracture reducing e.
staphylorrhaphy e.
straight periosteal e.
Sunday staphylorrhaphy e.
Swanson e.
Tegtmeier e.
Tenzel e.
T handle e.
Tronzo e.
von Langenbeck periosteal e.
Ward periosteal e.
Wiberg periosteal e.
wide periosteal e.
Willauer-Gibbon periosteal e.
Williger periosteal e.
Woodson e.
Yankauer periosteal e.
Yasargil e.

elevator-dissector
Freer e.-d.

elevator-periosteotome

elevatus
e. deformity
hallux e.
iatrogenic e.
metatarsus e.
metatarsus primus e.

Eligoy metal alloy
Elihorn Maze Test
elikian drainage
ELISA
enzyme-linked immunosorbent assay
Elite
E. Farley retractor for spinal
surgery
E. hip system
E. knee brace
E. posterior adjustable stop
E. posterior spring assist

Elizabethtown osteotomy
Elliott femoral condyle blade plate
ellipsoid joint
elliptical
e. incision
e. machine
e. overlap shadow
Ellis
E. classification
E. Jones peroneal tendon operation
E. skin traction technique
E. technique for Barton fracture
Ellis-Jones
E.-J. peroneal tendon displacement
E.-J. peroneal tendon technique
Ellison
E. fixation staple
E. iliotibial band tenodesis
E. lateral knee reconstruction
E. technique
Ellis-vanCreveld disease
Elmslie
E. peroneal tendon operation
E. peroneal tendon procedure
E. reconstruction
E. triple arthrodesis
Elmslie-Cholmely
E.-C. foot operation
E.-C. procedure
Elmslie-Trillat
E.-T. patellar operation
E.-T. patellar procedure
E.-T. patellar realignment method
E.-T. realignment
E.-T. transplant
elongation
ligament e.
peroneus brevis e.
e. property
repeated quick stretch from e.
(RQS-E)
elongation-derotation flexion
ELP
E. broach
E. femoral prosthesis
E. stem for hip arthroplasty
Ely test
Emagrin
emanate
embarrassment
circulatory e.

E

NOTES

191

embolic
> e. disease
> e. mononeuropathy

embolism, embolus
> air e.
> arterial gas e.
> fat e.
> pulmonary e.

embolization
embryology
embryonal rhabdomyosarcoma
EMED
> E. gait analysis
> E. insole

EMED-SF pedobarograph
Emerald implantation system
emergency closed manipulative measure
EMG
> electromyogram
> electromyography
>> Nordotrack motion EMG
>> Norotrack Motion Analyzer & EMG
>> scanning EMG
>> single-channel surface EMG
>> single fiber EMG
>> EMG 101T/201T

Emgel Topical
EMHI galvanic electrode stimulator
eminence
> hypothenar e.
> medial e.
> thenar e.
> tibial e.

EMLA
Emmon osteotomy
empirical
Empirin With Codeine
empty
> e. can syndrome
> e. can test

empyema
EMS 2000 neuromuscular stimulator
emulsified
en
> e. bloc
> e. bloc advancement
> e. bloc resection

Enbrel
encased screw
encephalitis
encephalopathy
encerclage
enchondral ossification
enchondroma
> e. of bone
> multiple e.
> solitary e.

enchondromatosis
> multiple e.

enclavement
> Regnauld e.

enclosure
> air-flow e.

encroachment
> bony e.
> cervical nerve root e.
> foraminal osteophyte e.
> osseous foraminal e.

end
> e. artery
> articulating bone e.
> bone e.
> bony distal e.
> e. corn
> e. cutter
> distal bone e.
> e. feel
> e.-feel palpation
> lateral e.
> medial e.
> e. plate
> e. play
> e. point
> e. range of motion
> e.-stage disruption
> e. vertebra

endarteritis obliterans
end-cutting
> end-weave anastomosis
> e.-c. reamer
> e.-c. reciprocating saw

Ender
> E. awl
> E. femoral fracture technique
> E. flexible medullary nail
> E. nail condylocephalic
> E. nail fixation
> E. nailing
> E. pin
> E. rod
> E. rod fixation
> E. rod fixation of fracture

ending
> A-delta nociceptor e.
> flower-spray e.
> nerve e.
> Ruffini e.

Endless Pool physical therapy pool
Endo
> E. button
> E. Multi-Mode stimulator
> E. rotating knee joint prosthesis

endoabdominal fascia

endochondral
    e. bone
    e. ossification
endochondromatosis
endocrine fracture
endogenous pain
Endolite prosthesis
Endo-Model
    E.-M. hinged knee prosthesis
    E.-M. rotating knee joint prosthesis
    E.-M. sled prosthesis
endomorph
endomysial
endomysium
endoneural tube
endoneurium degeneration
endoneurolysis
endoplasmic reticulum
endoprosthesis
    acetabular e.
    Atkinson e.
    Bio-Moore e.
    femoral e.
    F. R. Thompson e.
    nonporous-coated e.
    smooth e.
    tibial e.
    TPP hip e.
    tumor-replacement e.
endoprosthetic flange
Endoprothetik
    E. CSL-Plus cemented-hip system
    E. CS-Plus cemented-hip system
end-organ
    e.-o. disease
    Ruffini e.-o.
endorphin
β-endorphin
    plasma β-e.
endoscope
    Desormaux e.
    ETB e.
endoscopic
    e. anterior cruciate ligament
      reconstruction
    e. carpal tunnel instrumentation
    e. carpal tunnel release (ECTR,
      ECTRA)
    e. carpal tunnel release system
    e. plantar fasciotomy (EPF)
endoscopy
    fiberoptic intraosseous e.

    laser-assisted spinal e. (LASE)
    lumbar epidural e.
endoskeletal
    e. alignment system (EAS)
    solid-ankle flexible e. (SAFE)
    stationary attachment flexible e.
      (SAFE)
Endoskeleton
endosteal
    e. revascularization
    e. scalloping
    e. surface
    e. vessel
endosteum
endotenon
endothelial cell
endothelium
    vascular e.
endothoracic fascia
endotoxin
Endotrac
    E. blade system
    E. endoscopic carpal tunnel release
    E. system for carpal tunnel release
endotracheal intubation
endovaginal lipoma
endplate
    e. activity
    e. fragmentation
    e. invagination
    e. noise
    e. ossification
    posterior-superior e.
    e. potential (EPP)
    e. sclerosis
    e. spike
    e. zone
end-to-end
    e.-t.-e. anastomosis (EEA)
    e.-t.-e. suture
    e.-t.-e. tendon repair
end-to-side
    e.-t.-s. anastomosis
    e.-t.-s. repair
endurance
    e. exercise
    e. limit
Enduron acetabular liner
energetics
    Apex E.
energy
    e. absorption

E

NOTES

energy *(continued)*
    e. intake
    kinetic e.
    muscle e.
    E. Plus shoe insert
    strain e.
ENG
    electronystagmography
Engel
    E. angle
    E. plaster saw
Engelmann
    E. disease
    E. thigh splint
Engel-May nail
Engen
    E. palmar finger orthosis
    E. palmar wrist splint
Engh
    E. porous metal hip prosthesis
    E. total hip replacement
Engh-Glassman femoral stem
engine
    Acrotorque hand e.
Englehardt femoral prosthesis
English
    E. anvil nail nipper
    E. brace
English-McNab shoulder prosthesis
engram
enhancer cushion
enkephalin
enlarging bur
ENMG
    electroneuromyography
Enna classification
Enneking
    E. classification
    E. knee arthrodesis
    E. principle
    E. question
    E. resection-arthrodesis
    E. rod
    E. staging of malignant soft tissue
    tumor
enostosis
enoxacin
enoxaparin
Ensure-It dressing
entensile release
Enterobacter
    E. agglomerans
    E. cloacae
Enterobacteriaceae
Enterococcus
enterocutaneous fistula
enteropathic arthritis
enthesitis

enthesopathy
entrapment
    catheter e.
    lateral canal e.
    median nerve e.
    meniscoid e.
    nerve root e.
    popliteal fossa e.
    posterior interosseous nerve e.
    e. syndrome
Entrex small joint arthroscopy
    instrument set
entry point
entubulation
enucleate
enucleation
enucleator
    Marino transsphenoidal e.
    Rhoton e.
envelope
    e. arm sling
    capsuloperiosteal e.
    soft tissue e.
    e.-type arm sling
environmental illness
enzyme
    e.-linked immunosorbent assay
    (ELISA)
EO
    elbow orthosis
EOC goniometer
eosinophilia-myalgia syndrome
eosinophilic
    e. granuloma
    e. granuloma of bone
EPB
    extensor pollicis brevis
ependymoma
EPF
    endoscopic plantar fasciotomy
epiarticular osteochondromatous
    dysplasia
EPIC functional evaluation system
epicondylalgia
    radial e.
epicondylar
    e. avulsion fracture
    e. ridge
epicondyle
    femoral e.
    humeral e.
    lateral e.
    medial e.
epicondylectomy
    medial e.
epicondylitis
    e. of the elbow

lateral e.
medial e.
epicritic
e. pain
e. receptor
Epic wheelchair
epidemiology
epidermal inclusion cyst
epidermidis
Staphylococcus e.
epidermodysplasia
epidermoid cyst
epidermolysis bullosa
epidermolytic acanthoma
epidermophytid reaction
Epidermophyton floccosum
epidural
e. abscess evacuation
e. anesthesia
e. space
e. space infection
e. steroid
e. steroid injection
e. tumor evacuation
e. venography
epidurography
epifascicular epineurotomy
Epigard dressing
epilepsy
jacksonian e.
myoclonic e.
epiloia
epimysium
epinephrine
lidocaine and e.
Marcaine with e.
Xylocaine with e.
epineural
e. covering
e. repair
epineurectomy
interfascicular e.
epineurial
e. neuropathy
e. neurorrhaphy
e.-perineurial neuropathy
epineurium
epineurolysis
volar e.
epineurosis
epineurotomy
anterior e.

epifascicular e.
interfascicular e.
local e.
epiperineurial neuropathy
epiphyseal
e. arrest
e. artery
e. bar resection
e. closure
e. complex
e. dysgenesis
e. dysplasia
e. exostosis
e. growth plate
e. growth plate fracture
e. hyperplasia
e. injury
e. ischemic necrosis
e. line
e. osteochondritis
e. osteochondroma
e. oxygen
e. ring
e. slip fracture
e. staple
e. stapling
e. tibial fracture
epiphyseal-metaphyseal osteotomy
epiphyses (*pl. of* epiphysis)
epiphysiodesis
Abbott-Gill e.
Blount e.
bone peg e.
Heyman-Herndon e.
open bone graft e.
percutaneous e.
proximal phalangeal e.
screw e.
White e.
epiphysiolysis
femoral e.
proximal femoral e.
epiphysis, pl. epiphyses
capital e. (CE)
capital femoral e.
capitular e.
clavicular e.
distal humeral e.
femoral e.
humeral e.
iliac e.

E

NOTES

epiphysis *(continued)*
>Morrissy percutaneous fixation of slipped e.
>Perthes e.
>pressure e.
>slipped capital femoral e. (SCFE)
>stippled e.
>tibial e.
>traction e.

epiphysitis
>traction e.

EPI Sport epicondylitis clasp
epistemology of science
epitendineum
epitenon suture
epithelialization
epithelial membrane antigen (EEMA)
epithelioid sarcoma
epithelioma cuniculatum
Epitrain active elbow support
epitrochlea
epitrochlear
Epker osteotome
EPL
>extensor pollicis longus

epoetin alfa
eponychia
eponychium
EPP
>endplate potential

Eppright dial osteotomy
epsilon receptor
Epson salt soak
EPSP
>excitatory postsynaptic potential

Epstein
>E. bone rasp
>E. curette
>E. hip dislocation classification
>E. neurological hammer

Epstein-Thomas classification
EPTFE graft prosthesis
epX suspension sleeve
Equagesic
Equalizer
>E. air walker
>E. cast brace

equation
>Bloch e.
>Jackson-Pollock skinfold e.

Equilet
equilibratory ataxia
equilibrium
>protein-polysaccharide synthesis-depolymerization e.

Equilizer short leg walking cast
equina
>cauda e.

equine gait
equinocavovarus deformity
equinocavus foot
equinovalgus
>e. deformity
>e. foot
>spastic e.
>talipes e.

equinovarus
>congenital talipes e.
>e. foot
>e. hindfoot deformity
>talipes e. (TEV)
>Turco repair of talipes e.

equinus
>ankle e.
>compensated talipes e.
>e. contracture
>e. deformity
>e. foot
>forefoot e.
>gastrocnemius e.
>gastrosoleal e.
>heel e.
>metatarsus e.
>osseous e.
>pes e.
>e. position
>residual heel e.
>residual hindfoot e.
>spastic e.

equipment
>adaptive e.
>adjustment e.
>AquaMED dry hydrotherapy e.
>Austin Medical E. (AME)
>Baltimore Therapeutic E. (BTE)
>Body-Solid exercise e.
>Cybex back rehabilitation e.
>decompression e.
>DynaDisc exercise e.
>home medical e.
>insertion e.
>Invertrac e.
>OsteoStat single-use power surgical e.
>stainless steel e.
>Vitallium e.

E-R
>Indochron E-R

Erb
>E. muscular dystrophy
>E. point

Erb-Duchenne palsy
Erb-Goldflam disease
Erb-Landouzy disease
Erdheim-Chester disease

ERE
external rotation in extension
erector spinae
ERF
external rotation in flexion
Ergo
E. Cush back support
E. style flexion table
ergocalciferol
Ergociser
Cateye E.
E. exercise cycle
Ergoflex Premiere back support
ErgoForm contoured cold pack
ErgoLogic keyboard
ergometer
Concept II rowing e.
Cybex cycle e.
cycle e.
upper body e. (UBE)
ergonomic
e. assessment
e. assessment of risk and liability (EARLY)
e. chair
e. factor
ergoreceptor
ERGOS work simulator
Erhenfeld disease
Erichsen sign
Erich splint
Erickson-Leider-Brown technique
Eriksson
E. brachial block technique
E. cruciate ligament reconstruction
E. knee prosthesis
E. ligament technique
E. muscle biopsy cannula
ER/IR
external/internal rotation
ER/IR ratio
Erlenmeyer-flask shape
erogenic aid
erosion
e. of articular surface
bony e.
osteoclastic e.
erosive arthritis
erosonary
Eryderm Topical
Erygel Topical
Erymax Topical

erysipelas
erythema
e. ab igne
e. of joint
erythematosus
lupus e. (LE)
systemic lupus e. (SLE)
erythrocyte sedimentation rate (ESR)
erythroleukemia
erythromycin
e., topical
ES
electrotherapy system
Forte ES
Vicodin ES
eschar
escharotic
escharotomy
Escherichia coli
Esclim Transdermal
E-Series hip system
ESIN
elastic stable intramedullary nail
elastic stable intramedullary nailing
Esmarch
E. bandage
E. dressing
E. plaster knife
E. plaster shears
E. tourniquet
E. tube
E-Solve-2 Topical
esophageal perforation
ESR
erythrocyte sedimentation rate
essential fatty acid
Esser skin graft
Essex-Lopresti
E.-L. axial fixation technique
E.-L. calcaneal fracture classification
E.-L. calcaneal fracture technique
E.-L. fixation of calcaneal fracture
E.-L. injury
E.-L. joint depression fracture
E.-L. open reduction
ESSF
external spinal skeletal fixator
Essiac
established contracture
estazolam

E

NOTES

esterified
  estrogens, e.
Estersohn
  E. osteotomy for tailor's bunion
esthesia
esthesiometry
  Semmes-Weinstein monofilament
    pressure e.
estimated blood loss
Estinyl
Estok and Harris classification
Estrace Oral
Estraderm
  E. estradiol transdermal system
  E. Transdermal
estradiol
  ethinyl e.
Estra-L Injection
Estratab
Estratest H.S.
Estring
Estro-Cyp Injection
estrogen
estrogens
  e., conjugated
  e., esterified
  e. and medroxyprogesterone
  e. and methyltestosterone
etanercept
ETB endoscope
Ethafoam
ethambutol
ethanol
  anhydrous e.
ethchlorvynol
Ethibond suture
Ethiflex suture
Ethilon suture
ethinyl estradiol
ethmoid forceps
Ethrone implant material
ethyl
  e. chloride
  e. chloride and
    dichlorotetrafluoroethane
ethylene
  e. oxide
  e. oxide sterilization
etidocaine
etidronate
  e. disodium
  sodium e.
etiology
ETL
  echo train length
etodolac
etoposide

ETPS
  electrotherapeutic point stimulation
ETS-2% Topical
Eucalyptamint
eukinesia
Eulerian angle
Euler load
eumelanin
EuroCuff forearm crutch
Euroglide MKII slide board
European
  E. Chiropractic Union (ECU)
  E. compression technique (ECT)
  E.-style screwdriver
Eurotech table
evacuation
  epidural abscess e.
  epidural tumor e.
  nail bed hematoma e.
evacuator
  Hemo-Drain e.
evaluation
  baseline capacity e.
  Cyriax e.
  Doppler pulse e.
  Evans tenodesis e.
  Evolution hip prosthesis e.
  functional capacity e. (FCE)
  genitourinary e.
  Hughston knee e.
  job capacity e. (JCE)
  Mazur ankle e.
  pedicle e.
  physical capacity e. (PCE)
  preoperative e.
  Smith physical capacities e. (PCE)
  static e.
  toddler and infant motor e.
    (TIME)
evaluator
  Touch-Test sensory e.
Evan ankle joint instability operation
Evans
  E. ankle reconstruction technique
  E. anterior calcaneal osteotomy
  E. calcaneal lengthening
  E. intertrochanteric fracture
    classification
  E. lateral ankle reconstruction
  E. procedure
  E. tenodesis
  E. tenodesis evaluation
Evans-Burkhalter protocol
Evazote
  E. cushioning material
  E. foam
eventration
Eve reconstructive procedure

Ever-Flex insole
Evershears surgical instrument device
eversion
    ankle e.
    e.-external rotation deformity
    e. injury
    e. osteotomy
    e. stress test
evertor force
Everyday Objects ColorCards
Evista
evoked
    e. compound muscle action
        potential
    e. external urethral sphincter
        potential monitoring
    e. potential study
    e. response
Evolution
    E. hip prosthesis
    E. hip prosthesis evaluation
Ewald
    E. capitellocondylar total elbow
        arthroplasty
    E. elbow arthroplasty
    E. elbow arthroplasty rating system
    E. total elbow replacement
    E. unconstrained elbow prosthesis
Ewald-Walker
    E.-W. kinematic knee arthroplasty
    E.-W. knee arthroplasty
    E.-W. knee implant
EWHO
    elbow-wrist-hand orthosis
Ewing
    E. sarcoma
    E. tumor
E.X.
    Extra Strength Dynafed E.X.
exacerbated
exacerbation
Exact-Fit ATH hip replacement system
exaggeration reaction
exam (*See also* examination)
    Apley e.
    neurological nerve conduction
        velocity e.
examination (*See also* exam)
    arthroscopic e.
    BB to MM e.
    belly button to medial malleolus e.
    bench e.

Brodén stress e.
clinical e.
comparative radiographic e.
full spine radiographic e.
lateral full-spine radiographic e.
motor e.
palpatory e.
pedodynographic e.
reflex e.
sensory e.
stress e.
thermographic e.
Examiners
    National Board of Chiropractic E.
        (NBCE)
Ex-Balls
Excedrin
    E., Extra Strength
    E. P.M.
Excel Plus electrode
excision
    e. arthroplasty
    Bartlett nail fold e.
    bone cyst e.
    Bose nail fold e.
    bunionette e.
    cervical disk e.
    clavicle e.
    e.-curettage technique
    Curtin plantar fibromatosis e.
    Das Gupta scapular e.
    disk e.
    distal clavicular e.
    Ferciot e.
    Ferciot-Thomson e.
    Flatt e.
    funicular e.
    hemivertebral e.
    e. of intervertebral disk
    intralesional e.
    marginal e.
    McKeever-Buck fragment e.
    meniscal e.
    microlumbar disk e.
    e. of osteochondroma
    radical compartmental e.
    retropulsed bone e.
    ruptured disk e.
    split-thickness skin e. (STSE)
    Stewart distal clavicular e.
    Thompson e.
    ulnar head e.

E

NOTES

excision *(continued)*
 wide e.
 William microlumbar disk e.
excisional
 e. arthrodesis
 e. biopsy
excitability
excitation
excitatory postsynaptic potential (EPSP)
exclusion clamp
excoriation
excrescence
 bony e.
excursion
 hindfoot e.
 insertional e.
 range of e.
 tendon e.
Exelderm Topical
Exerball kit
ExerBand
Exerboard
 Velcro Hand E.
exercise
 active-assisted range-of-motion e.
 active range-of-motion e.'s
 aerobic e.
 anaerobic e.
 ankle-pump e.
 back e.
 e. band
 Buerger-Allen e.
 Calleja e.
 closed-chain e.
 closed kinetic chain progressive-
  resistance e.
 co-contraction e.
 Codman e.
 contracture e.
 Crane shoulder e.
 Daily Adjusted Progressive
  Resistance E. (DAPRE)
 DeLorme e.
 dynamic stump e.
 eccentric e.
 elevation e.
 endurance e.
 external rotation e.
 flexion-extension e.
 gastroc-resistive e.
 graded e.
 Gymnastik ball functional
  stabilization e.
 hamstring-setting e.
 heel cord stretching e.
 heel raises e.
 heel rocks e.
 hip abductor strengthening e.

hip extension e.
hook-lying pectoral stretch e.
horizontal shoulder abduction e.
increment after e.
internal rotation e.
inversion-eversion e.
e. ischemia
isokinetic e.
isometric e.
isotonic e.
kinesthetic e.
knee pump e.
McKenzie extension e.
muscle-setting e.
e. myopathy
open-chain e.
open kinetic chain e.
orthokinetic e.
passive range of motion e.
pendulum e.
e. physiology
plyometric e.
PNF e.
progressive-resistance e.
progressive-resistive e. (PR, PRE)
pulley e.
quadriceps-setting e.
quad strengthening e.
range of motion e.
Regen flexion e.
repetitive e.
resistive e.
rotation e.
E. Sandal
e. science
"six-pack hand" e.
stair-climbing e.
straight leg raising e.
Super-Seven e.
supported extension e.
Tai Chi Chuan e.
Thera-Band Max resistive e.
toe gripping e.
toe raises e.
unrestricted closed and open chain
 knee extension e.
volitional e.
wall-slide e.
Williams flexion e. (WFE)
work hardening e.
exerciser
 AccessTrainer e.
 animal beanbag e.
 ankle e.
 axial resistance e.
 bicycle e.
 Builder Grip hand e.
 Carpal Care E.

Cat's Paw E.
continuous anatomical passive e.
  (CAPE)
Cybex II, II+ isokinetic e.
Danniflex CPM e.
Digi-Flex finger e.
Digi-Flex hand e.
DynaFlex Gyro e.
Eggsercizer resistive hand e.
Exer-Cor e.
ExtendaFLEX e.
FiddleLink hand e.
finger e.
Finger Helper hand e.
Finger Platter hand e.
Flextender Plus hand e.
Grahamizer I e.
Gripp squeeze ball hand e.
hand e.
Hand Helper hand e.
isokinetic Unex III e.
Iso-Quadron e.
JACE shoulder e.
jaw e.
Jux-A-Cisor e.
KineTec clubfoot CPM e.
Knead-A-Ball e.
microcomputer upper limb e.
  (MULE)
MiniMedBall hand e.
Morpho E.
Motivator FTR2000 e.
MULE upper limb e.
Nelson finger e.
NordiCare Enabler e.
NordiCare Strider e.
NordicTrack ski e.
NuStep e.
Omni-Flexor wrist e.
Oppociser hand e.
Orthotron e.
pedal e.
plyo-sled e.
Powerflex CMP e.
Power Pogo stationary e
Power Web hand e.
Preston Traveler CPM e.
ProStretch e.
Pul-Ez e.
resistive e.
rickshaw rehab e.
rocky boat e.

Rotaflex e.
Roylan ergonomic hand e.
Seated Cable Row e.
soft touch hand e.
squeeze e.
strengthening e.
Stronghands hand e.
Stryker CPM e.
Stryker leg e.
Swanson Grip-X hand e.
Thera-Band ASSIST e.
Thera-Band resistive e.
Therabite jaw e.
Thera Cane shoulder e.
Theraflex wrist e.
Ther-A-Hoop e.
Thera-Loop e.
Toronto Medical CPM e.
Tuf Nex neck e.
Tunturi hand e.
Versa-Trainer e.
Walk-'n-Tone e.
Wilco ankle e.
Wristiciser e.
Zimmer continuous anatomical
  passive e.
Exer-Cor exerciser
Exercycle
Exer-Pedic cycle
exertion
  rated perceived e. (RPE)
  rating of perceived e.
exertional
  e. anterior compartment syndrome
  (EACS)
  e. compartment syndrome
  e. deep posterior compartment
  syndrome (EDPCS)
Exertools gymball
Exeter
  E. bone lavage
  E. cemented hip prosthesis
EX-FI-RE
  E.-F.-R. external fixation
  E.-F.-R. external fixation device
exhaustion
  postactivation e.
Exidine Scrub
Exo-Bed traction unit
exogenous
  e. fibrin clot
  e. reconstruction

E

NOTES

Exo-Overhead traction unit
exoskeletal
Exo-Static
    E.-S. cervical collar
    E.-S. traction
exostectomy
exostosis, pl. exostoses
    blocker's e.
    bony e.
    cuneiform-first metatarsal e.
    Dupuytren e.
    epiphyseal e.
    hereditary multiple e.
    hypertrophic e.
    impingement e.
    marginal e.
    metatarsal cuneiform e.
    metatarsocuneiform joint e.
    osteocartilaginous e.
    pump bump e.
    retrocalcaneal e.
    subungual e.
    tackler's e.
    talar neck e.
    talotibial e.
    traction e.
    turret e.
Exotec brace
expander
    acetabular e.
    Mentor tissue e.
    tissue e.
expanding reamer
Expandover athletic tape
expansile
    e. cyst
    e. lesion
expansion
    lateral extensor e.
    medial extensor e.
    e. screw
expansive laminaplasty
experimental threshold
explant
exploration
    e. and debridement
    e. and revision
exploratory incision
exploring electrode
explosion
    e. fracture
    e. injury
exposure
    Abbott-Gill epiphyseal plate e.
    anterior surgical e.
    extrapharyngeal e.
    Henry posterior interosseous
      nerve e.

    Kocher-Langenbeck e.
    radiation e.
    subperiosteal e.
    surgical e.
    thoracolumbar junction surgical e.
    thoracolumbar spine anterior e.
    transperitoneal e.
    upper cervical spine anterior e.
    vertebral e.
expulsion
    graft e.
exsanguinate
exsanguination tourniquet control
Exsel
exstrophy
ExtendaFLEX exerciser
extended
    e. ADLs
    e. iliofemoral approach
    e. maxillotomy
    e. medial shoe counter
    e. tibial in situ bypass
extended-counter shoe
extender
    Kalish Duredge wire e.
    nail e.
    Rousek e.
    Rush e.
    Superstabilizer cemented stem e.
    Superstabilizer press-fit stem e.
    Sven-Johansson e.
extending
Extend-It finger splint
Extend stem
extensibility
extensible
extensile approach
extension
    active knee e. (AKE)
    angle of greatest e. (AGE)
    e. block splint
    e. block splinting method
    e. body cast
    e. bone clamp
    e. bow
    brachioradialis transfer for wrist e.
    brake lever e.
    cast with dorsal toe plate e.
    cast with volar toe plate e.
    cervical rotation in e.
    compression e.
    e. contracture
    e. deformity
    distractive e.
    external rotation in e. (ERE)
    femoral-trunk e.
    flexion and e.
    e. gap

headrest e.
hip e.
Hittenberger halo e.
e. injury posterior atlantoaxial arthrodesis
e. instability
internal rotation in e. (IRE)
isokinetic knee e.
Legg-Perthes shoe e.
lumbar e.
e. malposition
Maquet table e.
NexGen offset stem e.
e. osteotomy
e. restriction
shoe e.
terminal knee e.
toe plate e.
e.-type cervical spine injury

extensive
e. neoplasm
e. posterior decompression

extensor
e. brevis arthroplasty
e. carpi radialis brevis (ECRB)
e. carpi radialis brevis muscle
e. carpi radialis brevis tendon
e. carpi radialis longus (ECRL)
e. carpi radialis longus muscle
e. carpi radialis longus tendon
e. carpi ulnaris (ECU)
e. carpi ulnaris muscle
e. carpi ulnaris tendon
e. comminicus muscle
e. digiti minimi (EDM)
e. digiti minimi muscle
e. digiti minimi tendon
e. digiti quinti (EDQ)
e. digiti quinti muscle
e. digiti quinti tendon
e. digitorum brevis (EDB)
e. digitorum brevis muscle
e. digitorum brevis tendon
e. digitorum communis (EDC)
e. digitorum communis muscle
e. digitorum communis tendon
e. digitorum longus (EDL)
e. digitorum longus muscle
e. digitorum longus tendon
e. digitorum transfer
e. hallucis
e. hallucis brevis muscle

e. hallucis longus (EHL)
e. hallucis longus muscle
e. hallucis longus strength
e. hallucis longus tendon
e. hallucis longus transfer
e. hood
e. hood mechanism
e. indicis proprius (EIP)
e. indicis proprius muscle
e. indicis proprius musculus
e. indicis proprius tendon
knee e.
e. lengthening
long e.
e. mechanism dysfunction
e. pollicis brevis (EPB)
e. pollicis brevis muscle
e. pollicis brevis tendon
e. pollicis longus (EPL)
e. pollicis longus muscle
e. pollicis longus tendon
e. quinti tendon
radial wrist e.
e. retinaculum
e. substitution
e. tendon injury
e. tendon repair
e. tenodesis
e. tenotomy
e. thrust reflex
toe e.
wrist e.

extensus
hallux e.

exteriorization

external
articulated e. fixator
e. elastic strap
e. fixator
e. fixator frame
e. ilium (EI)
e. ilium movement
e. immobilization
e. intercostal muscle
e. neurolysis
e. oblique muscle
posteroinferior e. (PIEx)
e. rotation
e. rotation-abduction stress test (EAST)
e. rotation contracture
e. rotation exercise

E

NOTES

external *(continued)*
    e. rotation in extension (ERE)
    e. rotation in flexion (ERF)
    e. rotation-recurvatum test
    e. rotation stress test
    e. rotator
    e. sequential pneumatic compression
      boot
    e. skeletal fixation apparatus
    e. spinal fixation
    e. spinal skeletal fixator (ESSF)
    e. support
    e. version
external-alignment compression jig
external-coil electrical stimulation
external/internal
    e. rotation (ER/IR)
    e. rotation ratio
externally rotated
externum
    os tibiale e.
exteroceptive sensation
exteroceptor
    postural e.
extirpation
extra
    Aspercin E.
    Buffinol E.
    E. Strength Adprin-B
    E. Strength Bayer Enteric 500
      Aspirin
    E. Strength Bayer Plus
    E. Strength Doan's
    E. Strength Dynafed E.X.
    e. toe
    Valorin E.
extraabdominal desmoid tumor
extraarticular
    e. ankylosis
    e. arthrodesis
    e. augmentation
    e. graft
    e. hip fusion
    e. knee ligament
    e. pain syndrome
    e. pigmented villonodular synovitis
    e. procedure
    e. pseudarthrosis
    e. reconstruction
    e. resection
    e. structure
    e. subtalar fusion
    e. subtalar joint
    e. technique
    e. tuberculosis
extrabursal approach
extracapsular
    e. ankylosis

    e. arterial ring
    e. dissection
    e. fracture
extracompartmental soft-tissue sarcoma
extract
    feverfew e.
extracting forceps
extraction pliers
extractor
    Austin Moore e.
    ball e.
    Bilos pin e.
    bone e.
    broach e.
    Cherry screw e.
    cloverleaf pin e.
    corkscrew femoral head e.
    femoral head e.
    femoral trial e.
    FIN e.
    Intraflex intramedullary pin e.
    Jewett e.
    Kalish Duredge wire e.
    Küntscher e.
    Mark II femoral component e.
    Mark II tibial component e.
    Massie e.
    Moore prosthesis e.
    Moreland femoral component e.
    e. nail drill
    Nicoll e.
    Sage e.
    Schneider e.
    Snap Lock wire/pin e.
    Southwick screw e.
    staple e.
    stem e.
    Take-Out E.
    T-C ring-handle pin and wire e.
    Universal modular femoral hip
      component e.
    Zimmer e.
extractor-driver
    Schneider e.-d.
extractor-impactor
    Fox e.-i.
extra-depth shoe
extradural granulation
extrafusal fiber contraction
extramedullary
    e. alignment
    e. alignment guide
    e. plasmacytoma
    e. tibial alignment jig
extra-octave
    e.-o. fracture
    e.-o. fracture of finger
extraosseous factor

extraperitoneal approach
extrapharyngeal
    e. approach
    e. exposure
extraskeletal
    e. chondroma
    e. chondrosarcoma
extravasation
    e. extremity
    e. extrusion
    e. injury
    e. irrigation solution
extremity
    elevation of e.
    extravasation e.
    left lower e. (LLE)
    left upper e. (LUE)
    lower e. (LE)
    e. mobilization strap
    e. mobilization technique
    e. pump
    right lower e. (RLE)
    right upper e. (RUE)
    upper e.
extrinsic
    e. entrapment test
    e. ligament
    e. muscle strength
    e. rearfoot post
extruded
    e. bar polyethylene
    e. disk

extrusion
    bone graft e.
    disk e.
    extravasation e.
extubation
    postoperative e.
exuberant
    e. granulation tissue
    e. synovium
exudate
exudation
exude
Exu-Dry
    E.-D. wound dressing
eye sign
Eyler flexorplasty
Eyre-Brook epiphyseal index
EZ
    EZ hand pump
    EZ Rider support chair
E-Z
    E-Z Flex jaw exercising device
    E-Z Reacher
    E-Z ROC anchor
Ezeform splint
EZ-Trac orthopaedic suspension device
Ezy
    Ezy Wrap lumbosacral support
    Ezy Wrap shoulder immobilizer

NOTES

E

FA
    false aneurysm
Fabco
    F. gauze bandage
    F. gauze dressing
fabella
fabellofibular
    f. complex
    f. ligament
faber
    flexion in abduction and external rotation
fabere
    f. sign
    f. test
Fabian screw
FABQ
    Fear Avoidance Beliefs Quest
fabric
    neoprene f.
    Staph-Chek Synergy f.
FAC
    Functional Ambulation Categories
facebow
    ‒Ortho-Yomy f.
facet
    f. angle
    f. anomaly
    f. apposition
    articular f.
    f. capsule
    f. capsule disruption
    f. dislocation
    f. excision technique
    f. fracture stabilization wiring
    fusion f.
    f. fusion
    inferior f.
    f. injection
    f. joint
    f. joint block
    f. joint disease (FJD)
    f. joint dysfunction
    f. joint irritation
    f. joint preparation
    f. joint syndrome
    lateral patellar f.
    oblique wiring f.
    f. plane
    posterior f.
    f. replacement
    f. screw system
    f. subluxation stabilization wiring
    f. synovial impingement
    f. tropism

facetectomy
    O'Donoghue f.
facial
    f. artery
    F. Disability Index (FDI)
    F. Grading System (FGS)
facies
    swan-neck f.
facilitate
facilitated
    f. spinal system
    f. subluxation
facilitation
    convergence f.
    Law of F.
    neuromuscular f.
    f. pattern
    postactivation f.
    posttetanic f.
    proprioceptive neuromuscular f.
        (PNF)
facilitatory technique
facioscapulohumeral muscle atrophy
    disease
factor
    biomechanical f.
    chemotactic f.
    coagulation f.
    F. Eleven: The Edge
    ergonomic f.
    extraosseous f.
    fibroblast growth f. (FGF)
    genetic f.
    granulocyte colony-stimulating f.
        (G-CSF)
    growth f.
    high-risk f.
    insulin-like growth f. (IGF)
    leg protection f. (LPF)
    neurotrophic f.
    platelet-derived growth f. (PDGF)
    RA f.
    rheumatoid arthritis f.
    F. Six: Sommaserene
    F. Ten: Femtrac
    transforming growth f. (TGF)
    f. VIII, IX deficiency
fadir
    flexion in adduction and internal rotation
    fadir sign
    fadir test
fad therapy
faecalis
    Streptococcus f.

F

Fahey
> F. approach
> F. pin
> F. retractor
> F. technique

Fahey-Compere pin
Fahey-O'Brien technique
fail arm
failed
> f. back surgery syndrome (FBSS)
> f. back syndrome (FBS)
> f. back syndrome with documented pseudarthrosis
> f. femoral osteotomy
> f. implant arthroplasty
> f. joint replacement
> f. procedure
> f. surgery
> f. surgery syndrome
> f. triple arthrodesis

fail-safe mechanism
failure
> congestive heart f.
> f. of conservative management
> differentiation f.
> fatigue f.
> Harrington rod instrumentation f.
> heart f.
> implant f.
> metal f.
> spinal implant load to f.
> stem f.

Fairbanks
> F. apprehension test
> F. sign
> F. technique
> F. technique with Sever modification

Fairbanks-Sever procedure
Fajersztajn crossed sciatic sign
FAL
> functional and anatomic loading
> Seipi FAL

falciparum
> *Plasmodium f.*

Fallat-Buckholz method
fallen-fragment sign
fallen-leaf sign
false
> f. acetabulum
> f. aneurysm (FA)
> f. ankylosis
> f.-negative result
> f. rib

familial
> f. dysautonomia
> f. lymphedema

> f. periodic paralysis
> f. shape

family management model
fan
> Schmitt f.
> f. sign

Fanconi syndrome
Farabeuf
> F. bone-hold forceps
> F. bone rasp
> F. periosteal elevator

Farabeuf-Collin rasp
Farabeuf-Lambotte
> F.-L. bone-holding forceps
> F.-L. raspatory

Farber disease
far fashion
far-field potential
Farmer
> F. operation
> F. technique

far-out syndrome
Farrior wire-crimping forceps
Fartlek training
fascia
> antebrachial f.
> anterior cervical f.
> Buck f.
> Camper f.
> cervical f.
> clavipectoral f.
> Colles f.
> crural f.
> cuff of f.
> deep f.
> deltoid f.
> endoabdominal f.
> endothoracic f.
> hypothenar f.
> infraspinous f.
> investing f.
> f. lata
> f. lata freeze-thawed graft
> lumbar f.
> lumbodorsal f. (LDF)
> medial geniculate f.
> palmar f.
> plantar f.
> quadratus femoris f.
> retrosacral f.
> Scarpa f.
> f. sheath
> Sibson f.
> f.-splitting incision
> transversalis f.
> vertebral f.

fascial
> f. arthroplasty

f. band
f. fibromatosis
f. graft
f.-muscle interface
f. plane
f. plexus
f. release
f. sheath covering
f. space
f. space infection
f. suture
fasciaplasty, fascioplasty
fasciatome (*var. of* fasciotome)
fascicle
motor f.
muscle f.
popliteomeniscal f.
sensory f.
silent f.
fascicular
f. neuropathy
f. repair
fasciculation
benign f.
contraction f.
malignant f.
f. potential
fasciculus, pl. **fasciculi**
f. cuneatus
f. gracilis
lateral plantar nerve f.
f. lenticularis
fasciectomy
dermal f.
limited f.
partial f.
radical palmar f.
fasciitis, fascitis
Dupuytren f.
iliotibial band f.
ITB f.
necrotizing f.
nodular f.
plantar f.
proliferative f.
recalcitrant plantar f.
fasciocutaneous
f. island flap
fasciodesis
fascio-fat graft
fasciogram
fascioplasty (*var. of* fasciaplasty)

fasciorrhaphy
fascioscapulohumeral dystrophy
fasciotome, fasciatome
intercompartment f.
Masson f.
Moseley f.
fasciotomy
compartment f.
decompression f.
decompression of f.
double-incision f.
endoscopic plantar f. (EPF)
Fronet f.
palmar f.
percutaneous plantar f. (PPF)
plantar f.
prophylactic f.
Rorabeck f.
single-incision f.
Skoog f.
subcutaneous palmar f.
Yount f.
fascitis (*var. of* fasciitis)
fashion
aseptic f.
Bunnell zigzag f.
cruciate f.
far f.
near-far f.
FASS
foot and ankle severity scale
FAST
fluoroallergosorbent test
Fast
F. Lanex rare earth screen
Snooze F.
FastIn threaded anchor
Fastlok implantable staple
FastOut device
Fas-Trac strip
fast-twitch muscle fiber
fat
aspirated f.
autogenous f.
f. embolism
f. embolism syndrome
f. and fat-free mass (FFM)
f. graft
f. pad
f. pad atrophy
f. pad of elbow

F

NOTES

fat *(continued)*
    f. pad retractor
    f. pad sign
fatigue
    f. failure
    f. fracture
    implant f.
    metal f.
    f. tolerance
    volitional f.
fatty
    f. tissue
    f. tissue tumor
Faulkner curette
fault
    dynamic f.
Favort-Feder test
Fazio-Londe
    F.-L. disease
    F.-L. syndrome
FB
    foreign body
    FB cast cushion
FBS
    failed back syndrome
FBSS
    failed back surgery syndrome
FCE
    functional capacity evaluation
FCER
    Foundation for Chiropractic Education
      and Research
FCR
    flexor carpi radialis
FCU
    flexor carpi ulnaris
FDB
    flexor digitorum brevis
FDC
    flexor digitorum communis
FDI
    Facial Disability Index
FDICT
    frequency-difference interferential current
      therapy
FDL
    flexor digitorum longus
FDMA
    first dorsal metatarsal artery
FDP
    flexor digitorum profundus
FDQB
    flexor digiti quinti brevis
FDS
    flexor digitorum sublimis
    flexor digitorum superficialis
Feagin shoulder dislocation test
Fear Avoidance Beliefs Quest (FABQ)

feasibility
    vocational f.
feeder
    offset suspension f.
    suspension f.
    Tumble Forms f.
feeding
    drip-tube f.
feel
    end f.
feet
    burning f.
    calcaneocavus f.
    flail f.
    planovalgus f.
    rockerbottom f.
Feiss line
Feldene
Feldenkrais
    F. cylinder
    F. foam roll
    F. method
Felix disease
fell on outstretched hand (FOOSH)
felon
    aseptic f.
    f. infection
felt
    f. apron Bowden cable suspension
      system
    f. collar splint
    orthopaedic f.
    f. padding
    rolled f.
    F. shears
Felty syndrome
female reamer
Femizole-7
Femizol-M
femoral
    f. aligner
    f. alignment jig
    f. antetorsion
    f. anteversion
    f. arteriography
    f. attachment
    f. canal
    f. circulation
    f. circumflex artery
    f. clamp
    f. component
    f. condylar shaving
    f. condylar template
    f. condyle
    f. cortex
    f. cortical perforation
    f. cortical ring allograft
    f. cortical window

f. cutaneous nerve
f. derotation osteotomy
f. diaphyseal allograft
f. diaphysis
f. distractor
f. drill bit
f. endoprosthesis
f. epicondyle
f. epiphysiolysis
f. epiphysis
f. groove
f. guidepin
f. guide pin
f. head
f. head amputation
f. head cork screw
f. head deformity
f. head driver
f. head dysplasia
f. head extractor
f. head line (FHL)
f. impactor
f. intermedullary guide
f. intertrochanteric fracture
f. metaphyseal shortening
f. metaphysis
f. nailing
f. neck
f. neck fracture
f. neck fracture reduction
f. neck prosthesis
f. neck version
f. nerve block
f. nerve stretch test
f. nerve traction test
f. notch guide
f. osteolysis
f. osteomyelitis
f. osteoporosis
f. plate
f. plug
f. prosthesis broach
f. prosthesis fixation
f. rasp
f. resection
f. retrotorsion
f. retroversion
f. sarcoma
self-articulating f. (SAF)
f. shaft
f. shaft axis
f. shaft fracture

f. shaft malunion
f. supracondylar fracture
f. trial extractor
f. tunnel
f. vein injury
femorale
calcar f.
femoral-trunk
f.-t. angle
f.-t. extension
f.-t. flexion
femoris
biceps f.
ligamentum capitis f.
linea aspera f.
profunda f.
quadratus f. (QF)
rectus f.
femorocrural graft
femorodistal
f. bypass
f. bypass procedure
femoroiliac thrombophlebitis
femoroischial transplantation
femorotibial
f. angle (FTA)
f. ligament tenodesis
f. torsion
Femtrac
Factor Ten: F.
femur
distal f.
f. graft
ligament of head of f.
proximal f.
Universal proximal f. (UPF)
fenamic acid
fence splint
fender fracture
fenestrated
f. drape
f. reamer
f. stem
fenestration
Fenlin total shoulder system
fenoprofen
fentanyl
droperidol and f.
F. Oralet
Fenton tibial bolt
Feochetti rib spreader

F

NOTES

Ferciot
- F. excision
- F. tiptoe splint

Ferciot-Thomson excision

Ferguson
- F. bone clamp
- F. bone holder
- F. hip reduction
- F. sacral base angle
- F. scoliosis measuring method
- F. view

Ferguson-Frazier suction tube

Ferguson-Thompson-King two-stage osteotomy

Fergusson
- F. forceps
- F. method for measuring scoliosis

Ferkel
- F. bipolar release
- F. torticollis technique

Fernandez
- F. extensile anterior approach
- F. osteotomy
- F. point-score wrist assessment system
- F. scale posttraumatic wrist assessment system

Ferno AquaCiser underwater treadmill system

Ferran awl

Ferrier coupler

Ferris
- F. Smith-Kerrison forceps
- F. Smith rongeur
- F. Smith rongeur forceps
- F. Smith-Spurling disk rongeur
- F. Smith tissue forceps

ferromagnetic metal plate

ferrous sulfate (FeSO₄)

FES
- functional electrical stimulation
- FES exercise bicycle

FeSO₄
- ferrous sulfate

festinating gait

fetal
- f. alcohol syndrome
- f. substantia nigra graft

fetalis
- chondrodystrophia f.

Fett prosthesis

fever
- fracture f.
- San Joaquin Valley f.
- f. of undetermined origin (FUO)

Feverall
- Infants F.
- F. Sprinkle Caps

feverfew extract

FF
- further flexion

FFC
- fixed flexion contracture

FFD
- focal film distance

FFM
- fat and fat-free mass

FGF
- fibroblast growth factor

FGS
- Facial Grading System

FHB
- flexor hallucis brevis

FHL
- femoral head line
- flexor hallucis longus

FHLD
- flexor hallucis longus dysfunction

FI
- fixator interne
- Functional Integration

fiber
- A-delta f.
- afferent f.
- annular f.
- carbon f.
- collagen f.
- f. density
- fast-twitch muscle f.
- intrafusal f.
- f.-metal peg
- myoclonic epilepsy with ragged-red f.'s
- ragged-red f.'s
- Sharpey f.
- f.-splitting incision
- tendinous f.
- f.-type disproportion

fiberglass
- f. bandage
- f. cast

fiberoptic
- f. arthroscope
- f. cable
- f. intraosseous endoscopy
- f. light source

fiber-region
- anterior f.-r.
- central f.-r.

fibrillar absorbable hemostat material

fibrillation
- f. potential
- synchronized f.

fibrin
- f. clot

f. debris
f. glue adhesive
fibrinogen
iodine-labeled f.
radioactive iodine-labeled f.
fibrinolysin
f. and desoxyribonuclease
fibrinolysis
fibrinolytic agent
fibroblast
f. growth factor (FGF)
regenerated f.
fibroblastic
f. phase
f. tumor
fibrocartilage
f. complex
triangular f.
fibrocartilaginous
f. disk
f. plate
fibrochondrocyte
fibrodysplasia
fibroepithelial polyp
fibroepithelioma of Pinkus
fibroepitheliomatous
fibrofatty infiltrate
fibroid tumor
fibrokeratoma
fibrolipomatosis
macrodactylia f.
fibroma
aponeurotic f.
calcifying aponeurotic f.
chondromyxoid f.
desmoid f.
desmoplastic f.
juvenile aponeurotic f.
Koenen periungual f.
f. molle
f. molluscum
nonossifying f. (NOF)
ossifying f.
osteogenic f.
periosteal f.
periungual f.
soft f.
subungual f.
fibromatosis
aggressive infantile f.
f. colli
congenital general f.

dermal f.
diffuse infantile f.
fascial f.
generalized f.
infantile dermal f.
irradiation f.
plantar f.
sternocleidomastoid muscle f.
subcutaneous pseudosarcomatous f.
fibromuscular disease
fibromyalgia syndrome (FMS)
fibromyalgic pain
fibromyositis
fibromyxoma
fibronectin
fibroosseous
f. pulley
f. ring of Lacroix
f. sheath
f. tunnel
fibropathic abnormality
fibroplasia
fibrosa
myositis f.
progressive myositis f.
fibrosarcoma
fibrosis
annular f.
intraneural f.
perineural f.
retroperitoneal f.
fibrositis
periarticular f.
fibrosus
annulus f.
lacertus f.
fibrotic
fibrous
f. adhesion
f. ankylosis
f. attachment
f. band
f. capsule
f. cortical defect
f. dysplasia
f. dysplasia ossificans progressiva
f. hamartoma
f. histiocytoma
f. lesion
f. loose body
f. scar tissue
f. spur

F

NOTES

213

fibrous *(continued)*
    f. talocalcaneal coalition
    f. tissue implant
    f. tumor
    f. xanthoma
fibrovascular connective tissue stroma
fibroxanthoma
fibula
    anterior ligament of head of f.
    diastasis f.
    distal f.
    dysplastic f.
    posterior ligament of head of f.
    f. protibial synostosis
    proximal f.
fibular
    f. anlage
    f. collateral ligament
    f. diaphyseal fracture
    f. groove
    f. head
    f. hemimelia
    f. metaphysis
    f. onlay-inlay graft
    f. ostectomy
    f. osteotomy
    f. peg
    f. pseudarthrosis
    f. sesamoid
    f. sesamoidal ligament
    f. sesamoidectomy
    f. strut graft
    f. transfer
    f. transplant
fibulare
    ligamentum collaterale f.
fibularis
    incisura f.
fibulectomy
    partial f.
fibulocalcaneal ligament
fibulotalar
    f. arthrodesis
    f. ligament
fibulotalocalcaneal (FTC)
    f. ligament
Ficat
    F. and Arlet classification
    F. and Arlet classification of
    stages of osteonecrosis
    F. and Arlet disease stage
    F. classification of femoral head
    osteonecrosis
    F. femoral head osteonecrosis
    classification
    F. procedure

    F. stage of avascular necrosis
    classification
    F. view
Ficat-Marcus grading system
Fick method
FID
    free induction decay
FiddleLink hand exerciser
field
    F. blade
    f. block
    bloodless f.
    f. of dissection
    f.-echo image
    pulsating electromagnetic f.
    pulsed electromagnetic f. (PEMF)
Fielding
    F. femoral fracture classification
    F. modification of Gallie technique
Fielding-Magliato
    F.-M. classification of
    subtrochanteric fracture
    F.-M. subtrochanteric fracture
    classification
fifth
    f. digit
    f. finger
    f. metacarpal
    f. metatarsal
    f. metatarsal base fracture
    f. metatarsophalangeal joint
    f. toe
fighter's fracture
figure-eight adjusting
figure-four position
figure-of-eight
    f.-o.-e. bandage
    f.-o.-e. brace
    f.-o.-e. cast
    f.-o.-e. dressing
    f.-o.-e. harness
    f.-o.-e. suture
    f.-o.-e. test
    f.-o.-e. thoracic orthosis
    f.-o.-e. wire loop
    f.-o.-e. wiring
figure-of-four test
file
    bone f.
    orthopaedic bone f.
    orthopaedic surgical f.
filgrastim
filiform
fill
    fit and f.
Fillauer
    F. bar
    F. bar foot orthosis

F. dorsiflexion assist ankle joint
F. endoskeletal alignment system
F. night splint
F. PDC ankle joint
F. prosthesis liner
F. Scottish Rite orthosis kit
F. silicone suspension liner

filler

f. block
nonosteoconductive bone-void f.
OsteoSet bone f.
ProOsteon implant 500 coralline
 hydroxyapatite bone void f.
shoe f.
Springlite toe f.

filleted graft
fillet local flap graft
film

scout f.
spot f.
stress f.

film-screen combination
filmy adhesion
filter

air f.
compensating f.
Greenfield inferior vena caval f.
high efficiency particulate air f.

filtration system
filum terminale syndrome
FIN

flexible intramedullary nail
FIN extractor
FIN pin guide
FIN system

finder

angle f.
canal f.
Dasco Pro angle f.
gravity-driven angle f.
pedicle f.

finding

constellation of clinical f.'s
thermographic f.

fine

f.-angled curette
f. curette
f. manipulation
f.-olive bur

finger

adduction stress to f.
baseball f.

claw f.
cloven-hoof fracture of f.
clubbing of f.
coach's f.
congenital trigger f.
f. cot
f. cot splint
Dasco Pro angle f.
f. deformity
f. exerciser
f. extension clockspring splint
extra-octave fracture of f.
fifth f.
F. Fitness Spring Ball
f. flap
f. flexion glove
f. flexion splint
f. flexor muscle
football f.
f. fracture
f. gauge
f. goniometer
F. Helper hand exerciser
f. hook
hypoplastic f.
index f. (2nd digit)
f. intrinsic
jammed f.
jersey f.
f. joint
f. joint arthroplasty
f. joint implant
f. joint implant prosthesis
f. ladder
little f. (5th digit)
long f. (3rd digit)
f. loop
lumbrical-plus f.
lumbrical syndrome f.
mallet f.
middle f.
multiple f.
paradoxical lumbrical-plus f.
F. Platter hand exerciser
f. pulp
f. ray
ring f. (4th digit)
sausage f.
f. separator
f. sling
spider f.
syndactylized f.

F

NOTES

finger *(continued)*
>   f.-to-nose test
>   f. tourniquet
>   trigger f.
>   f. tuft
>   f. web
>   webbed f.

fingerbreadth
Finger-Hugger splint
fingernail
>   base of f.
>   beak f.
>   f. drill

fingertip
>   f. amputation
>   f. cold intolerance
>   f. guard

fingertips-to-floor test
fingertrap
>   Chinese f.
>   Japanese f.
>   f. suspension
>   f. suture
>   f. traction

fin of the implant
finish bur
finisher
>   Küntscher f.

Finkelstein
>   F. maneuver
>   F. sign for synovitis
>   F. test
>   F. test for synovitis

Finney-Flexirod prosthesis
Finney prosthesis
Finn knee system
Finochietto
>   F. clamp carrier
>   F. rib retractor

Fiorinal with Codeine
firearm injury
Fired-Hendel procedure
firing
>   f. pattern
>   f. rate

FirmFlex
>   F. custom orthosis
>   F. custom orthotic

FIRST
>   FIRST knee prosthesis
>   FIRST total knee instrumentation

first
>   f. carpometacarpal joint fracture
>   f. cervical vertebra
>   f. cuneiform joint arthrodesis
>   f. cuneiform-navicular joint
>   arthrodesis
>   f. digit

>   f. dorsal metatarsal artery (FDMA)
>   f.-fifth intermetatarsal angle
>   f. intermetacarpal ligament
>   f. metacarpal
>   f. metatarsal
>   f. metatarsal-first cuneiform
>   arthrodesis
>   f. metatarsal head (FMH)
>   f. metatarsophalangeal joint
>   f. metatarsus rise test
>   f. plantar metatarsal artery (FPMA)
>   f. ray surgery
>   f. rib rasp
>   f. rib resection
>   f.-second intermetatarsal angle
>   f.-toe Jones repair
>   f. web space

Fisch
>   F. bone drill irrigator
>   F. drill

Fischer
>   F. pressure threshold meter
>   F. ring
>   F. tendon stripper
>   F. transfixing pin

Fish
>   F. cuneiform osteotomy
>   F. cuneiform osteotomy technique

Fisher
>   F. advancement flap
>   F. brace
>   F. exact test
>   F. guide
>   F. half pin
>   F. Protected Least Significant
>   Difference test
>   F. rasp

fishmouth
>   f. amputation
>   f. anastomosis
>   f. end-to-end suture
>   f. incision

fishtail
>   f. deformity
>   f. sign

Fiskars scissors
fissure fracture
fisticuffs
Fist-Palm-Side Test
Fist-Ring Test
fistula, pl. **fistulas, fistulae**
>   arteriovenous f. (AVF)
>   colocutaneous f.
>   enterocutaneous f.
>   Merland classification of
>   perimedullary arteriovenous fistulas
>   synovial f.
>   vesicocutaneous f.

fistulography
fit
    f. and fill
    interference f.
    press f.
    snap f.
    trial f.
Fit-Lastic therapy band
Fitness Safety Standards Committee
Fitnet joint testing system
Fitron
Fits-All sling
Fitstep
    F. II stair climber
    Universal F.
fitting
    immediate postsurgical f. (IPSF)
    prosthetic f.
    temporary prosthetic f.
    Velcro f.
five
    f. classifications of spondylolisthesis
    flexor wad of f.
    f.-hole plate
    f.-incision procedure
    f.-prong rake blade retractor
five-in-one
    f.-i.-o. knee ligament repair
    f.-i.-o. knee reconstruction
five-one
    f.-o. knee ligament repair
    f.-o. reconstruction
fixateur
    f. interne
    F. Interne fixation system
    F. Interne rod
    F. Interne screw
fixating apparatus
fixation
    abnormal f.
    Ace-Fischer f.
    Ace Unifix f.
    adjunctive screw f.
    Allen-Ferguson Galveston pelvic f.
    AMBI f.
    AMS intramedullary f.
    angled blade plate f.
    anterior internal f.
    anterior metallic f.
    anterior plate f.
    anterior screw f.
    anterior spinal f.

AO external f.
AO spinal internal f.
APR cement f.
arthroscopic screw f.
atlantoaxial rotatory f. (AARF)
Austin chevron osteotomy f.
axial f.
bar bolt f.
Barbour cervical f.
Barr open reduction and internal f.
Barr tibial fracture f.
bicortical screw f.
Biofix absorbable f.
biologic f.
blade plate f.
bolt f.
f. bolt
bone-ingrowth f.
bridge plate f.
buttressing in internal f.
Calandruccio f.
Campbell screw f.
cerclage wire f.
cervical spine internal f.
cervical spine screw-plate f.
chevron osteotomy with rigid
  screw f.
circumferential wire-loop f.
cloverleaf condylar plate f.
Cole tendon f.
compression plate f.
condylar screw f.
coracoclavicular screw f.
coracoclavicular suture f.
cross-screw f.
Denham external f.
dens anterior screw f.
Deverle f.
f. device
Dimon-Hughston fracture f.
dorsal wire-loop f.
dynamic compression plate f.
dynamic condylar screw f.
f. dysfunction of the lumbar spine
ECT internal fracture f.
Ender nail f.
Ender rod f.
EX-FI-RE external f.
external spinal f.
femoral prosthesis f.
four-bar external f.
four-point f.

F

NOTES

217

fixation *(continued)*
    fracture f.
    Gallie subtalar f.
    Galveston pelvic f.
    Georgiade visor halo f.
    Gouffon pin f.
    graft f.
    greenstick f.
    Hackethal intramedullary bouquet f.
    half-pin f.
    Halifax clamp posterior cervical f.
    Hammer external f.
    Harrington rod f.
    Herbert screw f.
    Hex-Fix external f.
    Hoffmann external f.
    hook-pin f.
    hook-plate f.
    iliac f.
    Ilizarov external f.
    f. imaging
    ingrowth f.
    interference fit f.
    intermedullary rod f.
    internal spinal f.
    interosseous wire f.
    intersegmental f.
    intramedullary rod f.
    intrapedicular f.
    f. jig
    Kavanaugh-Brower-Mann f.
    Kirschner pin f.
    Kirschner wire f.
    Kristiansen-Kofoed external f.
    Kronner external f.
    Kyle internal f.
    lag screw f.
    loop f.
    LPPS hydroxyapatite f.
    lumbar pedicle f.
    lumbar spine segmental f.
    lumbar spine transpedicular f.
    Luque-Galveston f.
    Luque loop f.
    Luque rod f.
    Luque segmental f.
    Magerl posterior cervical screw f.
    Matta-Saucedo f.
    McKeever medullary clavicle f.
    medial malleolus f.
    medullary nail f.
    Minerva f.
    minifragment plate f.
    monofilament wire f.
    Monticelli-Spinelli leg f.
    Morrissy percutaneous slipped
      epiphysis f.
    multiple-point sacral f.

    nail plate f.
    neutralization plate f.
    occipitocervical f.
    odontoid fracture internal f.
    Olerud transpedicular f.
    open reduction, internal f. (ORIF)
    Orthofix f.
    OrthoSorb pin f.
    pedicle f.
    pedicular f.
    f. peg
    pelvic f.
    percutaneous f.
    phalangeal fracture f.
    Phemister acromioclavicular pin f.
    f. pin
    pin f.
    pin-and-plaster f.
    plate f.
    plate-screw f.
    porous ingrowth f.
    posterior cervical f.
    posterior screw f.
    posterior segmental f.
    Precision Osteolock f.
    Press-Fit f.
    prophylactic skeletal f.
    provisional f.
    Rezaian external f.
    rigid internal f.
    rod sleeve f.
    Rogozinski spinal f.
    Roy-Camille posterior screw
      plate f.
    sacral pedicle screw f.
    sacral spine f.
    sacroiliac extension f.
    sacroiliac flexion f.
    sacrum fusion screw f.
    Schneider f.
    Schuind external f.
    scoliotic curve f.
    screw f.
    screw-and-plate f.
    screw-and-wire f.
    segmental f.
    Seidel intramedullary f.
    spinal f.
    spring f.
    staple f.
    static f.
    Steinmann pin f.
    strut plate f.
    sublaminar f.
    f. subluxation
    suprasyndesmotic f.
    suprasyndesmotic screw f.
    Suretac shoulder f.

suture f.
f. technique
tension band f.
TiMesh implantable hardware f.
transarticular screw f.
transarticular wire f.
transcapitellar wire f.
transiliac rod f.
transpedicular f.
transsyndesmotic screw f.
transverse f.
triangular external ankle f.
TSRH rod f.
tunnel-and-sling f.
Versa-Fx femoral f.
Vidal-Adrey modified Hoffmann f.
Volkov-Oganesian external f.
VSP f.
Ward-Tomasin-Vander-Griend f.
Warner-Farber ankle f.
Webb f.
white f.
Wilson-Jacobs tibial f.
wire loop f.
Wisconsin wire f.
Wolvek sternal approximation f.
Zickel nail f.
Zickel subtrochanteric fracture f.

fixator

Ace-Colles external f.
Ace-Fischer external f.
Agee-WristJack external f.
AO internal f.
articulated external f.
biplanar f.
carbon fiber f.
circular external f.
circular wire f.
Claiborne external f.
clamp f.
Clyburn Colles fracture f.
Clyburn external f.
DeBastiani external f.
dynamic axial f. (DAF)
EBI external f.
Edwards D-L modular f.
external f.
external spinal skeletal f. (ESSF)
f. frame
Ganz anti-shock pelvic f.
half-pin external f.

Herbert screw f.
Hex-Fix monolateral external f.
hinged articulated f.
Hoffmann C-series external f.
Hoffmann Dynamic external f.
Hoffmann-Vidal external f.
HTO f.
hybrid external f.
Ilizarov circular external f.
Ilizarov external ring f.
Ilizarov hybrid f.
f. interne (FI)
Jacquet f.
Kessler external f.
Lima external f.
Manuflex external f.
mini-Hoffmann external f.
mini-Orthofix f.
modified Hoffmann quadrilateral
  external f.
Monofixateur external f.
Monticelli-Spinelli f.
Olerud internal f.
one-plane bilateral external f.
one-plane unilateral external f.
Orthofix external f.
Orthofix monolateral femoral
  external f.
Oxford f.
Pennig dynamic wrist f.
pin external f.
Rezaian spinal f.
Richards Colles external f.
ring external f.
Roger Anderson external f.
spanning external f.
Stableloc Colles fracture external f.
thin-wire Ilizarov f.
Thomas f.
two-plane bilateral external f.
two-plane unilateral external f.
Vermont spinal f. (VSF)
Wagner device external f.
Wiltse f.

fixed

f. bearing knee implant
f. deformity
f. distraction
f. femoral head prosthesis
f. flexion contracture (FFC)
f.-offset guide

F

NOTES

fixed-angle
    f.-a. AO bladeplate
    f.-a. blade plate
FJD
  facet joint disease
flaccid
    f. cerebral palsy
    f. flatfoot
    f. gait
    f. paralysis
flaccidity
flag
    f. flap
    f. sign
Flagyl
flail
    f. digit
    f.-elbow hinge
    f. feet
    f. foot
    f. implant
    f. joint
    f. knee
    f. shoulder
    f. toe
flake fracture
flame-tip bur
Flanagan-Burem apposing hemicylindric graft
flange
  endoprosthetic f.
flap
  abdominal f.
  adductor magnus adductor f.
  adipofascial f.
  advancement f.
  anterior myocutaneous f.
  arm f.
  arterial f.
  Atasoy-Kleinert f.
  Atasoy triangular advancement f.
  Atasoy volar V-Y f.
  axial pattern f.
  axillary f.
  below-knee amputation using long posterior f.
  bilateral V-Y Kutler f.
  bilobed digital neurovascular island f.
  bilobed skin f.
  bipedicle dorsal f.
  brachioradialis f.
  buccinator myomucosal f.
  bursal f.
  capsular f.
  Chinese f.
  cocked-half f.
  composite groin fascial free f.

  f. congestion
  cross-arm f.
  cross-finger f.
  cross-leg f.
  cutaneous f.
  deltoid f.
  deltopectoral f.
  dorsal cross-finger f.
  dorsalis pedis f.
  DRAM f.
  fasciocutaneous island f.
  finger f.
  Fisher advancement f.
  flag f.
  foot first-web f.
  forearm f.
  free fasciocutaneous f.
  free latissimus dorsi f.
  free microsurgical f.
  free skin f.
  gastrocnemius f.
  Gilbert scapular f.
  gluteus maximus f.
  gracilis f.
  f. graft
  groin f.
  hemipulp f.
  horseshoe-shaped f.
  hypogastric f.
  iliac osteocutaneous f.
  iliofemoral pedicle f.
  intercostal f.
  inverted skin f.
  island adipofascial f.
  island skin f.
  Kutler double lateral advancement f.
  Kutler V-Y f.
  lateral arm f.
  lateral thigh f.
  lateral thoracic f.
  latissimus dorsi f.
  lazy-V deepithelialized turn-over fasciocutaneous f.
  Limberg f.
  medial plantar fasciocutaneous f.
  f. meniscal tear
  microvascular free f.
  Moberg advancement f.
  Morrison neurovascular free f.
  multistaged carrier f.
  muscle f.
  musculocutaneous free f.
  musculotendinous f.
  myocutaneous f.
  neurocutaneous hand f.
  neurovascular free f.
  nutrient f.

omental f.
osteocutaneous free f.
osteomusculocutaneous f.
osteoperiosteal f.
palmar advancement f.
palmar cross-finger f.
parascapular f.
pectoralis major f.
pedicle groin f.
perineal f.
plantar f.
posterior f.
pulp f.
radial-based f.
radial forearm f.
random pattern f.
rectus abdominis f.
rectus femoris f.
remote pedicle f.
reverse cross-finger f.
reverse forearm island f.
rhomboid f.
rotational f.
saphenous f.
scapular f.
serratus anterior f.
skew f.
skin f.
sliding f.
soft tissue f.
Steichen neurovascular free f.
supramalleolar f.
sural island f.
Tait f.
temporalis fascia f.
tensor fascia femoris f.
tensor fascia lata muscle f.
thenar f.
thoracoepigastric f.
transposition f.
triangular advancement f.
turn-down tendon f.
Urbaniak neurovascular free f.
Urbaniak scapular f.
vascularized free f.
V-Y advancement f.
V-Y Kutler f.
web space f.
wraparound neurovascular free f.

flare

f. of the condyle
foot f.

medial tibial f.
steroid f.

flared spinal rod
FlashCast
Delta-Lite F.

flat
f. back deformity
f. back syndrome
f. bone
f. bone graft
f.-bottomed Kerrison rongeur
f. drill
f. palpation
f. retractor
f. splint

flatfoot
acquired f.
calcaneovalgus f.
f. deformity
Durham f.
flaccid f.
hypermobile f.
Kidner f.
neonatal f.
peroneal spastic f.
pronated straight f.
rigid f.
rockerbottom f.
spastic f.

flatfooted
Flatt
F. classification
F. driver
F. excision
F. finger-joint prosthesis
F. finger prosthesis
F. finger-thumb prosthesis
F. implant
F. recess
F. self-retaining screwdriver
F. technique
F. tendon transfer

flattening of normal lordotic curve
F&L attenuating glove
flattop talus
flatware
Amefa F.
Cushion Grip F.
Melaware f.

flaval ligament
flavum, pl. **flava**
ligamentum f.

F

NOTES

Flaxedil
Fleck sign
flesh
    proud f.
Fletching femoral hernia implant
  material
flex
    f. against gravity
    F. Foam brace
    F. Foam orthosis
Flexall gel
Flexaphen
Flexderm
    F. wound dressing
flexed
    plantar f.
    f. position
Flexeril
Flex-Foam bandage
Flex-Foot prosthesis
Flexform
flexibility
    Cotrel-Dubousset rod f.
    f. training
flexible
    f. bandage
    f. digital implant
    f. hammertoe
    f. hinge implant
    f. hinge suspension
    f. intramedullary nail (FIN)
    f. medullary nail
    f. medullary reamer
    f. pes planus
    f. pes valgus
    f. socket
    f. sound
    f. talipes
Flexicair bed
FLEXIGRID dressing
Flexilite conforming elastic bandage
Flexinet dressing
flexing
flexion
    f. in abduction and external
      rotation (faber)
    f., abduction, external rotation
      contracture
    active f.
    f.-adduction
    f. in adduction and internal
      rotation (fadir)
    f. angle
    angle of greatest f. (AGF)
    f. axis
    f. body cast
    f. body jacket
    f. bumper

    f.-burst fracture
    cervical specific rotation in f.
    compression f.
    f.-compression fracture
    f. compression spine injury
      stabilization
    f. contracture
    f. creaking
    f. distraction
    distractive f.
    dorsiflexion f.
    elongation-derotation f.
    f. and extension
    external rotation in f. (ERF)
    femoral-trunk f.
    forward f.
    full fist f.
    further f. (FF)
    f. gap
    f. glove
    hip f.
    f. injury posterior atlantoaxial
      arthrodesis
    f. instability
    internal rotation in f. (IRF)
    f.-internal rotational deformity
    knee f.
    lateral f.
    left lateral f.
    lumbar lateral f.
    lumbosacral f.
    f. malposition
    f. osteotomy
    palmar f.
    passive plantar f.
    plantar f.
    resisted active f.
    f. restriction
    right lateral f.
    Riordan finger f.
    f.-rotation-compression maneuver
    f.-rotation-drawer knee instability
      test
    Schober test of lumbar f.
    shelf f.
    sitting f.
    f. spinal radiography test
    spine f.
    standing f.
    transverse axis knee f.
    f. valgus deformity
flexion-distraction
    f.-d. fracture
    f.-d. injury
    f.-d. table
flexion-extension
    f.-e. arc
    f.-e. axis

f.-e. control cervical orthosis
f.-e. exercise
f.-e. gap
hip f.-e.
knee f.-e.
f.-e. maneuver
f.-e. MRI
f.-e. plane
f.-e. radiography
Flexirule
Flexisplint
    F. flexed arm board
    F. flexed armboard
FlexiSport orthotic
Flexi-Therm diabetic diagnostic insole
FlexiTherm Thermographic System
FlexLite hinged knee support
Flex-Master bandage
flexometer
    Moeltgen f.
flexor
    anterior long toe f.
    f. cap
    f. carpi radialis (FCR)
    f. carpi radialis muscle
    f. carpi radialis tendon
    f. carpi ulnaris (FCU)
    f. carpi ulnaris muscle
    f. carpi ulnaris syndrome
    f. carpi ulnaris tendon
    f. digiti quinti brevis (FDQB)
    f. digiti quinti muscle
    f. digitorum brevis (FDB)
    f. digitorum communis (FDC)
    f. digitorum communis tendon
    f. digitorum longus (FDL)
    f. digitorum longus muscle
    f. digitorum longus tendon
    f. digitorum longus tendon transfer
    f. digitorum profundus (FDP)
    f. digitorum profundus muscle
    f. digitorum profundus tendon
    f. digitorum slip
    f.-digitorum sublimis (FDS)
    f. digitorum sublimis muscle
    f. digitorum sublimis tendon
    f. digitorum superficialis (FDS)
    f. digitorum superficialis muscle
    f. digitorum superficialis tendon
    f. glove
    f. groove
    f. hallucis brevis (FHB)

f. hallucis brevis muscle
f. hallucis brevis tendon
f. hallucis longus (FHL)
f. hallucis longus dysfunction
  (FHLD)
f. hallucis longus muscle
f. hallucis longus tendon
f. hallucis longus tendon release
f. hallucis longus tenosynovitis
f.-hinge hand-splint brace
f. hinge splint
long f.
long toe f.
f. mechanism
f. origin syndrome
f. phase
f. plate
f. pollicis brevis (FPB)
f. pollicis brevis muscle
f. pollicis brevis tendon
f. pollicis longus (FPL)
f. pollicis longus abductor-plasty
f. pollicis longus muscle
f. pollicis longus tendon
f. profundus tendon
f. pronator slide
f. retinaculum
f. retinaculum of hand
f. skin crease
snapping thumb f.
f. sublimis tendon
f. tendon anastomosis
f. tendon graft
f. tendon laceration
f. tendon repair
f. tendon rupture
f. tendon sheath
f. tenosynovectomy
f. tenotomy
f. wad
f. wad of five
f. withdrawal reflex
X-TEND-O knee f.
flexorplasty
    Bunnell modification of Steindler f.
    Eyler f.
    Steindler f.
flexor-pronator
    f.-p. origin
    f.-p. origin release
Flextender Plus hand exerciser
flexural concavity

F

NOTES

flexus
  hallux f.
Flick-Gould technique
Flip-Flop pillow
flipper hand
flip test
FLOAM ankle stirrup brace
floating
  f. arch fracture
  f. clavicle
  f. elbow
  f. gait
  f. knee
  f. ligament
  f. rib
  f. thumb
  f. toe
  f. traction
floccosum
  Epidermophyton f.
flocculent foci of calcification
Flo-Fit Comfortseat
FloFit cushion
floor
  f. of the acetabulum
  f.-reaction ankle-foot orthosis
  f. sitter
floppy
  f. infant
  f. toe
flora
  bacterial f.
Floralax
Florical
florid
  f. callus
  f. reactive periostitis
  f. rickets
  f. synovitis
Florida
  F. back brace
  F. cervical brace
  F. contraflexion brace
  F. extension brace
  F. hyperextension brace
  F. J-24, J-35, J-45, J-55 brace
  F. post-fusion brace
  F. spinal brace
Flotan thumb
Flo-Tech prosthetic socket
Flo-Trol drinking cup
flottant
  pouce f. (floating thumb)
flow
  axoplasmic f.
  blood f.
  laminar air f.
flower-spray ending

flowmeter
  Doppler ultrasound f.
flowmetry
  laser Doppler f. (LDF)
Flowtron
  F. DVT
  F. pneumatic compression system
    BioCryo system
FLP
  Functional Limitation Profile
fluctuation test
flucytosine
fluff dressing
FLUFTEX gauze roll
fluid
  f. balance
  bursal f.
  cerebrospinal f. (CSF)
  f. homeostasis
  interstitial f.
  f. sign
  synovial f.
FluidAir bed
Fluidotherapy sterile dry heat modality
fluorescein
  f. dye test
  f. perfusion monitoring
  f. study
fluoride
Fluori-Methane Topical Spray
fluormethane
fluoroallergosorbent test (FAST)
fluorometholone
fluoroquinolone
  f.-associated Achilles tendon
    disorder
FluoroScan
fluoroscope
  C-arm f.
  Xi-scan f.
fluoroscopic table
fluoroscopy
  C-arm f.
  intraoperative f.
  portable C-arm image intensifier f.
  two-plane f.
  Xi-scan f.
flurazepam
flurbiprofen
Fluro-Ethyl Aerosol
flush
  heparinized saline f.
  peroxide f.
fluted
  f. medullary rod
  f. reamer
  f. Sampson nail
  f. titanium nail

flutes of cannulated screw
Flutex
FLX flexible treatment coilette
Flynn
    F. femoral neck fracture reduction
    F. technique
FMH
    first metatarsal head
FMS
    fibromyalgia syndrome
    FMS Intracell stick
FO
    foot orthosis
foam
    Evazote f.
    gelatin f.
    hi-density f.
    Neoplush f.
    f. padding
    Pedilen polyurethane f.
    Plastazote f.
    polyethylene f.
    prosthetic f.
    f. ring
    f. slant
    f. tape
    Temper f.
    f. tubing
FOAMART Foot Impression System
focal
    f. deficiency
    f. dystonia
    f. film distance (FFD)
    f. nodular myositis
    f. pigmented villanodular synovitis
focus, pl. foci
    foci of hyaline cartilage detritus
Foerster forceps
fold
    asymmetric skin f.
    Bartlett nail f.
    nail f.
    f.-over finger splint
    synovial f.
Folex PFS
Foley catheter
folic acid
fomentation therapy
Fomon
    F. chisel
    F. periosteal elevator

    F. periosteotome
    F. rasp
Fonar
    F. QUAD MRI scanner
FONAR Stand-Up MRI
FOOSH
    fell on outstretched hand
    FOOSH injury
foot
    Aftate for Athlete's F.
    f. angle
    f. and ankle severity scale (FASS)
    athlete's f.
    ball of the f.
    basketball f.
    calcaneocavus f.
    calcaneovalgus f.
    Carbon Copy II light f.
    cavovarus f.
    cavus f.
    Charcot f.
    Cirrus composite prosthetic f.
    clavus f.
    clawfoot f.
    cleft f.
    f. collapse
    College Park TruStep f.
    f. cosmesis
    C-shaped f.
    dangling f.
    f. decompression
    diabetic Charcot f.
    f. drop
    f. drop night splint
    dropped f., dropfoot
    Dr Scholl's Athlete's F.
    Dycor prosthetic f.
    equinocavus f.
    equinovalgus f.
    equinovarus f.
    equinus f.
    f. first-web flap
    flail f.
    f. flare
    Friedreich f.
    F. Hugger foot support
    hypermobile f.
    f. imprinter
    inferior extensor of f.
    insensate f.
    interpositional arthroplasty of f.
    f. ischemia

NOTES

F

foot (*continued*)
    ischemic f.
    Kingsley Steplite f.
    lateral spring ligament of f.
    F. Levelers custom orthotic
    F. Levelers orthosis
    lobster f.
    f. magnet
    malodorous f.
    march f.
    f. model
    Morton f.
    multiaxis f.
    neuroarthropathic f.
    neuropathic f.
    numb f.
    f. orthosis (FO)
    f. orthotic
    Otto Bock 1A30 Greissinger
      Plus f.
    Otto Bock 1D25 Dynamic Plus f.
    paralytic f.
    Persian slipper f.
    f. pillow
    f. placement test
    plantigrade f.
    f. plate
    polydactylous cleft f.
    f. pound
    f.-progression angle
    pronated f.
    pronation of the f.
    f. prosthesis
    f. puncture wound
    Quantum f.
    Re-Flex VSP artificial f.
    f. rest
    rheumatoid f.
    rigid f.
    rockerbottom f.
    f. rotation
    SACH f.
    SAFE f.
    serpentine f.
    single-axis Syme DYCOR f.
    sole of f.
    solid ankle, cushioned heel f.
    f. stabilizer
    stairclimbers f.
    f. stool
    f. strike phase of gait
    superior extensor retinaculum of f.
    supination of the f.
    Sure-Flex III prosthetic f.
    Syme Dycor prosthetic f.
    tabetic f.
    tripod f.
    Trowbridge TerraRound f.
    f. type
    University of California, Berkeley
      SACH f.
    valgus f.
    f. volumeter
    z f.

foot-ankle
    f.-a. assembly
    f.-a. brace

football
    f. ankle
    f. finger

footbrush
    Dr. Joseph's f.

footdrop
    f. brace
    f. gait

Foot-Fitter

footgear

footpiece
    Bunker f.
    traction f.

footplate
    metal f.
    Springlight f.

footprint
    f. analysis
    Cavanaugh-Rogers classification
      of f.'s
    tibial f.

footrest

Foot-Station 3-D foot imaging system

foot-thigh axis

FootTrak testing

footwear
    Ambulator conform f.

forage
    f. core biopsy
    f. procedure

foramen, pl. **foramina**
    arcuate f.
    intravertebral f. (IVF)
    f. magnum
    neural f.
    open exit f.
    sciatic f.
    f. transversarium

foraminal
    f. compression test
    f. encroachment subluxation
    f. osteophyte encroachment
    f. stenosis

foraminotomy
    neural f.

Forbes
    F. modification of Phemister graft
      technique
    F. onlay bone graft

force

    activation f.
    f. application
    contact f.
    f.-couple splint reduction
    distraction f.
    dynamic joint f.
    evertor f.
    forefoot f.
    gravity ground reaction f.
    ground reaction f.
    hamstring f.
    invertor f.
    isometric f.
    joint f.
    knee f.
    lateral compression f.
    moment of f.
    Newton f.
    f. nucleus
    patellofemoral joint reaction f.
    f. plate
    f. plate foot analysis
    prehension f.
    reaction f.
    subthreshold f.
    tensile f.
    tension f.
    torque f.
    f. transducer
    translatory f.
    weightbearing ground reaction f.
forced
    f. flexion injury
    f. vital capacity (FVC)
forceps
    Acland clamp-applying f.
    Acufex curved basket f.
    Acufex rotary biting basket f.
    Adson drill guide f.
    Adson hypophyseal f.
    adventitial f.
    Aesculap f.
    Aesculap bipolar cautery f.
    alligator grasping f.
    Allis tissue f.
    Angell James hypophysectomy f.
    angled-down f.
    angled-up f.
    anterior f.
    AO reduction f.
    Arrowsmith-Clerf pin-closing f.

    arthroscopy basket f.
    arthroscopy grasping f.
    Asch f.
    Babcock f.
    baby Lane f.
    Backhaus towel f.
    Baer bone-cutting f.
    Bane rongeur f.
    Bardeleben bone-holding f.
    basket f.
    bearing-seating f.
    Beasley-Babcock f.
    Berens muscle clamp f.
    biopsy f.
    bipolar f.
    Bircher-Ganske cartilage f.
    blunt f.
    Boies f.
    bone-biting f.
    bone-breaking f.
    bone-cutting f.
    bone-grasping f.
    bone-holding f.
    bone punch f.
    bone-splitting f.
    Brand tendon-holding f.
    Brand tendon-passing f.
    Brown-Adson f.
    Brown-Cushing f.
    Brown tissue f.
    bulldog clamp-applying f.
    Cairns hemostatic f.
    Carroll bone-holding f.
    Carroll dressing f.
    Carroll tendon-pulling f.
    Carroll tissue f.
    cartilage f.
    cervical punch f.
    Chandler spinal perforating f.
    Charnley wire-holding f.
    Citelli punch f.
    clamp f.
    Cleveland bone-cutting f.
    clip-applying f.
    clip-bending f.
    clip-cutting f.
    clip-introducing f.
    coagulating f.
    cupped grasping f.
    curved basket f.
    cutting f.
    Dawson-Yuhl-Kerrison rongeur f.

F

NOTES

forceps *(continued)*
  Dawson-Yuhl-Leksell rongeur f.
  Dawson-Yuhl rongeur f.
  Dingman bone-holding f.
  disk f.
  Dreyfus prosthesis f.
  drill guide f.
  Echlin rongeur f.
  ethmoid f.
  extracting f.
  Farabeuf bone-hold f.
  Farabeuf-Lambotte bone-holding f.
  Farrior wire-crimping f.
  Fergusson f.
  Ferris Smith-Kerrison f.
  Ferris Smith rongeur f.
  Ferris Smith tissue f.
  Foerster f.
  Friedman rongeur f.
  gall duct f.
  Gardner bone f.
  Gildenberg biopsy f.
  glenoid-reaming f.
  grasping f.
  Greene f.
  Gruppe wire prosthesis-crimping f.
  Gunderson bone f.
  Gunderson muscle f.
  Guppe f.
  Hajek-Koffler bone punch f.
  Harrington clamp f.
  Harrison bone-holding f.
  Hartmann mosquito f.
  Heermann alligator f.
  hemostatic f.
  Hibbs bone-cutting f.
  Hinderer cartilage f.
  Hirsch hypophysis punch f.
  Hoen f.
  Horsley bone-cutting f.
  Horsley-Stille bone-cutting f.
  Horsley-Stille rib shears f.
  Housepan clip-applying f.
  Howmedica Microfixation System f.
  Hudson f.
  Hurd bone-cutting f.
  implant f.
  Jackson broad-blade staple f.
  Jackson dressing f.
  Jackson tendon-seizing f.
  Jacobson mosquito f.
  James wound f.
  Jansen monopolar f.
  Jarell f.
  Jarit tendon-pulling f.
  jeweler's f.
  Juers-Lempert rongeur f.
  Kelly f.

  Kern bone-holding f.
  Kern-Lane bone f.
  King wound f.
  Kleinert-Kutz rongeur f.
  Kleinert-Kutz tendon f.
  knotting f.
  Kocher f.
  Lalonde hook f.
  Lambotte bone-holding f.
  Landolt spreading f.
  Lane bone-holding f.
  Lane screw-holding f.
  Lane self-retaining bone-holding f.
  Langenbeck bone-holding f.
  Larsen tendon-holding f.
  Leibinger Micro System plate-
    holding f.
  Leksell rongeur f.
  Lempert rongeur f.
  LeRoy clip-applying f.
  Lester muscle f.
  Lewin bone-holding f.
  Lewin spinal perforating f.
  ligamentum flavum f.
  lion f.
  lion-jaw f.
  Liston bone-cutting f.
  Liston-Key bone-cutting f.
  Liston-Littauer bone-cutting f.
  Liston-Stille bone-cutting f.
  Littauer-Liston bone-cutting f.
  Llorente dissecting f.
  long-jaw basket f.
  Lore suction tube and tip-
    holding f.
  Love-Gruenwald alligator f.
  Love-Kerrison rongeur f.
  Lowman bone-holding f.
  Luer rongeur f.
  Luer-Whiting rongeur f.
  Luhr Microfixation System plate-
    holding f.
  Malis-Jensen microbipolar f.
  Malis jeweler bipolar f.
  Mantis retrograde f.
  Markwalder rib f.
  Martin cartilage f.
  Mayfield f.
  McCain TMJ f.
  McGee-Priest wire f.
  McGee wire-crimping f.
  McIndoe rongeur f.
  meniscus f.
  Micro-One dissecting f.
  Micro-Two f.
  Mixter f.
  mosquito-tip grasping f.
  nail-pulling f.

Nicola f.
Niro bone-cutting f.
Niro wire-twisting f.
Olivecrona clip-applying and
  removing f.
orthopaedic f.
Overholt clip-applying f.
perforating f.
Perman cartilage f.
pick-up f.
pin-seating f.
plain tissue f.
plate-holding f.
Poppen f.
Potts-Smith dressing f.
Preston ligamentum flavum f.
punch f.
Raimondi hemostatic f.
rat-tooth f.
reduction f.
rib f.
Riches artery f.
ring f.
Rochester-Carmalt f.
Rochester-Ochsner f.
Rochester-Pean f.
rongeur f.
rotary basket f.
Rowe disimpaction f.
Rowe glenoid-reaming f.
Rowe-Harrison bone-holding f.
Rowe modified-Harrison f.
Ruskin bone-splitting f.
Ruskin-Liston bone-cutting f.
Ruskin rongeur f.
Ruskin-Rowland bone-cutting f.
Russian f.
Samuels f.
Sauerbruch rib f.
Schlesinger cervical punch f.
Schlesinger rongeur f.
Schwartz clip-applying f.
Schwartz temporary clamp-
  applying f.
screw-holding f.
Seaber f.
seizing f.
self-retaining bone-holding f.
Selverstone rongeur f.
Semb bone f.
Semb rib f.
septal f.

sequestrum f.
Shutt Mantis retrograde f.
side-cutting basket f.
Smithwick clip-applying f.
smooth-tipped jeweler's f.
spatula f.
Spence rongeur f.
sponge-holding f.
spreading f.
Spurling-Kerrison rongeur f.
Steinmann tendon f.
Stevenson alligator f.
Stevenson grasping f.
Stille-Horsley rib f.
Stille-Liston bone-cutting f.
Stille-Luer rongeur f.
Stiwer bone-holding f.
Storz Microsystems plate-holding f.
straight basket f.
Synthes Microsystems plate-
  holding f.
tack-and-pin f.
Takahashi f.
Take-apart f.
taper-jaw f.
tenaculum-reducing f.
tendon f.
tendon-braiding f.
tendon-holding f.
tendon-passing f.
tendon-pulling f.
tendon-retrieving f.
tendon-seizing f.
tendon-tunneling f.
Thompson hip prosthesis f.
three-edge cutting f.
thumb f.
tissue f.
titanium microsurgical bipolar f.
Toennis tumor f.
toothed tissue f.
Tudor-Edwards bone-cutting f.
tumor-grasping f.
tying f.
Ulrich bone-holding f.
Ulrich-St. Gallen f.
upbiting basket f.
upcurved punch f.
Utrata f.
Van Buren sequestrum f.
vascular f.
Verbrugge bone-holding f.

F

NOTES

forceps *(continued)*
    Walter-Liston f.
    Walton-Ruskin f.
    Walton wire-pulling f.
    Weller cartilage f.
    Wiet cup f.
    Wilde ethmoid f.
    Wilde rongeur f.
    wire-cutting f.
    wire-extracting f.
    wire-holding f.
    wire prosthesis-crimping f.
    wire-pulling f.
    wire-tightening f.
    wire-twisting f.
    X-long cement f.
    Zimmer-Hoen f.
    Zimmer-Schlesinger f.
force-time integral (FTI)
Ford triangulation technique
forearm
    f. amputation
    carrying angle of f.
    f. compartment syndrome
    f. complex
    f. contracture
    distal f.
    f. flap
    f. fracture
    f. lift-assist prosthesis
    one-bone f.
    f. splint
    f. supination test
    three-bone f.
    f. tourniquet
forefoot
    f. abduction deformity
    f. abductus
    f. adductovarus
    f. adductus
    f. angulation
    f. arthroplasty
    f. block
    f. digital amputation
    f. equinus
    f. force
    Larmon f.
    f. splaying
    f. valgus
    f. varus
foreign
    f. body (FB)
    f. body granuloma
    f. body response
    f. body screw
forequarter amputation
Forest-Hastings technique

Forestier
    F. bowstring sign
    F. disease
fork strap prosthetic support
form
    f. constancy
    IKDC f.
    International Knee Documentation
      Committee f.
    Jettmobile positioning and
      tumble f.
    SF-36 patient assessment f.
    Vestibulator positioning tumble f.
formal hemipelvectomy
formation
    adhesion f.
    beaklike osteophyte f.
    bunion f.
    callous f.
    Cyclops f.
    intramembranous f.
    lappet f.
    osteophyte f.
    procallus f.
    rouleaux f.
    scar f.
    spur f.
    trellis f.
Formatray mandibular splint
forme fruste
formula
    Bayer Select Pain Relief F.
    Dreyer f.
Forrester
    F. cervical collar brace
    F. splint
Forrester-Brown
    F.-B. collar
    F.-B. head halter
Fortaz
Forte
    Aristocort F.
    Citanest F.
    F. ES
    F. harness
    Norgesic F.
    Parafon F.
    Triam F.
fortuitum
    Mycobacterium f.
forward
    f. bending
    f.-cutting knife
    f. flexion
    f. flexion posture
    f. head posture
Fosamax
Fosnaugh nail biopsy

fossa
> antecubital f.
> glenoid f.
> intercondylar f.
> ischiorectal f.
> lower fossa active, lateral knee pain, and long leg on the side ipsilateral to the weak f. (LLL)
> olecranon f.
> f. ovalis
> popliteal f.
> sphenoidal f.
> upper fossa active, medial knee pain, and short leg on the side ipsilateral to the week f. (UMS)

FossFill Health Pillow

Foster
> F. bed
> F. splint
> F. turning frame

Foster-Kennedy maneuver

Foucher classification of epiphyseal injury

foundation
> F. for Chiropractic Education and Research (FCER)
> level f.
> Musculoskeletal Transplant F. (MTF)

four
> f.-corner midcarpal fusion
> f.-flanged nail
> f.-incision procedure
> f.-limb Z-plasty
> f.-prong finger splint
> f.-star exercise program
> f.-tap screw
> f.-wire trochanter reattachment

four-bar
> f.-b. external fixation
> f.-b. external fixation apparatus
> f.-b. linkage on knee prosthesis
> f.-b. linkage prosthetic knee mechanism
> F.-b. Polycentric knee prosthesis

four-hole side plate

Fourier
> F. analysis
> F. pulsatility index
> F. transform infrared spectroscopy

four-in-one
> f.-i.-o. arthroplasty
> f.-i.-o. block

Fournier test

four-part
> f.-p. fracture
> f.-p. variant

four-point
> f.-p. cervical brace
> f.-p. fixation
> f.-p. gait
> f.-p. walker

four-poster
> f.-p. cervical brace
> f.-p. cervical orthosis
> f.-p. frame

fourth
> f. carpometacarpal joint fracture
> f. digit
> f. metatarsophalangeal joint

fovea

foveal fat pad

Fowler
> F. central slip tenotomy
> F. knee system
> F. maneuver
> F. osteotomy
> F. position
> F. procedure
> F. spread
> F. technique
> F. tendon transfer
> F. tenodesis

Fowler-Philip
> F.-P. angle
> F.-P. approach
> F.-P. incision

Fowles
> F. dislocation technique
> F. open reduction

Fox
> F. clavicular splint
> F. extractor-impactor
> F. impactor-extractor
> F. internal fixation apparatus
> F. internal fixation device
> F. wrench

Fox-Blazina knee procedure

FP5000 pump system

FPB
> flexor pollicis brevis

NOTES

F

FPL
    flexor pollicis longus
FPMA
    first plantar metatarsal artery
Frac-Sur splint
fract
    fracture
fraction
    linear f.
    motor unit f.
fractional
    f. curve
    f. lengthening
fractionation
Fractomed splint
Fractura
    F. Flex bandage
    F. Flex cast
fracture (fract, fx)
    abduction-external rotation f.
    acetabular posterior wall f.
    acetabular rim f.
    acute avulsion f.
    adduction f.
    Aebi-Etter-Coscia fixation dens f.
    agenetic f.
    AIIS avulsion f.
    Aitken classification of
      epiphyseal f.
    Allen open reduction of
      calcaneal f.
    alveolar bone f.
    anatomic location of f.
    Anderson-Hutchins unstable tibial
      shaft f.
    angulated f.
    angulation f.
    ankle mortise f.
    anterior calcaneal process f.
    anterior column f.
    anterolateral compression f.
    AO classification of ankle f.
    AO-Denis-Weber classification of
      ankle f.
    apophyseal f.
    arch f.
    articular mass separation f.
    articular pillar f.
    Ashhurst-Bromer ankle f.
      classification
    Atkin epiphyseal f.
    atlas f.
    atrophic f.
    avulsion chip f.
    avulsion stress f.
    backfire f.
    Bankart f.
    Barton f.

basal neck f.
baseball finger f.
basilar femoral neck f.
basocervical f.
bayonet position of f.
beak f.
bedroom f.
Bennett comminuted f.
Berndt-Hardy classification of
  transchondral f.
bicondylar T-shaped f.
bicondylar Y-shaped f.
bicycle spoke f.
bimalleolar ankle f.
bipartite f.
birth f.
f. blister
blow-in f.
blow-out f.
f. boot
boot-top f.
Bosworth f.
both-bone f.
both-column f.
bowing f.
boxer's f.
Boyd type II f.
f. bracing
Broberg-Morrey f.
bucket-handle f.
buckle f.
bumper f.
bunk bed f.
Burkhalter-Reyes method
  phalangeal f.
burst f.
butterfly f.
buttonhole f.
calcaneal avulsion f.
calcaneal displaced f.
f. callus
f. callus loading
Canale-Kelly talar neck f.
capitellar f.
capitulum radiale humeri f.
carpal bone stress f.
carpal navicular f.
carpal scaphoid bone f.
carpometacarpal joint f.
cartwheel f.
cemental f.
cementum f.
central f.
cephalomedullary nail f.
cerebral palsy pathologic f.
cervical trochanteric f.
cervicotrochanteric displaced f.
Chance vertebral f.

Chaput f.
chauffeur's f.
chip f.
chiropractic treatment of f.
chisel f.
circumferential f.
f. classification
clavicular birth f.
clay shoveler's f.
cleavage f.
closed-reak f.
coccyx f.
Colles f.
collicular f.
combined flexion-distraction injury
  and burst f.
combined radial-ulnar-humeral f.
comminuted intraarticular f.
complete f.
complex f.
composite f.
condylar femoral f.
congenital f.
Conrad-Bugg trapping of soft
  tissue in ankle f.
contrecoup f.
f. by contrecoup
controlled comminuted f.
coracoid f.
corner f.
coronal split f.
coronoid process f.
cortical f.
Cotton ankle f.
cough f.
crack f.
craniofacial dysjunction f.
crush f.
"crushed eggshell" f.
cuboid f.
cuneiform f.
Danis-Weber f.
Darrach-Hughston-Milch f.
dashboard f.
Delbet splint for heel f.
Denis Browne sacral f.
  classification
Denis Browne spinal f.
  classification
Denis spinal f.
dens f.
dentate f.

depressed f.
depression f.
de Quervain f.
Descot f.
diacondylar f.
diametric pelvic f.
diaphyseal f.
diastatic f.
dicondylar f.
die punch f.
f. disease
dislocation f.
displaced intraarticular f.
distal femoral epiphyseal f.
distal humeral f.
distal radial f.
distraction of f.
dogleg f.
dome f.
dorsal wing f.
double f.
Dupuytren f.
Duverney f.
dyscrasic f.
El-Ahwany classification of humeral
  supracondylar f.
elbow f.
electrostimulation for nonunion
  of f.
elementary f.
Ellis technique for Barton f.
f. en coin
Ender rod fixation of f.
endocrine f.
f. en rave
epicondylar avulsion f.
epiphyseal growth plate f.
epiphyseal slip f.
epiphyseal tibial f.
Essex-Lopresti fixation of
  calcaneal f.
Essex-Lopresti joint depression f.
explosion f.
extracapsular f.
extra-octave f.
fatigue f.
femoral intertrochanteric f.
femoral neck f.
femoral shaft f.
femoral supracondylar f.
fender f.
f. fever

F

NOTES

fracture *(continued)*
    fibular diaphyseal f.
    Fielding-Magliato classification of
      subtrochanteric f.
    fifth metatarsal base f.
    fighter's f.
    finger f.
    first carpometacarpal joint f.
    fissure f.
    f. fixation
    f. fixation device
    flake f.
    flexion-burst f.
    flexion-compression f.
    flexion-distraction f.
    floating arch f.
    forearm f.
    four-part f.
    fourth carpometacarpal joint f.
    f. frame
    Freiberg f.
    Frykman radial f.
    fulcrum f.
    Gaenslen f.
    Galeazzi f.
    f. gap
    Garden femoral neck f.
    Gartland humeral supracondylar f.
      classification
    glenoid rim f.
    Gosselin f.
    Grantham classification of femur f.
    greater trochanteric femoral f.
    greenstick f.
    grenade-thrower's f.
    gross f.
    Guérin f.
    gunshot f.
    Gustilo-Anderson open clavicular f.
    Hahn-Steinthal f.
    hairline f.
    hamate tail f.
    hangman's f.
    Hansen classification of f.
    Hawkins classification of talar f.
    head-splitting humeral f.
    f. healing
    heat f.
    hemicondylar f.
    Henderson f.
    Herbert scaphoid bone f.
    Hermodsson f.
    hickory-stick f.
    high-energy f.
    Hill-Sachs f.
    hip f.
    hockey-stick f.
    Hoffa f.

Holstein-Lewis f.
hoop stress f.
horizontal f.
humeral head-splitting f.
humeral physeal f.
humeral shaft f.
humeral supracondylar f.
Hutchinson f.
hyperflexion f.
ice skater's f.
idiopathic f.
impacted f.
impacted articular f.
implant f.
impression f.
incomplete f.
indirect f.
inflammatory f.
infraction f.
Ingram-Bachynski hip f.
    classification
insufficiency f.
intercondylar femoral f.
intercondylar humeral f.
intercondylar tibial f.
internally fixed f.
interperiosteal f.
intertrochanteric femoral f.
intertrochanteric four-part f.
intraarticular calcaneal f.
intraarticular proximal tibial f.
intracapsular f.
intraoperative f.
intraperiosteal f.
inverted-Y f.
ipsilateral femoral neck f.
ipsilateral femoral shaft f.
irreducible f.
Jefferson f.
Jeffery radial f. classification
joint depression f.
Jones f.
juvenile Tillaux f.
juxtaarticular f.
juxtacortical f.
Kapandji f.
Key-Conwell classification of
    pelvic f.
Kilfoyle humeral medial
    condylar f. classification
knee f.
Kocher f.
Kocher-Lorenz f.
Kocher-Lorenz classification of
    capitellum f.
LaGrange humeral supracondylar f.
    classification
laminar f.

lap seatbelt f.
lateral column calcaneal f.
lateral condylar humeral f.
lateral humeral condyle f.
laterally displaced f.
lateral malleolus f.
lateral mass f.
lateral talar process f.
lateral tibial plateau f.
Lauge-Hansen ankle f. classification
Lauge-Hansen stage II supination-
  eversion f.
Laugier f.
lead pipe f.
Le Fort fibular f.
LeFort II f.
Le Fort mandible f.
Le Fort-Wagstaffe f.
lesser trochanter f.
f. line
linear f.
f. line consolidation
Lisfranc f.
Lloyd-Roberts open reduction of
  Monteggia f.
long bone f.
longitudinal f.
long oblique f.
loose f.
lorry driver's f.
low-energy f.
low lumbar spine f.
low T humerus f.
lumbar spine burst f.
lumbosacral junction f.
lunate f.
Maisonneuve fibular f.
Malgaigne pelvic f.
malleolar f.
mallet f.
malunited calcaneus f.
malunited forearm f.
malunited radial f.
mandibular f.
March f.
marginal f.
Mason f.
Mathews olecranon f. classification
maxillary f.
medial column calcaneal f.
medial epicondyle humeral f.
medial malleolar f.

metacarpal neck f.
metaphyseal tibial f.
metatarsal f.
Meyers-McKeever tibial f.
  classification
middle tibial shaft f.
midfacial f.
midfoot f.
midshaft f.
Milch classification of humeral f.
minimally displaced f.
mini-pilon f.
missed f.
Moberg-Gedda f.
monomalleolar ankle f.
Monteggia forearm f.
Montercaux f.
Moore f.
Mouchet f.
Mueller classification of humerus f.
multangular ridge f.
multilevel f.
multipartite f.
multiple f.
multiray f.
navicular f.
naviculocapitate f.
f. of necessity
neck f.
Neer-Horowitz classification of
  humeral f.
neoplastic f.
neurogenic f.
neuropathic f.
neurotrophic f.
Newman radial neck and head f.
  classification
nightstick f.
nonarticular distal radial f.
noncontiguous f.
nondisplaced f.
nonphyseal f.
nonrotational burst f.
f. nonunion
nonunited f.
nutcracker f.
oblique f.
O'Brien classification of radial f.
obturator avulsion f.
occipital condyle f.
occult f.
odontoid condyle f.

F

NOTES

fracture *(continued)*
  old f.
  olecranon f.
  one-part f.
  open-book f.
  open-break f.
  OrthoGen implantable stimulator for nonunion of f.
  os calcis f.
  osteochrondral slice f.
  Ovadia-Beals classification of tibial plafond f.
  Pais f.
  Papavasiliou olecranon f. classification
  paratrooper f.
  parry f.
  pars interarticularis f.
  patellar sleeve f.
  pathologic f.
  Pauwels f.
  pedicle f.
  pelvic avulsion f.
  pelvic ring f.
  pelvic straddle f.
  penetrating f.
  perforating f.
  periarticular f.
  periprosthetic f.
  peritrochanteric f.
  PER-IV f.
  pertrochanteric f.
  phalangeal diaphyseal f.
  physeal f.
  Piedmont f.
  pillow f.
  pilon f.
  ping-pong f.
  Pipkin classification of femoral f.
  plafond f.
  plastic bowing f.
  Poland epiphyseal f. classification
  pond f.
  Posada f.
  posterior arch f.
  posterior column f.
  posterior element f.
  posterior talar process f.
  posterior wall f.
  postirradiation f.
  postmortem f.
  postoperative f.
  Pott ankle f.
  prevention of f.
  profundus artery f.
  pronation-abduction f.
  pronation-eversion f.
  pronation-external rotation f.

  proximal femoral f.
  proximal humeral f.
  proximal tibial f.
  proximal tibial metaphyseal f.
  pulsing current for nonunion of f.
  puncture f.
  pyramidal f.
  Quinby pelvic f. classification
  radial head f.
  radial neck f.
  radial styloid f.
  f. reducing elevator
  f. reduction
  reduction of f.
  f. repair
  resecting f.
  retrodisplaced f.
  reverse Barton f.
  reverse Colles f.
  reverse Monteggia f.
  rib f.
  ring f.
  Riseborough-Radin intercondylar f. classification
  Rockwood classification of clavicular f.
  Rolando f.
  rotation f.
  rotational f.
  rotational burst f.
  Ruedi f.
  Ruedi-Allgower tibial plafond f.
  Russell traction for femoral f.
  sacral f.
  sacroiliac f.
  sacrum f.
  Sakellarides calcaneal f. classification
  Salter f.
  Salter-Harris classification of epiphyseal f.
  Salter-Harris-Rang classification of epiphyseal f.
  Salter-Harris f. (type I–VI)
  scaphoid f.
  secondary f.
  segmental f.
  Segond f.
  Seinsheimer femoral f. classification
  sentinel f.
  SER-IV f.
    supination-external rotation IV fracture
  shaft f.
  shear f.
  Shepherd f.
  short oblique f.
  sideswipe elbow f.

silver-fork f.
f. site
skier's f.
Skillern f.
sleeve f.
small f.
Smith f.
Sneppen talar f.
Sorbie calcaneal f. classification
spinal f.
spinous process f.
spiral oblique f.
f. splint
split f.
split-heel f.
splitting f.
spontaneous f.
sprain f.
Springer f.
sprinter's f.
stability of f.
f. stabilization
stable burst f.
stairstep f.
Steinert classification of
  epiphyseal f.
stellate f.
step-off of f.
Stieda f.
straddle f.
strain f.
stress f.
stress-type f.
subcapital f.
subcutaneous f.
subperiosteal f.
subtrochanteric femoral f.
supination-adduction f.
supination-eversion f.
supination-external rotation IV f.
  (SER-IV fracture)
supracondylar humeral f.
supracondylar Y-shaped f.
suprasyndesmotic f.
surgical neck f.
sustentaculum tali f.
T f.
f. table
talar avulsion f.
talar neck f.
talar osteochondral f.
tarsal bone f.

T-condylar f.
teacup f.
teardrop f.
teardrop-shaped flexion-
  compression f.
temporal bone f.
tension f.
thalamic f.
Thompson-Epstein classification of
  femoral f.
thoracic spine f.
thoracolumbar burst f.
three-part f.
through-and-through f.
thrower's f.
tibial bending f.
tibial condyle f.
tibial diaphyseal f.
tibial open f.
tibial plafond f.
tibial plateau f.
tibial shaft f.
tibial triplane f.
tibial tuberosity f.
tibiofibular f.
Tillaux f.
Tillaux-Chaput f.
Tillaux-Kleiger f.
toddler's f.
tongue f.
tongue-type f.
torsion f.
torsional f.
torus f.
traction f.
transcapitate f.
transcervical femoral f.
transchondral f.
transcondylar f.
transcutaneous fixation of f.
transepiphyseal f.
transhamate f.
transiliac f.
transsacral f.
transscaphoid dislocation f.
transtriquetral f.
transverse process f.
trapezium f.
trimalleolar ankle f.
triplane tibial f.
triquetral f.

F

NOTES

fracture *(continued)*
Tronzo classification of
  intertrochanteric f.
trophic f.
tuft f.
two-part f.
type I, II, III, IIIA, IIIB, IIIC
  open f.
ulnar f.
uncinate process f.
undisplaced f.
unicondylar f.
unstable f.
ununited f.
vertebral body f.
vertebral stable burst f.
vertebral wedge compression f.
vertebra plana f.
vertical shear f.
volar shear f.
Volkmann f.
Vostal classification of radial f.
wagon wheel f.
Wagstaffe f.
Walther f.
Watson-Jones classification of tibial
  tubercle avulsion f.
Weber C f.
wedge compression f.
wedge-shaped uncomminuted tibial
  plateau f.
"western boot" in open f.
Wilkins radial f. classification
willow f.
Wilson f.
Winquist-Hansen classification of
  femoral f.
f. with scoliosis
Y f.
Y-T f.
Zickel f.
ZMC f.
fractured bone mobility
fracture-dislocation
atlantoaxial f.-d.
Bennett f.-d.
carpometacarpal f.-d.
Galeazzi f.-d.
Lisfranc f.-d.
perilunate f.-d.
posterior f.-d.
f.-d. reduction
Rowe and Lowell classification
  system for f.-d.
tarsalmetatarsal f.-d.
tarsometatarsal f.-d.
thoracolumbar f.-d.
thoracolumbar spine f.-d.

tibial plateau f.-d.
transcapitate f.-d.
transhamate f.-d.
transtriquetral f.-d.
unstable f.-d.
volar plate arthroplasty
  technique f.-d.
f.-d. with anterior ligament
fragilis
osteosclerosis f.
fragilitans
osteitis f.
fragilitas ossium congenita
Fragmatome tip
fragment
alignment of fracture f.
articular f.
avascular f.
avulsion f.
bone f.
bony f.
butterfly fracture f.
capital f.
chondral f.
cortical f.
depression of f.
disk f.
distal f.
free f.
free-floating cartilaginous f.
hinged f.
hypervascular f.
intraarticular f.
loose f.
osteochondral f.
retrolisthesed f.
retropulsed bony f.
sustentacular f.
tuberosity f.
wedge-shaped uncomminuted f.
fragmental bone
fragmentation
endplate f.
graft f.
Fragmin
Frahur cartilage clamp
frame
Ace-Colles fracture f.
Ace-Fischer fracture f.
Ace-Fischer ring f.
Alexian Brothers overhead f.
Andrews spinal surgery f.
anterior quadrilateral triplane f.
f. application
Balkan fracture f.
bilateral f.
Böhler-Braun f.
Böhler fracture f.

Böhler reducing f.
Bradford f.
Bradford fracture f.
Braun f.
Brooker f.
Chalet f.
Charest head f.
Chick CLT operating f.
CircOlectric f.
claw-type basic f.
Cole fracture f.
Cole hyperextension f.
Crawford head f.
delta f.
DePuy rainbow f.
DePuy reducing f.
double-ring f.
Elekta stereotactic head f.
external fixator f.
fixator f.
Foster turning f.
four-poster f.
fracture f.
fusion f.
Gardner-Wells fixation f.
Goldthwait f.
Granberry f.
Hastings f.
Heffington lumbar seat spinal f.
Herzmark f.
Hibbs f.
Hitchcock stereotactic
  immobilization f.
Hoffmann f.
Hoffmann-Vidal-Adrey f.
Hoffmann-Vidal double f.
Ilizarov f.
Janes f.
Jones abduction f.
Kessler traction f.
laminectomy f.
Lex-Ton spinal f.
Maddacrawler Crawler f.
Malcolm-Lynn C-RXF cervical
  retractor f.
Mayfield fixation f.
Monticelli-Spinelli f.
one-plane bilateral f.
one-plane unilateral f.
Pearson attachment to Thomas f.
phantom f.
Pittsburgh pelvic f.

quadrilateral f.
rectangular f.
Relton-Hall f.
Risser f.
scoliosis operating f.
Slätis pelvic fracture f.
sling f.
spinal turning f.
spine f.
Stealth f.
Stryker fracture f.
Stryker turning f.
Taylor spinal f.
tent f.
Thomas f.
Thompson f.
triangular ankle fusion f.
triangulate triple f.
triple f.
two-plane bilateral f.
two-plane unilateral f.
vasocillator f.
Wagner f.
Watson-Jones f.
Weber f.
Whitman f.
Wilson convex f.
Wingfield f.
Wolfson f.
Zimmer fracture f.
Zimmer laminectomy f.
Framer
  F. finger extension bow
  F. splint
  F. tendon passer
  F. tendon-passing needle
frank dislocation
Fränkel
  F. neurologic deficit classification
  F. sign
  F. white line
Franz-O'Rahilly classification
fray
frayed meniscus
Frazier-Adson
  F.-A. osteoplastic flap clamp
Frazier-Sachs clamp
Frazier suction tip
FRD
  flexion-rotation-drawer
  FRD test

F

NOTES

freckle
Hutchinson f.
free
f. body diagram
f. fasciocutaneous flap
f. fat graft
f. flap of cartilage
f. flap transfer
f. fragment
f. gracilis muscle transfer
f. induction decay (FID)
f. knee joint
f. latissimus dorsi flap
f. microsurgical flap
f. revascularized autograft
f. skin flap
f. skin graft
f. speed
f.-spinning probe
f.-swinging knee gait
f. tie
f. tissue transfer
f. vascularized bone transplant
Freebody
F. pin
F. stay-retractor
Freebody-Bendall-Taylor
F.-B.-T. fusion technique
Freebody-Steinmann retractor
FREEDOM
F. Arthritis Support
F. Back Support
F. Elastic Long Wrist Support
F. Neutral Position Splint
F. Omni Progressive Splint
F. Palm Guard
F. Progressive Resting Splint
F. Sportsfit Splint
F. Thumbkeeper
F. Thumb Spica
F. Thumb Stabilizer
F. Ultimate Grip Splint
F. USA Wristlet
freedom
F. arthritis support for hand
degrees of f. (DOF)
F. Micro Pro stimulator
f. of movement
free-floating
f.-f. cartilaginous fragment
f.-f. osteotomy
freehand
f. CT-guided biopsy
f. cut
f. suturing technique
Freeman
F. calcaneal fracture classification

F. clamp
F. modular total hip prosthesis
Freeman-Samuelson knee prosthesis
Freeman-Sheldon syndrome
Freeman-Swanson
F.-S. knee prosthesis
F.-S. knee system
freer
F. chisel
dental f.
F. dissector
F. elevator-dissector
F. periosteal elevator
F. septal elevator
Free-Up massage cream
freeze-dried
f.-d. bone
f.-d. graft
freeze-drying
freeze-thawed graft
Freiberg
F. cartilage knife
F. disease
F. fracture
F. infraction
F. meniscectomy knife
F. traction
Freiberg-Kohler disease
Frejka
F. cast
F. jacket
F. pillow
F. pillow orthosis
F. pillow splint
F. traction
fremitus
French
F. adapter
F. fracture technique
F. lateral closing-wedge osteotomy
F. rod bender
F. scale
F. supracondylar fracture operation
frenectomy
frenulum, pl. **frenula**
frequency
f. analysis
f.-difference interferential current
therapy (FDICT)
discharge f.
onset f.
recruitment f.
fresh
f. frozen allograft
f. frozen graft
freshening of bone
freshen the surface
Fresnel prism

fretting corrosion
Frey syndrome
friable
Friatec manual arthroscopy instrument
fricative
friction
    f. artifact
    coefficient of f.
    cross f.
    f. lock pin
    f. massage
    patient-on-table f.
frictional torque
friction-reduced
    f.-r. examination table
    f.-r. segmented table
Fried-Green
    F.-G. foot operation
    F.-G. foot procedure
Fried-Hendel
    F.-H. tendon operation
    F.-H. tendon technique
Friedman
    F. bone rongeur
    F. brace
    F. rongeur forceps
    F. support
Friedreich
    F. ataxia
    F. disease
    F. foot
    F. sign
Friedrich clamp
Friedrich-Petz clamp
Fries
    F. score for rheumatoid arthritis
    F. score for rheumatoid arthritis
      classification
fringe
    f. of osteophyte
    synovial f.
frog-leg
    f.-l. lateral view
    f.-l. position
    f.-l. splint
frog splint
Fröhlich adiposogenital dystrophy
Frohse
    arcade of F.
    F. arcade of the elbow
    arch of F.

Froimson
    F. procedure
    F. splint
    F. technique
Froimson-Oh
    F.-O. arm procedure
    F.-O. repair
Froment paper sign
Fromm triangle orthopaedic device
frond
    synovial f.
Fronet fasciotomy
frontal
    f. bossing
    f. motion
    f. plane
    f. plane growth abnormality
    f. plane (XY)
frontal plane correction
    Kilsyn-Evans principle of f. p. c.
front-entry guide
fronting of velar
Frost
    F. foot procedure
    F. H-block
    F. posterior tibialis technique
    F. posterior tibialis tendon
      lengthening
    F. stitch
frostbite
    f. of hand
    f. injury
frostnip
frozen shoulder
Fruehevald splint
fruste
    forme f.
Frykman
    F. distal radius fracture
      classification
    F. radial fracture
F-Scan foot force and gait analysis
  system
FSI
    Functional Status Index
FSQ
    Functional Status Questionnaire
FSU
    functional spinal unit
FT03C transducer
FTA
    femorotibial angle

F

NOTES

FTC
  fibulotalocalcaneal
    FTC ligament
FTI
  force-time integral
FTSG
  full-thickness skin graft
Fukuda humeral head retractor
fulcrum
  f. distance
  f. fracture
  joint f.
  f. test
fulcruming
Fulford procedure
fulgurate
Fulkerson
  F. functional knee score
  F. osteotomy
full
  f.-circle goniometer
  f. curve
  f.-curved clamp
  f. fist flexion
  f.-hand splint
  f. interference pattern
  f. lateral position
  f.-occlusal splint
  f. spine radiographic examination
  f. thumb spica cast
  f. weightbearing (FWB)
Fuller shield dressing
full-radius
  f.-r. resector
  f.-r. resector knife
full-thickness
  f.-t. cuff tear
  f.-t. skin graft (FTSG)
fully constrained tricompartmental knee prosthesis
fulminans
  purpura f.
fulminate
Fulvicin
  F. P/G
  F. U/F
fumigatus
  Aspergillus f.
function
  adrenergic vagal f.
  ambulatory f.
  bundle f.
  Charnley classification of f.
  cholinergic vagal f.
  concentric f.
  eccentric f.
  intrinsic f.
  Jebsen assessment of hand f.

  motor f.
  perverted f.
  position of f.
  reflex f.
  sensory f.
  splinted in position of f.
  subtalar joint f. (SJF)
  sudomotor f.
  throwing f.
  tibialis posterior f.
functional
  f. activity
  f. ambulation
  F. Ambulation Categories (FAC)
  f. and anatomic loading (FAL)
  f. axial rotation
  f. back pain
  f. capacity assessment
  f. capacity evaluation (FCE)
  f. capacity measurement
  f. electrical stimulation (FES)
  f. fracture brace
  f. instability
  F. Integration (FI)
  f. intermetatarsal angle
  f. leg length inequality
  F. Limitation Profile (FLP)
  f. neuromuscular stimulation
  f. orthotic
  f. performance
  f. refractory period
  f. restoration
  f. scoliosis
  f. short leg
  f. spinal unit (FSU)
  F. Status Index (FSI)
  F. Status Questionnaire (FSQ)
  f. subluxation
  f. technique
functionally debilitating symptom
fungal
  f. arthritis
  f. infection
Fungoid
  F. AF Topical Solution
  F. Creme
fungoides
  mycosis f.
funicular excision
funiculitis
funiculus
funnelization of metaphysis
Funsten supination splint
Funston syndrome
FUO
  fever of undetermined origin
Furacin gauze dressing
Furlong tendon stripper

Furnas bayonet osteotome
Furnas-Haq-Somers technique
Furness-Clute pin
furrowing
    scarring and f.
further flexion (FF)
fuse
fused hip
fusiform
    f. defect
    f. periosteal new bone
fusimotor
    f. neuron
    f. system
fusion
    Adkins spinal f.
    Albee lumbar spinal f.
    Anderson ankle f.
    ankle f.
    anterior cervical f. (ACF)
    anterior cervical body f.
    anterior cervical diskectomy and f.
    (ACDF)
    anterior lumbar interbody f.
    anterior lumbar vertebral
     interbody f.
    anterior and posterior f.
    anterior spinal f.
    AP f.
    atlantoaxial f.
    atlantooccipital f.
    Bailey-Badgley cervical spine f.
    bilateral lateral f.
    Blair ankle f.
    Bohlman triple-wire f.
    Bosworth lumbar spinal f.
    Bradford f.
    Brooks cervical f.
    Brooks-Gallie cervical f.
    Brooks-Jenkins atlantoaxial f.
    Brooks-Jenkins cervical f.
    Brooks-type f.
    buried K-wire fixation in digital f.
    f. cage
    calcaneotibial f.
    cervical interbody f.
    cervical spine posterior f.
    cervicooccipital f.
    Chandler hip f.
    Charnley compression-type knee f.
    chevron f.
    Chuinard-Peterson ankle f.

Cloward anterior spinal f.
Cloward back f.
CMC f.
Coltart calcaneotibial f.
convex f.
Copeland-Howard scapulothoracic f.
4-corner midcarpal f.
Davis f.
degenerative lumbar spine f.
degenerative spondylosis
  decompression and f.
Dewar posterior cervical f.
diaphyseal-epiphyseal f.
DIP f.
diskectomy with Cloward f.
distal tibiofibular f.
dowel spinal f.
extraarticular hip f.
extraarticular subtalar f.
facet f.
f. facet
four-corner midcarpal f.
f. frame
Gallie atlantoaxial f.
Gallie cervical f.
Gallie subtalar ankle f.
Gallie wire f.
Glissane ankle f.
Goldstein spinal f.
f. graft
Hall facet f.
hammer toe correction with
  interphalangeal f.
Harris-Smith cervical f.
Hatcher-Smith cervical f.
Henry-Geist spinal f.
H-graft f.
Hibbs-Jones spinal f.
Hibbs spinal f.
Horwitz-Adams ankle f.
Horwitz ankle f.
hyperostotic bony f.
interbody spinal f.
interfacet wiring and f.
interphalangeal f.
interspinous process f.
intertransverse f.
intraarticular knee f.
joint f.
Kellogg-Speed lumbar spinal f.
King intraarticular hip f.
knee f.

NOTES

fusion *(continued)*
    Langenskiöld f.
    lateral f.
    f. limit determination
    long segment spinal f.
    lower cervical spine f.
    lumbar spine f.
    lumbar vertebral interbody f.
    lumbosacral f.
    lunotriquetral f.
    Marcus-Balourdas-Heiple ankle f.
    McKeever metatarsophalangeal f.
    metatarsocuneiform joint f.
    metatarsophalangeal joint f.
    multilevel f.
    naviculocuneiform f.
    f. nonunion rate
    occipitoatlantoaxial f.
    occipitocervical f.
    pantalar f.
    f. plate
    posterior cervical f.
    posterior lumbar interbody f. (PLIF)
    posterior spinal f.
    posterolateral interbody f. (PLIF)
    posterolateral lumbosacral f.
    radiolunate f.
    radioscaphoid f.
    Robinson anterior cervical f.
    Robinson cervical spine f.
    Robinson-Southwick f.
    Robins-Riley spinal f.
    Rowe f.
    sacral spine f.
    scaphocapitate f.
    scapulothoracic f.
    screw f.
    selective thoracic spine f.
    short segment spinal f.
    Simmons cervical spine f.
    single-level spinal f.
    in situ spine f.
    Smith-Petersen sacroiliac joint f.
    Smith-Robinson anterior f.
    Smith-Robinson cervical f.
    Smith-Robinson interbody f.
    Soren ankle f.
    Stamm procedure for intra-articular hip f.
    Steffee plates and screws for lumbar f.
    f. stiffness
    subastragalar f.
    subaxial posterior cervical spinal f.
    subtalar distraction bone block f.
    symmetric vertebral f.
    talocalcaneal f.
    talocrural f.
    talonavicular f.
    f. technique
    thoracic facet f.
    thoracic spinal f.
    tibiocalcaneal f.
    tibiofibular f.
    tibiotalar f.
    tibiotalocalcaneal f.
    transfibular f.
    trapeziometacarpal f.
    triple tarsal f.
    triple-wire f.
    triscaphe f.
    two-stage hip f.
    upper cervical spine f.
    Watkins f.
    Watson scaphotrapeziotrapezoidal f.
    White posterior ankle f.
    Wilson ankle f.
    Wiltse bilateral lateral f.
    Winter convex f.
    Zielke instrumentation for scoliosis spinal f.

Fusobacterium nucleatum
Futrex body fat analyzer
Futureplex Flower Essence Combinations
Futuro
    F. splint
    F. wrist brace
    F. wrist support
FVC
    forced vital capacity
F wave
FWB
    full weightbearing
fx
    fracture
FyBron dressing

G5

    G5 Fleximatic massage/percussion unit
    G5 Porta-Plus muscle stimulator
    G5 Vibracare massager/percussor
    G5 Vibramatic massage/percussion unit

GABA

    gamma aminobutyric acid

gadolinium-diethylenetriamine pentaacetic acid

gadolinium-labeled diethylenetriamine pentaacetic acid

gadopentetate-dimeglumine-enhanced magnetic resonance imaging

GADS

    gas atomized dispersion strengthened
    GADS technology

Gaenslen

    G. fracture
    G. osteomyelitis
    G. sign
    G. split-heel incision
    G. split-heel technique
    G. test

Gaffney

    G. ankle prosthesis
    G. joint

gag

    Dingman mouth g.

Gage

    G. distal transfer
    G. sign

Gagnon splint

gain

    Body Oscillation Integrates Neuromuscular G. (BOING)
    body oscillation neuromuscular g. (BOING)

GAIT

    great toe arthroplasty implant technique

gait

    abductor lurch g.
    G. Abnormality Rating Scale (GARS)
    G. Abnormality Rating Scale Modified version (GARS-M)
    adult g.
    analysis of g.
    g. analysis
    angle of g.
    antalgic g.
    apraxic g.
    arthrogenic g.
    astasia-abasia g.

batrachian g.
g. belt
biomechanical evaluation of foot function during stance phase of g.
broad-based g.
cadence of g.
calcaneal g.
calcaneus g.
Charlie Chaplin type of g.
choreatic g.
clumsy g.
cogwheel g.
component of g.
crab g.
cross-leg g.
cross-legged g.
crouch g.
g. cycle
dancing g.
dancing bear g.
dorsiflexor g.
double-leg stance phase of g.
double-step g.
double-tap g.
drag-to g.
dromedary g.
drop-foot g.
drunken sailor g.
duck waddle g.
dystrophic g.
equine g.
festinating g.
flaccid g.
floating g.
footdrop g.
foot strike phase of g.
four-point g.
free-swinging knee g.
gastrocnemius-soleus g.
glue-footed g.
gluteus maximus g.
gluteus medius g.
heel g.
heel-and-toe g.
heel contact phase of g.
heel-off phase of g.
heel-toe g.
heel-to-toe g.
hemiplegic or hemiparetic g.
hip extensor g.
hobbling g.
hyperextended knee g.
hysterical g.
instability g.

G

gait *(continued)*

    intermittent double-step g.
    internal rotational g.
    intoeing g.
    jerky g.
    g. laboratory
    listing g.
    g. lock splint (GLS)
    lurching g.
    marche à petits pas g.
    midstance period of g.
    narrow-base g.
    Oppenheim g.
    opposite foot strike phase of g.
    opposite toe-off phase of g.
    painful g.
    parkinsonian g.
    g. pathomechanics
    g. pattern
    penguin g.
    Petren g.
    pigeon-toeing g.
    g. plate
    propulsion g.
    push-off phase of g.
    quality of g.
    reeling g.
    retropulsion of g.
    reversal of fore-aft shear phase
      of g.
    rigid g.
    scissor-leg g.
    scissors g.
    scraping toe g.
    shuffling g.
    slap foot g.
    slapping g.
    speed of g.
    stable g.
    staggering g.
    stance phase of g.
    g. and station
    station and g.
    stiff-knee g.
    stiff-legged g.
    stride length of g.
    strike phase of g.
    stuttering of g.
    swaying g.
    swing phase of g.
    swing-through g.
    swing-to g.
    tabetic g.
    tandem g.
    Thorazine shuffle g.
    three-point g.
    tiptoe g.
    toeing-in g.
    toeing-out g.
    toe-off phase of g.
    toe-walking g.
    tottering g.
    Tracto-Halter g.
    g. training
    Trendelenburg g.
    Tubersitz amputee g.
    two-point g.
    uncoordinated g.
    unsteadiness of g.
    unsteady g.
    waddling g.
    wide-based g.

gaiter cast
Galant
    G. sign
    G. test
Galante hip prosthesis
Galaxy
    G. McManis hylo table
Galeazzi
    G. fracture
    G. fracture-dislocation
    G. patellar operation
    G. realignment
    G. sign
    G. test
Galen scoliosis
Gallagher rasp
gallamine triethiodide
Gallannaugh plate
gall duct forceps
Gallie
    G. ankle arthrodesis
    G. atlantoaxial arthrodesis
    G. atlantoaxial fusion
    G. atlantoaxial fusion technique
    G. cervical fusion
    G. fusion-using cable
    G. needle
    G. procedure
    G. subtalar ankle fusion
    G. subtalar fixation
    G. wire fusion
    G. wiring technique
gallium-67 scan
gallium citrate scan
Gallo traction
Gallows splint
Galt hand drill
galvanic
    g. bath
    g. electrode stimulator
    high-voltage pulsed g.
    g. skin response
    g. stimulation

galvanism
    high-volt g.
    high-voltage g.
Galveston
    G. fixation with TSRH crosslink
    G. metacarpal brace
    G. pelvic fixation
    G. plate
    G. splint
    G. technique
gambiense
    Trypanosoma g.
game
    Boloxie OT Prehension G.
    Cone checkers g.
    g. knee
gamekeeper's
    g. injury
    g. thumb
    g. thumb dislocation
gamma
    g. aminobutyric acid (GABA)
    g. camera
    g. camera imaging
    g. locking nail
gammopathy
    monoclonal g.
ganciclovir
ganglion, pl. ganglia
    Acrel g.
    g. block
    g. cyst
    dorsal root g. (DRG)
    intraosseous g.
    periosteal g.
ganglionectomy
    dorsal root g.
ganglioneuroma
ganglionic cyst in synovial tendon sheath
gangrene
    dry g.
    gas g.
    ischemic g.
    Meleney synergistic g.
    peripheral g.
    postnatal g.
    vascular g.
    wet g.
gangrenosum
    pyoderma g.
gangrenous necrosis

Ganley
    G. modification of Keller arthroplasty
    G. splint
    G. technique
Gant
    G. hip arthrodesis
    G. osteotomy
Ganz anti-shock pelvic fixator
gap
    extension g.
    flexion g.
    flexion-extension g.
    fracture g.
    g. healing
    g. nonunion
    scapholunate g.
Garamycin Topical
Garceau
    G. cheilectomy
    G. tendon technique
Garceau-Brahms arthrodesis
garden
    G. alignment index
    G. angle
    G. femoral neck fracture
    G. femoral neck fracture classification
    g. spade deformity
Gardner
    G. bone forceps
    G. chair
    G. elevator
    G. operation
    G. syndrome
Gardner-Wells
    G.-W. fixation frame
    G.-W. tongs
    G.-W. tong traction
garment
    antishock g.
    g. hook
    pneumatic g.
    pneumatic antishock g. (PASG)
    PresSsion pneumatic g.
Garré
    G. disease
    G. sclerosing osteomyelitis
Garrod disease
GARS
    Gait Abnormality Rating Scale

G

NOTES

GARS-M
   Gait Abnormality Rating Scale Modified
    version
garter strapping
Gartland
   G. humeral supracondylar fracture
    classification
   G. procedure
   G. Universal radial fracture
    classification
GAS
   General Adaption Syndrome
gas
   g. atomized dispersion strengthened
    (GADS)
   g. gangrene
   g.-producing streptococcal infection
gastrocnemius
   g. equinus
   g. flap
   lateral head of g.
   g. lengthening
   g. muscle
   g. recession
   g. soleus
   g. tendon
   g. tendon transfer
gastrocnemius-soleus
   g.-s. complex
   g.-s. fascial strip
   g.-s. gait
   g.-s. junction
   g.-s. muscle group
gastroc-resistive exercise
gastroc-soleus
   g.-s. complex
   g.-s. contractures
   g.-s. muscle
   g.-s. stretching
   g.-s. tendon
gastrointestinal
   g. obstruction
   g. tract
gastrosoleal equinus
Gatch bed
gatched bed
gate control theory of pain
Gatellier-Chastang
   G.-C. ankle approach
   G.-C. incision
   G.-C. posterolateral approach
Gates-Glidden drill
Gatlin gun drill guide
gator plastic orthosis
Gaucher disease
gauge
   acetabular g.
   aneroid g.

14-g. Angiocath
B&L pinch g.
bone screw depth g.
bone screw ruler g.
Charnley femoral condyle radius g.
Charnley socket g.
Cloward depth g.
Cobb g.
CTS g.
depth g.
Durkan CTS g.
finger g.
isometric strain g.
Jamar hydraulic pinch g.
measuring g.
orthopaedic depth g.
pain threshold g.
Philips toe force g.
pinch g.
Preston pinch g.
Rocabado posture g.
Rosette strain g.
screw depth g.
socket g.
spanner g.
strain g.
tourniquet g.
Vernier caliber g.
gauntlet
   g. anesthesia
   g. cast
   Jobst g.
   wrist g.
gauze
   Adaptic g.
   Cover-Roll g.
   g. dressing
   iodoform g.
   Kerlix g.
   g. packing
   petrolatum g.
   plain g.
   pledget of g.
   Safe-Wrap g.
   g. sponge
   Surgitube tubular g.
   Telfa g.
   g. wrap
Gaynor-Hart
   G.-H. position
   G.-H. x-ray position of carpal
    tunnel
GCS
   Glasgow Coma Score
G-CSF
   granulocyte colony-stimulating factor
GCT
   giant cell tumor

GDLH posterior spinal system
GD Regainer System
gear
    shoe g.
gearbox
gearshift probe
Geckler screw
GED
    General Education Development
    GED Scale
Gedda-Moberg incision
Geibel blade plate
Geiger counter
Geissling rating scale
"Gel"
    Sit-Straight wheelchair cushion with antidecubitus "Gel"
gel
    Adcon adhesive control g.
    Adcon-L anti-adhesion barrier g.
    Aquasonic Transmission G.
    Biofreeze topical analgesic g.
    Carrington Dermal wound g.
    Ceres Secret aloe vera g.
    Crystal polymer g.
    g. cushion
    Dermaflex G.
    Flexall g.
    Gel Care self-adhesive g.
    H.P. Acthar G.
    Iamin hydrating g.
    Keralyt G.
    g. pack
    Regranex G., 0.01%
    silicone g.
    Silipos g.
    Silosheath g.
    G.-Sole shoe insert
    g. stump sock
    g. suspension sleeve
    g. tubing
    Uni-Patch electrode g.
    g. warmer
    g. wrap
gelatin
    g. compression boot
    g. foam
gelatinosa
    substantia g.
gelatinous
gelatin-resorcin-formalin glue
GelBand arm band

Gelfoam
    G. cookie
    G. pledget
    G. stamp
    thrombin-soaked G.
Gel-Foam Ultra-Wedge cushion
Geliperm dressing
Gelman foot procedure
Gelocast cast
Gelpi retractor
Gelpirin
GELS
    gravity extension locking system
gemellus, pl. gemelli
Gemini
    G. cup
    G. hip system prosthesis
Genahist Oral
Genapap
Genaspor
Gencalc 600
general
    G. Adaption Syndrome (GAS)
    g. adjustment
    g. capsular stretch
    G. Education Development (GED)
    g. endotracheal anesthesia
    g. thrust manipulation
    G. Well-Being Schedule
generalized fibromatosis
Generation
    G. II KAFO
    G. II knee brace
generator
    electrosurgical g.
generic screening
Genesis
    G. II total knee system
    G. knee prosthesis
    G. unicompartmental knee
genetic
    g. disease
    g. factor
genicula (pl. of geniculum)
genicular
    g. artery
    g. neuralgia
geniculate
    g. artery
    medial g.
    g. neuralgia
geniculum, pl. genicula

G

NOTES

genital system
genitofemoral nerve
genitourinary
    g. evaluation
    g. infection
Genpril
gentamicin
    g. bead
    g. implant
gentle traction
genu
    g. recurvatum
    g. valgum
    g. valgum deformity
    g. valgus
    g. varum
    g. varum deformity
    g. varus
Genucom
    G. ACL laxity analysis system
    G. arthrometer
    G. knee flexion analysis system
genus
    ligamenta cruciata g.
    ligamentum cruciatum anterius g.
    ligamentum cruciatum posterius g.
    ligamentum transversum g.
Genutrain
    G. knee brace
    G. PE patellar realignment
    G. P3 knee support
geode
Geo-Matt contour cushion
Geomedic
    G. system
    G. total knee prosthesis
geometric
    g. extension osteotomy
    g. supracondylar extension
    osteotomy
    G. total knee prosthesis
George
    G. line
    G. test
Georgiade
    G. fixation device
    G. visor cervical traction
    G. visor halo fixation
    G. visor halo fixation apparatus
Gerard
    G. prosthesis
    G. resurfacing procedure
Gerbert-Mellilo method
Gerbert osteotomy
Gerdy
    G. ligament
    G. tubercle
geriatric chair trunk support

germinal matrix
Gerota capsule
Gerson diet
Gerster
    G. bone clamp
    G. traction bar
Ger technique
Gertie ball
Gerzog bone mallet
Get-A-Grip grip
Getty
    G. decompression
    G. decompression technique
Ghajar guide
GHL
    glenohumeral ligament
Ghon-Sachs complex
Ghon tubercle
Ghormley
    G. arthrodesis
    G. shelf procedure
Giannestras
    G. metatarsal oblique osteotomy
    G. modification of Lapidus
    technique
    G. oblique metatarsal osteotomy
    G. step-down modified osteotomy
giant
    g. cell reaction
    g. cell reparative granuloma
    g. cell tumor (GCT)
    g. motor unit action potential
    g. synovial cyst
Gianturco
    G. macrocoil
    G. prosthesis
GIA staple
gibbus deformity of the spine
Gibney
    G. bandage
    G. boot
    G. taping
Gibson
    G. approach
    G. bandage
    G. splint
Gibson-Piggott osteotomy
Giertz rib shears
Giertz-Shoemaker rib shears
Giertz-Stille scissors
Gifford mastoid retractor
gigantomastia
Gigli
    G. saw
    G. saw blade
    G. saw guide
    G. saw osteotomy
Gigli-Strully saw

GII

GII KAFO
GII Unloader ADJ knee brace

Gilbert

G. disease
G. harvesting
G. scapular flap

Gilbert-Tamai-Weiland technique
Gilchrist

G. splint
G. test

Gildenberg biopsy forceps
Gilfillan humeral prosthesis
Giliberty

G. acetabular prosthesis
G. apparatus
G. bipolar femoral head
G. device
G. femoral neck prosthesis
G. hip prosthesis

Gill

G. arthrodesis
G. massive sliding graft
G. modification of Campbell ankle operation
G. modification of Campbell ankle procedure
G. posterior bone block
G. shelf procedure
G. sliding graft technique

Gillespie syndrome
Gillet marching test
Gillette

G. brace
G. double-flexure ankle joint system
G. joint
G. joint orthosis
G. joint prosthesis
G. modification of ankle-foot orthosis

Gilliat-Summer nerve-damaged hand
Gillies

G. bone graft
G. bone hook
G. pollicization
G. prosthesis

Gillies-Dingman hook
Gillies-Millard

G.-M. cocked-hat technique
G.-M. metacarpal lengthening

Gillis suture

Gill-Manning-White

G.-M.-W. spondylolisthesis
G.-M.-W. spondylolisthesis technique

Gillquist

G. procedure
G. suction curette
G. suction tube

Gill-Stein arthrodesis
Gilmer splint
Gilquist arthroscopy
gimpy knee
ginglymoarthrodial
ginglymoid joint
ginglymus
ginkgo biloba
Girard keratoprosthesis prosthesis
girdle

Cadenza g.
limb g.
pectoral g.
pelvic g.
shoulder g.

Girdlestone

G. hip procedure
G. pseudarthrosis
G. resection
G. resection arthroplasty
G. tendon transfer

Girdlestone-Taylor procedure
give-way phenomenon
giving way of knee
glabella
Glacier

G. ceramic 4-in-1 cutting guide
G. ceramic knee cutting guide
G. Pack

gland

eccrine sweat g.
haversian g.
thyroid g.

Glasgow

G. Coma scale
G. Coma Score (GCS)
G. screw

glass

magnifying g.

Glass-Bessen transfixion screw
Glasscock ear dressing
Glassman-Engh-Bobyn trochanteric slide
Gledhill technique

NOTES

G

Gleich
    G. osteotomy
    G. osteotomy for pes valgo planus
G-lengthening of semitendinosus tendon
glenohumeral
    g. adhesive capsulitis
    g. arthrodesis
    g. dislocation repair
    g. joint
    g. joint cohesion
    g. joint disease
    g. joint dislocation
    g. joint stability
    g. joint subluxation
    g. ligament (GHL)
    g. pain
glenohumeralia
    ligamenta g.
glenoid
    g. alignment peg
    g. cartilage
    g. cavitary
    g. cavity
    g. component
    g. concavity
    g. drill
    g. drill guide
    g. fixation screw
    g. fossa
    g. implant base impactor
    g. labrum
    lip of g.
    g. metal tray
    g. neck
    g. osteotomy
    g. point
    g.-reaming forceps
    g. rim
    g. rim fracture
    g. slot
glenoplasty
    posterior g.
    Scott g.
    Scott posterior g.
Gliadel implant
glide
    anterior g.
    anterior-posterior g.
    cervical dorsal g.
    craniocaudal g.
    dorsal g.
    inferior g.
    mushroom walker g.
    patellar g.
    posterior g.
    posterior-anterior g.
    superior g.
    volar g.

gliding
    g. hinge joint
    g. hole
    g.-hole-first technique
    g. layer
    g. mechanism
    g. principle
glioma
Glissane
    G. ankle fusion
    G. arthrodesis
    G. crucial angle
    G. spike
Glisson sling
Global
    G. total shoulder arthroplasty
    G. total shoulder arthroplasty system
    G. total shoulder implant
globose
globulin
    immune g.
    tetanus immune g.
glomangiosarcoma
glomus tumor
glossodynia
glossopharyngeal neuralgia
glove
    AliFleece g.'s
    antivibration g.
    Biobrane g.
    compression g.
    electrode g.
    finger flexion g.
    F&L attenuating g.
    flexion g.
    flexor g.
    Handeze fingerless g.
    impact g.
    Isotoner g.
    Jobst g.
    Kevlar g.
    Kid G.'s
    Life Liner stick and cut-resistant g.
    Maxxus orthopaedic latex surgical g.
    Medak g.
    Medarmor puncture-resistant g.
    Necelon surgical g.
    peripheral nerve g.
    pressure g.
    Push-Ease wheelchair g.
    radial nerve g.
    surgical g.
    vibration g.

GLS
gait lock splint
GLS brace
glubionate
calcium g.
Gluck rib shears
GlucoBalance
glucocorticoid
gluconate
chlorhexidine g.
glucosamine sulfate
glucose
blood g.
glucosteroid
glue
cyanoacrylate g.
g.-footed gait
gelatin-resorcin-formalin g.
skin g.
Tisseel fibrin g.
glutamic-oxaloacetic transaminase
glutamic-pyruvic transaminase
glutaraldehyde
glutaraldehyde-prepared bovine
pericardium
gluteal
g. artery
g. bonnet
g. cleft
g. lurch
g. nerve
glutethimide
gluteus
g. maximus flap
g. maximus gait
g. maximus muscle
g. maximus tensing test
g. medius gait
g. medius muscle
g. medius paralysis
g. minimus muscle
glycation
nonenzymatic connective tissue g.
glycol
salicylic acid and propylene g.
glycosaminoglycan
Glynn-Neibauer technique
GMFM
Gross Motor Function Measure
G-myticin Topical
goblet incision
Gohil-Cavolo method

Golaski graft
gold
g.-handled chuck
g. probe
g. salt
g. sodium thiomalate
g. weight and wire spring implant
material
Goldberg technique
Golden
G. closing-wedge osteotomy
G. Comfort orthotic
G. Fitness orthotic
G. mean testing system
Goldenhar syndrome
Goldman-Fristoe test of articulation
Goldmar opponensplasty
Goldner
G. reconstruction
G. spinal arthrodesis
Goldner-Clippinger technique
Goldner-Hayes procedure
gold-paneled chisel
GoldPoint brace
Goldstein
G. spinal fusion
G. spinal fusion technique
Goldthwait
G. brace
G. frame
G. sign
Goldthwait-Hauser procedure
Golfers
Thera-Band Exercise System for G.
golfer's
g. elbow
g. elbow test
Golf Exercise System
Golgi
G. device
G. membrane
G. tendon
G. tendon organ
gonarthrosis
gonial angle
goniometer
electronic g.
EOC g.
finger g.
full-circle g.
O'Brien g.
orthopaedic g.

G

NOTES

goniometer *(continued)*
    Polk finger g.
    Sammons biplane g.
    Scerratti g.
    Sedan g.
    universal full-circle manual g.
    Zimmer g.
goniometric
goniometry
Goniopora
    coralline hydroxyapatite G. (CHAG)
gonococcal septic arthritis
gonorrheal heel
gonorrhoeae
    Neisseria g.
Gonstead
    G. pelvic marking system
    G. technique
Gooch splint
Goodman orthopaedic bed
Good 'N Bed wedge
Goodpasture syndrome
Goodwin bone clamp
Goody's Headache Powders
gooseneck gouge
Gordon
    G. approach
    G. joint injection technique
    G. knee phenomenon
    G. reflex
    G. splint
    G. squeeze test
gordonae
    Mycobacterium g.
Gordon-Broström technique
Gordon-Taylor
    G.-T. hindquarter amputation
    G.-T. technique
Gore
    G. bit
    G. smoother
    G. smoother crucial tool
Gore-Tex
    G.-T. anterior cruciate ligament
    G.-T. knee prosthesis
    G.-T. nonabsorbable suture
    G.-T. vascular graft
    G.-T. waterproof cast liner
Gorham disease
Gorlin syndrome
GO scope
Gosselin fracture
Gottron
    G. papule
    G. sign
Gouffon
    G. hip pin
    G. pin fixation

gouge
    Abbott g.
    Acufex g.
    Alexander g.
    Andrews g.
    Army bone g.
    arthroplasty g.
    Aufranc g.
    Bishop g.
    bone g.
    Buch-Gramcko g.
    Campbell g.
    Capner g.
    Cobb spinal g.
    curved g.
    Dawson-Yuhl g.
    Duray-Reed g.
    gooseneck g.
    Guy g.
    Hibbs g.
    Hoen g.
    Jewett g.
    Killian g.
    Lexer g.
    Lucas g.
    Metzenbaum g.
    Meyerding g.
    Moe g.
    Murphy g.
    orthopaedic g.
    oscillating g.
    Partsch g.
    Read g.
    Ruben g.
    Sheehan g.
    Smith-Petersen curved g.
    Smith-Petersen straight g.
    Stagnara g.
    Stille bone g.
    straight g.
    swan-neck g.
    tendon g.
    U.S. Army g.
    Watson-Jones bone g.
    West bone g.
    Zielke g.
    Zimmer g.
Gould procedure
gout
    acute g.
    chronic tophaceous g.
    latent stage of g.
    tophaceous g.
gouty
    g. arthritis
    g. node
    g. pain

g. tophaceous deposit
g. tophus

Gowers
G. maneuver
G. muscular dystrophy
G. sign

grab
g. bar
g. sign

grabber
arthroscopic g.
disk g.
Tab G.

Grace
G. method of ratio of metatarsal length
G. plate 4-hole adapter

gracilis
fasciculus g.
g. flap
g. muscle
g. muscle graft
g. procedure
g. tendon
g. test

grade
g. A, B, C1, C2, D mantle
g. I, II oscillation
Risser g.

graded
g. exercise
g. exercise test (GXT)
g. Gore-Tex tape
g. spinal anesthesia

grades of mobilization (grade 1–5)
grading
activity g.
g. of manipulation

graduated-height block
Graflex material
Graf stabilization system
graft
AAA bone g.
acetabular augmentation g.
ACL g.
advancement flap g.
Albee bone g.
allogenic bone g.
allogenous bone g.
alloplastic g.
antebrachial fascial g.
anterior sliding tibial g.

anterosuperior iliac spine g.
arterial g.
autochthonous g.
autogenous bone g.
autogenous fibular g.
autogenous patellar-ligament g.
autogenous semitendinosus-gracilis g.
autologous reverse g.
Banks bone g.
bicondylar g.
bicortical iliac bone g.
bicortical ilial strip g.
bifid g.
BioPolyMeric g.
Blair-Brown skin g.
bone autogenous g.
bone chip g.
bone marrow g.
bone peg g.
bone-tendon-bone g.
bone-to-bone g.
Bonfiglio g.
bovine collagen g.
Boyd dual-onlay bone g.
BPB autologous g.
BPTB g.
Braun skin g.
bridge g.
bulk g.
cadaver bone g.
Calcitite g.
Campbell onlay bone g.
cancellous chip bone g.
cancellous and cortical bone g.
cancellous insert g.
cancellous morselized bone g.
carbon fiber g.
cartilage g.
chip g.
Chuinard autogenous bone g.
Clancy patellar tendon g.
clothespin spinal fusion g.
Codivilla bone g.
composite rib g.
composite skin g.
consolidated g.
cortical bone g.
cortical strut g.
corticocancellous bone g.
corticocancellous chip g.
cranial bone g.

NOTES

G

graft *(continued)*

cutaneous g.
Dacron g.
Daniel iliac bone g.
Davis muscle-pedicle g.
delayed g.
demineralized bone g.
dermal g.
devitalized bone g.
diamond-inlay g.
discrete blood supply to a bone g.
double-looped gracilis g.
Douglas skin g.
dowel bone g.
Dragstedt skin g.
g. driver
dual-onlay cortical bone g.
dura mater g.
Esser skin g.
g. expulsion
extraarticular g.
fascial g.
fascia lata freeze-thawed g.
fascio-fat g.
fat g.
femorocrural g.
femur g.
fetal substantia nigra g.
fibular onlay-inlay g.
fibular strut g.
filleted g.
fillet local flap g.
g. fixation
Flanagan-Burem apposing
    hemicylindric g.
flap g.
flat bone g.
flexor tendon g.
Forbes onlay bone g.
g. fragmentation
free fat g.
free skin g.
freeze-dried g.
freeze-thawed g.
fresh frozen g.
full-thickness skin g. (FTSG)
fusion g.
Gillies bone g.
Gill massive sliding g.
Golaski g.
Gore-Tex vascular g.
gracilis muscle g.
Haldeman bone g.
hamstring g.
Harris superior acetabular g.
g. harvest
Hemashield enhanced g.
hemicondylar g.

hemicylindrical bone g.
Henderson onlay bone g.
Henry bone g.
heterodermic g.
heterogeneous g.
heterogenous g.
Hey-Groves-Kirk bone g.
H-graft bone g.
Hoaglund bone g.
homogeneous g.
homogenous g.
homologous g.
H-shaped g.
Huntington bone g.
iliac crest bone free g.
iliac crest-inlay g.
iliac slot g.
iliac strut bone g.
iliotibial band g.
g. impingement
Inclan bone g.
inlay bone g.
insert g.
interbody g.
intercalary g.
interfascicular Millesi nerve g.
interposition bone g.
intramedullary g.
island g.
isologous g.
Isotec patellar tendon g.
Judet g.
Jump g.
keystone g.
Krause-Wolfe skin g.
Kutler V-Y flap g.
Langenskiöld bone g.
lateral patellar autologous g.
Lee anterosuperior iliac spine g.
Lee bone g.
ligament g.
load-bearing g.
lyophilized bone g.
Massie sliding g.
massive sliding g.
matchstick g.
g. material alternative
Matti-Russe bone g.
McFarland bone g.
McMaster bone g.
medullary bone g.
meniscus g.
mesh g.
Meyers quadratus muscle-pedicle
    bone g.
Millesi nerve g.
Moberg dowel g.
morcellized bone g.

Mueller patellar tendon g.
multiple cancellous chip g.
muscle pedicle bone g.
nail bed g.
nerve g.
neurovascular island g.
Nicoll cancellous bone g.
Nicoll cancellous insert g.
nonisometric g.
nontubed closed distant flap g.
nontubed open distant flap g.
Ollier thick split free g.
Ollier-Thiersch skin g.
onlay bone g.
onlay cancellous iliac g.
osteoarticular g.
osteocartilaginous g.
osteochondral g.
osteoperiosteal bone g.
Overton dowel g.
Papineau g.
particulate cancellous bone g.
patellar tendon g.
pedicle bone g.
pedicle fat g.
peg bone g.
percutaneous autogenous dowel
  bone g.
pericardium g.
peroneus brevis g.
Phemister onlay bone g.
pie-crusting skin g.
pinch skin g.
plantaris tendon g.
porcine skin g.
porous polyethylene g.
postage stamp skin g.
posterior bone g.
posterior cruciate ligament g.
posterolateral bone g.
powdered bone g.
g. preparation
prophylactic bone g.
prosthetic femorodistal g.
PTFE g.
reanastomosis of blood supply to
  bone g.
revascularization of g.
Reverdin epidermal free g.
rib g.
Russe bone g.
Ryerson bone g.

sandwiched iliac bone g.
scapular g.
segmental tendon g.
semitendinosus-gracilis g.
semitendinous g.
single-condylar g.
single-onlay cortical bone g.
single-stage tendon g.
in situ vein g.
skin bone free g.
sliding bone g.
sliding inlay bone g.
sliding tibial bone g.
Soto-Hall bone g.
split calvarial bone g.
split-thickness skin g. (STSG)
split thin g.
Stark g.
g. strength
structural bone g.
g. structure
strut g.
subclavius tendon g.
Tait g.
Taylor-Townsend-Corlett iliac crest
  bone g.
temporal fascia g.
tendon g. (TG)
g. tension
tension-free Millesi nerve g.
tension-free nerve g.
Thiersch medium split free g.
Thiersch thin split free g.
Thomas extrapolated bar g.
tibial bone g.
tricortical iliac crest bone g.
tricortical ilial strip g.
tube flap g.
tubularization of the g.
tumbler g.
vascularized bone g.
vascularized fibular g.
vascularized osteoseptocutaneous
  fibular autogenous g.
vascularized rib strut g.
vein g.
wedge g.
Weiland iliac crest bone g.
Whitecloud-LaRocca fibular strut g.
Wilson bone g.
Wilson-Jacobs patellar g.
Windson-Insall-Vince bone g.

G

NOTES

graft *(continued)*
    Wolfe-Kawamoto bone g.
    Wolf full-thickness free g.
    wraparound flap bone g.
    zooplastic g.
    Z-plasty local flap g.
graft-bony tunnel wall abrasion
grafting vein
Graftmaster device
Graham
    G. ankle arthrodesis
    G. muscle hook
    G. nerve hook
    G. traction
Grahamizer I exerciser
Gram-negative
Gram-positive
Gram stain
Granberg cervical traction system
Granberry
    G. frame
    G. splint
    G. traction
Grand Stand support stand
Grantham
    G. classification of femur fracture
    G. femur fracture classification
Grant-Small-Lehman supracondylar extension osteotomy
Granuflex dressing
granular
    g. cell myoblastoma
    g. histiocytosis
granulation
    extradural g.
    g. phase
    g. tissue
granule
    ProOsteon Implant 500 g.
Granulex
granulocyte colony-stimulating factor (G-CSF)
granuloma
    eosinophilic g.
    foreign body g.
    giant cell reparative g.
    pyogenic g.
    reparative g.
    subungual g.
    swimming pool g.
    tubercular g.
granulomatosis
    Langerhans cell g.
    Wegener g.
granulomatous
    g. fungal infection
    g. myositis

graph
    Moseley bone age g.
    Moseley straight line g.
Graphic Rating Scale (GRS)
Graphton putty
grasp
    pinch g.
    thumb-pinch g.
grasper
    Acufex g.
    loose body g.
    pituitary g.
grasper-cutter
    Questus leading edge g.-c.
grasping
    g. forceps
    g. power
    g. suture
Grasshopper positioner
Grass neurostimulator
grate
grater
    g. reamer
    g.-type reamer with Zimmer-Hudson shank
gravis
    myasthenia g.
    Tensilon test for myasthenia g.
gravitational
    g. insecurity
    g. line
    g. proprioception
gravity
    center of g. (COG)
    g. drawer test
    g.-driven angle finder
    g. extension locking system (GELS)
    flex against g.
    g. ground reaction force
    g. line
    line of g.
    g. method of Stimson
    g. stress test
gray
    G. bone drill
    g. matter
    periaqueductal g. (PAG)
    G. ramus communicans
    G. revision instrument system
Grayson
    G. ligament
    G. ligament in hand
grease gun injury
great
    g. toe
    g. toe arthroplasty implant technique (GAIT)

g. toe implant
g. toe implant prosthesis
g. toe push-off
g. vessel
greater
g. multangular
g. multangular bone
g. multangular ridge
g. rhomboid muscle
g. trochanter
g. trochanteric apophyseal arrest
g. trochanteric femoral fracture
g. tuberosity
Green
G. muscle hook
G. procedure
G. transfer
Green-Anderson growth table
Green-Banks
G.-B. technique
G.-B. transfer
Greenberg clamp
Greene forceps
Greenfield
G. inferior vena caval filter
G. osteotomy
G. spinocerebellar ataxia
classification
Green-Laird modification of the Reverdin osteotomy
Green-O'Brien evaluation system
Green-Reverdin osteotomy
greenstick
g. dorsal proximal metatarsal
osteotomy
g. fixation
g. fracture
Green-Watermann osteotomy
Greissinger
G. foot prosthesis
G. Multi-Axis joint
Grelot
image en G.
grenade-thrower's
g.-t. arm
g.-t. fracture
Greulich-Pyle
G.-P. bone age
G.-P. technique
Grice
G. extraarticular subtalar arthrodesis

G. incision
G. procedure
Grice-Green
G.-G. extraarticular subtalar
arthrodesis
G.-G. technique
grid
g. cabinet
g. maze board
g. maze set
radiographic g.
Shar-Tek foot positioning g.
Grierson
G. meniscal shaver
G. tendon stripper
Griffith incision
Grifulvin V
grimace test
grinder
DePuy calcar g.
grinding test
grip
dowel g.
Get-A-Grip g.
key g.
g. lock
polly power g.
Posey g.
Skil-Care cushion g.
syringe g.
g. tester
ulnar side g.
Grip-Ease device
Gripp
G. squeeze ball
G. squeeze ball hand exerciser
Gripper acetabular cup prosthesis
Grisactin Ultra
Grisel syndrome
griseofulvin
Gris-PEG
Gristina-Webb
G.-W. total shoulder arthroplasty
Griswold distraction machine
Gritti-Stokes
G.-S. amputation
G.-S. distal thigh procedure
G.-S. knee prosthesis
groin
g. flap
g. pain
g.-to-ankle cast

G

NOTES

grommet
  g. bone liner
  circumferential g.
  Press-Fit circumferential g.
  titanium circumferential g.
groove
  annular g.
  biceps g.
  bicipital g.
  deltopectoral g.
  g. distal tibia
  femoral g.
  fibular g.
  flexor g.
  intercollicular g.
  intercondylar g.
  intertubercular g.
  nail g.
  parasagittal g.
  patellar g.
  patellofemoral g.
  peroneal g.
  g. of Ranvier
  spiral humeral g.
  trochlear g.
grooved
  g. director
  g. dissector
  G. Pegboard Test
  g. protector
grooving osteotome
gross
  g. fracture
  g. manipulation
  G. Motor Function Measure
    (GMFM)
Grosse-Kempf
  G.-K. interlocking medullary nail
  G.-K. interlocking medullary nailing
  G.-K. locking nail
  G.-K. tibial technique
ground
  g. electrode
  purchase and press the g.
  g. reaction
  g. reaction force
group
  activity g.
  adductor muscle g.
  ancillary muscle g.
  AO g.
  g. fascicular repair
  gastrocnemius-soleus muscle g.
  g. handling
  levator ani g.
  quadriceps muscle g.

grouped
  g. discharge
  g. fascicular repair
Grover
  G. meniscotome
  G. meniscus knife
Groves-Goldner technique
Groves opponensplasty
growing pains
growth
  anchorage-dependent g.
  g. arrest
  g. arrest line
  asymmetrical g.
  bone g.
  chondroosseous g.
  g. factor
  g. hormone
  g. hormone resistance
  latitudinal g.
  physeal g.
  g. plate
  g.-plate abscess
  g. plate injury
  g. prediction
  g. retardation
  g. zone
GRS
  Graphic Rating Scale
Gruca
  G. lower leg procedure
  G. stabilization
Gruca-Weiss spring
Gruen
  G. mode
  G. zone
Gruppe
  G. wire prosthesis
  G. wire prosthesis-crimping forceps
GSB
  Gschwind-Scheier-Bahler
  GSB elbow prosthesis
  GSB expanded version for knee
    prosthesis
Gschwind-Scheier-Bahler (GSB)
  G.-S.-B. elbow prosthesis
GSR/Temp2
G suit
**Guam amyotrophic lateral sclerosis-
  parkinsonism dementia**
Guard
  FREEDOM Palm G.
  Progressive Palm G.
guard
  Cloward cervical drill g.
  drill g.
  fingertip g.
  Kneed-It knee g.

McDavid ankle g.
McDavid hinged knee g.
Omed vented instrument g.
palm g.
pin g.
Ullrich drill g.
guarded osteotome
Guardian walker
guarding
muscle g.
Guardsman femoral interference screw
Gudas
G. scarf Z-plasty
G. scarf Z-plasty osteotomy
Guepar hinged knee prosthesis
Guérin fracture
Guhl
G. distraction
G. technique
guide
Accu-Line g.
acetabular cup peg drill g.
ACL drill g.
Acufex alignment g.
Acufex tibial g.
Adapteur multi-functional drill g.
adjustable angle g.
Adson drill g.
Adson saw g.
alignment g.
angel wing g.
AO-stopped drill g.
axis g.
Bailey-Gigli saw g.
Bailey saw g.
ball-tipped Küntscher g.
barrel g.
Blair saw g.
Bow & Arrow cannulated drill g.
Bullseye femoral g.
g. bushing
calibrated pin g.
Cloward drill g.
contoured anterior spinal plate
drill g.
Cushing-Gigli saw g.
Cushing saw g.
Davis saw g.
Delta Recon proximal drill g.
DePuy femoral acetabular
overlay g.
distal femoral cutting g.

drill g.
Duopress g.
eccentric drill g.
extramedullary alignment g.
femoral intermedullary g.
femoral notch g.
FIN pin g.
Fisher g.
fixed-offset g.
front-entry g.
Gatlin gun drill g.
Ghajar g.
Gigli saw g.
Glacier ceramic 4-in-1 cutting g.
Glacier ceramic knee cutting g.
glenoid drill g.
handheld drill g.
Hewson cruciate g.
Hewson ligament drill g.
Hoffmann pin g.
g. hole
humeral cutting g.
intercondylar drill g.
intermedullary g.
Lebsche saw g.
Levin drill g.
ligature g.
Lipscomb-Anderson drill g.
long axial alignment g.
long nail-mounted drill g.
MOD femoral drill g.
nail-driving g.
nail rotational g.
neutral drill g.
notch cutting g.
nut alignment g.
patellar drill g.
patellar reamer g.
patellar resection g.
PCA cutting g.
PCA medullary g.
picket fence g.
pin g.
g. pin
Poppen Gigli saw g.
ProTrac alignment g.
Puddu drill g.
Raney saw g.
reamer g.
rear-entry ACL drill g.
Reece osteotomy g.
Richards angle g.

G

NOTES

guide *(continued)*
    Richards drill g.
    g. rod
    saw g.
    scaphoid screw g.
    Scott-RCE osteotomy g.
    screw angle g.
    Stader pin g.
    stationary angle g.
    Synthes wire g.
    targeting drill g.
    T-bar g.
    telescopic view g.
    tibial cutter g.
    tibial cutting g.
    Todd-Wells g.
    tube g.
    tunnel drill g.
    tunnel locator g.
    Tworek screw g.
    Uslenghi drill g.
    g. wire
    wire and drill g.
    wound measuring g.
    XMB tibial reaming g.
    Yasargil ligature g.
guideline
    Böhler g.
    Hartel g.
    Letournel g.
guidepin, guide pin
    AO g.
    ball g.
    ball-point g.
    ball-tip g.
    beaded reamer g.
    calibrated g.
    femoral g.
    lateral g.
    nonbeaded g.
    precurved ball-tipped g.
    Rica wire g.
    Synthes g.
    threaded g.
    tibial g.
    Watson-Jones g.
guidewire
    beaded g.
    drill-tipped g.
Guilford cervical brace
Guilford-Wright prosthesis
Guillain-Barré syndrome
Guilland sign
guillotine
    g. amputation
    Charnley femoral inlay g.
Guldmann Overhead Trac System
Guleke bone rongeur

Guleke-Stookey approach
Gulick Anthropometric Tape
Guller resection
Gumley seat beat injury classification
gum rubber Martin bandage
gun
    g. barrel sign
    Biofix arrow g.
    cement injection g.
    CMW cement g.
    Harris cement g.
    heat g.
    Lidge cement g.
    Reflex G.
    rivet g.
    staple g.
    g. stock deformity
Gunderson
    G. bone forceps
    G. muscle forceps
Gunning splint
Gunn jaw winking
gunshot
    g. fracture
    g. wound
GunSlinger shoulder orthosis
Gunston
    G. arthroplasty
    G. polycentric knee prosthesis
Gunston-Hult knee prosthesis
Guppe forceps
Gurd
    G. procedure
    G. resection
gurney
Gustilo
    G. classification of puncture wound
    G. fracture classification system
    G. hip prosthesis
    G. knee prosthesis
    G. puncture wound classification
Gustilo-Anderson
    G.-A. open clavicular fracture
    G.-A. open fracture classification
Gustilo-Kyle
    G.-K. cementless total hip
      arthroplasty
    G.-K. femoral component
gutter
    g. cast
    g. splint
Guttmann
    G. subtalar arthrodesis
    G. technique
guy
    G. gouge
    g. suture

Guyon
>G. canal
>G. tunnel release

G/W Heel Lift, Inc. orthosis
GXT
>graded exercise test

gym
>g. ball
>hand g.
>limb g.
>total g.
>Zuni g.

gymball
>Exertools g.

Gymnastik
>G. ball
>G. ball functional stabilization
>exercise

gymnast's wrist
Gymnic ball
Gyne-Lotrimin
Gynogen L.A. Injection
Gypsona
>G. cast
>G. cast material

gyrectomy
Gyroscan superconducting MRI

NOTES

G

H

per hypodermic
- H region
- H wave

H2 blocker

HA

hallux abductus
hydroxyapatite
- HA 65101 implant metal
- HA 65101 implant metal prosthesis

Haacker sling

Haas
- H. disease
- H. osteotomy
- H. paralysis

Haber-Kraft osteotomy

habitual
- h. control
- h. dislocation

habituation

Hackethal
- H. intramedullary bouquet fixation
- H. nail
- H. stacked nailing technique

hacksaw

HA-coated hip implant

Haddad metatarsal osteotomy

Haddad-Riordan arthrodesis

Hadfield hand board

Hadley S-curve

Haemophilus
- *H. influenzae*
- *H. parainfluenzae*

Hafnia alvei

Hagie
- H. hip pin
- H. pin nail
- H. sliding nail plate

HAGL

humeral avulsion of the glenohumeral
ligament

Hagl lesion

Haglund
- H. deformity
- H. syndrome

Haglund-Stille plaster spreader

Hahn
- H. bone nail
- H. cleft
- clefts of H.
- H. screw

Hahn-Steinthal
- H.-S. capitellum fracture
  classification
- H.-S. fracture
- H.-S. fracture of capitellum

Haid
- H. cervical plate
- H. UBP system
- H. Universal bone plate

Haight-Finochietto rib spreader

**Haines-McDougall medial sesamoid
ligament**

hairline fracture

Hajek
- H. chisel
- H. mallet

Hajek-Koffler bone punch forceps

halazepam

Halcion

Haldeman bone graft

Halder locking nail

Haldol

Haldrone

half
- h.-and-half nail
- h.-circle plate
- h. Jimmie
- h. ring
- h.-shell splint

half-pin
- h.-p. external fixator
- h.-p. fixation

Halfprin 81

Halifax
- H. clamp posterior cervical fixation
- H. interlaminar clamp
- H. interlaminar clamp kit

Hall
- H. air drill
- H. air-driven oscillating saw
- H. bur
- H. double-hole spinal stapler
- H. driver
- H. facet fusion
- H. mandibular implant system
- H. Micro-Aire drill
- H. modular acetabular reamer
  system
- H. Neurairtome
- H. power drill
- H. sagittal saw
- H. screwdriver
- H. series 4 large bone instrument
- H. spinal screw
- H. step-down drill
- H. technique
- H. Versipower drill
- H. Versipower oscillating saw

H

Hall *(continued)*
    H. Versipower reamer
    H. Versipower reciprocating saw
Hall-Dundar drill
Halle bone curette
Hall-effect strain transducer
Hallister heel cup
Hall-Pankovich medullary nail
hallucal sesamoid
hallucis
    h. brevis tenodesis
    extensor h.
    hyperdynamic abductor h.
    h. longus laceration
hallux
    h. abductovalgus (HAV)
    h. abductus (HA)
    h. abductus valgus
    h. dolorosa
    h. dorsiflexion angle (DFA)
    h. elevatus
    h. extensus
    h. flexus
    h. interphalangeal joint arthrodesis
    h. interphalangeus
    intrinsic minus h.
    h. IP joint
    h. limitus deformity
    h. malleus
    h. migrati
    h. migration
    h. nail
    h. rigidus
    h. rigidus arthrodesis
    h. sesamoid
    h. valgus
    h. valgus angle (HVA)
    h. valgus deformity
    h. valgus interphalangeus angle
    h. valgus-metatarsus primus varus
      complex
    h. valgus night splint
    h. valgus procedure
    h. varus
    h. varus correction
halo
    h. body jacket
    h. brace
    h. cast
    h.-cast distraction
    h. cervical orthosis
    h. cervical traction system
    h.-dependent traction
    h. extension orthosis
    h.-extension traction
    h.-gravity traction device
    h.-hyperextension traction

    h.-Ilizarov distraction
      instrumentation
    h. immobilization
    h. nevus
    h. pedestal
    pericellular h.
    Perry-Nickel cranial h.
    h. pin
    h. ring
    h. sign
    h. traction jacket
    h. traction orthosis
    Twin Cities Lo-Profile h.
    h. vest
    h. vest apparatus
    h. vest device
    h.-vest orthosis
    h.-wheelchair traction
halo-femoral
    h.-f. distraction
    h.-f. traction
halogen lamp
halo-pelvic
    h.-p. distraction
    h.-p. traction
haloprogin
Halotex
Halsey
    H. nail scissors
    H. needle holder
Halsted maneuver
halter
    Cerva Crane h.
    DePuy h.
    Diskard head h.
    Forrester-Brown head h.
    head h.
    Redi head h.
    Repro head h.
    TMJ h.
    h. traction
    Upper 7 head h.
    Zimfoam head h.
    Zimmer head h.
Haltran
hamartoma
    cartilaginous h.
    fibrous h.
    lipofibromatous h.
hamartomatous lesion
Hamas
    H. technique
    H. upper limb prosthesis
hamate
    h. bone
    hook of the h.
    h. hook
    h. hook nonunion

h. ligament
h. tail fracture
hamate-lunate joint
Hambly procedure
Hamby twist drill
Hamilton
H. apparatus
H. bandage
H. pelvic traction screw tractor
H. Rating Scale for Depression
H. ruler test
H. screw
H. traction
Hamman sign
hammer
Babinski h.
Berliner percussion h.
Buck neurological h.
cervical/lumbar h.
Cloward h.
h. digit syndrome
Epstein neurological h.
H. external fixation
Küntscher h.
orthopaedic h.
reflex h.
slap h.
sliding h.
Taylor percussion h.
h. toe correction with
interphalangeal fusion
h. toe deformity
hammertoe, hammer toe (HT)
flexible h.
Hammond splint
Hammon foot procedure
hamstring
h. force
h. graft
h. lengthening
h. ligament augmentation
medial h.
h. muscle
h. release
h.-setting exercise
h. tendon
h. tightness
hamstrung knee
hand
all-median nerve h.
all-ulnar nerve h.
h. amputation

h. anomaly
ape h.
apelike h.
bear's paw h.
h. block
h. board
h. brace
Breuerton x-ray view of h.
h. chuck
cleft h.
Cleland ligament in the h.
h. cock-up splint
h. cone
h. cuff
h. dominance
dorsum of h.
h. drill
h. evaluation set
h. exercise ball
h. exerciser
fell on outstretched h. (FOOSH)
flexor retinaculum of h.
flipper h.
h.-foot syndrome
Freedom arthritis support for h.
frostbite of h.
Gilliat-Summer nerve-damaged h.
h. grasp strength
Grayson ligament in h.
h. grip dynamometer
h. grip strength
h. gym
H. Helper
H. Helper hand exerciser
hemiplegic h.
hypoplastic h.
h. infection
lobster-claw h.
mirror h.
mitten h.
Myobock artificial h.
oath h.
obstetrician's h.
opera-glass h.
h.-operated drill
h. orthosis (HO)
Otto Bock system electric h.
pancake h.
h. paralysis
h. placement
h. prosthesis
psychoextended h.

NOTES

H

hand *(continued)*
    psychoflexed h.
    h. reconstruction
    h. saw
    spastic h.
    spread h.
    symbrachytactylous h.
    tangential h.
    vaginal ligament of h.
    Volkmann claw h.
    h. volumeter
    web area of h.
    web border of h.
handbag muscle
handbreadth
HandClens ultra antiseptic spray
handedness
Handeze fingerless glove
handheld
    h. drill guide
    h. dynamometer (HHD)
    h. retractor
handicap
    International Classification of
      Impairments, Disabilities, H.'s
      (ICIDH)
handicapped
handle
    Bard-Parker h.
    Barton traction h.
    Beaver blade h.
    Charnley brace h.
    cup holder h.
    Dynagrip blade h.
    multisided blade h.
    Ortho-Grip silicone rubber h.
    stone basket screw mounted h.
    surgical knife h.
    Thera-Band h.
    Therap-Loop door h.
    T-pin h.
    traction h.
    h.-type reamer
handlebar palsy
handling
    group h.
handpiece
    Coopervision irrigation/aspiration h.
    Max 3 electric h.
    reciprocating power h.
Hand-Schüller-Christian disease
Hands Free Knee Retractor System
handshake cast
Handy-Buck traction
hanging
    h. arm cast
    h. cast sling
    h. heel sign

    h. hip
    h. hip operation
    h. of limb
    h. toe operation
hangman's fracture
Hankin reduction
Hanna night splint
Hannover classification
Hansen
    H. classification of fracture
    H. disease
    H. fracture classification
Hansen-Street
    H.-S. driver-extractor
    H.-S. nail
    H.-S. pin
    H.-S. plate
Hanslik patellar prosthesis
Hansson
    Lars Ingvar H. (LIH)
Hapad
    H. longitudinal metatarsal arch pad
    H. medial arch pad
    H. metatarsal arch
    H. metatarsal insole
    H. scaphoid arch
    H. shoe insert
Hara infiltration block
hard
    h. callus stage
    h. collar
    h. corn
    h. socket
Hardcastle
    H. classification
    H. classification of tarsometatarsal
      joint injury
hardening
    work h.
Hardinge
    H. femoral approach
    H. lateral approach
    H. technique
    H. vastus lateralis procedure
Hardt-Delima osteotome
hardware
    orthopaedic h.
    h. photopenia
Hardy
    H. aluminum crutch
    H. hypophysial curette
Hardy-Clapham sesamoid classification
Hardy-Joyce triangle
Hare
    H. apparatus
    H. compact traction splint
    H. pin

H. splint device
H. traction
Harken prosthesis
Hark foot procedure
Harloff cart
Harlow plate
Harmon
H. cervical approach
H. chisel
H. hip reconstruction
H. modified posterolateral approach
H. posterolateral approach
H. procedure
H. shoulder approach
H. transfer
H. transfer technique
Harm posterior cervical plate
Harms-Moss anterior thoracic instrumentation
harness
figure-of-eight h.
Forte h.
Pavlick h.
Pavlik h.
weight-relieving Forte h.
Zuni h.
Harold Crowe drill
Harpenden
H. caliper
H. dynamometer
Harriluque
H. sublaminar wiring modification
H. technique
Harrington
H. clamp forceps
H. compression rod
H. distraction instrumentation
H. distraction outrigger
H. distraction rod
H. flat wrench
H. hook clamp
H. hook driver
H. outrigger splint
H. pedicle (bifid) hook
H. rod fixation
H. rod and hook system
H. rod instrumentation
H. rod instrumentation compression
H. rod instrumentation distraction outrigger device
H. rod instrumentation failure

H. rod instrumentation force application
H. spinal elevator
H. spreader
H. total hip arthroplasty
Harrington-Kostuik
H.-K. distraction device
H.-K. instrumentation
Harris
H. anterolateral approach
H. bolt
H. brace-type reamer
H. broach
H. cemented hip prosthesis
H. cement gun
H. center-cutting acetabular reamer
H. condylocephalic nail
H. condylocephalic nailing
H. condylocephalic rod
H. criteria
H. criteria for implant loosening
H. design (HD)
H. Design femoral prosthesis
H. Design-2 implant
H. femoral component removal
H. four-wire trochanter reattachment
H. growth arrest line
H. Hemi Arm Sling
H. hip nail
H. hip scale
H. hip score
H. hip status system
H. Infant Neuromotor Test (HINT)
H. lateral approach
H. medullary nail
H. Micromini prosthesis
H. plate
H. scope
H. splint
H. splint sling
H. superior acetabular graft
H. view
H. wire tier
Harris-Aufranc device
Harris-Beath
H.-B. arthrodesis
H.-B. axial calcaneus view
H.-B. projection
Harris-CDH hip prosthesis
Harris-Galante
H.-G. acetabular cup

NOTES

H

Harris-Galante *(continued)*
    H.-G. hip replacement acetabular component
    H.-G. I porous-coated acetabular component
    H.-G. porous hip prosthesis
    H.-G. stem
Harris-Mayo hip score
Harrison bone-holding forceps
Harrison-Nicolle polypropylene peg
Harris-Smith
    H.-S. anterior interbody drill
    H.-S. cervical fusion
Hartel guideline
Hart extension finger splint
Hartmann
    H. bone rongeur
    H. mosquito forceps
Hartshill rectangle
harvest
    graft h.
    h. site
harvesting
    Gilbert h.
    Tamae h.
    Weiland h.
Harvey wire-cutting scissors
Hass
    H. disease
    H. osteotomy
    H. procedure
Hassmann-Brunn-Neer elbow technique
Hastings
    H. bipolar hemiarthroplasty
    H. frame
    H. hip prosthesis
    H. open reduction
Hatcher pin
Hatcher-Smith cervical fusion
hatchet-face
hatchet-head deformity
Hatfield
    H. bone curette
Hauser
    H. ambulation index
    H. bunionectomy
    H. heel cord procedure
    H. patellar realignment technique
    H. patellar tendon procedure
    H. realignment
    H. tendo calcaneus lengthening
Hausmann
    H. Velcro-Lock mat platform
    H. weight rack
    H. Work-Well work hardening system
Hausted orthopaedic bed
Hautant test

HAV
    hallux abductovalgus
haversian
    h. bone remodeling
    h. canal
    h. gland
    h. system
    h. vessel
Hawiva test
Hawkeye
    H. suture needle
    H. suture needle for arthroscopy
Hawkins
    H. classification of talar fracture
    H. impingement sign
    H. line
    H. procedure
    H. talar fracture classification
    H. test
hawthorn
Hayes retractor
Haygarth node
Hay-Groves shelf procedure
Hay lateral approach
Haynes-Griffin mandibular splint
Haynes pin
Haynes-Stellite (HS)
    H.-S. 21 implant metal
    H.-S. implant metal prosthesis
Hays hand retractor
H-block
    Frost H.-b.
HBO
    hyperbaric oxygen
    HBO therapy
HC
    Bancap H.
HCA
    heel cord advancement
HCl
    hydrochloride
        Cleocin HCl
        cyclobenzaprine HCl
        Isocaine HCl
        tacrine HCl
        terbinafine HCl
        tramadol HCl
HCMI
    Health Care Manufacturing Inc.
    HCMI Chiropractic System
HCTU
    home cervical traction unit
HD
    Harris design
    heloma durum
HD-2 cemented hip prosthesis
head
    Aequalis h.

h.-at-risk sign
h. brace
cartilaginous cap of phalangeal h.
cobalt-chromium h.
collared femoral h.
core decompression of femoral h.
countersink screw h.
DePuy hip prosthesis with
  Scuderi h.
femoral h.
fibular h.
first metatarsal h. (FMH)
Giliberty bipolar femoral h.
h. halter
h.-halter traction
H. hip arthroplasty
humeral h.
infrared h.
h. injury
ischemic necrosis of femoral h.
  (INFH)
long h.
Matroc femoral h.
met h.
metatarsal h.
Phillips screw h.
pseudometatarsal h.
radial h.
screw h.
Series-II humeral h.
H. & Shoulders Intensive
  Treatment
h.-splitting humeral fracture
h.-stem offset
terminal h.
ulnar h.
V40 forged femoral h.
Vitox femoral h.
Ziramic femoral h.
Zirconia orthopaedic prosthetic h.
Zyranox femoral h.
headache
  cervicogenic h.
headholder
  Aesculap h.
headlight
  Cogent LightWear h.
Headmaster collar
headrest
  doughnut h.
  h. extension
  Mayfield neurosurgical h.

McConnell orthopaedic h.
pin h.
three-prong h.
Healey revision acetabular component
healing
  bone h.
  cartilage h.
  contact h.
  fracture h.
  gap h.
  per primam h.
  h. retardation
  h. shoe
  soft tissue h.
  spiritual h.
Health Care Manufacturing Inc.
  (HCMI)
Healthflex orthotic
Healthier seating cushion
Health O Meter Scale
heart
  h.-and-hand syndrome
  h. failure
  h. rate (HR)
  h.-shaped buttocks
Heartline
heat
  h. application
  h.-cured acrylic femoral head
    prosthesis
  h. fracture
  h. gun
  moist h.
  h.-molded petroplastic ankle-foot
    orthosis
  h.-molder petroplastic ankle-foot
    orthosis
  h. therapy
Heath mallet
heave
  parasternal h.
heavy
  h. cross-slot screwdriver
  h. side plate
heavy-duty
  h.-d. femur plate
  h.-d. two-tooth retractor
HeavyMed ball
Heberden node
hebosteotomy
hebotomy
Hebra blade

NOTES

H

Heck screw
hectobar
Hedblom rib retractor
Hedley-Hungerford hip prosthesis
heel
> h.-and-toe gait
> anterior h.
> black-dot h.
> h. contact phase of gait
> h. cord
> h. cord advancement (HCA)
> h. cord lengthening
> h. cord stretch
> h. cord stretching exercise
> h. counter
> cucumber h.
> h. cup
> h. cushion
> cushion h.
> h. equinus
> h. fat pad
> H. Free splint
> h. gait
> gonorrheal h.
> high-prow h.
> H. Hugger therapeutic heel
>   stabilizer
> h. lift
> h. pad pathology
> painful h.
> h.-palm test
> h. posting
> prominent h.
> h. raises exercise
> reverse Thomas h.
> h. rocks exercise
> rubber walking h.
> SACH orthopaedic h.
> h. sleeve
> h. and sole insert
> solid ankle, cushioned h. (SACH)
> h.-spike
> h. spur
> h. spur/plantar fasciitis syndrome
> H. Spur Special
> h. spur syndrome
> h. stand
> h.-strike
> tennis h.
> h. tension
> Thomas h.
> h.-tip test
> h. and toe walking
> h.-to-knee test
> h.-to-shin test
> h.-to-toe gait
> h. valgus
> h. varus

> h. varus sign
> walking h.
> wedge adjustable cushioned h.

Heelbo decubitus heel/elbow protector
HeelCup
> Sof Gel H.

Heelift suspension boot
heel-off
> h.-o. phase of gait

heel-toe
> h.-t. gait
> h.-t. runners

Heerfort syndrome
Heermann alligator forceps
Heffington lumbar seat spinal frame
Hefty-bite pin cutter
Hegge pin
Heifetz procedure
height
> intervertebral disk h.

Hein rongeur
Heiple arthrodesis
Heiss soft tissue retractor
Helal
> H. flap arthroplasty
> H. modification
> H. osteotomy

Helbing sign
Helenca
> H. bandage
> H. binder

Helfet test
helical computed tomography
Heliodorus bandage
heloma
> h. durum (HD)
> h. molle (HM)

Helparm
> Swedish H.

Helper
> Hand H.

hemangiectasia
> Klippel-Trenaunay
>   osteohypertrophic h.

hemangioendothelioma
hemangioendotheliosarcoma
hemangioma
> capillary h.
> cavernous h.

hemangiomatosis
hemangiopericytoma
hemangiosarcoma
hemarthrosis
> acute traumatic h.
> posttraumatic h.

Hemashield enhanced graft
hematocrit

hematogenous
  h. infection
  h. osteomyelitis
hematoma
  iliopsoas muscle h.
  intramedullary h.
  sciatic nerve palsy h.
  subgluteal h.
  subungual h.
hematuria
hemiambulator walker
hemianopsia
  homonymous h.
hemiarm sling
hemiarthroplasty
  Austin Moore h.
  Bateman h.
  Hastings bipolar h.
  I-beam hip h.
  large humeral-head h.
  Miller-Galante I h.
  Neer h.
  prosthetic h.
  Smith-Petersen h.
hemichondrodiasthesis
hemicondylar
  h. fracture
  h. graft
hemicylindrical bone graft
hemidiaphyseal debridement
hemidystonia
hemiepiphysiodesis
hemihypertrophy
hemi-implant
  Dow Corning titanium h.-i.
hemi-interpositional implant
hemijoint arthroplasty
hemiknee
  Savastano h.
hemilaminectomy knife
hemimelia
  Achterman-Kalamachi fibular h.
  dysplasia epiphysealis h.
  fibular h.
  paraxial h.
  radial h.
  tibial h.
hemiparetic
hemipelvectomy
  formal h.
  internal h.
hemipelvis

hemiphalangectomy
  Johnson h.
hemipiphysiodesis
  transpedicular convex anterior h.
hemiplegia
  bilateral h.
  double h.
  spastic h.
hemiplegic
  h. hand
  h. or hemiparetic gait
hemiprosthesis
  single-stemmed silicone h.
hemipulp flap
hemiresection interposition arthroplasty
hemisection
  triple h.
hemi/semi-laminotomy
Hemi-Silastic implant
hemispherical pusher
hemivertebra
  balanced h.
  congenital h.
  unbalanced h.
hemivertebral excision
hemochromatosis
Hemo-Drain evacuator
hemogenesis
hemolymphangioma
hemophilia
  h. A, B
hemophiliac arthritis
hemopneumothorax
hemorrhage
  retroperitoneal h.
hemosiderin
hemostasis
hemostat
  blunt nose h.
  Crile h.
  Kelly h.
  mosquito h.
  orthopaedic h.
  Surgicel fibrillar h.
  Surgicel Nu-Knit absorbable h.
hemostatic
  h. forceps
  h. thoracic clamp
hemothorax
Hemovac
  H. Hydrocoat drain
  H. suction tube

NOTES

H

273

Henahan elevator
Hendel guided osteotome
Henderson
  H. arthrodesis
  H. clamp approximator
  H. classification
  H. fracture
  H. lag screw
  H. onlay bone graft
  H. posterolateral approach
  H. posteromedial approach
  H. skin incision
Henderson-Jones chondromatosis
Hendler unitunnel technique
Henle ligament
Hennessy knee brace
Henning
  H. cast spreader
  H. inside-to-outside technique
  H. instrument set
  H. mallet
  H. meniscal retractor
  H. plaster spreader
Henry
  H. acromioclavicular technique
  H. anterior strap approach
  H. anterolateral approach
  H. bone graft
  H. extensile approach
  H. incision
  H. knot
  knot of H.
  leash of H.
  master knot of H.
  H. paralysis
  H. posterior interosseous nerve
    approach
  H. posterior interosseous nerve
    exposure
  H. radial approach
  H. resection
Henry-Geist spinal fusion
Henschke-Mauch
  H.-M. saw
  H.-M. SNS knee prosthesis
  H.-M. SNS lower limb prosthesis
Hensen plane
heparin
  reconstituted depolymerized h.
heparinized
  h. Ringer lactate solution
  h. saline flush
hepatitis B
hepatotoxicity
herb
  ayurvedic h.'s
herbal therapy

Herbert
  H. bone screw
  H. and Fisher fracture classification
    system
  H. knee prosthesis
  H. saw
  H. scaphoid bone fracture
  H. scaphoid bone fracture
    classification
  H. scaphoid screw
  H. screw fixation
  H. screw fixator
Herbert-Fisher fracture system
  classification
Herbert-Whipple bone screw
Hercules
  H. plaster shears
  H. TM drop-adjusting table
Herczel
  H. rib elevator
  H. rib rasp
hereditary
  h. multiple exostosis
  h. neuropathic disease
  h. neuropathy of infancy
  h. sensory motor neuropathy
  h. sensory motor neuropathy, type
    III (HSMN III)
  h. spinocerebellar ataxia
heredopathia atactica polyneuritiformis
Heritage hip system
Herman-Gartland osteotomy
Hermes
  H. Evolution tricompartmental knee
    system
  H. total knee system
Hermodsson
  H. fracture
  H. internal rotation
  H. internal rotation technique
  H. tangential view
Hernandez-Ros bone staple
Herndon-Heyman
  H.-H. foot operation
  H.-H. foot procedure
Herndon hip classification system
hernia
  inguinal h.
  muscle h.
  sliding abdominal h.
herniated
  h. cervical disk
  h. contained disk
  h. disk disease
  h. intervertebral disk (HID)
  h. nucleus pulposus (HNP, HPN)
herniation
  central h.

cervical midline disk h.
disk h.
intervertebral disk h.
intraspongy nuclear disk h.
midline disk h.
phalangeal h.
posterolateral h.
synovial h.
traumatic cervical disk h.

herpes simplex
herpetic

h. infection
h. whitlow

Herring lateral pillar classification
hertz (Hz)
Herzenberg bolt
Herzmark frame
HESSCO 300, 500 series
Hessel-Nystrom pin
Hessing brace
heterodermic graft
heterogeneous graft
heterogenesis
heterogenous graft
heterograft
heterotopic

h. bone
h. calcification
h. ossification
h. ossification prevention

heterotrophic ossification bridging
Heuter-Volkmann law
Hewson

H. breakaway pin
H. cruciate guide
H. drill
H. ligament button
H. ligament drill guide
H. suture passer

HEX

HEX heat applicator

hex

h. handle curette
h. screw
h. wrench

hexachlorophene
Hexadrol Phosphate
hexagonal slot-cap screw
Hexalite plastic
Hexcel

H. knee prosthesis

H. total condylar knee system
H. total condylar prosthesis

Hexcelite

H. cast
H. sheet splint

Hex-Fix

H.-F. Add-A-Clamp
H.-F. external fixation
H.-F. monolateral external fixator
H.-F. Universal swivel clamp

hexhead

h. bolt
h. pin
h. screwdriver

Heyer-Schulte

H.-S. antisiphon device
H.-S. wound drain

Hey-Groves

H.-G. fascia lata technique
H.-G. ligament reconstruction
technique

Hey-Groves-Kirk

H.-G.-K. bone graft
H.-G.-K. technique

Heyman

H. hip classification system
H. procedure

Heyman-Herndon

H.-H. clubfoot operation
H.-H. epiphysiodesis
H.-H. procedure
H.-H. release

Heyman-Herndon-Strong

H.-H.-S. capsular release
H.-H.-S. technique

HFOV

high-frequency oscillatory ventilation

HG

HG multilock hip prosthesis
HG multilock hip stem

hGH

human growth hormone

H-graft

H-g. bone graft
H-g. fusion

HHD

handheld dynamometer

Hi

All-Purpose Boot Hi
Hi Speed Pulse lavage

HIAD

high-impact aerobic dance

NOTES

H

hiatus
> adductor h.
> popliteal h.

Hibbs
> H. arthrodesis
> H. blade
> H. bone-cutting forceps
> H. chisel
> H. chisel elevator
> H. curette
> H. curved osteotome
> H. frame
> H. gouge
> H. mallet
> H. metatarsocalcaneal angle
> H. procedure
> H. retractor
> H. spinal fusion
> H. straight osteotome
> H. tendosuspension
> H.-type retractor

Hibbs-Jones spinal fusion
hibernoma
Hibiclens
> H. scrub
> H. solution
> H. Topical

Hibistat Topical
hickory-stick fracture
Hicks lugged plate
HID
> herniated intervertebral disk

hi-density foam
hidroacanthoma simplex
hierarchical scales of ADLs
high
> h.-air-loss bed
> h. efficiency particulate air filter
> h.-frequency oscillatory ventilation (HFOV)
> h. heel shoe
> h.-impact aerobic dance (HIAD)
> h.-Knight brace
> h. median-high radial palsy
> h. median-high ulnar palsy
> h. molecular weight polyethylene (HMWPE)
> h. muscular resistance bed
> h. performance silicone elastomer
> h.-prow heel
> h.-resolution analysis
> h.-riding patella
> h.-risk factor
> h. tibial osteotomy (HTO)
> h.-toe box
> h.-torque bur
> h. ulnar-high radial palsy

> h. velocity/low amplitude
> h.-volt galvanism

high-energy
> h.-e. fracture
> h.-e. trauma

high-grade
> h.-g. spondylolisthesis
> h.-g. surface osteogenic sarcoma

high-speed
> h.-s. bur
> h.-s. twist drill

high-voltage
> h.-v. galvanism
> h.-v. pulsed galvanic
> h.-v. pulse galvanic stimulation (HVPGS)
> h.-v. therapy (HVT)

HIHA tendon implant
hila (*pl. of* hilum)
hilar
Hilgenreiner
> H. angle
> H. brace
> H. horizontal Y line

Hilgenreiner-Pauwels line
Hilgenreiner-Perkins (H-P)
> H-P line

Hill Air-Drop HA90C table
Hill-Nahai-Vasconez-Mathes technique
Hillock arch
Hill-Rom orthopaedic bed
Hill-Sachs
> H.-S. deformity
> H.-S. fracture
> H.-S. shoulder dislocation
> H.-S. shoulder lesion
> H.-S. sign
> H.-S. view

hi-lo
> h.-l. rehab bed
> h.-l. table

hilum, pl. **hila**
hilus
> neurovascular h.
> h. of tendon

Hinderer
> H. cartilage forceps
> H. malar prosthesis

hindfoot
> h. anatomic variation
> h. arthrodesis
> h. deformity
> h. excursion
> h. instability
> h. joint complex
> h. kinematics
> lateral h.
> h. motion

h. orthosis
spastic varus h.
h. valgus
varus h.
hindfoot-midfoot collapse
hindquarter amputation
hinge
h. abduction
Adjusta-Wrist h.
AHSC-Volz h.
Arizona Health Sciences Center-
Volz h.
Bahler h.
Camber axis h. (CAH)
Compass h.
Dee elbow h.
elbow h.
flail-elbow h.
implant h.
h. joint
Kinematic rotation h.
Kudo h.
Lacey h.
medial/plantar h.
Noiles h.
offset h.
Quengel h.
Rancho swivel h.
h. rod
rotating h.
soft tissue h.
stabilizing h.
hinged
h. articulated fixator
h. brace
h. constrained knee prosthesis
h. cylinder cast
h. cylinder splint
h. fragment
h. great toe replacement prosthesis
h. implant
h. implant prosthesis
h. joint
h. Thomas splint
h. total knee prosthesis
hinging
HINT
Harris Infant Neuromotor Test
HIO
hole-in-one
HIO technique

hip
h. abduction
h. abductor strengthening exercise
anthropometric total h. (ATH)
h. arthroplasty
biologically designed h. (BDH)
h. bump
h. capsule joint
h. click
h. compression screw
congenital dislocation of h. (CDH)
congenital dysplasia of h. (CDH)
h. contusion
cup-on-cup arthroplasty of the h.
developmental dislocated h. (DDH)
developmental dysplasia of the h.
(DDH)
h. disarticulation prosthesis
h. dislocation
dysplasia of h.
h. extension
h. extension exercise
h. extension range of motion
h. extensor gait
h. flexion
h. flexion-extension
h. flexor contracture
h. fracture
fused h.
hanging h.
h. joint angle (HJA)
h. joint aspiration under
fluoroscopic control
h. joint syndrome
Link anatomical h.
h. mobility
h. orthosis (HO)
h. pinning
h. pointer
Precision total h.
h. reduction
h. replacement
revision of total h.
h. roll
h. rotation
Senegas approach to h.
h. skid
snapping h.
h. spica
h. spica cast
h. subluxation
tuberculosis of h.

NOTES

H

hip (*continued*)
    windblown h.
    windswept h.
hipGRIP
    h. pelvic positioning system
hip-knee-ankle-foot orthosis (HKAFO)
Hipokrat bimodular shoulder system
Hippocrates
    H. bandage
    H. manipulation
Hippocratic maneuver
hipRAP
Hirayma osteotomy
HiRider motorized/lift wheelchair
Hiroshim transfer
Hirsch
    H. hypophyseal punch
    H. hypophysis punch forceps
Hirschberg
    H. reflex
    H. sign
Hirschhorn
    H. compression approach
    H. compression technique
Hirschtick utility shoulder splint
hirudin
Hirudo medicinalis
His-Haas
    H.-H. muscle transfer
    H.-H. procedure
histiocytic tumor
histiocytoma
    angiomatoid malignant fibrous h.
      (AMFH)
    fibrous h.
    malignant fibrous h.
    nevoid h.
    pleomorphic fibrous h.
histiocytosis
    granular h.
    sinus h.
    h. X group of diseases
Histoacryl glue adhesive
histochemistry
Histofreezer cryosurgical system
histogenesis
    distraction h.
histologically
histomorphometry
Histoplasma capsulatum
histoplasmosis
history (hx)
    natural h.
histotoxin
hitch
    ankle h.
    spinal h.

Hitchcock
    H. arm procedure
    H. stereotactic immobilization frame
    H. tendon technique
Hi-Top
    H.-T. foot/ankle brace
    H.-T. foot/ankle walker
    H.-T. shoe
Hittenberger
    H. halo extension
    H. prosthesis
HIV
    human immunodeficiency virus
Hivid
HJA
    hip joint angle
HJD total hip system
HKAFO
    hip-knee-ankle-foot orthosis
HLA
    human leukocyte antigen
    human lymphocyte antigen
HLA-B27 blood antigen
HM
    heloma molle
HMWPE
    high molecular weight polyethylene
HNA
    hypothalamoneurohypophyseal axis
HNP
    herniated nucleus pulposus
HO
    hand orthosis
    hip orthosis
Hoaglund bone graft
Hoaglund-States classification
hoarseness
hobbling gait
Hobb view
hockey-stick
    h.-s. fracture
    h.-s. incision
Hodgen
    H. hip splint
    H. leg splint
Hodge plane
Hodgkinson acetabular component loosening criteria
Hodgkin tumor
Hodgson technique
Hodor-Dobbs procedure
Hoek-Bowen cement removal system
Hoen
    H. clamp
    H. forceps
    H. gouge
    H. periosteal elevator
    H. retractor

H. rongeur
H. skull plate

Hoffa
H. fat pad
H. fracture
H. massage
H. syndrome
H. tendon shortening
H. test

Hoffer
H. ankle procedure
H. split transfer

Hoffer-Daimler
H.-D. cast spreader

Hoffmann
H. apex fixation pin
H. approach
H. C-series external fixator
H. Dynamic external fixator
H. external fixation
H. external fixation system
H. fixation device
H. frame
H. ligament clamp
H. metatarsal operation
H. metatarsal procedure
H. panmetatarsal head resection
H. pin guide
H. reflex
H. sign
H. syndrome
H. test
H. transfixion pin

Hoffmann-Clayton procedure
Hoffmann-Vidal
H.-V. double frame
H.-V. external fixation apparatus
H.-V. external fixation device
H.-V. external fixator

Hoffmann-Vidal-Adrey frame
Hogg chair
Hohl
H. fracture classification system
H. tibial condylar fracture
classification

**Hohl-Luck tibial plateau fracture
classification**
Hohl-Moore
H.-M. classification
H.-M. technique

Hohmann
H. osteotomy

H. procedure
H. retractor

Hoke
H. Achilles tendon lengthening
H. Achilles tendon lengthening
operation
H. lumbar brace
H. lumbar brace/corset
H. lumbar corset
H. osteotome
H. procedure for tibial palsy
H. tibial palsy procedure
H. triple arthrodesis
H. triple-section method

Hoke-Kite technique
Hoke-Martin traction
Hoke-Miller procedure
Hold-and-Hold positioner
Holdaway ratio
holder
acetabular cup h.
Alvarado knee h.
arm h.
Ayers needle h.
Barraquer needle h.
Böhler-Steinmann pin h.
bone h.
Castroviejo needle h.
Charnley trochanter h.
clamp h.
Crile-Wood needle h.
cup h.
DeMartel-Wolfson clamp h.
Donaghy angled suture needle h.
Drummond hook h.
Ferguson bone h.
Halsey needle h.
hook h.
hookbar h.
Jacobson needle h.
knee h.
leg h.
limb h.
Malis needle h.
Mayo-Hegar needle h.
microneedle h.
needle h.
neonatal trach tube h.
octopus h.
pin h.
Rhoton needle h.
rod h.

NOTES

H

holder *(continued)*
>Ryder needle h.
>Sarot needle h.
>Schmidt rod h.
>shoulder h.
>staple h.
>thigh h.
>tibial track h.
>trochanter h.
>TSRH hook h.
>Wangensteen needle h.
>washer h.
>Watanabe pin h.
>Webster needle h.
>well-leg h.
>Yasargil needle h.

holding mitt

hold-relax
>h.-r. method
>h.-r. technique

Holdsworth spinal fracture classification

hole
>acetabular seating h.
>anchor h.
>anchoring h.
>10-h. blade plate
>blind anchorage h.
>bur h.
>centering h.
>drill h.
>gliding h.
>guide h.
>lag screw thread h.
>offset drill h.
>11-h. plate
>17-h. plate
>h. preparation method

hole-in-one (HIO)
>h.-i.-o. technique

holism

Hollander clog

Hollister Hot/Ice knee blanket

hollow
>h. mill Asnis cannulated screw
>h. mill drill
>h. mill instrumentation
>h. mill reamer

Hollywood
>H. bed
>H. bed extension hook set

holmium YAG laser

Holscher
>H. knee retractor
>H. root retractor

Holstein fracture of humerus

Holstein-Lewis fracture

Holt
>H. bolt

>H. nail
>H. nail plate

Holter traction

Holt-Oram atriodigital dysplasia

Holzheimer retractor

Homan retractor

Homans
>H. sign
>H. test

home
>h. cervical traction unit (HCTU)
>h. medical equipment
>H. Ranger
>h. spinal stabilization program

homeopathy

homeostasis
>fluid h.
>osseous h.

HomeTrac
>Saunders cervical H.

homogeneous
>h. graft
>h. screen

homogenous graft

homograft
>h. implant material
>h. prosthesis

homologous graft

homonymous hemianopsia

homunculus

Honda jack

hood
>dorsal h.
>extensor h.
>retinacular h.

hoof bottom

hook
>Acufex nerve h.
>anatomic h.
>André anatomical h.
>h. approximator
>APRL prosthetic h.
>Austin Moore h.
>Barr h.
>h. blade
>h. blocker
>Bobechko sliding barrel h.
>bone h.
>Boyes-Goodfellow h.
>button h.
>buttressed h.
>canted finger h.
>Carroll skin h.
>C-D h.
>closed Cotrel-Dubousset h.
>closed transverse process TSRH h.
>compression h.
>cranial Jacobs h.

Culler h.
h. dislodgment
distraction h.
h. distractor
double-open h.
down-angle h.
downsized circular laminar h.
drop-entry (closed body) h.
Drummond h.
Edwards h.
Edwards-Levine h.
Effler-Groves h.
h.-end intramedullary pin
finger h.
garment h.
Gillies bone h.
Gillies-Dingman h.
Graham muscle h.
Graham nerve h.
Green muscle h.
hamate h.
h. of the hamate
h. of hamate bone
Harrington pedicle (bifid) h.
H. hemi-harness shoulder
  immobilizer
h. holder
h. hollow-ground connection design
Hosmer Dorrance h.
h. impactor
intermediate C-D h.
Isola spinal implant system h.
Jameson muscle h.
Jannetta h.
Joseph h.
Keene compression h.
Kennerdell-Maroon h.
Kilner h.
Kirby muscle h.
Knodt rod and h.
Krayenbuehl h.
Küntscher nail-extracting h.
Lambotte bone h.
laminar C-D h.
Leatherman h.
h.-lying pectoral stretch exercise
lyre-shaped finger h.
meniscus h.
Moe alar h.
Moss h.
multispan fracture h.
h.-nail deformity

nerve h.
neutral h.
O'Brien rib h.
Oesch h.
open C-D h.
Osher irrigating implant h.
PCL-oriented placement marking h.
pediatric C-D h.
pediatric TSRH h.
pedicle C-D h.
h. pin
h.-pin fixation
h. plate
h.-plate fixation
prosthetic h.
h. pusher
ribbed h.
Rogozinski h.
h. rotary scissors
Selby II h.
sharp worm h.
side-opening laminar h.
h. site
skin h.
sliding barrel h.
split-finger h.
square-ended h.
T-handled h.
top-entry (open body) h.
h.-to-screw L4-S1 compression
  construct
Trautman Locktite prosthetic h.
h. trial set screw
TSRH buttressed laminar h.
TSRH circular laminar h.
TSRH pedicle h.
TSRH trial h.
Tyrell h.
UCLA CAPP TD h.
up-angle h.
h. V-groove connection design
Vilex Ouchless H.
Volkmann bone h.
Yasargil spring h.
Zielke bifid h.
Zuelzer h.
hookbar holder
hooked
      h. intramedullary nail
      h. knife
      h. medullary nail
Hookian region

NOTES

H

hook-rod
> Cotrel-Dubousset h.-r.
> Isola h.-r.
> TSRH h.-r.

hoop stress fracture
Hoover
> H. sign
> H. test

hop
> h. index
> h. test

Hopkins plaster knife
Hoppenfeld-Deboer
> H.-D. approach
> H.-D. technique

Hori technique
horizontal
> h. cleavage
> h. external rotation
> h. fracture
> h. gantry cut
> h. mattress suture
> h. meniscal tear
> h. osteotomy
> h. pedicle diameter
> h. plane
> h. position
> h. shoulder abduction exercise

hormone
> adrenocorticotropic h. (ACTH)
> growth h.
> human growth h. (hGH)
> sex h.
> thyrotropin-releasing h.

horn
> anterior h.
> bone graft shoe h.
> central h.
> cutaneous h.
> posterior h.

Horner syndrome
horse
> charley h.
> h.-hoof fracture nonunion

horseback
> h. rider's knee
> h. riding accident

horse's foot callus
horseshoe
> h. abscess
> h. appearance
> h. heel pad

horseshoe-shaped
> h.-s. felt pad
> h.-s. flap

Horsley
> H. bone cutter
> H. bone-cutting forceps

> H. bone saw
> H. bone wax

Horsley-Stille
> H.-S. bone-cutting forceps
> H.-S. rib shears forceps

Horwitz
> H. ankle arthrodesis
> H. ankle fusion
> H. transmalleolar arthrodesis

Horwitz-Adams
> H.-A. ankle fusion
> H.-A. arthrodesis

HOS
> human osteogenic sarcoma

hose
> TED h.
> Venosan support h.

hosiery
Hosmer
> H. above knee rotator
> H. Dorrance hook
> H. single axis friction knee
> H. single axis locking knee
> H. VC four-bar knee orthosis
> H. WALK prosthesis
> H. weight activated locking knee

Hosmer-Dorrance voluntary control four-bar knee mechanism
Hospital
> H. for Special Surgery knee score
> H. for Special Surgery scale
> Texas Scottish Rite H. (TSRH)
> H. Trauma Index

host-allograft junction
host tolerance
hot
> h. dog technique
> h. fomentation therapy
> h. knife
> h. pack (HP)
> h. plate
> h. water bath
> h. weld

hot-cross-bun
> h.-c.-b. skull
> h.-c.-b. skull sign

Hot/Ice
> H./I. System III
> H./I. System III knee blanket

Houghton-Akroyd
> H.-A. fracture technique
> H.-A. open reduction

Houle test
hourglass
> h. constriction
> h. deformity

House-Dieter malleus nipper
housemaid's knee

Housepan clip-applying forceps
House reconstruction
Houston
    H. halo cervical support
    H. halo cervical traction
Hovanian
    H. latissimus dorsi muscle transfer
    H. procedure
    H. transfer technique
Howard
    H. bone block
    H. technique
Howmedica
    H. cement
    H. cerclage
    H. Duracon implant
    H. ICS screw
    H. Kinematic II knee prosthesis
    H. knee instrumentation
    H. knee system
    H. Microfixation System drill bit
    H. Microfixation System forceps
    H. Microfixation Sytem plate cutter
    H. monotube
    H. monotube external rotator
    H. total ankle system
    H. Vitallium staple
Howorth
    H. approach
    H. procedure
    H. prosthesis
Howorth-Keillor procedure
Howse-Coventry prosthesis
Howse total hip replacement
Howship lacuna
Hoyer
    H. lift
    H. traction
H-P
    Hilgenreiner-Perkins
    H-P line
HP
    hot pack
    Vicodin HP
HPA
    hypothalamic-pituitary-adrenal
H.P. Acthar Gel
HPC-device
HPN
    herniated nucleus pulposus
HPS II total hip prosthesis

HR
    heart rate
H-reflex
HS
    Haynes-Stellite
H.S.
    Estratest H.S.
H-shaped
    H-s. capsular incision
    H-s. graft
    H-s. plate
HSMN III
    hereditary sensory motor neuropathy,
      type III
HSS total condylar knee prosthesis
Hsu-Hsu percutaneous tendo calcaneus
  lengthening
HT
    hammertoe
    Hubbard tank
5-HT
    serotonin
HTO
    high tibial osteotomy
    HTO fixator
Hubbard
    H. bolt
    H. physical therapy tank
    H. plate
    H. tank (HT)
Hubbard-Nylok bolt
hubbed needle
Huber
    H. abductor digiti quinti transfer
    H. adductor digiti quinti
      opponensplasty
    H. transfer of abductor digiti
      quinti
Hubscher maneuver
Huckstep nail
huck towel
Hudson
    H. bone drill
    H. brace with bur
    H. chuck adapter
    H. forceps
    H. Hydrofloat Cushion
    H. TLSO brace
Hudson-Jones knee-cage brace
Hueter
    H. bandage

NOTES

H

Hueter (continued)
    H. line
    H. sign
Hughston
    H. classification
    H. external rotation recurvatum test
    H. knee evaluation
    H. knee jerk test
    H. knee score
    H. plica test
    H. posterolateral drawer test
    H. posteromedial drawer test
    H. procedure
    H. realignment
    H. view
Hughston-Degenhardt reconstruction
Hughston-Hauser procedure
Hughston-Jacobson
    H.-J. lateral compartment
      reconstruction
    H.-J. technique
Hughston-Losee jerk test
Hugh Young pedicle clamp
Hui-Linscheid procedure
human
    h. bite infection
    h. growth hormone (hGH)
    h. immunodeficiency virus (HIV)
    h. leukocyte antigen (HLA)
    h. lymphocyte antigen (HLA)
    h. osteogenic sarcoma (HOS)
Humby knife
humeral
    h. avulsion of the glenohumeral
      ligament (HAGL)
    h. canal
    h. circumflex vessel
    h. component
    h. condyle
    h. cutting guide
    h. epicondyle
    h. epiphysis
    h. fracture abduction splint
    h. fracture malunion
    h. head
    h. head retractor
    h. head-splitting fracture
    h. impactor
    h. neck
    h. physeal fracture
    h. reamer
    h. saw
    h. shaft fracture
    h. supracondylar fracture
    h.-ulnar angle
humeri (pl. of humerus)
humeroperoneal muscular dystrophy
humeroradial articulation

humerothoracic abduction
humeroulnar
    h. articulation
    h. joint
humerus, pl. **humeri**
    articulatio humeri
    distal h.
    Holstein fracture of h.
    periarthrosis humeri
    proximal h.
humoral immunity
hump
    buffalo h.
    dowager's h.
humpback deformity
humpbacked spinal curvature
Humphrey
    ligament of H.
hunchback
Hungerford-Krackow-Kenna knee arthroplasty
Hungerford technique
hung-up knee jerk
Hunter
    H. canal
    H. open cord tendon implant
    H. Silastic prosthesis
    H. Silastic rod
    H. syndrome
    H. tendon prosthesis
Hunter-Boyes II
hunting reaction
Huntington
    H. bone graft
    H. chorea
    H. sign
    H. tibial technique
Hurd bone-cutting forceps
Hurler syndrome
Hutchinson
    H. fracture
    H. freckle
    melanotic Whitlow of H.
    H. teeth
HV
    HV NightSplint splint
    HV SoftSplint splint
HVA
    hallux valgus angle
HVO splint
HVPGS
    high-voltage pulse galvanic stimulation
HVT
    high-voltage therapy
hx
    history
Hyalgan
hyaline cartilage

hyalinization
hyaluronate
    sodium h.
hyaluronidase
hybrid
    h. external fixator
    h. fixation of hip replacement
      component
    h. total hip replacement
HybridFit
    H. total hip system
    H. total knee system
Hycort
Hydra-Cadence
    H.-C. gait-control unit
    H.-C. knee prosthesis
Hydragrip clamp insert
hydrate
    chloral h.
hydraulic
    h. knee unit
    h. knee unit prosthesis
    h. test system
Hydrisinol
    H. creme
    H. lotion
hydrocephalus
Hydrocet
hydrochloride (HCl)
    alfentanil h.
    naloxone h.
    oxycodone h.
    oxymorphone h.
    pentazocine h.
    phencyclidine h. (PCP)
    propoxyphene h.
    tramadol h.
hydrocodone
    h. and acetaminophen
    h. and aspirin
    h. bitartrate and ibuprofen
    h. and ibuprofen
Hydrocol
    H. dressing
    H. wound dressing
hydrocollator
    CMO h.
    H. heating unit
    H. pad
    H. steam pack
hydrocolloid
    h. occlusive dressing

Hydrocort
hydrocortisone
    bacitracin, neomycin, polymyxin B,
      and h.
    neomycin and h.
    neomycin, polymyxin B, and h.
    h. phonophoresis
Hydrocortone
    H. Acetate
    H. Phosphate
hydro cushion
hydrofloat cushion
Hydrogel
    Lido-Gel topical anesthetic H.
    H. wound dressing
hydrogen
    h. peroxide
    h. washout method
Hydrogesic
hydrolyze disc content
hydromassage table
hydromelia
hydromorphone
Hydron Burn Bandage
hydrops canal
Hydro Soothe recliner
Hydro-Splint II
hydrostatic pressure
HydroStat IR
hydrosyringomyelia
    communicating h.
hydrotherapy
    AquaMED dry h.
    dry h.
Hydro-Tone Bell
Hydrotrack underwater treadmill
Hydroxial hip prosthesis
hydroxyapatite (HA)
    h. adhesive
    APS h.
    h. bone
    h. bone replacement material
    calcium h.
    coralline h.
    h. deposition disease
    h. implant material
    LLPS h.
hydroxyapatite-coated stem
hydroxychloroquine
25-hydroxyvitamin D
hydroxyzine

NOTES

H

hygroma
    cystic h.
Hylamer
    H. acetabular liner
    H. orthopaedic bearing polymer
Hyland's Leg Cramps with Quinine
Hylin rasp
hyoid bone
HypaFix wound dressing
hypalgesia
Hypaque contrast media
hyperabduction
    h. maneuver
    h. syndrome test
hyperactive
    h. reflex
    h. response
hyperactivity
    physiological h.
hyperalgesia
hyperalimentation
hyperbaric
    h. oxygen (HBO)
    h. oxygen therapy
hypercalcemia
hypercortisolism
hyperdynamic abductor hallucis
hyperemia
hyperemic
hyperesthesia
hyperesthetic
hyperextend
hyperextended knee gait
hyperextensibility of joint
hyperextension
    h. brace
    h. cast
    cruciform anterior spinal h.
     (CASH)
    h. deformity
    h. injury
    intraoperative neck h.
    rebound h.
    recurrent h.
    segmental h.
    h. stress
    h. test
    h. trauma
Hyperex thoracic orthosis
hyperflexion
    h. fracture
    h. injury
    h. trauma
hypergammaglobulinemia
    polyclonal h.
hyperhidrosis, hyperidrosis
hyperkeratosis, pl. hyperkeratoses

hyperkeratotic lesion
hyperkyphoscoliosis
    neuropathic h.
hyperkyphosis
hyperlordosis
hypermobile
    h. flatfoot
    h. foot
    h. joint
hypermobility
    compensatory h.
    joint h.
hypernephroma
hyperosteoidosis
hyperostosis
    ankylosing spinal h.
    Caffey h.
    diffuse idiopathic sclerosing h.
     (DISH)
    diffuse idiopathic skeletal h.
     (DISH)
    infantile cortical h.
    h. syndrome
    h. triangularis ilii
hyperostotic bony fusion
hyperparathyroidism
    brown tumor of h.
    h. tumor
hyperplantarflexion injury
hyperplasia
    epiphyseal h.
hyperplastic
hyperpolarization
hyperpronation
hyperpyrexia
    malignant h.
hyperreflexia
hypertension
    calf h.
hyperthermia
    malignant h.
hyperthermic
hypertonia
hypertonicity
hypertonus
hypertrophic
    h. chondrocyte
    h. exostosis
    h. granulation tissue
    h. ligament
    h. synovitis
    h. vital nonunion
hypertrophy
    cartilage h.
    cartilaginous h.
    ligamentous-muscular h.
    uncinate h.

hypervascular
  h. fragment
  h. nonunion
hypesthesia, hypoesthesia
Hy-Phen
hypnoanalgesia
hypnoanesthesia
hypnopedia
hypnoplasty
hypnosis
hypnotherapy
hypnotic
  h. amnesia
  h. displacement
  h. dissociation
  h. reinterpretation
  h. replacement
  h. time disorientation
hypoactive deep tendon reflex
hypoaldosteronism
  hyporeninemic h.
Hypobaric
  H. micro-valve
  H. transfemoral system
  H. transtibial system
hypochondriac region
hypochondriasis
hypocycloidal ankle tomography
hypodermic
  per h. (H)
hypoesthesia (*var. of* hypesthesia)
hypofibrinolysis
hypogastric
  h. artery
  h. flap
hypoglossal nerve
hypoglycemia
hypokinetic aberration
hypokyphosis
  right thoracic curve with h.
  thoracic h.
hypolordosis
  cervical h.
hypomobile
hypomobility
hyponychium
hypoparathyroidism

hypophalangism
  pedal h.
hypophosphatasia
hypophosphatemic bone disease
hypophysial curette
hypoplasia
  cartilage-hair h.
  phalangeal h.
  skeletal h.
hypoplastic
  h. disk space
  h. finger
  h. first rib
  h. hand
  h. thumb
hyporeninemic hypoaldosteronism
hypotension
hypotensive
  h. anesthesia
  h. surgery
hypothalamic-pituitary-adrenal (HPA)
  h.-p.-a. axis
hypothalamoneurohypophyseal axis (HNA)
hypothenar
  h. eminence
  h. fascia
  h. hammer syndrome
  h. muscle
hypothermic
hypothyroidism
hypotonia
  congenital h.
hypotonus
hypotrophic arthritis
hypovitaminosis
hypovolemic shock
hypoxemia
hypoxia
hysteresis
hysterical
  h. gait
  h. scoliosis
Hytakerol
Hyzine-50
Hz
  hertz

NOTES

H

IADL
    instrumental activities of daily living
Iamin hydrating gel
iatrogenic
    i. dural tear
    i. elevatus
    i. injury
    i. lumbar kyphosis
    i. osteomyelitis
IB
    Dynafed IB
    Midol IB
    Motrin IB
    Sine-Aid IB
I-beam
    I-b. cement punch
    I-b. hemiarthroplasty hip prosthesis
    I-b. hip hemiarthroplasty
    I-b. hip operation
    Jergesen I-b.
IBF
    Insall-Burstein-Freeman
    IBF knee instrument
IBM
    inclusion body myositis
IBU
    ibuprofen
Ibuprin
ibuprofen (IBU)
    hydrocodone and i.
    hydrocodone bitartrate and i.
    pseudoephedrine and i.
Ibuprohm
ICC
    interclass correlation coefficient
ice
    i. application
    i. massage
    N'ice Stretch night splint
      suspension system with Sealed I.
    i. pack
    i. skater's fracture
    I. Wedge hot/cold therapy wrap
Icecross silicone socket
I.C.E. Down cold pack
ICE-Magic pain reduction kit
Iceross
    I. Comfort Plus silicone gel liner
ICEROSS sleeve
ICEX socket
ICIDH
    International Classification of
    Impairments, Disabilities, Handicaps
ICLH
    ICLH ankle prosthesis

    ICLH double cup arthroplasty
    ICLH knee prosthesis
ICN
    inferior calcaneonavicular ligament
ICS
    inferior capsular shift
    intercostal space
ICT
    intermittent cervical traction
I&D
    incision and drainage
    irrigation and debridement
IDCN
    intermediate dorsal cutaneous nerve
IDDM
    insulin-dependent diabetes mellitus
Ideal spinal implant
Ideberg glenoid fracture classification
Identifit hip prosthesis
idiopathic
    i. avascular necrosis
    i. fracture
    i. genu valgum (IGV)
    i. hallux valgus
    i. juvenile osteoporosis
    i. osteonecrosis
    i. polymyositis myopathy
    i. scoliosis
    i. skeletal
    i. skeletal hyperostosis syndrome
    i. transient osteoporosis
idiopathica
    osteopsathyrosis i.
IDK
    internal derangement of the knee
id reaction
IGF
    insulin-like growth factor
IGF-binding protein
IGHL
    inferior glenohumeral ligament
    IGHL insertion
igne
    erythema ab i.
IGV
    idiopathic genu valgum
IHS
    International Headache Society
IHW
    inner heel wedge
IKDC
    International Knee Documentation
      Committee
    IKDC form
    IKDC score

I

Ikuta
  I. clamp approximator
  I. fixation device
  I. pectoralis major transfer
ileus
  bladder i.
  intestinal i.
  paralytic i.
Ilex
  Biofreeze with I.
Ilfeld
  I. brace
  I. splint
  I. splint orthosis
Ilfeld-Gustafson splint
iliac
  i. apophysis
  i. apophysis sign
  i. apophysitis
  i. artery
  i. artery injury
  i. buttressing procedure
  i. clamp
  i. compression test
  i. crest
  i. crest bone free graft
  i. crest bone graft stabilization
  i. crest bridge
  i. crest-inlay graft
  i. crest ossification
  i. epiphysis
  i. fixation
  i. oblique view
  i. osteocutaneous flap
  i. osteotomy
  i. post
  i. screw
  i. slot graft
  i. spine
  i. strut bone graft
  i. vein
  i. wing
  i. wing resection
iliacus muscle
ilial
ilii
  hyperostosis triangularis i.
iliococcygeus muscle
iliocostalis lumborum syndrome
iliocostal muscle
iliofemoral
  i. approach
  i. flap artery
  i. ligament
  i. pedicle flap
  i. thrombosis
iliofemorale
  ligamentum i.

iliohypogastric nerve
ilioinguinal
  i. acetabular approach
  i. nerve
  i. syndrome
iliolumbale
  ligamentum i.
iliolumbar
  i. artery
  i. ligament
  i. vein
iliopatellar
  i. band
  i. ligament
iliopsoas
  i. bursitis
  i. muscle
  i. muscle hematoma
  i. recession
  i. tendon
  i. test
  i. transfer
iliosacral
  i. and iliac fixation construct
  i. screw
iliotibial (IT)
  i. band (ITB)
  i. band fasciitis
  i. band friction syndrome
  i. band graft
  i. band graft augmentation
  i. band tenodesis
  i. band transfer
  i. tract
ilium
  AS i.
  ASEx i.
  ASIn i.
  i. drainage
  external i. (EI)
  In-Ex i.
  PIEx i.
  PIIn i.
  piriform sclerosis i.
  wing of i.
Ilizarov
  I. ankle arthrodesis
  I. apparatus
  I. circular external fixator
  I. corticotomy
  I. device
  I. distractor
  I. external fixation
  I. external ring fixator
  I. frame
  I. hybrid fixator
  I. leg lengthening
  I. limb lengthening

I. limb-lengthening system
I. limb-lengthening technique
I. method
I. ring
I. screw
I. wire

ILL
inequality in length of legs
illness
I. Behavior Questionnaire
I. Depression Questionnaire
environmental i.
illuminator
Cogent XL i.
IM
intermetatarsal
intermetatarsal angle
intermuscular
intramedullary
intramuscular
IM joint
IMA
intermetatarsal angle
image
axial multiplanar gradient
refocused i.
axial multiplanar gradient refocused
magnetic resonance i.
i. control
i. en Grelot
field-echo i.
i. intensification
i. intensifier
multiplanar gradient recall i.
sagittal T1-weighted spin-echo i.
spin-echo i.
transaxial gradient recalled i.
transaxial spoiled gradient
recalled i.
T1-weighted i.
T2-weighted i.
Xi-scan i.
Image-I analysis software
imaging
cine-magnetic resonance i. (cine-
MRI)
color duplex i.
contrast medium-enhanced magnetic
resonance i. (CME-MRI)
delayed bone i.
diagnostic i.
dipyridamole thallium i.

dynamic magnetic resonance i.
fixation i.
gadopentetate-dimeglumine-enhanced
magnetic resonance i.
gamma camera i.
magnetic resonance i. (MRI)
magnetic source i. (MSI)
multiple line-scan i. (MLSI)
radionucleotide i.
sagittal-plane i.
Tc 99m sestamibi myocardial
perfusion i.
imbalance
isokinetic torque i.
muscle i.
imbricate
imbrication
capsular i.
MacNab line for facet i.
medial i.
medial capsular i.
medialis obliquus i.
IMEX scleral implant
imipenem and cilastatin
imipramine
IML
intermetacarpal ligament
immediate
i. postoperative prosthesis (IPOP)
i. postoperative prosthesis dressing
i. postsurgical fitting (IPSF)
immersion
immitis
Coccidioides i.
immobilization
cast i.
i. degeneration
external i.
halo i.
i. jacket
joint i.
i. method
postoperative i.
Rowe-Zarins shoulder i.
sling i.
sternal-occipital-mandibular i.
(SOMI)
Velcro i.
Webril i.
immobilize
immobilizer
ankle i.

NOTES

immobilizer *(continued)*
    Comfort wrist i.
    Ezy Wrap shoulder i.
    Hook hemi-harness shoulder i.
    knee i.
    long leg i.
    OEC knee i.
    Plastizote-Kydex cervical i.
    QuickCast wrist i.
    Raymond shoulder i.
    sateen knee i.
    shoulder i.
    shoulder abduction i.
    sternooccipitomanubrial i.
    Tab-Strap knee i.
    Trimline knee i.
    Velcro i.
    Velpeau shoulder i.
    Watco knee i.
    Westfield acromioclavicular i.
    Y-strap knee i.
    Zimmer knee i.
    Zinco thumb-wrist i.
immobilizing bandage
immovable joint
immune
    i. globulin
    i. system
immunity
    cell-mediated i.
    humoral i.
immunocompetence
immunogenicity
immunoglobulin
Immunomount
immunotherapy
IMN
    intramedullary nailing
IMP
    Innovative Medical Products
    IMP bone screw targeter
    IMP knee positioning triangle
    IMP Steri-Clamp
    IMP surgical leg pedestal
    IMP turnstile casting stand
    IMP Universal knee positioner
    IMP Universal lateral positioner
impact
    i. biomechanics
    i. glove
    i. mitt
    I. modular porous prosthesis
    I. modular total hip system
impacted
    i. articular fracture
    i. fracture

impaction
    atlantoaxial i.
    digital i.
impactor
    Austin Moore i.
    bone i.
    Cloward bone graft i.
    Cohort spinal i.
    Dawson-Yuhl i.
    femoral i.
    glenoid implant base i.
    hook i.
    humeral i.
    Küntscher i.
    Moe bone i.
    mushroom i.
    orthopaedic i.
    i. rod
    shell i.
    Smith-Petersen i.
    vertebral body i.
impactor-extractor
    Fox i.-e.
impairment
    neurovascular i.
    physical i.
    sensory i.
IMP-Capello slimline abduction pillow
impedance
    bioelectrical i.
    i. plethysmography
imperfecta
    dentinogenesis i.
    osteogenesis i. (OI)
impinge
impingement
    anterior ankle i.
    anterior cord i.
    anterior soft tissue i.
    i. exostosis
    facet synovial i.
    I.-Free Tibial Guide System
    graft i.
    lateral i.
    i. pain
    i. rod
    roof i.
    i. sign
    i. syndrome
    i. test
    tibiotalar i.
    ulnocarpal i.
implant
    i. alloy aluminum
    AO-ASIF orthopaedic i.
    i. arthroplasty
    articulated chin i.
    artificial joint i.

Bannon-Klein i.
bicompartmental i.
Bicoral i.
i. biocompatibility
Biodel i.
Biofix biodegradable i.
Biomet custom i.
BioSphere suture anchor i.
i. blank
bone i.
bovine collagen i.
Calnan-Nicolle finger i.
carbon i.
cartilage i.
Cartwright i.
i.-cement interface
ceramic i.
Charnley i.
chromium i.
chromium-cobalt-alloy i.
CKS i.
    Continuum knee system implant
coated i.
cobalt i.
cobalt-chromium i.
i. collar
condylar i.
Continuum knee system i. (CKS
    implant)
Corail HA-coated stem hip i.
CUI dorsal i.
CUI malar i.
curvilinear chin i.
Custodis i.
custom i.
Cutter i.
DePuy orthopaedic i.
dorsal columella i.
dorsal column stimulator i.
double-stem i.
DTT i.
Duracon knee i.
Durallium i.
Durapatite i.
DynaGraft i.
electrical i.
Ewald-Walker knee i.
i. failure
i. fatigue
fibrous tissue i.
fin of the i.
finger joint i.

fixed bearing knee i.
flail i.
Flatt i.
flexible digital i.
flexible hinge i.
i. forceps
i. fracture
gentamicin i.
Gliadel i.
Global total shoulder i.
great toe i.
HA-coated hip i.
Harris Design-2 i.
hemi-interpositional i.
Hemi-Silastic i.
HIHA tendon i.
i. hinge
hinged i.
Howmedica Duracon i.
Hunter open cord tendon i.
Ideal spinal i.
IMEX scleral i.
Insall-Burstein intracondylar knee i.
Insall-Burstein total knee i.
Interpore i.
joint i.
Koenig total great toe i.
LaPorte great toe i.
Lawrence first metatarsophalangeal
    joint i.
LCS i.
Low-Contact Stress i.
i. material
McCutchen hip i.
metacarpophalangeal i.
i. metal
metal-backed acetabular component
    hip i.
metal-backed patellar i.
metal hemi-toe i.
metallic i.
metal orthopaedic i.
methyl methacrylate beads i.
Microloc knee i.
Miragel i.
mobile bearing knee i.
modular i.
Neer II total shoulder system i.
NexGen knee i.
Nexus i.
Niebauer i.
Niebauer-Cutter i.

NOTES

implant *(continued)*
    orthotic attachment i.
    OsteoGen resorbable osteogenic bone-filling i.
    Osteonics HA femoral i.
    Partnership i.
    patellar resurfacing i.
    pectoralis muscle i.
    pedicle i.
    percutaneous dorsal column stimulator i.
    permanent i.
    pin i.
    plastic ball i.
    PLLA i.
    PMMA i.
    polyglycolide i.
    polylactide i.
    polymethyl methacrylate i.
    processed carbon i.
    ProOsteon I. 500
    i. reaction
    i. removal
    Scottish Rite Hospital spinal i.
    Seeburger i.
    Septacin i.
    Sgarlato toe i.
    Ship hammertoe i.
    SHIP-Shaw rod hammertoe i.
    Silastic finger i.
    Silastic toe i.
    silicone breast i.
    silicone elastomer rubber ball i.
    silicone MP i.
    single-stemmed toe i.
    Sinterlock i.
    Smart Screw bioabsorbable i.
    i. stage
    i. stem
    supraspinatus i.
    Surgibone i.
    Surgicel i.
    i. survival rate
    Sutter i.
    Swanson carpal lunate i.
    Swanson carpal scaphoid i.
    Swanson finger joint i.
    Swanson great toe i.
    Swanson metacarpophalangeal i.
    Swanson radial head i.
    Swanson radiocarpal i.
    Swanson small joint i.
    Swanson trapezium i.
    Swanson ulnar head i.
    Swanson wrist joint i.
    Swiss MP joint i.
    Syed-Neblett i.
    Syed template i.

    Techmedica i.
    TheraSeed i.
    titanium i.
    titanium-alloy i.
    tobramycin-impregnated PMMA i.
    toe i.
    trial i.
    tricompartmental i.
    TSRH i.
    unicompartmental knee i.
    Unilab Surgibone surgical i.
    Vitallium i.
    Weber hip i.
    Weil i.
    Weil-modified Swanson i.
    Zang metatarsal cap i.
    Zeichner i.
    Zymderm collagen i.

implantation
    collared Press-Fit femoral stem i.
    noncollared Press-Fit femoral stem i.
    screw i.

implanted bone growth stimulator

Implast
    I. adhesive
    I. bone cement

impression
    basilar i.
    i. defect
    i. fracture

imprinter
    foot i.

impulse
    afferent nerve i.
    i.-based nerve transmission
    efferent nerve i.
    i. inertial exercise trainer
    mobilization with i.
    venous i.

IMSC
    intramedullary supracondylar
    IMSC five-hole nail
    IMSC multihole nail

Imuran

ImuranAgent

In
    internal

in
    4-i.-1 positioning block system
    i. situ arthrodesis
    i. situ spine fusion
    i. situ vein graft
    i. vivo study

inactivity
    electrical i.

InCare brace

incarnatus
    unguis i.
Incavo wire passer
incidence
    myelopathy i.
    nonunion i.
incise drape
incised wound
incision
    abdominal i.
    anteromedial i.
    Banks-Laufman i.
    battledore i.
    bifrontal i.
    bikini skin i.
    Brockman i.
    Bruner i.
    Brunner modified i.
    Brunner palmar i.
    Bruser skin i.
    Burns-Haney i.
    Burwell-Scott modification of
      Watson-Jones i.
    capsular i.
    Chang-Miltner i.
    Charnley i.
    chevron i.
    Cincinnati i.
    circumscribing i.
    Colonna-Ralston i.
    coronal i.
    coronal scalp i.
    Couvelaire i.
    Crawford i.
    Cubbins i.
    Curtin i.
    curved i.
    curvilinear i.
    deltoid-splitting i.
    i. dilator
    dorsal linear i.
    dorsal longitudinal i.
    dorsal transverse i.
    dorsomedial i.
    double i.
    i. and drainage (I&D)
    DuVries i.
    Dwyer i.
    elliptical i.
    exploratory i.
    fascia-splitting i.
    fiber-splitting i.

    fishmouth i.
    Fowler-Philip i.
    Gaenslen split-heel i.
    Gatellier-Chastang i.
    Gedda-Moberg i.
    goblet i.
    Grice i.
    Griffith i.
    Henderson skin i.
    Henry i.
    hockey-stick i.
    H-shaped capsular i.
    inverted-Y i.
    Jergesen i.
    J-shaped skin i.
    Kocher collar i.
    Koenig-Schaefer i.
    lateral utility i.
    lazy-C i.
    lazy-S i.
    L-curved i.
    Leslie-Ryan modified axillary i.
    Loeffler-Ballard i.
    longitudinal i.
    L-shaped capsular i.
    Ludloff i.
    Mayfield i.
    McLaughlin-Ryder i.
    medial parapatellar i.
    median parapatellar i.
    midaxillary line i.
    midline oblique i.
    Moberg-Gedda i.
    muscle-splitting i.
    Nicola i.
    Ober i.
    oblique i.
    Ollier i.
    palmar i.
    paramedial i.
    parapatellar i.
    parathenar i.
    Picot i.
    plantar longitudinal i.
    posterior i.
    posterolateral costotransversectomy i.
    Pridie i.
    racquet-shaped i.
    relaxing i.
    relieving i.
    right-sided submandibular
      transverse i.

NOTES

incision *(continued)*
    S i.
    saber-cut i.
    serpentine i.
    S-flap i.
    skin i.
    skived i.
    split i.
    split-heel i.
    S-shaped i.
    stab i.
    standard retroperitoneal flank i.
    straight i.
    subfascial i.
    Sutherland-Rowe i.
    tangential i.
    "Texas T" i.
    thoracoabdominal i.
    transverse i.
    T-shaped i.
    universal i.
    upright-Y i.
    U-shaped i.
    vertical midline i.
    volar midline oblique i.
    volar zigzag finger i.
    V-shaped i.
    Wagner skin i.
    Watson-Jones i.
    webspace i.
    Westin-Hall i.
    Y i.
    Y-shaped i.
    Y-V-plasty i.
    zigzag finger i.
    Z-plasty i.
incisional
    i. biopsy
    i. neuroma
Incisor arthroscopic blade
incisura fibularis
Inclan
    I. bone graft
    I. modification of Campbell ankle
      operation
    I. modification of Campbell ankle
      procedure
    I. posterior bone block
Inclan-Ober procedure
inclination
    i. angle
    angle of thoracic i.
inclinaton
    sacral i.
inclinometer
inclusion
    i. body myositis (IBM)
    i. cyst

incomplete
    i. amputation
    i. coalition
    i. dislocation
    i. fracture
    i. luxation
    i. paraplegia
    i. reduction
    i. syndactyly
    i. tear
incongruity
    angle of i.
incontinence
    urinary i.
incorporation
    bone graft i.
increased
    i. carrying angle
    i. depolymerization
    i. insertional activity
    i. lateral joint space
increment after exercise
incremental response
incrementing response
incubation period
incurvated
incurvatum reflex
independent
    i. exercise program
    i. transfer
Inderal
index, pl. **indices**
    acetabular i.
    acromial spur i. (ASI)
    ADL indices
    indices of ADLs
    alignment i.
    ankle-arm blood pressure i.
    ankle-arm ischemic i.
    ankle-brachial i. (ABI)
    ankle-brachial blood pressure i.
    arch i.
    Arthritis Helplessness I. (AHI)
    Barthel ADL i.
    Benink tarsal i.
    body mass i. (BMI)
    Caregiver Strain I. (CSI)
    Chippaux-Smirak arch i.
    Convery polyarticular disability i.
    cortical i.
    creatine:height i.
    cyst i.
    Eyre-Brook epiphyseal i.
    Facial Disability I. (FDI)
    i. finger (2nd digit)
    i. finger abduction
    Fourier pulsatility i.
    Functional Status I. (FSI)

Garden alignment i.
Hauser ambulation i.
hop i.
Hospital Trauma I.
Insall-Salvati patellar height i.
ischemic i.
Jette Functional Status i.
Katz ADL i.
Keitel i.
Kenny ADL i.
I. Knobber II massage tool
Life Satisfaction I. (LSI)
Lucas and Drucker Motor I.
McDowell Impairment I. (MII)
McMurtry kinematic i.
i. metacarpophalangeal joint
  reconstruction
Motricity I.
Northwick Park Index of
  Independence in ADL i.
notch width i. (NWI)
Nottingham Extended ADL i.
Oswestry i.
PICA i.
pipe stemming of ankle-brachial i.
poststress ankle-arm Doppler i.
Quetelet i.
i.-ray amputation
Reimers hip position migration i.
Reimers instability i.
Reintegration to Normal Living i.
resting ankle-arm Doppler i.
Ritchie i.
Rivermead ADL i.
Rivermead Mobility I. (RMI)
sciatic function i. (SFI)
Singh osteoporosis i.
Spinal Cord Motor Index and
  Sensory Indices
Takakura i.
talocalcaneal i.
Waddell Chronic Back Pain
  Disability i.
Western Ontario and McMaster
  University osteoarthritis i.
Zung Depression I.
Indiana
  I. conservative prosthesis
  I. reamer
  I. tome carpal tunnel syndrome
    release system
indifferent electrode

indirect
  i. fracture
  i. hypnotic suggestion
  i. manipulation
  i. reduction
  i. triangulation
indium-111
  i.-labelled leukocyte bone scanning
  i. scintigraphy
Indochron E-R
Indocin
  I. I.V.
  I. SR
indoleacetic acid
indomethacin
Indong Oh hip prosthesis
indoprofen
induction
  pain i.
indurated plantar keratoma (IPK)
induration
industrial
  i. physical therapist (IPT)
  I. Work brace
inelastic
inequality
  anatomic leg length i.
  functional leg length i.
  leg length i. (LLI)
  i. in length of legs (ILL)
Inerpan flexible burn dressing
inertia
  moment of i.
In-Ex ilium
inextensibility
inf
  inferior
infancy
  hereditary neuropathy of i.
infant
  i. abduction splint
  i. clown cast shoe
  I.'s Feverall
  floppy i.
  Movement Assessment of I.'s
    (MAI)
  premature i.
  very low birth weight i.
infantile
  i. cortical hyperostosis
  i. dermal fibromatosis
  i. idiopathic scoliosis

NOTES

infantile *(continued)*
    i. spinal muscular atrophy
    i. tibia vara (ITV)
    i. trigger digit
Infants' Silapap
infarct
    bone i.
infarction
    bone i.
    myocardial i.
infected
    i. bone
    i. nondraining nonunion
infection
    aerobic i.
    anaerobic i.
    aspergillosis i.
    blood-borne i.
    bone i.
    clostridial i.
    coccidioidomycosis i.
    cryptococcal i.
    deep delayed i.
    deep wound i.
    epidural space i.
    fascial space i.
    felon i.
    fungal i.
    gas-producing streptococcal i.
    genitourinary i.
    granulomatous fungal i.
    hand i.
    hematogenous i.
    herpetic i.
    human bite i.
    Meleney i.
    musculoskeletal i.
    mycobacterial i.
    mycotic i.
    nontuberculous mycobacterial i.
    percutaneous bone marrow i.
    pin tract i.
    postoperative i.
    i. prevention
    Pseudomonas i.
    pyogenic spinal i.
    spinal i.
    superficial i.
    suppurative joint i.
    tarsal joint i.
    unusual i.
    web space i.
infectious arthritis
infera
    patella i.
inferential therapy
inferior (inf)
    i. angle

    i. band cruciform ligament
    i. calcaneonavicular ligament (ICN)
    i. capsular shift (ICS)
    i. extensor of foot
    i. facet
    i. glenohumeral ligament (IGHL)
    i. glenohumeral ligament insertion
    i. glide
    i. ilioischial ligament
    i. laryngeal nerve
    i. leaf
    i. movement
    i. peroneal retinaculum
    i. process
    i. spurring
    i. thyroid artery
    i. TV ligament of scapula
    i. vena cava
    i. vertebra
inferius
    ligamentum transversum scapulae i.
InFerno moist heat therapy
INFH
    ischemic necrosis of femoral head
infiltrate
    fibrofatty i.
infiltration
    root i.
Infinity
    I. femoral component
    I. hip system
    I. modular hip prosthesis
inflame
inflamed synovial pouch
inflammation
    bursal i.
    polyarticular symmetric tophaceous
     joint i.
    prepatellar bursa i.
    tendon i.
inflammatory
    i. arthropathy
    i. fracture
    i. myositis
    i. phase
    i. tenovaginitis
inflatable elbow splint
inflexion point
inflow
    i. cannula
    vascular i.
influenzae
    Haemophilus i.
information
    ballistic i.
infracalcaneal bursitis
infraclavicular triangle

I

infraction
    i. fracture
    Freiberg i.
infraganglionic injury
infragluteal
    i. creaking
    i. crease
infraisthmal
infrapatellar
    i. bursitis
    i. contracture syndrome (IPCS)
    i. fat pad
    i. ligament
    i. plica
    i. tendinitis
    i. tendon
    i. tendon rupture
    i. view
infrapedicle
infrared
    i. applicator
    i. head
    i. light (IR)
    i. light-emitting diode
    i. therapy
    i. thermography
infraspinatus
    i. muscle
    i. tendinitis
    i. tendon
infraspinous fascia
Infumorph Injection
Infusible pressure infusion bag
Inge
    I. retractor
    I. spreader
Ingebrightsen traction
Inglis-Cooper
    I.-C. release
    I.-C. technique
Inglis-Pellicci elbow arthroplasty rating system
Inglis-Ranawat-Straub
    I.-R.-S. elbow synovectomy
    I.-R.-S. technique
Inglis triaxial total elbow arthroplasty
Ingram
    I. bony bridge resection
    I. osteotomy
    I. procedure
Ingram-Bachynski
    I.-B. hip fracture classification

Ingram-Canle-Beaty epiphyseal-metaphyseal osteotomy
Ingram-Withers-Speltz motor test
ingrown toenail
ingrowth
    bone i.
    i. fixation
inguinal
    i. approach
    i. hernia
    i. ligament
    i. ligament syndrome
    i. TEPP repair
inguinale
    ligamentum i.
inhalant anesthesia
inhalation anesthesia
inherent motion
inheritable disease
inhibition test
inhibitive
    i. cast
    i. traction
inhibitor
    αa_2-plasmin i.
    shoulder subluxation i. (SSI)
inhibitory postsynaptic potential (IPSP)
inion bump
initiation
    rhythmic i. (RI)
initiator drill
injection
    Adlone I.
    alcohol i.
    Alfenta I.
    A-methaPred I.
    Articulose-50 I.
    Astramorph PF I.
    Ben-Allergin-50 I.
    Bicillin C-R 900/300 I.
    Black peroneal tendon sheath i.
    Calciferol I.
    Calcimar I.
    cervical nerve root i.
    chymopapain i.
    Cibacalcin I.
    Cipro I.
    corticosteroid i.
    cortisone i.
    Cytoxan I.
    depGynogen I.
    depMedalone I.

NOTES

injection *(continued)*
Depo-Estradiol i.
Depogen I.
Depoject I.
Depo-Medrol I.
Depopred I.
Dioval I.
D-Med I.
Duralone I.
Duramorph I.
epidural steroid i.
Estra-L I.
Estro-Cyp I.
facet i.
Gynogen L.A. I.
Infumorph I.
i. injury
intramuscular i.
Kefurox I.
Key-Pred I.
Key-Pred-SP I.
Lovenox I.
lumbar facet i.
lumbar nerve root i.
Medralone I.
Miacalcin I.
M-Prednisol I.
Nafcil I.
Nallpen I.
Neosar I.
nerve root i.
Novocain I.
Octocaine I.
Oncovin i.
Osteocalcin I.
peroneal bupivacaine i.
peroneal tendon sheath i.
Pontocaine With Dextrose I.
Predcor-TBA I.
Prednisol TBA I.
procaine-phenol motor point i.
Salmonine I.
Sandimmune I.
Seconal I.
Solu-Medrol I.
steroid I.
Sublimaze i.
Sufenta i.
i. technique
tenosynovial i.
thecal i.
Toposar I.
Toradol I.
trigger point i.
Unipen I.
VePesid I.
Vincasar PFS I.

Zinacef I.
zygapophyseal joint i.

injury
abdominal i.
acceleration/deceleration i.
accessory nerve i.
acquired brain i. (ABI)
acromioclavicular joint i.
acute stretch i.
i. algorithm
ankle i.
annular i.
athletic i.
avulsion i.
axial compression i.
axial loading i.
axillary nerve i.
ballistic i.
barked i.
bending toward the side of i.
bicycle i.
birth i.
bladder i.
brachial artery i.
brachial plexus i.
brachial plexus traction i. (BPTI)
brain i.
Brief Test of Head I. (BTHI)
burst i.
Callahan extension of cervical i.
cervical nerve root i.
cervical spinal i.
Chopart osseous joint i.
closed soft tissue i.
cocking i.
cold i.
compression-plus-torque theory of cervical i.
compressive flexion i.
compressive hyperextension i.
contrecoup i.
crush i.
cuneiform i.
Danis-Weber classification of ankle i.
dashboard i.
degloving i.
de Quervain i.
diffuse axonal i. (DAI)
discoligamentous i.
distal tibial epiphyseal i.
distraction i.
dye punch i.
elbow i.
electrical i.
epiphyseal i.
Essex-Lopresti i.
eversion i.

explosion i.
extension-type cervical spine i.
extensor tendon i.
extravasation i.
femoral vein i.
firearm i.
flexion-distraction i.
FOOSH i.
forced flexion i.
Foucher classification of
  epiphyseal i.
frostbite i.
gamekeeper's i.
grease gun i.
growth plate i.
Hardcastle classification of
  tarsometatarsal joint i.
head i.
hyperextension i.
hyperflexion i.
hyperplantarflexion i.
iatrogenic i.
iliac artery i.
infraganglionic i.
injection i.
interosseous nerve i.
inversion i.
Klumpke i.
knee ligamentous i.
laryngeal nerve i.
lateral compartment i.
lateral compression i.
lawn mower i.
ligamentous i.
Lisfranc i.
liver i.
long thoracic nerve i.
low back i.
lower plexus i.
lumbar plexus i.
lunate facet dye punch i.
MacKinnon nerve i.
matrix i.
medial brachial cutaneous nerve i.
medial compartment i.
median nerve i.
meniscal i.
metatarsophalangeal joint i.
midcarpal i.
middle column i.
missile i.
multiple i.

muscle-tendon i.
musculocutaneous nerve i.
nerve i.
neural i.
neurovascular i.
nuclear i.
obturator nerve i.
Ontario Cohort of Running-
  Related i.
open-book pelvic i.
osteochondral i.
overuse i.
paint gun i.
paint thinner i.
pelvic i.
P-ER i.
perihamate i.
peripheral nerve i.
peripisiform i.
peritrapezial i.
peritrapezoidal i.
peroneal nerve i.
physeal i.
pitching i.
plantarflexion i.
pleural i.
Poland classification of physeal i.
posterior ligamentous i.
i. potential
predictor of i.
pronation i.
pronation-abduction i.
pronation-eversion i.
pronation-eversion-external
  rotation i.
pseudogamekeeper's i.
pudendal nerve i.
Pugil stick i.
radial artery i.
radial nerve i.
radioulnar joint i.
recurrent laryngeal nerve i.
reperfusion i.
repetition strain i. (RSI)
Rockwood classification of
  acromioclavicular i.
roller i.
Rosenthal classification of nail i.
running-related i.
sacral plexus i.
sacroiliac joint i.

NOTES

injury *(continued)*
 Sage-Salvatore classification of acromioclavicular joint i.
 Salter-Harris epiphyseal i.
 Salter-Harris tibial-fibular i.
 sand toe i.
 Scales of Cognitive Ability for Traumatic Brain I. (SCATBI)
 scaphoid tuberosity i.
 scapuloclavicular i.
 sciatic nerve i.
 seat belt i.
 self-induced i.
 sesamoid i.
 I. Severity Score (ISS)
 shearing i.
 shotgun i.
 sideswipe i.
 skier's i.
 softball sliding i.
 soft tissue i.
 soft tissue ankle i.
 spinal accessory nerve i.
 spinal cord i. (SCI)
 spleen i.
 sports i.
 stable cervical spine i.
 sternoclavicular joint i.
 straddle i.
 strain-sprain i.
 stress i.
 stretch i.
 subclavian artery i.
 subclavian vein i.
 subscapular artery i.
 subscapular nerve i.
 supination i.
 supination-adduction i.
 supination-eversion i.
 supination-external rotation i.
 supination-inversion i.
 supination-inversion rotation i.
 supination-outward rotation i.
 supination-plantarflexion i.
 supraganglionic i.
 suprascapular nerve i.
 tarsometatarsal joint i.
 thermal i.
 thoracic duct i.
 thoracic nerve i.
 thoracoabdominal artery i.
 thoracodorsal nerve i.
 thoracolumbar spinal i.
 thoracolumbar spine flexion-distraction i.
 three-column cervical spine i.
 throwing i.
 tibial nerve i.

 tornado i.
 tracheal i.
 trampoline i.
 transcutaneous crush i.
 translation i.
 turf toe i.
 two-column cervical spine i.
 ulnar artery i.
 ulnar collateral ligament i.
 ulnar nerve i.
 unstable cervical spine i.
 ureter i.
 urologic i.
 vascular i.
 vertebrobasilar i.
 Weber classification of physeal i.
 weight-bearing rotation i.
 wind-up i.
 wringer i.
 Zlotsky-Ballard classification of acromioclavicular i.

Inland Super Multi-Hite orthopaedic bed
inlay bone graft
inlet view
innate intelligence
inner
 i. heel wedge (IHW)
 I. Lip Plate
 i. table
innervation
 reciprocal i.
Innomed
 I. arthroplasty measuring system
 I. Assistant Free surgical instrument
 I. bone curette
innominate
 anterior i.
 i. bone
 i. bone resection
 left i.
 i. movement
 i. osteotomy
 posterior i.
 right posterior i.
 i. vein
Innovar
Innovative
 I. Medical Products (IMP)
 I. Medical Products Steri-Clamp
Inronail finger or toenail prosthesis
Insall
 I. anterior cruciate ligament reconstruction
 I. criteria
 I. ligament reconstruction technique
 I. patella alta method

I. patellar injury classification
I. procedure
I. proximal realignment
Insall-Burstein
I.-B. II modular knee system
I.-B. intracondylar knee implant
I.-B. semiconstrained
tricompartmental knee prosthesis
I.-B. total knee implant
Insall-Burstein-Freeman (IBF)
I.-B.-F. knee arthroplasty
Insall-Hood reconstruction technique
Insall-Salvati
I.-S. measurement
I.-S. patellar height index
I.-S. ratio
insecurity
gravitational i.
insensate foot
insert
AliMed i.
angled bearing i.
articular i.
cancellous i.
clamp i.
cushioned shoe i.
Energy Plus shoe i.
Gel-Sole shoe i.
i. graft
Hapad shoe i.
heel and sole i.
Hydragrip clamp i.
Johnson & Johnson PFC cruciate-
substituting i.
New York University i.
NYU orthosis i.
Orthex Relievers shoe i.
orthotic shoe i.
Osteonics Scorpio i.
Poly-Dial i.
polypropylene i.
POWERPoint orthotic shoe i.
Profix confirming tibial i.
ROHO solid seat i.
shoe i.
silicone gel socket i.
sole i.
Spenko shoe i.
S-ROM Poly-Dial i.
thermomoldable i.
tibial i.
UCB shoe i.

University of California,
Berkeley i. (UCBI)
Urbanwalkers shoe i.
viscoelastic heel i.
warm-and-form i.
inserter
Buck cement restrictor i.
Buck femoral cement restrictor i.
CDH cup i.
cement restrictor i.
cement spacer i.
cerclage wire i.
C-wire i.
DDT lock screw i.
deluxe FIN pin i.
Kirschner wire i.
Massie i.
Moon-Robinson prosthesis i.
Robinson-Moon prosthesis i.
Shaffner orthopaedic i.
spacer i.
staple i.
T-shaped i.
TSRH hook i.
inserter-extractor
compression i.-e.
insertion
i. activity
anatomic i.
anomalous i.
Bosworth bone peg i.
C-D rod i.
i. equipment
IGHL i.
inferior glenohumeral ligament i.
lag screw i.
ligamentous i.
oblique screw i.
pedicle screw i.
percutaneous pin i.
Pierrot-Murphy advancement i.
rerouting i.
screw i.
i. tendinopathy
insertional excursion
inside-out
i.-o. Bankart shoulder instability
operation
i.-o. technique for establishing
ankle portal
inside-to-outside technique
insidious

NOTES

Insight knee positioning and alignment system
insole
> Aliplast i.
> Apex i.
> Comf-Orthotic 3/4 length i.
> Comf-Orthotic sports replacement i.
> Darco moldable i.
> Diab-A-Foot rocker i.
> Diab-A-Pad i.
> Diab-A-Sole i.
> diabetic i.
> Diabetic Diagnostic i.
> D-Soles i.
> EMED i.
> Ever-Flex i.
> Flexi-Therm diabetic diagnostic i.
> Hapad metatarsal i.
> Kinetic Wedge molded i.
> molded postpartum i.
> Orthex reliever i.
> PAL Diasole i.
> Plastazote i.
> Plexidure i.
> Poron 400 i.
> PPT flat i.
> PPT MXL soft moulded i.
> PPT Plastazote i.
> PPT RX firm moulded i.
> PumpPals i.
> silicone i.
> Spenco i.
> S-Soles i.
> Viscoped S i.

instability
> i. of the ankle
> ankle i.
> anterior i.
> anterolateral-anteromedial rotary i.
> anterolateral rotary i. (ALRI)
> anterolateral rotary knee i.
> anteromedial-posteromedial rotary i.
> anteromedial rotary i.
> articular i.
> atlantoaxial i.
> atraumatic multidirectional i.
> atraumatic, multidirectional, bilateral i. (AMBRI)
> axial i.
> capitate-lunate i.
> carpal i.
> chronic functional i.
> collateral ligament i.
> combined i.
> congenital atlantoaxial i.
> distal intercalated segment i. (DISI)
> dorsal intercalary segment i. (DISI)

> dorsiflexed intercalated segment i. (DISI, DISMAL)
> DRUJ i.
> extension i.
> flexion i.
> functional i.
> i. gait
> hindfoot i.
> intercalated segment i.
> inversion i.
> joint i.
> knee i.
> lateral rotatory ankle i.
> ligamentous repair of the knee for rotatory i.
> lumbar spine i.
> lunotriquetral i.
> mechanical i.
> medial column i.
> membrane i.
> midcarpal i. (MCI)
> multidirectional i. (MDI)
> one-plane i.
> osseous i.
> patellar i.
> pelvic i.
> perilunar i.
> posterior i.
> posterolateral rotary i.
> posteromedial rotary i.
> progressive perilunar i.
> push-pull i.
> radiocarpal i.
> repair of the knee for rotatory i.
> rotary ankle i.
> rotational i.
> sagittal plane i.
> scapholunate i.
> shoulder i.
> spinal i.
> straight lateral i.
> subtalar i.
> traumatic anterior i.
> triquetrolunate i.
> valgus i.
> varus-valgus i.
> vertebral i.
> volar flexed intercalated segment i. (VISI)

installation procedure
install method
Insta-Nerve device
instantaneous axis of rotation
instant cold pack
institutionalized patient
Instron machine
instrument
> Accu-Line knee i.

activating adjusting i. (AAI)
Acufex arthroscopic i.
Acufex MosaicPlasty i.
Arthrex arthroscopy i.
arthroscopic laser i.
Atlas orthogonal percussion i.
back range-of-motion i.
battery-powered i.
Bone Grafter i.
cervical range-of-motion i. (CROM)
Collis TDR i.
Command instrument system
  surgical i.
Corb bone biopsy i.
Cotrel-Dubousset spinal i.
Dreyfus prosthesis placement i.
Dyonic arthroscopic i.
ECTRA carpal tunnel i.'s
electrosurgical i.
Friatec manual arthroscopy i.
Hall series 4 large bone i.
IBF knee i.
Innomed Assistant Free surgical i.
Kirschner surgical i.
LAM i.
laser i.
I. Makar biodegradable interference
  screw
microsurgical i.
Midas Rex pneumatic i.
i. migration
Mitek SuperAnchor i.
Monogram total knee i.
Nicolet Compass EMG i.
orthopaedic cutting i.
OrthoVise orthopaedic i.
paraspinal skin temperature
  thermocouple i.
Partnership i.
Rancho external fixation i.
reciprocal planing i.
RingLoc i.
Schema Assessment i. (SAI)
ScoliTron i.
Shea prosthesis placement i.
single reference point i. (SRP
  instrument)
SRP i.
  single reference point instrument
Steffee i.
thermocouple i.
Wiet graft-measuring i.

instrumental
  i. activities of daily living (IADL)
  i. ADLs
instrumentation
Accu-Line knee i.
Acufex arthroscopic i.
anterior distraction i.
anterior Zielke i.
AO fixateur interne i.
AO notched i.
Apofix cervical i.
Arthrotek Ellipticut hand i.
bone-holding i.
cable-hook compression i.
Caspar anterior i.
C-D i.
compression Harrington i.
compression U-rod i.
Cotrel-Dubousset pedicle screw i.
Cotrel-Dubousset pedicular i.
distraction i.
double Zielke i.
Drummond spinal i.
Dwyer spinal i.
dynamic compression plate i.
Edwards i.
endoscopic carpal tunnel i.
FIRST total knee i.
halo-Ilizarov distraction i.
Harms-Moss anterior thoracic i.
Harrington distraction i.
Harrington-Kostuik i.
Harrington rod i.
hollow mill i.
Howmedica knee i.
Jacobs locking hook spinal rod i.
Kambin and Gellman i.
Kaneda anterior spinal i.
Kostuik-Harrington spinal i.
locking hook i.
Louis i.
lumbar spine i.
lumbosacral spine transpedicular i.
Luque II segmental spinal i.
Luque semirigid segmental spinal i.
Mayfield i.
McElroy i.
modular i.
Moreland total hip revision i.
Moss i.
multiple hook assembly C-D i.
Passport i.

NOTES

instrumentation *(continued)*
> posterior cervical spinal i.
> posterior distraction i.
> posterior hook-rod spinal i.
> Putti-Platt i.
> sacral spine modular i.
> sacral spine Universal i.
> segmental spinal i. (SSI)
> Sielke i.
> skin-contact i.
> Smith-Richards i.
> spinal i.
> Steffee spinal i.
> Stryker power i.
> i. system
> total knee i.
> TSRH i.
> Universal i.
> variable screw placement system i.
> VSP plate i.
> Wisconsin interspinous segmental spinal i.
> Zielke pedicular i.

instrument, sponge, and needle count
insufficiency
> abductor i.
> active i.
> capsular length i.
> deep vein i. (DVI)
> i. fracture
> ligamentous i.
> mechanical i.
> muscle i.
> passive i.
> peripheral vascular i.
> transverse plane motion i.
> vertebrobasilar i.

insufflate
insulin
> i.-dependent diabetes mellitus (IDDM)
> i.-like growth factor (IGF)
> i.-like growth factor I
> nasal i.

intact
> cranial nerves II-XII i.
> I. dressing
> neurologically i.
> neurovascularly i.
> i. neurovascular status
> peripheral pulses symmetrical and i.
> i. spinous lamina
> i. spinous process

intake
> energy i.

integral
> force-time i. (FTI)

> I. hip system
> I. Interlok femoral prosthesis
> pressure-time i. (PTI)

integrated
> i. electromyography
> i. shape and imaging system (ISIS)

integration
> body side i.
> Functional I. (FI)
> sensory i.

integrity
> I. acetabular cup
> I. acetabular cup prosthesis
> I. acetabular cup screw
> i. and alignment
> soft tissue i.

Intelect
> I. Legend stimulator
> I. 600MP microcurrent stimulator

InteliJet fluid management system
intelligence
> innate i.
> universal i.

intensification
> image i.

intensifier
> image i.

intention
> primary i.
> i. tremor

intentional rotation
Inteq small joint suturing system
interaction
> near-infrared i.

interarticularis
> pars i.

interarticular ligament of head of rib
interbody
> i. arthrodesis
> i. graft
> i. spinal fusion

intercalary
> i. allograft procedure
> i. diaphyseal allograft
> i. graft
> i. resection
> i. segmental replacement

intercalated segment instability
intercarpal
> i. arthrodesis
> i. articulation
> i. joint
> i. ligament

intercellular
interclass correlation coefficient (ICC)
interclaviculare
> ligamentum i.

interclavicular ligament
intercollicular groove
intercompartment fasciotomy
intercondylar
    i. drill guide
    i. femoral fracture
    i. fossa
    i. groove
    i. humeral fracture
    i. notch
    i. roof
    i. space
    i. tibial fracture
intercostal
    i. artery
    i. flap
    i. nerve
    i. neuralgia
    i. restriction
    i. space (ICS)
    i. vein
intercostobrachial nerve
intercritical time
intercuneiforme
    os i.
interdigital
    i. corn
    i. ligament
    i. neoplasm
    i. nerve
    i. neuroma
interdischarge interval
interdisciplinary vocational evaluation
    program
interepicondylar axis
interexaminer
interface
    acetabular prosthetic i.
    bone-cement i.
    bone-implant i.
    bone-peg i.
    bony i.
    cement i.
    cement-bone i.
    cup-cement i.
    fascial-muscle i.
    implant-cement i.
    long-term bone-instrumentation i.
    patient-table i.
    pin-bone i.
    prosthesis i.
    prosthesis-cement i.

    ShearGuard low-friction i.
    shoe-foot i.
    soft tissue i.
interfacet
    i. wiring
    i. wiring and fusion
interfacial porosity
interfascicular
    i. epineurectomy
    i. epineurotomy
    i. Millesi nerve graft
interference
    i. fit
    i. fit fixation
    nerve i.
    i. pattern
    i. screw
    i. screw technique
    vertebrogenic i.
interferential
    i. current
    i. electrical stimulation
    i. stimulator
    i. therapy
interfragmental compression
interfragmentary
    i. compression
    i. lag screw
    i. plate
    i. wire
intergluteal cleft
interilioabdominal amputation
interinnominate asymmetry
interinnominoabdominal
    i. amputation
    i. cleft
interlaminar
    i. clamp
interleukin-1 beta release
interline
    Lisfranc articular i.
interlocking
    distal i.
    i. medullary nail
    i. nailing
    proximal i.
intermediate
    i. bundle
    i. cast
    i. C-D hook
    i. dorsal cutaneous nerve (IDCN)

NOTES

intermediate *(continued)*
   i. interference pattern
   i. phalangectomy
Intermedics
   I. natural hip system
   I. Natural-Knee knee prosthesis
intermedius
   vastus i.
intermedullary
   i. guide
   i. nailing
   i. rod fixation
intermetacarpal
   i. articulation
   i. ligament (IML)
intermetatarsal (IM)
   i. angle (IM, IMA)
   i. angle I or II
   i. angle-reducing operation
   i. angle-reducing procedure
   i. ligament
   i. nerve
   i. space
intermetatarseum
   os i.
intermetatarsophalangeal
   i. bursa
   i. bursitis
intermittens
   myotonia i.
intermittent
   i. casting
   i. cervical traction (ICT)
   i. double-step gait
   i. extremity pump
   i. impulse compression
   i. paresthesia
   i. traction
intermuscular (IM)
   i. septum
internal (In)
   i. carotid artery
   i. derangement
   i. derangement of the knee (IDK)
   i.-external rotation
   i. fixation apparatus
   i. fixation, closed reduction
   i. fixation compression arthrodesis
     of the ankle
   i. fixation plate-screw system
   i. fixation spring
   i. hemipelvectomy
   i. iliac artery
   i. iliac vein
   i. jugular vein
   i. microneuroanalysis
   i. movement
   i. neurolysis

   i. oblique muscle
posteroinferior i. (PIIn)
   i. rotation
   i. rotational gait
   i. rotation deformity
   i. rotation exercise
   i. rotation in extension (IRE)
   i. rotation in flexion (IRF)
   i. rotator
   i. spinal fixation
   i. tibial torsion (ITT)
   i. tibial torsion brace
   i. tibiofibular torsion
   i. topography
   i. version
internally
   i. fixed fracture
   i. rotated
International
   Chi'Am I.
   I. Classification of Impairments,
     Disabilities, Handicaps (ICIDH)
   I. Headache Society (IHS)
   I. Knee Documentation Committee
     (IKDC)
   I. Knee Documentation Committee
     form
   I. Knee Documentation Committee
     knee scale
   I. Listing System
   Sacro Occipital Research Society I.
     (SORSI)
   I. 10-20 System
interne
   AO-ASIF fixateur i.
   AO fixateur i.
   Dick AO fixateur i.
   fixateur i.
   fixator i. (FI)
internervous plane
"intern's triangle" in hip spica cast
internus
   metatarsus i.
interoceptor
   postural i.
interossea
   ligamenta cuneometatarsalia i.
   ligamenta intercarpalia i.
   ligamenta intercuneiformia i.
   ligamenta metacarpalia i.
   ligamenta metatarsalia i.
   ligamenta sacroiliaca i.
   ligamenta tarsi i.
   ligamentum intercarpalia dorsalia i.
interosseous
   i. anastomosing channel
   i. branch
   i. compartment

i. cuneocuboid ligament
i. cuneometatarsal ligament
i. intercarpal ligament
i. intercuneiform ligament
i. ligaments of tarsus
i. membrane (IOM)
i. metacarpal ligament
i. metatarsal ligament
i. muscle
i. nerve
i. nerve injury
i. sacroiliac ligament
i. syndrome
i. talocalcaneal ligament
i. tendon
i. wire fixation

interosseum
ligamentum cuneocuboideum i.
ligamentum talocalcaneum i.

interpeak interval
interpediculate
interpeduncular
i. notch
i. space

interpelviabdominal amputation
interperiosteal fracture
interphalangeal (IP)
i. amputation
i. articulation
distal i. (DIP)
i. fusion
i. joint (IPJ)
i. joint dislocation
proximal i. (PIP)
i. tenodesis

interphalangealium
ligamenta palmaria articulationum i.

interphalangectomy
interphalangeus
hallux i.

Interpore
I. bone
I. bone replacement material
I. implant

interposition
i. bone graft
i. membrane
soft tissue i.

interpositional
i. arthroplasty of foot
i. elbow arthroplasty

i. shoulder arthroplasty
i. toe arthroplasty

interpositioned
interpotential interval
interregional displacement
Inter-Royal frame orthopaedic bed
interrupted suture
interscalene block
interscapular
i. aching
i. amputation

interscapulothoracic amputation
Interseal acetabular cup
intersection syndrome
intersegmental
i. fixation
i. mobility
i. motion
i. movement
i. range of motion palpation (IRMP)
i. rotation
I. table

intersesamoidal
intersesamoid ligament
interspace (IS)
atlantodental i.
atlantoodontoid i.

interspinalia
ligamenta i.

interspinal ligament
interspinous
i. cable
i. ligament
i. process fusion
i. pseudarthrosis
i. segmental spinal instrumentation technique (ISSI)
i. wiring

interstices
bone i.

interstitial
i. fluid
i. meniscal tear
i. myofasciitis

interteardrop line
intertransversaria
ligamenta i.

intertransversarii
i. laterales musculi
i. mediales lumborum musculi

NOTES

intertransverse
    i. fusion
    i. ligament
    i. process arthrodesis
intertrigo
intertrochanteric
    i. femoral fracture
    i. four-part fracture
    i. plate
    i. varus osteotomy
Intertron therapy microprocessor
intertubercular
    i. groove
    i. plane
interval
    acromiohumeral i. (AHI)
    anterior atlantoodontoid i.
    atlantodens i. (ADI)
    atlantodental i. (ADI)
    atlas-dens i.
    confidence i. (CI)
    deltopectoral i.
    interdischarge i.
    interpeak i.
    interpotential i.
    posterior atlantoodontoid i.
    recruitment i.
    response i.
    scaphocapitate i.
    Scheffé i.
    trapeziodeltoid i.
intervening
    i. connective tissue
    i. muscle
intervention
    late i.
intervertebral
    i. disk
    i. disk disorder
    i. disk height
    i. disk herniation
    i. disk narrowing
    i. disk nucleus signal
    i. joint
    i. motor unit
    i. notch
intervolar plate ligament
intestinal ileus
intoeing gait
intolerance
    cold i.
    fingertip cold i.
intorsion
intraabdominal pressure
intraacetabular
intraarticular
    i. adhesion
    i. arthrodesis

    i. calcaneal fracture
    i. cautery
    i. cautery device
    i. clavicle
    i. disk ligament
    i. dislocation
    i. fragment
    i. knee fusion
    i. loose body
    i. osteochondroma
    i. osteoid osteoma
    i. osteotomy
    i. procedure
    i. proximal tibial fracture
    i. reconstruction
    i. structure
intraarticulare
    ligamentum capitis costae i.
intracapsular
    i. ankylosis
    i. fracture
    i. osteoid osteoma
    i. osteotomy
Intracath needle
Intracell
    I. mechanical muscle device
    I. myofascial trigger-point device
    I. Sprinter stick
intracellulare
    Mycobacterium i.
intracompartmental
    i. edema
    i. ischemia
    i. pressure
Intracone intramedullary reamer
intracortical
    i. fibrous dysplasia
    i. osteogenic sarcoma
intractable plantar keratosis (IPK)
intracuticular stitch
intradermal suture
intradiscal pressure
intradural
    i. dorsal spinal root rhizotomy
    i. tumor surgery
intraepiphyseal osteotomy
intraexaminer
Intraflex
    I. intramedullary pin
    I. intramedullary pin extractor
intraforaminal approach
intrafusal fiber
intralesional
    i. excision
    i. resection
intramedullary (IM)
    Ace i. (AIM)
    i. alignment jig

i. alignment rod
i. bar
i. canal
i. drill
i. graft
i. hematoma
i. lesion
i. nailing (IMN)
i. pin
i. rod fixation
i. saw
i. stem
i. supracondylar (IMSC)
i. supracondylar multihole nail
intramembranous formation
intramuscular (IM)
i. injection
i. lengthening
i. nerve transposition
i. recording
intraneural
i. fibrosis
i. lipofibroma
intraoperative
i. Cell Saver
i. complication
i. dural tear
i. fluoroscopy
i. fracture
i. neck hyperextension
i. roentgenography
i. stress-relaxation
i. view
i. x-ray
intraorganically induced
intraosseous
i. abscess
i. ganglion
i. gouty invasion
i. lipoma
i. membrane
i. nerve transposition
i. osteosarcoma
i. probe
i. tophaceous gouty invasion
i. tumor
i. vascular congestion
i. venography
i. wire
i. wiring
intrapedicular fixation
intrapelvic protrusio acetabulum

intraperiosteal fracture
intraprosthetic
intrascaphoid angle
Intrasite dressing
intraspinous muscle
intraspongy nuclear disk herniation
intratendinous
intrathecal
i. anesthesia
Lioresal i.
intrathecally enhanced CT scan
intravenous
i. block anesthesia
i. pyelogram
i. regional anesthesia (IVRA)
i. therapy
intravertebral foramen (IVF)
intrinsic
i. contracture
finger i.
i. function
i. minus deformity
i. minus hallux
i. minus position
i. muscle
i. muscle strength
i. paralysis
i. plus deformity
i. restoration
i. test
i. transverse connector
i. transverse connector role
i. vascular disease
introducer
Dumon-Gilliard prosthesis i.
staple i.
intubation
endotracheal i.
Invacare
I. APM mattress
I. padded shower chair
I. vinyl transfer bench
I. wheelchair
invagination
basilar i.
endplate i.
invalid
i. cushion
i. ring
invasion
intraosseous gouty i.

NOTES

invasion *(continued)*
    intraosseous tophaceous gouty i.
    vascular i.
inventory
    Beck Depression I.
    Millon Behavioral Health I.
        (MBHI)
    Minnesota Multiphasic
        Personality I. (MMPI)
    Westhaven Yale Multidimensional
        Pain I. (WHYMPI)
inversion
    i. ankle sprain
    i. ankle stress view
    i. injury
    i. instability
    i. of muscle action
    restricted i.
    i. stress test
inversion-eversion
    i.-e. exercise
    i.-e. rotation
invert
inverted
    i. champagne bottle leg
    i. skin flap
    i. smile
inverted-Y
    i.-Y fracture
    i.-Y incision
inverting knot technique
invertor force
Invertrac equipment
investing fascia
involucrum
involuntary activity
involvement
    tumorous i.
    vertebral artery i.
inward rotation
Inyo nail
Iodex
    I.-p
iodine
    i.-labeled fibrinogen
    i. starch test
iodoform
    i. gauze
    i.-impregnated plastic sheet
iodophor solution
iohexol contrast media
IOM
    interosseous membrane
ion-bombarded cobalt-chromium
iontophoresis
    Dynaphor i.
    i. electrode

ion transfer
Iowa
    I. degenerative change
    I. hip score
    I. hip status system
    I. implant material
    I. internal prosthesis
    I. stem
    I. total hip prosthesis
    I. University periosteal elevator
IP
    interphalangeal
I-Paracaine
IPCS
    infrapatellar contracture syndrome
IPJ
    interphalangeal joint
IPK
    indurated plantar keratoma
    intractable plantar keratosis
I-plate
I-Plus humeral brace
IPOP
    immediate postoperative prosthesis
ipos
    i. arch support system
    i. heel relief orthosis
    i. heel relief shoe
IPSF
    immediate postsurgical fitting
ipsilateral
    i. approach
    i. femoral neck fracture
    i. femoral shaft fracture
    i. nerve root lesion
IPSP
    inhibitory postsynaptic potential
IPT
    industrial physical therapist
IR
    infrared light
    isotonic reversal
    HydroStat IR
IRE
    internal rotation in extension
IRF
    internal rotation in flexion
iris scissors
IRMP
    intersegmental range of motion palpation
iron
    Jewett bending i.
irradiation fibromatosis
irreducible
    i. dorsal dislocation of the
        metatarsophalangeal joint
    i. fracture

I

irregular
    i. potential
    i.-shaped lesion
irregularity
    tendon i.
irrigating solution
irrigation
    i. bulb
    i. burn
    closed i.
    i. and debridement (I&D)
    Pulsavac i.
    i. solution
    i. suction
    Systec i.
    i. system
    i. tube
    Water Pik i.
    wound i.
irrigator
    Arthro-Flo i.
    Baumrucker clamp i.
    Fisch bone drill i.
    jet i.
    ophthalmic i.
    pulse i.
irritability
    nerve root i.
    soft tissue i.
irritable
    i. lesion
    i. symptom
irritation
    i. callus
    facet joint i.
    nerve root i.
    sciatic nerve i.
Irvine ankle arthroplasty
Irwin osteotomy
IS
    interspace
Isaacs syndrome
Isch-Dish Plus cushion
ischemia
    capillary i.
    critical limb i. (CLI)
    exercise i.
    foot i.
    i. foot ulcer
    intracompartmental i.
    muscle i.
    myoneural i.

    tourniquet i.
    vasospastic i.
    Volkmann i.
    warm i.
ischemic
    i. compression
    i. contracture
    i. disease
    i. foot
    i. forearm exercise test
    i. gangrene
    i. index
    i. lesion
    i. limb
    i. myositis
    i. necrosis of femoral head (INFH)
    i. tourniquet technique
    i. ulcer
ischial
    i.-bearing seat
    i. containment socket
    i. spine
    i. tuberosity
    i. weightbearing leg brace
    i. weightbearing prosthesis (IWP)
    i. weightbearing ring
ischial-gluteal weightbearing socket
ischiofemorale
    ligamentum i.
ischiofemoral ligament
ischiogluteal
    i. bursa
    i. bursitis
ischiopubica
    osteochondritis i.
ischiorectal fossa
ischium
Iselin disease
Isherwood projection
Ishihara Color Blindness Test
Ishizuki unconstrained elbow prosthesis
ISIS
    integrated shape and imaging system
    ISIS screening
island
    i. adipofascial flap
    i. adipofascial flap in Achilles
    tendon resurfacing
    bone i.
    bony i.
    i. graft
    i. skin flap

NOTES

Isobex dynamometer
Isocaine HCl
isochrone
isodynamic
isoelastic pelvic prosthesis
isograft
    bone i.
isoinertial
isokinetic
    i. dynamometry
    i. exercise
    i. joint apparatus
    i. knee extension
    i. movement
    i. performance
    i. testing
    i. torque imbalance
    i. Unex III exerciser
Isola
    I. fixation system
    I. hook-rod
    I. spinal implant system
    I. spinal implant system accessory
    I. spinal implant system anchor
    I. spinal implant system application
    I. spinal implant system eye rod
    I. spinal implant system hook
    I. spinal implant system iliac post
    I. spinal implant system iliac
      screw
    I. spinal implant system plate-rod
      combination
    I. spinal instrumentation system
    I. vertebral screw
    I. wire
isolated
    i. avulsion
    i. dislocation
    i. paralysis
    i. zone
isologous graft
Isoloss AC material
isometer
    I. bone graft placement site
      detector
    CA-5000 drill-guide i.
    tension i.
isometheptene mucate
isometric
    i. cervical extension strength
    i. contraction
    i. device
    i. exercise
    i. force
    i. point
    i. resistance
    i. strain gauge

    i. strength testing
    i. technique
isometricity
isoniazid
isophendylate
Isoprene plastic splint
isoproterenol
Isoptin
Iso-Quadron exerciser
Isostation B200
Isotechnologies B-200 low back machine
Isotec patellar tendon graft
Isotoner glove
isotonic
    combination of i.'s (COI)
    i. contraction
    i. exercise
    i. machine
    i. resistance
    i. reversal (IR)
Israel retractor
ISS
    Injury Severity Score
Isseis-Aussies scoliosis operation
ISSI
    interspinous segmental spinal
      instrumentation technique
isthmic spondylolisthesis
isthmus
isuprel
IT
    iliotibial
ITB
    iliotibial band
      ITB fasciitis
Itch
    Absorbine Jock I.
    Aftate for Jock I.
    Tinactin for Jock I.
itraconazole
Itrel
    I. II, III spinal cord stimulation
      system
    I. programmed transmitter-receiver
ITT
    internal tibial torsion
ITV
    infantile tibia vara
Ivalon prosthesis
IVF
    intravertebral foramen
ivory bone
IVRA
    intravenous regional anesthesia
Iwashi clamp approximator
IWP
    ischial weightbearing prosthesis

J

J board
J pad
J septum
J sign

J-55

J. postfusion brace
J. postfusion orthosis

J-24 cervical orthosis
J2 cushion
J-35 hyperextension orthosis
J-45 contraflexion orthosis
J-59 Florida brace
Jaboulay amputation
Jaccoud

J. arthropathy
J. syndrome

JACE

JACE hand continuous passive
  motion unit
JACE shoulder exerciser
JACE W550 CPM wrist device

jack

J. Frost hot/cold pack
Honda j.
Joint J.
turnbuckle j.

jacket

body j.
Boston soft body j.
cervicothoracic j.
flexion body j.
Frejka j.
halo body j.
halo traction j.
immobilization j.
Kydex body j.
Lexan j.
Low Profile plastic body j.
LS^4 custom spinal j.
Minerva cervical j.
Orfizip body j.
Orthoplast j.
plastic body j.
Prenyl j.
Royalite body j.
underarm body j.
Vitrathene j.
von Lackum transection shift j.
Wilmington plastic j.

jackknife

j. position
j. test

The Jacknobber II

Jackson

J. bone clamp
J. bone-extension clamp
J. bone-holding clamp
J. broad-blade staple forceps
J. compression test
J. disk rongeur
J. dressing forceps
J. intervertebral disk rongeur
J. spinal surgery and imaging table
J. syndrome
J. tendon-seizing forceps

Jackson-Gorham syndrome
jacksonian epilepsy
Jackson-Pollock skinfold equation
Jackson-Pratt drain
Jacksonville sling
Jackson-Weiss syndrome
Jacobs

J. chuck
J. chuck adapter
J. chuck drill
J. chuck drive
J. distraction rod
J. locking hook spinal rod
J. locking hook spinal rod
  instrumentation
J. locking hook spinal rod
  instrumentation modification
J. locking hook spinal rod
  technique

Jacob shift test
Jacobson

J. bulldog clamp
J. mosquito forceps
J. needle holder
J. system

Jacoby

J. bunion splint
J. heel splint

Jacquet fixator
Jaddassohn-Lewandowsky syndrome
Jaffe

J. disease
J. procedure

Jaffe-Capello-Averill hip prosthesis
Jahss

J. ankle dislocation classification
J. classification of ankle dislocation
J. maneuver
J. metatarsophalangeal joint
  dislocation classification
J. ninety-ninety method
J. procedure

Jakob test

J

Jamaica Sandalthotics orthotic
Jamar
    J. grip tester
    J. hydraulic hand dynamometer
    J. hydraulic pinch gauge
    J. test
James
    J. position
    J. splint
    J. wound forceps
Jameson
    J. muscle clamp
    J. muscle hook
jammed finger
Jamshidi needle
Janecki-Nelson
    J.-N. shoulder girdle resection
    J.-N. shoulder operation
Janes frame
Jannetta
    J. duckbill elevator
    J. hook
Jansen
    J. bone curette
    J. metaphyseal dysostosis
    J. monopolar forceps
    J. test
Jansey
    J. procedure
    J. technique
Jan van Breemen Function Questionnaire (JVBF)
Japanese
    J. fingertrap
    J. Orthopaedic Association (JOA)
Japas
    J. osteotomy
    J. V-osteotomy
Jarcho-Levin syndrome
Jarell forceps
Jarit
    J. anterior resection clamp
    J. cartilage clamp
    J. meniscal clamp
    J. pin cutter
    J. small bone-holding clamp
    J. tendon-pulling forceps
JAS
    joint activated system
    JAS elbow motion device
javelin thrower's elbow
jaw
    j. exerciser
    j. opening reflex (JOR)
Jay
    J. basic cushion
    J. combi cushion
    J. J2 wheelchair

    J. Rave cushion
    J. Triad cushion
    J. Xtreme cushion
JCE
    job capacity evaluation
Jeanie
    J. Rub
    J. Rub Massager
Jebsen
    J. assessment of hand function
    J. hand test
Jebsen-Taylor hand function test
Jefferson
    J. fracture
    J. fracture of atlas
Jeffery
    J. radial fracture classification
    J. technique
Jelanko splint
Jendrassik maneuver
Jenet sign
Jergesen
    J. I-beam
    J. I-beam plate
    J. incision
    J. tapered plate
    J. tube
jerk
    Achilles j.
    ankle j. (AJ)
    biceps j. (BJ)
    elbow j. (EJ)
    hung-up knee j.
    knee j. (KJ)
    patellar j. (PJ)
    quadriceps j.
    j. sign
    supinator j.
    tendon j.
    j. test
    triceps j. (TJ)
    triceps surae j.
jerky gait
jersey finger
jet
    j. irrigator
    j. lavage
    Ortholav j.
    J. Vac cement dispenser
Jet-Air splint
Jette Functional Status index
Jettmobile
    J. positioning and tumble form
jeweler's
    j. forceps
    j. thumb
Jewett
    J. bending iron

J. contraflexion brace
J. contraflexion orthosis
J. driver
J. extractor
J. gouge
J. hyperextension brace
J. hyperextension orthosis
J. nail
J. nail overlay plate
J. pick-up screw
J. post-fusion brace
J. post-fusion orthosis
J. prosthesis
J. thoracolumbosacral orthosis
Jewett-Benjamin
    J.-B. cervical brace
    J.-B. cervical orthosis
JIDC
    juvenile intervertebral disk calcification
jig
    chamfer cut j.
    Charnley tibial onlay j.
    cutting j.
    drill j.
    drilling j.
    external-alignment compression j.
    extramedullary tibial alignment j.
    femoral alignment j.
    fixation j.
    intramedullary alignment j.
    Miller-Galante j.
    Osteonics j.
    Plexiglas j.
    precompression j.
    spacer-tensor j.
    tibial j.
Jimmie
    half J.
jitter
J&J
    J&J postoperative shoe
    J&J Ulcer dressing
JOA
    Japanese Orthopaedic Association
    JOA Scale
job capacity evaluation (JCE)
Jobe-Glousman capsular shift procedure
Jobst
    J. air band
    J. appliance
    J. athrombotic pump
    J. brassiere

J. gauntlet
J. glove
J. prosthesis
J. stockings
Joerns orthopaedic bed
jogging in place test
Johannesberg staple
Johannson
    J. hip nail
    J. lag screw
Johannson-Barrington arthrodesis
John
    J. Barnes myofascial release
    J. C. Wilson arthrodesis
Johner-Wruhs tibial fracture
classification
Johns Hopkins bulldog clamp
Johnson
    J. chevron osteotomy
    J. hemiphalangectomy
    J. & Johnson PFC cruciate-substituting insert
    J. medial meniscal suturing
    J. pelvic fracture technique
    J. procedure
    J. pronator advancement
    J. resection arthroplasty
    J. screwdriver
    J. staple technique
Johnson-Boseker
    J.-B. scale
    J.-B. scale classification
Johnson-Jahss
    J.-J. classification of posterior tibial tendon tear
    J.-J. posterior tibial tendon tear classification
Johnson-Spiegl
    J.-S. hallux varus correction
    J.-S. procedure
    J.-S. tendon transfer
Johnson-Zuck-Wingate motor test
join
    PIP j.
joint
    AC j.
    acromioclavicular j.
    j. activated system (JAS)
    adjustable dynamic j. (ADJ)
    anterior sternoclavicular j.
    apophyseal j.
    j. arthrodesis

J

NOTES

joint *(continued)*
  j. arthropathy
  j. aspiration
  atlantoaxial j.
  atlantooccipital j.
  atlantoodontoid j.
  bail-lock knee j.
  ball-and-socket j.
  basal j.
  calcaneocuboid j.
  calcaneonavicular j.
  Cam Lock knee j.
  capitate-hamate j.
  capitate-lunate j.
  j. capsule
  j. capsule mechanoreceptor
  carpal-intercarpal j.
  carpometacarpal j.
  carpophalangeal j.
  j. cavitation
  j. cavity
  CC j.
  cervical j.
  Charcot j.
  Chopart midtarsal j.
  chronic recurrent dislocation of the
    ankle j.
  j. cinch
  CMC j.
  j. congruency
  congruent metatarsophalangeal j.
  j. congruity
  coracoclavicular j.
  costochondral j.
  costotransverse j.
  costovertebral j.
  coxofemoral j.
  cracking of j.
  cubonavicular j.
  cuneiform j.
  j. debris
  j. deformity
  j. degeneration
  Delrin j.
  deltoid insertion over j.
  j. depression fracture
  diarthrodial j.
  DIP j.
  j. disarticulation
  j. dislocation
  j. disruption
  distal interphalangeal j. (DIPJ)
  distal radioulnar j. (DRUJ)
  distal tibiofibular j.
  j. distraction
  j. distraction cuff
  j. distractor
  double-stem silicone lesser MP j.

j. dysfunction
j. effusion
ellipsoid j.
erythema of j.
extraarticular subtalar j.
facet j.
fifth metatarsophalangeal j.
Fillauer dorsiflexion assist ankle j.
Fillauer PDC ankle j.
finger j.
first metatarsophalangeal j.
flail j.
j. force
fourth metatarsophalangeal j.
free knee j.
j. fulcrum
j. fusion
Gaffney j.
Gillette j.
ginglymoid j.
glenohumeral j.
gliding hinge j.
Greissinger Multi-Axis j.
hallux IP j.
hamate-lunate j.
hinge j.
hinged j.
hip capsule j.
humeroulnar j.
hyperextensibility of j.
hypermobile j.
j. hypermobility
IM j.
j. immobilization
immovable j.
j. implant
j. instability
intercarpal j.
interphalangeal j. (IPJ)
intervertebral j.
irreducible dorsal dislocation of the
  metatarsophalangeal j.
J. Jack
knee j.
lap j.
lateral ligament of ankle j.
j. lavage
j. laxity
lesser metatarsophalangeal j.
limited-motion metal ankle j.
j. line
j. line pain
j. line tenderness
Lisfranc j.
locking of j.
LT j.
lumbar facetal and interbody j.
Luschka j.

j. manipulation
j. meniscoid
metacarpocapitate j.
metacarpocarpal j.
metacarpohamate j.
metacarpophalangeal j. (MPJ)
metacarpotrapezial j.
Metasul j.
metatarsal j.
metatarsocuboid j.
metatarsocuneiform j.
metatarsophalangeal j. (MTPJ)
j. mice
midcarpal j.
midfoot j.
midtarsal j.
j. mobility
j. mobilization
j. model
mortise and tenon j.
MTP j.
multiple axis knee j.
naviculocuneiform j.
neuropathic tarsal-metatarsal j.
neurotrophic j.
noncongruent metatarsophalangeal j.
nonsubluxated metatarsophalangeal j.
oblique metatarsocuneiform j.
occipital-axis j.
occipitoatlantoaxial j.
Oklahoma ankle j.
Otto Bock 3R65 children's
  hydraulic knee j.
Otto Bock 3R45 modular knee j.
patellofemoral j.
pisotriquetral j.
pivot j.
plastic limited-motion j.
j. play
j. position sense (JPS)
proximal interphalangeal j. (PIPJ)
proximal tibiofibular j.
radiocapitellar j.
radiocarpal j.
radiohumeral j.
radiolunate j.
radioscaphoid j.
radioscapholunate j.
radioulnar j.
j. reconstruction
Regnauld degeneration of MTP j.
j. release

j. rice
sacroiliac j.
saddle j.
scaphocapitate j.
scapholunate j.
scapulothoracic j.
Scotty stainless ankle j.
Select j.
septic finger j.
sesamoidometatarsal j.
SI j.
Silastic finger j.
single-axis ankle j.
solid-ankle j.
j. spacer
sternoclavicular j.
j. stiffness
STT j.
subluxated metatarsophalangeal j.
subtalar j. (STJ)
Surgeon's tarsal j.
Swanson finger j.
j. swelling
synovial j.
talocalcaneal j.
talocalcaneonavicular j.
talocrural j.
talofibular j.
talonavicular j.
Tamarack flexure j.
tarsal j.
tarsometatarsal j.
temporomandibular j. (TMJ)
tenotomy of metatarsophalangeal j.
tibiofemoral j.
tibiofibular j.
tibiotalar j.
total replacement j.
track-bound j.
transverse tarsal j.
trapeziometacarpal j.
trapeziotrapezoidal j.
triscaphe j.
ulnocarpal j.
ulnohumeral j.
Ultraflex Dynamic J.
uncovertebral j.
unstable j.
Virtual hip j.
j. warmth
weightbearing j.
j. wound

J

NOTES

joint *(continued)*
 j. wrap
 zygapophyseal j.
Joint-Jack finger splint
joker
 j. dissector
 j. periosteal elevator
Jolly test
Jonas prosthesis
Jonathan Livingston Seagull patellar prosthesis
Jonell
 J. countertraction finger splint
 J. thumb splint
Jones
 J. abduction frame
 J. arm splint
 J. brace
 J. classification of congenital tibial deficiency
 J. cock-up toe operation
 J. compression pin
 J. compression plate
 J. congenital tibial deficiency classification
 J. diaphyseal fracture classification
 J. dressing
 J. first-toe repair
 J. forearm splint
 J. fracture
 J. metacarpal splint
 J. position
 J. procedure
 J. resection arthroplasty
 J. scissors
 J. screw
 J. suspension traction
 J. tendosuspension
 J. thoracic clamp
 J. towel clamp
 J. traction splint
 J. transfer
 J. view
Jones-Barnes-Lloyd-Roberts classification
Jones-Brackett technique
Jones-Ellison ACL reconstruction
Joplin
 J. bunionectomy
 J. toe prosthesis
JOR
 jaw opening reflex
Jordan-Day drill
Joseph
 J. disease
 J. hook
 J. osteotome
 J. periosteal elevator
 J. periosteotome

 J. rasp
 J. splint
joule
Jousto dropfoot splint, skid orthosis
J-periosteal elevator
JPS
 joint position sense
Jr.
 Caltrate Jr.
 Children's Dynafed Jr.
JRA
 juvenile rheumatoid arthritis
J. R. Moore procedure
J-shaped skin incision
judder
Judet
 J. graft
 J. hip status system
 J. pelvic x-ray view
 J. Press-Fit hip prosthesis
 J. quadricepsplasty
 J. radiograph
Juers-Lempert rongeur forceps
jugal suture
jump
 J. graft
 j. sign
 J. Start Rehab
jumper's
 j. knee
 j. knee position
jumping leg
junction
 allograft-host j.
 atlantooccipital j.
 beaked cervicomedullary j.
 cervicothoracic j.
 gastrocnemius-soleus j.
 host-allograft j.
 lumbosacral j.
 meniscocapsular j.
 meniscosynovial j.
 metaphyseal-diaphyseal j.
 metaphysial-diaphyseal j.
 musculotendinous j.
 myotendinous j.
 occipitocervical j.
 tarsometatarsal j.
 thoracolumbar j.
junctional kyphosis
junctura, pl. **juncturae**
 juncturae tendinum
Junior
 J. Strength Motrin
 J. Strength Panadol
Jurgan
 J. pin
 J. pin ball

J. Pin Ball pin protector
J. pin-ball system
jury-rig
Juvara
J. foot operation
J. procedure
juvenile
j. aponeurotic fibroma
j. bunion
j. discitis
j. flatfoot pathomechanics
j. hallux valgus
j. idiopathic scoliosis
j. intervertebral disk calcification (JIDC)
j. muscular dystrophy
j. plantar dermatosis
j. polyarthritis
j. rheumatoid arthritis (JRA)
j. Tillaux fracture
j. xanthogranuloma
juvenilis
osteochondritis j.
Jux-A-Cisor exerciser
juxtaarticular
j. bone cyst
j. fracture
j. lesion
juxtaarticulation
juxtacortical
j. chondroma
j. fracture
juxtacubital reconstruction
J-Vac closed drainage system
JVBF
Jan van Breemen Function Questionnaire

NOTES

Kadian Capsule
Kaessmann
    K. nail
    K. screw
KAFO
    knee-ankle-foot orthosis
    Generation II KAFO
    GII KAFO
    PRAFO KAFO
Kager triangle
Kahre-Williger periosteal elevator
Kalamchi classification
Kalamchi-Dawe classification of
    congenital tibial deficiency
Kaleidoscope chair
Kalish
    K. Duredge wire cutter
    K. Duredge wire extender
    K. Duredge wire extractor
    K. osteotomy
Kallassy
    K. ankle support
    K. brace
    K. orthosis
Kaltenborn system of joint mobilization
Kaltostat dressing
Kambin and Gellman instrumentation
Kampe corset
KAM Super Sucker
kanamycin
Kanavel
    K. cock-up splint
    K. sign
Kaneda
    K. anterior spinal instrumentation
    K. distraction device
    K. rod
kansasii
    Mycobacterium k.
Kantrex
Kantrowitz thoracic clamp
Kapandji
    K. fracture
    K. fracture of radius
    K. technique
Kapandji-Sauvé arthrodesis
Kapel elbow dislocation technique
Kaplan
    K. oblique line
    K. open reduction
    K. osteotomy
    K. sign
    K. technique
    K. test

Kaplan-Meier
    K.-M. analysis
    K.-M. survivorship
    K.-M. survivorship analysis system
    K.-M. time-to-event analysis
        method
Kaposi sarcoma
kappa receptor
Karakousis-Vezeridis
    K.-V. procedure
    K.-V. resection
Karfoil splint
Karlsson procedure
Kasabach-Merritt syndrome
Kasdan retractor
Kashin-Bek disease
Kashiwagi
    K. resection
    K. technique
Kast-Maffucci syndrome
kastRAP wrap
KAT
    Kinesthetic Ability Trainer
Kates
    K. forefoot arthroplasty
Kates-Kessel-Kay technique
Katz
    K. ADL index
    K. index of activities of daily
        living
Kaufer tendon technique
Kaufmann technique
Kavanaugh-Brower-Mann fixation
kava root
Kawaii-Yamamoto procedure
Kawamura
    K. dome osteotomy
    K. pelvic osteotomy
Kawasaki disease
Kayser-Fleischer ring
Kazanjian splint
KB
    knee-bearing
K blade
K-Cap
Keane Mobility bed
Kearns-Sayre syndrome
Keasbey lesion
Kech and Kelly osteotomy
KED
    Kendrick extrication device
keel
    All Poly Deltafit k.
    Deltafit K.
    k. of glenoid component

K

Keene
> K. compression hook
> K. obturator

Keen sign

Keesay treatment

Kefurox Injection

Kefzol

Kehr sign

Keitel index

Keithley clamp kit

Keith needle

Kelikian
> K. classification of nail deformity
> K. foot dressing
> K. modified Z bunionectomy
> K. modified Z osteotomy
> K. modified Z
> osteotomy/bunionectomy
> K. nail deformity classification
> K. procedure

Kelikian-Clayton-Loseff
> K.-C.-L. surgical syndactyly
> K.-C.-L. technique

Kelikian-McFarland procedure

Kelikian-Riashi-Gleason
> K.-R.-G. patellar tendon repair
> K.-R.-G. technique

Kellam-Waddel classification

Keller
> K. bunionectomy
> K. foot operation
> K. hallux valgus operation
> K. procedure
> K. resection arthroplasty

Keller-Blake
> K.-B. half-ring splint
> K.-B. leg splint

Keller-Brandes procedure

Keller-Lelièvre arthroplasty

Keller-Lelièvre-Hoffman procedure

Keller-Mann resection arthroplasty

Kellgren-Lawrence grading system

Kellgren sign

Kellogg-Speed
> K.-S. fusion technique
> K.-S. lumbar spinal fusion

Kelly
> K. clamp
> K. forceps
> K. hemostat
> K. and Kelly osteotomy

Kelly-Keck osteotomy

keloid

Kelsey unloading exercise therapy

Kelvin body

Kempf-Grosse-Abalo Z-step osteotomy

Kemp test

Kemron

Ken
> K. driver
> K. driver-extractor
> K. screwdriver
> K. sliding nail

Kenacort

Kenaject-40

Kenalog
> K.-10, -40
> K. H

Kendall A-V impulse system

Kendrick
> K. extrication device (KED)
> K. procedure

Kendrick-Sharma-Hassler-Herndon technique

Kenna Knee Scale

Kennedy
> K. LAD
> K. ligament augmenting device
> K. ligament technique
> K. spillproof cup

Kennerdell-Maroon
> K.-M. elevator
> K.-M. hook

Kenney Self-Care Questionnaire

Kenny ADL index

Kenny-Howard
> K.-H. shoulder sling
> K.-H. splint

Keolar implant material

Keralyt Gel

Kerasal ointment

keratinization

keratoacanthoma

keratoderma

keratolysis

keratolytic agent

keratoma
> indurated plantar k. (IPK)

keratome Beaver blade

keratophilic

keratosis, pl. keratoses
> actinic k.
> arsenical k.
> intractable plantar k. (IPK)
> k. palmaris et plantaris
> plantar k.
> k. punctata

Kerlix
> K. bandage
> K. cast pad
> K. cast padding
> K. dressing
> K. gauze
> K. wrap

Kern
- K. bone-holding clamp
- K. bone-holding forceps

Kernig
- K. sign
- K. test

Kern-Lane bone forceps
Kerpel bone curette
Kerr
- K. abduction splint
- K. electro-torque drill
- K. hand drill
- K. sign

Kerrison
- K. chisel
- K. curette
- K. downbiting rongeur
- K. punch

Kerr-Lagen abdominal support
Kessel-Bonney
- K.-B. extension osteotomy
- K.-B. procedure

Kessel plate
Kessler
- K. external fixator
- K. grasping suture
- K. metacarpal distractor
- K. metacarpal lengthening
- K. posterior tibial tendon transfer
- K. posterior tibial tendon transfer operation
- K. prosthesis
- K. repair
- K. stitch
- K. suture technique
- K. traction
- K. traction frame

Kessler-Tajima suture
Ketac cement
ketamine
ketoconazole
ketoprofen
ketorolac tramethamine
ketorolac tromethamine
Kevlar glove
Kevorkian curette
key
- k. the cement
- k. grip
- K. intraarticular knee arthrodesis
- K. periosteal elevator
- k. pinch

- K. rasp
- k. release

keyboard
- ErgoLogic k.
- Kinesis k.
- wave k.

Keyboarders
- MouseMitt K.

Key-Conwell
- K.-C. classification of pelvic fracture
- K.-C. pelvic fracture classification

key-grip tenodesis
keyhole
- k. approach
- k. method
- k. punch
- k. tenodesis
- k. tenodesis technique

Key-loc wrench
Key-Pred Injection
Key-Pred-SP Injection
Keys-Kirschner traction
keystone
- k. of the calcar arch
- k. graft
- K. splint
- k. structure

keyway
- OEC lag screw component with k.

K-Fix Fixator system
KFS
- Klippel-Feil syndrome

Khan-Lewis phonological analysis
Khodadad clip
Kickaldy-Willis arthrodesis
kick bucket
kick-point
Kid-Dee-Lite orthosis
Kid Gloves
Kidner
- K. dissector
- K. flatfoot
- K. foot procedure
- K. lesion
- K. procedure for accessory navicular

kidney
- k. dysfunction
- liver, spleen, k. (LSK)
- k. rest

Kiehn-Earle-DesPrez procedure

K

NOTES

Kiel bone
Kienböck
    K. disease
    K. dislocation
Kiene bone tamp
Kikuchi-MacNap-Moreau approach
Kilfoyle
    K. humeral medial condylar
        fracture classification
Killian gouge
Kilner hook
Kiloh-Nevin ocular form of progressive
  muscular dystrophy
kilopond
kilovoltage potential (kVP)
Kilsyn-Evans
    K.-E. principle of frontal plane
        correction
Kimerle anomaly
Kimura disease
KinAir bed
Kinamed Exact-Fit ATH system
Kinast indirect reduction
KinCom electromechanical dynamometer
Kin-Con
    K.-C. device
    K.-C. isokinetic exercise system
kinematic
    K. fully constrained
        tricompartmental knee prosthesis
    k. gait pattern change
    hindfoot k.'s
    K. II condylar and stabilizer total
        knee system
    K. II rotating hinge knee system
    K. II rotating hinge total knee
        prosthesis
    k. indices of McMurtry
    k. linkage
    K. rotation hinge
    k. study
Kinemax
    K. modular condylar and stabilizer
        total knee system
    K. Plus knee prosthesis
    K. Plus total knee system
    K. removable fixation peg
    K. spacer
Kinemetric guide system
kinesiology
    applied k. (AK)
    k. of the knee
kinesiopathologic component
kinesiopathology
Kinesis keyboard
kinesthesia
kinesthesiometer

kinesthetic
    K. Ability Trainer (KAT)
    k. awareness
    k. exercise
KineTec
    K. clubfoot CPM exerciser
    K. hip CPM machine
kinetic
    k. chain
    k. energy
    k. energy theory
    k. foot pain
    k. rehab device (KRD)
    k. splint
    K. Wedge molded insole
    K. Wedge orthotic
kinetics
Kinetix instrument for carpel tunnel
  release
Kinetron muscle strengthening
  apparatus
King
    K. cervical brace
    K. cervical traction
    K. classification of thoracic
        scoliosis
    K. intraarticular hip fusion
    K. open reduction
    K. scoliosis (type I–V)
    K. technique
    K. type IV curve posterior
        correction
    K. type thoracic and lumbar curve
        (type I–IV)
    K. wound forceps
King-Moe scoliosis
King-Richards dislocation technique
Kingsley Steplite foot
King-Steelquist
    K.-S. hindquarter amputation
    K.-S. technique
kinking
    catheter k.
    pedicular k.
Kinnier-Wilson disease
Kinsbourne syndrome
Kirby muscle hook
Kirk
    K. distal thigh amputation
    K. distal thigh operation
    K. orthopaedic mallet
Kirkaldy-Willis three phases of
  degeneration
Kirmission periosteal elevator
Kirner deformity
Kirschenbaum retractor
Kirschner
    K. bone drill

K. device
K. II-C shoulder system
K. integrated shoulder system
K. Medical Dimension hip
 replacement
K. Medical Dimension prosthesis
K. pin fixation
K. skeletal traction
K. stem
K. surgical instrument
K. tightener
K. total shoulder prosthesis
K. traction bow nut
K. wire (K-wire)
K. wire bow
K. wire cutter
K. wire drill
K. wire driver
K. wire fixation
K. wire inserter
K. wire pin
K. wire placement
K. wire tensioner
kissing
 k. sequestrum
 k. spine
Kistler force platform
kit
 Alpha suction attachment block k.
 BFO K.
 carpal tunnel surgery relief k.
 diabetic orthosis k.
 Digital Care k.
 DynaPak electrode k.
 Elastafit tubing k.
 Exerball k.
 Fillauer Scottish Rite orthosis k.
 Halifax interlaminar clamp k.
 ICE-Magic pain reduction k.
 Keithley clamp k.
 Merit Final Flexion K.
 modular temPPTthotic k.
 palmar swab k.
 parallel pin k.
 pelvic reconstruction k.
 Posey bar k.
 PPT temPPThotics k.
 Quick-Sil starter k.
 resistive chair exercise k.
 sensory stimulation k.
 Skin Care k.

 Tacticon peripheral neuropathy k.
 Unna-Flex Plus venous ulcer k.
 VersaFlex tubing k.
Kitaoka clinical rating scale
**Kitaoka-Leventen medial displacement
 metatarsal osteotomy**
Kite
 K. angle
 K. clubfoot cast
 K. metatarsal cast
 K. slipper
KJ
 knee jerk
Kjolbe technique
Klagsbrun harvesting technique
klapping
Klebsiella
 K. oxytoca
 K. pneumoniae
Kleiger test
Klein
 K. drainage
 K. technique
Kleine-Levin syndrome
Kleinert
 K. modification
 K. postoperative traction brace
 K. repair
 K. splint
Kleinert-Kutz
 K.-K. bone cutter
 K.-K. bone rongeur
 K.-K. clamp approximator
 K.-K. rasp
 K.-K. rongeur forceps
 K.-K. synovectomy rongeur
 K.-K. tendon forceps
 K.-K. tendon retriever
Kleinert-Ragdell retractor
Kleinmant test
Klemm-Schellman nail
Klengall brace
Klenzak
 K. double-upright splint
 K. orthosis
 K. spring brace
Klinefelter syndrome
Kling
 K. adhesive dressing
 K. cervical brace
 K. elastic bandage

K

NOTES

Klippel-Feil
    K.-F. segmentation defect
    K.-F. syndrome (KFS)
Klippel-Trenaunay
    K.-T. osteohypertrophic
      hemangiectasia
    K.-T. syndrome
Klippel-Trenaunay-Weber syndrome
Klisic-Jankovic technique
Kloehn craniofacial remodeling
   technique
Klumpke
    K. injury
    K. palsy
KMC
    KMC femoral stem prosthesis
    KMC hip system
KMP
    KMP femoral stem
    KMP femoral stem prosthesis
KMW hip system
KMW/PC femoral prosthesis
knavel table
Knead-A-Ball exerciser
kneading massage
knee
    above k. (AK)
    ACL-deficient k.
    anatomic modular k. (AMK)
    k. anatomy
    anterior cruciate deficit k.
    anterior cruciate ligament of k.
    k. arthrodesis
    k. arthroplasty
    biocompartmental replacement of k.
    k. bolster
    k. brace
    k. brace splint
    breaststroker's k.
    cadaveric k.
    k. cage brace
    k. complex
    constant-friction k.
    constrained condylar k.
    cruciate ligaments of k.
    deficient k.
    dislocated k.
    k. dislocation
    k. extension assist
    k. extension orthosis
    k. extensor
    flail k.
    k. flexion
    k. flexion-extension
    floating k.
    k. force
    k. fracture
    k. fusion

game k.
Genesis unicompartmental k.
gimpy k.
giving way of k.
hamstrung k.
k. holder
horseback rider's k.
Hosmer single axis friction k.
Hosmer single axis locking k.
Hosmer weight activated locking k.
housemaid's k.
k. immobilizer
k. immobilizer splint
k. instability
internal derangement of the k.
  (IDK)
k. jerk (KJ)
k. jerk reflex
k. jerk reflex test
k. joint
jumper's k.
kinesiology of the k.
49er k. brace
Korn Cage k.
k. laxity test
k. ligamentous injury
k. lock
locked k.
Mauch Swing and Stance
  hydraulic k.
k. MD brace
Miller-Galante k.
motorcyclist's k.
neuropathic k.
Noiles posterior stabilized k.
Noiles rotating hinge k.
k. orthosis (KO)
Otto Bock modular rotary
  hydraulic k.
Otto Bock 3R60 EBS k.
Otto Bock 3R80 modular rotary
  hydraulic k.
Otto Bock Safety constant-
  friction k.
PC Performer k.
K. Pillo
pneumatic 4-bar linkage k.
PolymerFriction total k.
porous-coated anatomic total k.
k. positioner
k. positioning triangle
posterior cruciate ligament of k.
Press-Fit Condylar Total k.
ProAdvantage k.
k. prosthesis
k. pump
k. pump exercise
Q angle of the k.

reefing of the medial retinaculum
of the k.
k. rotation
runner's k.
k. saver
self-aligning k. (SAL)
septic k.
k. signature system
single-axis friction k. (SAFK)
single-axis locking k. (SALK)
k. sleeve
k. stability
total condylar k.
Total Knee 2100 prosthetic k.
transverse ligament of k.
trick k.
USMC stance locking safety k.
valgus k.
varus k.
k. varus-valgus
voluntary control 4-bar k.
weight-activated locking k.
  (WALK)
windblown k.
wrenched k.
knee-ankle-foot orthosis (KAFO)
knee-bearing (KB)
kneecap stabilizer
knee-chest
  k.-c. push
  k.-c. rocking
  k.-c. table
knee-control orthosis pad
KneeCrank
Kneed-It
  K.-I. knee guard
  K.-I. kneeguard
kneeGRIP
kneeguard
  Kneed-It k.
kneeling
  k. position
  90-90 k. position
kneeRAP wrap
knife
  acetabular k.
  ACL graft k.
  amputation k.
  arthroscopic k.
  backward-cutting k.
  Ballenger swivel k.
  banana k.

Bard-Parker k.
bayonet k.
Beaver cataract k.
Beaver-DeBakey k.
Bircher meniscus k.
k. blade
Blair k.
Blount k.
Bovie k.
C k.
cast k.
Castroviejo bladebreaker k.
Catlin amputating k.
chondroplasty k.
Collin amputating k.
cutting current k.
DeMarneffe meniscotomy k.
Down epiphyseal k.
Downing cartilage k.
Esmarch plaster k.
forward-cutting k.
Freiberg cartilage k.
Freiberg meniscectomy k.
full-radius resector k.
Grover meniscus k.
hemilaminectomy k.
hooked k.
Hopkins plaster k.
hot k.
Humby k.
Krull acetabular k.
Langenbeck flap k.
Langenbeck resection k.
Lindvall-Stille k.
Liston amputating k.
Liston amputation k.
Liston phalangeal k.
Lowe-Breck cartilage k.
Lowe-Breck meniscectomy k.
Maltz cartilage k.
McKeever cartilage k.
meniscectomy k.
meniscus k.
Midas Rex k.
Neff meniscus k.
Oretorp retractable k.
orthopaedic k.
Reiner plaster k.
retrograde-cutting hook-shaped k.
Ridlon plaster k.
rocker k.
Salenius meniscus k.

K

NOTES

knife *(continued)*
    sculp k.
    semilunar cartilage k.
    serrated fine-cutting k.
    sheathed k.
    skiving k.
    Smillie-Beaver k.
    Smillie cartilage k.
    Smillie meniscal k.
    Smith cartilage k.
    Stryker cartilage k.
    tenotomy k.
    upward-cutting triangular k.
    Weck k.
    Yamanda myelotomy k.
Knight back brace
Knight-Taylor
    K.-T. thoracic brace
    K.-T. thoracolumbosacral orthosis
    K.-T. and Williams spinal orthosis
Knirk-Jupiter elbow evaluation scale
Knit-Rite suspension sleeve
Knobber
    The Original Index K. II
Knobble massager
Knobby-Clark procedure
knock-knee
    k.-k. brace
    k.-k. deformity
Knodt
    K. rod
    K. rod and hook
knot
    Henry k.
    k. of Henry
    PDS k.
    k. pusher
    Revo k.
    sliding k.
    surfer's k.
    wire k.
knotting forceps
Knott rod distraction device
Knowles
    K. hip pin
    K. pin nail
    K. pinning
knuckle
    K. Benders
    k.-bender splint
    k. pad
    k. shaped
KO
    knee orthosis
Kocher
    K. clamp
    K. classification
    K. collar incision

    K. curved L approach
    K. dissector
    K. elevator
    K. forceps
    K. fracture
    K. lateral J approach
    K. maneuver
    K. method
    K. retractor
Kocher-Cushing sign
Kocher-Debré-Semelaigne syndrome
Kocher-Gibson posterolateral approach
Kocher-Langenbeck
    K.-L. approach
    K.-L. exposure
Kocher-Lorenz
    K.-L. classification of capitellum
        fracture
    K.-L. fracture
    K.-L. fracture of capitellum
Kocher-McFarland hip arthroplasty
Koch-Mason dressing
Kodel knee sling
Kodex drill
Koenen periungual fibroma
Koenig
    K. metatarsal broach
    K. metatarsophalangeal joint
        arthroplasty
    K. MPJ implant and arthroplasty
    K. MPJ prosthesis
    K. nail-splitting scissors
    K. rasp
    K. total great toe implant
Koenig-Schaefer
    K.-S. incision
    K.-S. medial approach
Kofoed scoring system
Köhler
    K. disease
    K. lines
Kohs block
koilonychia
Kold Wrap
Kollagen dressing
Kolmogorov-Smirov test
König disease
Konstram angle
Kool Kit cold therapy pack
koolPAK
koolRAP
Korex cork sheet
Korn
    K. Cage knee
    K. Cage knee brace
Kortzeborn
    K. hand operation
    K. procedure

Kostuik-Alexander arthrodesis
Kostuik-Errico
    K.-E. classification of spinal
       stability
    K.-E. spinal stability classification
Kostuik-Harrington
    K.-H. distraction system
    K.-H. spinal instrumentation
Kostuik screw
Kotz-Salzer rotationplasty
Koutsogiannis
    K. calcaneal displacement
       osteotomy
    K. procedure
Koutsogiannis-Fowler-Anderson
    osteotomy
Krackow
    K. HTO blade staple
    K. maneuver
    K. point
Krackow-Cohn technique
Krackow-Thomas-Jones technique
Kramer-Craig-Noel basilar femoral neck
    osteotomy
Kramer modification of Hohmann
    osteotomy
Krankendonk pin
Kraske position
Krause
    suture of K.
Krause-Wolfe
    K.-W. prosthesis
    K.-W. skin graft
Krayenbeuhl hook
KRD
    kinetic rehab device
    KRD L2000 rehab device
Krempen-Craig-Sotelo tibial nonunion
    technique
Krempen-Silver-Sotelo nonunion
    operation
Kretschmer syndrome
Kreuscher bunionectomy
Kristiansen eyelet lag screw
Kristiansen-Kofoed external fixation
Kronendonk pin
Kronfeld pin
Kronner
    K. external fixation
    K. external fixation apparatus
    K. external fixation device

Krukenberg
    K. hand operation
    K. hand reconstruction
    K. procedure
Krull acetabular knife
Kruskal-Wallis test
KSO brace
KT
    Orudis KT
    KT side-to-side difference
KT1000
    KT1000 foot stabilizer
    KT1000 knee ligament arthrometer
KT2000 knee ligament arthrometer
KT1000/s surgical arthrometer
Kuda shaver
Kudo
    K. hinge
    K. unconstrained elbow prosthesis
Kugelberg reconstruction
Kugelberg-Welander disease
Kuhlman
    K. cervical traction device
    K. traction
Kumar
    K. application
    K. spica cast technique
Kumar-Cowell-Ramsey technique
Kümmell disease
Küntscher
    K. awl
    K. condylocephalic rod
    K. drill
    K. extractor
    K. finisher
    K. hammer
    K. humeral prosthesis
    K. impactor
    K. medullary nailing
    K. nail
    K. nail driver
    K. nail-extracting hook
    K. ossimeter
    K. pin
    K. reamer
    K. technique
    K. traction apparatus
    K. traction device
Küntscher-Hudson brace
Kunzel
    nerve of K.
Kunzli orthopaedic sports shoe

K

NOTES

Kurlander orthopaedic wrench
Kurosaka interference-fit screw
Kurtzke score
Kutes arthroplasty
Kutler
    K. double lateral advancement flap
    K. V-Y flap
    K. V-Y flap graft
kVP
    kilovoltage potential
K-wire
    Kirschner wire
    K-wire driver
    K-wire placement
Kydex
    K. body jacket
    K. brace
Kyle
    K. fracture classification system
    K. internal fixation
Kyle-Gustilo classification
Kyle-Gustilo-Premer classification
kyphectomy
    Sharrard-type k.
kyphometer
    Debrunner k.
kyphoscoliosis
    neurofibromatosis k.
    k. secondary to neurofibromatosis
    severe k.
    thoracolumbar k.
kyphosing scoliosis
kyphosis
    acute angular k.

adolescent k.
anterior k.
apprentice k.
k. brace
congenital k. (type I, II)
k. correction
k. creation
iatrogenic lumbar k.
junctional k.
long-radius k.
lumbar k.
lumbosacral k.
Luque rod fixation for k.
k. muscularis
myelodysplastic k.
paralytic k.
postlaminectomy k.
postradiation k.
posttraumatic k.
right thoracic curve with
    junctional k.
rotational k.
sagittal k.
Scheuermann juvenile k. (SJK)
short-radius k.
thoracic k.
thoracolumbar k.
kyphos resection
kyphotic
    k. angulation
    k. curve
    k. deformity
    k. deformity pathomechanics

L
  L plate
  L rod
LA
  Dexone LA
L.A.
  L.A. cervical orthosis
  Dalalone L.A.
  Dexasone L.A.
  Solurex L.A.
labium
laboratory
  Army Prosthetics Research L.
    (APRL)
  gait l.
labral
  l. avulsion
  l. lesion
  l. tear
labrum
  acetabular l.
  anterior glenoid l.
  articular l.
  glenoid l.
  posterior glenoid l.
LAC
  long arm cast
lace
  no-tie stretch l.
  spyrolace shoe l.
lace-on brace
laceration
  burst-type l.
  chevron l.
  flexor tendon l.
  hallucis longus l.
  stellate l.
lacertus fibrosus
Lacey
  L. fully constrained
    tricompartmental knee prosthesis
  L. hinge
  L. hinged knee prosthesis
Lachman
  L. maneuver
  L. sign
  L. test
Lac-Hydrin lotion
lacinate ligament
lacing ankle brace
lacrimal duct dilator
Lacroix
  fibroosseous ring of L.
  osseous ring of L.
  L. osseous ring

lactate
  calcium l.
  Ringer l.
  l. threshold (LT)
lactic
  l. acidosis
  l. acidosis threshold (LAT)
Lactinol-E creme
Lactinol lotion
Lactobacillus
lacuna
  Howship l.
LAD
  ligament augmentation device
  Kennedy LAD
ladder
  finger l.
  shoulder l.
Lafayette skinfold caliper
lag
  interfragmentary l. screw
  l. screw
  l. screw fixation
  l. screw insertion
  l. screw thread hole
Lagenbeck bone saw
**LaGrange humeral supracondylar
  fracture classification**
LaGrange-Letoumel hip prosthesis
lag-screw
Lahey clamp
Laing
  L. concentric hip cup
  L. hip cup prosthesis
  L. plate
Lalonde
  L. bone clamp
  L. hook forceps
  L. tendon approximator
LAM
  laminotomy and diskectomy
  limb accurate measurement
  LAM instrument
lam
  laminectomy
Lambert cosine law
**Lambert-Eaton myasthenic syndrome
  (LEMS)**
Lambert-Lowman
  L.-L. bone clamp
  L.-L. chisel
Lamb-Marks-Bayne technique
Lamb muscle transfer
lamboid suture

L

Lambotte
- L. bone-holding clamp
- L. bone-holding forceps
- L. bone hook
- L. elevator
- L. osteotome
- L. principle

Lambrinudi
- L. arthrodesis
- L. drop foot operation
- L. osteotomy
- L. splint
- L. technique

lamb's wool pad

lamella, pl. **lamellae**
- concentric l.

lamellar
- l. bone
- l. pattern
- l. separation

lamellated bone

lamellation

lami

lamina, pl. **laminae**
- l. elevator
- intact spinous l.

laminaplasty, laminoplasty
- expansive l.
- Tsuji l.
- l. with extended foraminoplasty for cervical myelopathy

laminar
- l. air flow
- l. bone
- l. C-D hook
- l. cortex posterior aspect
- l. fracture
- l. spreader

laminectomized spine

laminectomy (lam)
- cervical spine l.
- decompression l.
- l. frame
- multilevel l.
- osteoplastic l.
- radial l.

laminoforaminotomy

laminoplasty (*var. of* laminaplasty)

laminotomy and diskectomy (LAM)

Lamisil
- L. Cream
- L. Oral

Lamis patellar clamp

lamp
- halogen l.
- Wood l.

Lanceford prosthesis

lancinating pain

lancing

land
- no man's l. (in hand)

Landers-Foulks prosthesis

landmark
- bony l.
- pedicle l.

Landolt spreading forceps

Landouzy-Dejerine disease

Landsmeer ligament

Lane
- L. bone-holding clamp
- L. bone-holding forceps
- L. bone lever
- L. bone screw
- L. periosteal elevator
- L. plate
- L. procedure
- L. screwdriver
- L. screw-holding forceps
- L. self-retaining bone-holding forceps

Lanex screen

Lange
- L. Achilles tendon reconstruction
- L. bone retractor
- L. hip reduction
- L. procedure
- L. skinfold caliper
- L. tendon lengthening
- L. tendon lengthening and repair

Lange-Hohmann bone retractor

Langenbeck
- L. bone-holding forceps
- L. flap knife
- L. metacarpal saw
- L. periosteal elevator
- L. rasp
- L. resection knife
- L. retractor
- L. triangle

Langenskiöld
- L. bone graft
- L. bony bridge resection
- L. classification (stage I–VI)
- L. fusion
- L. grading system
- L. procedure

Langer
- L. arch
- L. line
- L. muscle

Langerhans cell granulomatosis

Langoria sign

language
- mind l.

lanula
- os l.

lap
    laparotomy
        lap joint
        lap seatbelt fracture
laparotomy (lap)
    l. sheet
    l. sponge
Lapidus
    L. alternating air-pressure mattress
    L. bed
    L. bunionectomy
    L. hammertoe technique
LAPOC prosthesis
LaPorte
    L. great toe implant
    L. total toe prosthesis
lappet formation
L'Aprina topical spray
LapTop cushion
large
    l.-bore inflow cannula
    l. callus podi-burr
    l. composite allograft
    l.-head humeral component
    l. humeral-head hemiarthroplasty
    l. nail podi-burr
    l.-nail spicule bur
Largon
Larmon
    L. forefoot
    L. forefoot arthroplasty
    L. forefoot procedure
Laron dwarfism
Larsen
    L. syndrome
    L. tendon-holding forceps
Lars Ingvar Hansson (LIH)
Larson
    L. hip status system
    L. ligament reconstruction
    L. syndrome
    L. technique
laryngeal nerve injury
LAS
    local adaptation syndrome
LASA
    Lisfranc articular set angle
Laschal suture scissors
LASE
    laser-assisted spinal endoscopy
        LASE probe

Lasègue
    L. rebound test
    L. sign
laser
    ArthroProbe arthroscopic l.
    l. arthroscopy
    l.-assisted spinal endoscopy (LASE)
    carbon dioxide l.
    l. Doppler flowmetry (LDF)
    l. Doppler probe
    holmium YAG l.
    l. image custom arthroplasty
      (LICA)
    l. instrument
    l. nucleotomy
    red light neon l.
    Surgilase CO_2 l.
    Trimedyne Omnipulse homium l.
    VersaPulse holmium l.
Laserflo BPM
lashing suture
last normal vertebra (LNV)
LAT
    lactic acidosis threshold
lat
    lateral
        lat men
        lat pulldown
lata
    fascia l.
    tensor fascia l. (TFL)
Latarjet procedure
LATC
    lateral talocalcaneal angle
late
    l. intervention
    l. response
    l. stance
latency
    l. of activation
    distal l.
    motor l.
    onset l.
    peak l.
    proximal l.
    residual l.
    sensory peak l.
    terminal l.
latent
    l. period
    l. stage of gout
lateral (lat)

L

NOTES

lateral *(continued)*
l. acromial border
l. ankle sprain
l. antebrachial cutaneous nerve
l. anterior thoracic nerve
l. arm flap
l. aspiration
l. atlantooccipital ligament
l. band
l. band mobilization
l. bending
l. canal entrapment
l. capsular release
l. capsular sign
l. closing wedge osteotomy
l. collateral ligament (LCL)
l. column calcaneal fracture
l. compartment
l. compartment disruption
l. compartment injury
l. compartment reconstruction
l. compression (LC)
l. compression force
l. compression injury
l. condylar humeral fracture
l. cord
l. cortex
l. costotransverse ligament
l. decompression
l. decubitus position
l. deltoid splitting approach
l. deviation
l. deviation angle
l. disk protrusion
l. displacement osteotomy
l. drainage
l. electrical surface stimulation
   (LESS)
l. end
l. epicondyle
l. epicondylitis
l. extensor expansion
l. extensor release
l. femoral condyle
l. femoral cutaneous nerve
l. flexion
l. flexion dynamic visual analysis
l. flexion malposition
l. flexion restriction
l. full-spine radiographic
   examination
l. fusion
l. Gatellier-Chastung approach
l. guidepin
l. head of gastrocnemius
l. hindfoot
l. hip arthroscopy
l. humeral condyle fracture

l. hyperpressure syndrome
l. impingement
l. interosseous ligament
l. J approach
l. joint line
l. joint space
l. Kocher approach
l. ligament of ankle joint
l. listhesis
l. lumbar shift
l. malleolus
l. malleolus fracture
l. mass fracture
l. meniscal cyst
l. meniscectomy (lat men)
l. meniscus
l. oblique view
l. Ollier approach
l. opening wedge osteotomy
l. parapatellar approach
l. park-bench position
l. patellar autologous graft
l. patellar compression syndrome
l. patellar facet
pelvic l.
l. pivot shift
l. pivot shift test
l. plantar metatarsal angle
l. plantar nerve
l. plantar nerve fasciculus
l. process
l. projection (LC)
l. quadruple complex
l. recess
l. recess spinal stenosis
l. recess stenosis (LRS)
l. retinaculum release
l. rhachotomy
l. roentgenogram
l. root pressure
l. rotary displacement
l. rotatory ankle instability
l. sacrococcygeal ligament
l. screw
l. sesamoidectomy
l. shear
l. shelf
l. sling procedure
l. slip
l. spring ligament
l. spring ligament of foot
l. squeeze pinch
l. stability
l. step-up
l. sway
l. talar process fracture
l. talocalcaneal angle (LATC)
l. talocalcaneal ligament (LTC)

l. tarsometatarsal angle
l. tear
l. thigh flap
l. thoracic flap
l. tibial condyle
l. tibial plateau fracture
l. tibial tubercle
l.-to-medial thrust
l. transfer
l. transmalleolar portal
l. trap suture
l. trunk shift
l. utility incision

laterale
ligamentum atlanto-occipitale l.
ligamentum costotransversarium l.
ligamentum sacrococcygeum l.
ligamentum talocalcaneare l.

lateralis
vastus l. (VL)

laterality
atlas l.

lateralization
laterally displaced fracture
laterolisthesis
lateropulsion
latex
l. allergy
l. anaphylaxis
l. cushion

latissimus
l. dorsi
l. dorsi flap
l. dorsi muscle

latitudinal growth
latticework
latus
metatarsus l.

Lauenstein procedure
Lauge-Hansen
L.-H. ankle fracture classification
L.-H. stage II supination-eversion
fracture

Laugier
L. fracture
L. sign

Lauren view
Laurin angle
lavage
angled showerhead l.
bone l.
Exeter bone l.

Hi Speed Pulse l.
jet l.
joint l.
Ortholav jet l.
pulsatile jet l.
pulsatile pressure l.
Pulsavac l.
pulsed l.
Simpulse pulsing l.
Simpulse S/I l.

lavender
Lavine reduction
law
all or none l.
L. of Facilitation
Heuter-Volkmann l.
Lambert cosine l.
Sherrington l.
von Schwann l.
Wolff l.

lawn mower injury
Lawrence first metatarsophalangeal joint implant
Lawson-Thornton plate
laxity
ankle l.
joint l.
ligamentous l.
radioscaphocapitate ligament l.
l. to varus stress

layer
capsular l.
gliding l.
parietal tendon sheath l.
periosteal cambium l.

Lazepen-Gamidov anteromedial approach
LazerSporin-C solution
lazy-C incision
lazy-S incision
lazy-V deepithelialized turn-over fasciocutaneous flap
L-bolt
TSRH L.-b.

LBP
low back pain

LBW
lean body weight

LC
lateral compression
lateral projection

LCL
lateral collateral ligament

L

NOTES

LCPD
Legg-Calvé-Perthes disease
LCS
low contact stress
LCS implant
LCS mobile bearing knee system
LCS New Jersey knee prosthesis
LCT
liquid crystal thermography
L-curved incision
LDF
laser Doppler flowmetry
lumbodorsal fascia
LE
lower extremity
lupus erythematosus
Le
Le Dentu suture
Le Fort fibular fracture
Le Fort mandible fracture
Le Fort-Wagstaffe fracture
LEA
lower-extremity amputation
Leach-Igou step-cut medial osteotomy
Leach-Schepsis-Paul augmentation
lead
l. line
l.-line scan
l. pipe fracture
l. poisoning
l. synovitis
Leadbetter
L. hip manipulation
L. maneuver
L. technique
leaders and trailers
leaf
inferior l.
l. splint
superior l.
leaf-spring
AFO posterior l.-s.
l.-s. brace
plastic l.-s. (PLS)
leakage
bony slurry l.
chylous l.
Leake Dacron mandible prosthesis
lean
antalgic l.
l. body weight (LBW)
Leander
L. chiropractic table
L. motorized flexion table
L. 79- Series distraction table
leaning hop test
LEAP
Lewis expandable adjustable prosthesis

learning
spinal l.
leash of Henry
leather
l. ankle corset
l. cuff
l. orthosis
Leatherman hook
Lebsche
L. rongeur
L. saw guide
L. wire saw
LeCocq brace
lederhosen disease
Ledraplastic exercise ball
Lee
L. anterosuperior iliac spine graft
L. bone graft
L. procedure
L. reconstruction
L. technique
Leeds spinal procedure
Lefferts rib shears
leflunomide
LeFort II fracture
left
l. erector spinae musculature
l. innominate
l. lateral flexion
l. lower extremity (LLE)
l. lower limb (LLL)
l. lumbar convexity
l.-right leg displacement
l. rotation
l. side bending
l. thoracolumbar major curve pattern
l. upper extremity (LUE)
l. upper limb (LUL)
left-hand
l.-h. dominance
l.-h. dominant
left-sided
l.-s. nail
l.-s. thoracotomy
leg
anatomic short l.
l. axis
badger l.
baker's l.
bandy l.
bayonet l.
bow l.
l. brace
l. compartment release
l. decompression
functional short l.
l. holder

inequality in length of l.'s (ILL)
inverted champagne bottle l.
jumping l.
l. length
l. length determination
l. length discrepancy (LLD)
l. length inequality (LLI)
l. positioner
l. press
l. protection factor (LPF)
restless l.
short l.
l. shortening
l. sling
stork l.
table short l.
tennis l.
l. walking cast
Legasus support CPM device
leg-curl
ankle joint l.-c.
Legg-Calvé-Perthes disease (LCPD)
Legg-Perthes
L.-P. disease
L.-P. disease orthosis
L.-P. shoe extension
L.-P. sling
legholder
Alvarado l.
Arthroplasty Products Consultants
foot and l.
arthroscopic l.
Bickel l.
Cherf l.
LH1000 arthroscopic l.
lithotomy l.
Low Profile l.
operative l.
OSI Arthroscopic l.
Prep-Assist l.
Surbaugh l.
SurgAssist surgical l.
Zollinger l.
leg-holding
l.-h. apparatus
l.-h. device
leg press
CamStar power l. p.
Lehman technique
Leibinger
L. Micro System drill bit
L. Micro System plate cutter

L. Micro System plate-holding
forceps
L. Profyle hand system
Leibolt technique
Leichtenstern sign
Leinbach
L. device
L. femoral prosthesis
L. hip prosthesis
L. olecranon screw
L. osteotome
Leksell
L. rongeur
L. rongeur forceps
Leksell-Stille thoracic rongeur
Lelièvre osteotomy
Lema strap
Lemmon
L. rib contractor
L. sternal approximator
L. sternal spreader
Lempert
L. bone curette
L. bone rongeur
L. periosteal elevator
L. rongeur forceps
LEMS
Lambert-Eaton myasthenic syndrome
Lenart-Kullman technique
length
echo train l. (ETL)
Grace method of ratio of
metatarsal l.
leg l.
pedicle screw cord l.
pedicle screw path l.
resting l.
l. of stay (LOS)
step l.
l.-tension curve
lengthening
Achilles tendon l.
aponeurotic l.
Armistead ulnar l.
Codivilla tendon l.
Compere l.
l. contraction
DeBastiani femoral l.
distraction l.
Evans calcaneal l.
extensor l.
fractional l.

L

NOTES

lengthening *(continued)*
    Frost posterior tibialis tendon l.
    gastrocnemius l.
    Gillies-Millard metacarpal l.
    hamstring l.
    Hauser tendo calcaneus l.
    heel cord l.
    Hoke Achilles tendon l.
    Hsu-Hsu percutaneous tendo
      calcaneus l.
    Ilizarov leg l.
    Ilizarov limb l.
    intramuscular l.
    Kessler metacarpal l.
    Lange tendon l.
    limb l.
    limb-girdle l.
    metacarpal l.
    percutaneous heel cord l.
    reverse undercutting l.
    Silfverskiöld Achilles tendon l.
    Silver-Simon l.
    Spencer tendon l.
    step-cut l.
    Strayer l.
    subscapularis-capsular l.
    Tachdjian fractional l.
    Tachdjian hamstring l.
    Tajima metacarpal l.
    tendo Achilles l. (TAL)
    tendon l.
    tibial l.
    transiliac l.
    ulnar l.
    Vulpius l.
    Vulpius-Compere gastrocnemius l.
    Wagner femoral l.
    Wagner tibial l.
    Warren White Achilles tendon l.
    white tendo calcaneus l.
    Z-slide l.
Lenox
    L. bucket
    L. Hill derotational knee brace
    L. Hill knee orthosis
    L. Hill Spectralite knee brace
lens
    Nikon SMZ 2T magnifying l.
lenticularis
    fasciculus l.
lentigo, pl. **lentigines**
    l. maligna
    l. maligna melanoma
Lentulo spiral drill
Leo Bathlifter
Leone expansion screw
leopard syndrome
Lepird procedure

L'Episcopo hip reconstruction
L'Episcopo-Zachary procedure
leprosy
leptomeninges
Lere bone mill
Leriche syndrome
Leri sign
Lerman
    L. hinge brace
    L. multiligamentous knee control
      orthosis
LeRoy clip-applying forceps
Leser-Trelat sign
lesion
    acute traumatic l.
    ALPSA l.
    anterior labrum periosteum shoulder
      arthroscopic l. (ALPSA)
    articular cartilage l.
    atlantoaxial l.
    Bankart shoulder l.
    Bennett l.
    biceps interval l. (BIL)
    bony l.
    Brown-Séquard l.
    callosal l.
    cartilaginous l.
    chiropractic l.
    cleavage l.
    complete common peroneal nerve l.
    cyclops l.
    cystic bone l.
    desmoid l.
    destructive l.
    disk l.
    DREZ l.
    dysarthric l.
    expansile l.
    fibrous l.
    Hagl l.
    hamartomatous l.
    Hill-Sachs shoulder l.
    hyperkeratotic l.
    intramedullary l.
    ipsilateral nerve root l.
    irregular-shaped l.
    irritable l.
    ischemic l.
    juxtaarticular l.
    Keasbey l.
    Kidner l.
    labral l.
    lytic bone l.
    Monteggia equivalent l.
    Morel-Lavele l.
    morphea-like l.
    muscular l.
    nerve root l.

neuromechanical l.
nonlinear l.
occult talar l.
Osgood-Schlatter l.
osteocartilaginous l.
osteochondral l.
osteopathic l.
pedal hyperpigmented l.
Perthes l.
Perthes-Bankart l.
postfracture l.
retroacetabular l.
reverse Hill-Sachs l.
rotator cuff l.
Sinding-Larsen-Johansson l.
skin l.
soft tissue l.
Stener l.
striatal l.
subchondral l.
superior labrum anterior and
  posterior l. (SLAP)
transient l.
traumatic, unidirectional instability
  and Bankart l. (TUBS)
tuberculous l.
uncommitted metaphyseal l.
upper motor neuron l.
vertebral l.
Wolin meniscoid l.
Woofry-Chandler classification of
  Osgood-Schlatter l.
Wrisberg l.

Leslie-Ryan
L.-R. anterior axillary approach
L.-R. modified axillary incision

LESS
lateral electrical surface stimulation

lesser
l. metatarsal
l. metatarsophalangeal joint
l. multangular
l. multangular bone
l. tarsal arthrodesis
l. toe
l. trochanter
l. trochanter fracture
l. tuberosity

Lester muscle forceps

Letournel
L. guideline
L. plate

Letournel-Judet
L.-J. acetabular fracture
  classification
L.-J. approach

Letterer-Siwe disease

Leukeran

leukocyte
neutrophilic l.
polymorphonuclear l.
l. scan

leukocytosis

leukodystrophy
Canavan l.

Leukotape
L. P sportstape

leukotriene

Leung thumb loss classification

levator
l. ani group
l. scapulae muscle
l. scapulae syndrome

level
l. of activity
comfort l.
l. foundation
myoinositol l.
segmental l.
sorbitol l.
spinal l.
vertebral l.

lever
l. arm
Lane bone l.

levering

Leveron door opener

Levin drill guide

Levine patellar tendon strap

Levis arm splint

levodopa

Levo-Dromoran

Levoprome

levorotary scoliosis

levorphanol
l. tartrate

levoscoliosis scoliosis

Levy & Rappel foot orthosis

Lewin
L. baseball-finger splint
L. bone-holding clamp
L. bone-holding forceps
L. bunion dissector
L. collar

L

NOTES

Lewin *(continued)*
L. punch test
L. reverse Lasègue test
L. snuff test
L. spinal perforating forceps
L. standing test
L. supine test
Lewin-Gaenslen test
Lewin-Stern
L.-S. finger splint
L.-S. thumb splint
Lewis
L. expandable adjustable prosthesis (LEAP)
L. intercalary resection
L. nail
L. periosteal elevator
L. rasp
L. Trapezio prosthesis
L. upper limb cardiovascular disease
Lewis-Chekofsky resection
Lewis-Prusik test
Lewit stretch technique
Lexan jacket
Lexer
L. chisel
L. gouge
L. osteotome
Lex-Ton spinal frame
Leyal arm
Leyla bar
LFAC
low-frequency alternating current
LFIT
low-friction ion treatment
LH1000 arthroscopic legholder
Lhermitte sign
liability
ergonomic assessment of risk and l. (EARLY)
LIAD
low-impact aerobic dance
Liberty spinal system
Librium
LICA
laser image custom arthroplasty
Lichtblau osteotomy
Lichtman
L. staging system
L. technique
Lidge cement gun
LIDO
LIDO lift and work set
LIDO WorkSET work simulator
Lido
L. Active Multijoint System
L. isokinetic dynamometer

L. lift
L. Passive Multijoint System
Lidoback isokinetic dynamometry system
lidocaine
bacitracin, neomycin, polymyxin B, and l.
l. and epinephrine
l. and prilocaine
Lido-Gel
L.-G. topical anesthetic Hydrogel
Liebolt radioulnar technique
life
L. Liner stick and cut-resistant glove
quality of l.
L. Satisfaction Index (LSI)
LIFEC
lumbar intersomatic fusion expandable cage
Lifestride treadmill
lifestyle
l. education (LSE)
sedentary l.
lift
BTE dynamic l.
DiPalma shoe l.
heel l.
Hoyer l.
Lido l.
M/L l.
shoe l.
VuRyser monitor l.
LiftALERT
lifting
biomechanics of l.
lift-off
l. test
tibial l.
varus-valgus l.
LiftStation
lig
ligament
ligature
Ligaclip applier
ligament (lig)
accessory atlantoaxial l.
accessory collateral l.
accessory lateral collateral l.
acromioclavicular l.
acromiocoracoid l.
alar l.
allograft reconstruction of fibular collateral l.
annular l.
anterior collateral l.
anterior cruciate l. (ACL)
anterior longitudinal l. (ALL)

anterior meniscofemoral l.
anterior oblique l. (AOL)
anterior sacrococcygeal l.
anterior sacroiliac l.
anterior talofibular l. (ATFL)
anterior tibiofibular l.
anterior tibiotalar l.
apical dental l.
arcuate l.
arcuate popliteal l.
artificial l.
atlantal transverse l.
atlantoaxial l.
atlantooccipital l.
l. augmentation device (LAD)
avulsed l.
l. avulsion
avulsion fibular collateral l.
Barkow l.
beak l.
bifurcate l.
l.-bone complex
l. button
calcaneoclavicular l.
calcaneocuboid l.
calcaneofibular l. (CFL)
calcaneonavicular l.
calcaneotibial l.
capital l.
capsular l.
carpal l.
cervical mover l.
CH l.
checkrein l.
Chrisman-Snook reconstruction of
  ankle l.
l. clamp
Cleland l.
collateral fibular l.
collateral radial l.
collateral tibial l.
collateral ulnar l.
congenital laxity of l.
conoid l.
coracoacromial l.
coracoclavicular l.
coracohumeral l.
coronary l.
corporotransverse inferior l.
corporotransverse superior l.
costoclavicular l.
costotransverse l.

cruciate l.
deep collateral l.
deep posterior sacrococcygeal l.
deep transverse carpal l.
deep transverse metacarpal l.
deep TV metatarsal l.
deltoid l.
deltotrapezius fascial l.
dorsal calcaneonavicular l.
dorsal carpometacarpal l.
dorsal cuboideonavicular l.
dorsal cuneocuboid l.
dorsal cuneonavicular l.
dorsal intercarpal l.
dorsal intercuneiform l.
dorsal metacarpal l.
dorsal metatarsal l.
dorsal radiocarpal l.
dorsal tarsometatarsal l.
dorsoradial l. (DRL)
dural l.
l. elongation
extraarticular knee l.
extrinsic l.
fabellofibular l.
fibular collateral l.
fibular sesamoidal l.
fibulocalcaneal l.
fibulotalar l.
fibulotalocalcaneal l.
first intermetacarpal l.
flaval l.
floating l.
fracture-dislocation with anterior l.
FTC l.
Gerdy l.
glenohumeral l. (GHL)
Gore-Tex anterior cruciate l.
l. graft
Grayson l.
Haines-McDougall medial
  sesamoid l.
hamate l.
l. of head of femur
Henle l.
humeral avulsion of the
  glenohumeral l. (HAGL)
l. of Humphrey
hypertrophic l.
iliofemoral l.
iliolumbar l.
iliopatellar l.

L

NOTES

ligament *(continued)*
  inferior band cruciform l.
  inferior calcaneonavicular l. (ICN)
  inferior glenohumeral l. (IGHL)
  inferior ilioischial l.
  infrapatellar l.
  inguinal l.
  intercarpal l.
  interclavicular l.
  interdigital l.
  intermetacarpal l. (IML)
  intermetatarsal l.
  interosseous cuneocuboid l.
  interosseous cuneometatarsal l.
  interosseous intercarpal l.
  interosseous intercuneiform l.
  interosseous metacarpal l.
  interosseous metatarsal l.
  interosseous sacroiliac l.
  interosseous talocalcaneal l.
  intersesamoid l.
  interspinal l.
  interspinous l.
  intertransverse l.
  intervolar plate l.
  intraarticular disk l.
  ischiofemoral l.
  lacinate l.
  Landsmeer l.
  lateral atlantooccipital l.
  lateral collateral l. (LCL)
  lateral costotransverse l.
  lateral interosseous l.
  lateral sacrococcygeal l.
  lateral spring l.
  lateral talocalcaneal l. (LTC)
  limited proteoglycan matrix of l.
  Lisfranc l.
  longitudinal l.
  long plantar l. (LPL)
  LRL l.
  LT l.
  lumbocostal l.
  lunotriquetral l.
  medial capsular l.
  medial collateral l. (MCL)
  medial patellofemoral l. (MPFL)
  medial talocalcaneal l.
  meniscofemoral l.
  meniscotibial l.
  metacarpal l.
  metacarpoglenoidal l.
  metacarpophalangeal l.
  middle glenohumeral l.
  midline l.
  natatory l.
  naviculocuneiform l.
  nuchal l.

  oblique popliteal l.
  oblique retinacular l.
  orbicular l.
  ossification of the posterior
    longitudinal l. (OPLL)
  palmar carpometacarpal l.
  palmar intercarpal deltoid l.
  palmar metacarpal l.
  palmar radiocarpal l.
  palmar ulnocarpal l.
  patellar l.
  patellofemoral l.
  patellomeniscal l.
  patellotibial l.
  petroclinoid l.
  pisiform metacarpal l.
  pisohamate l.
  pisometacarpal l.
  plantar calcaneocuboid l.
  plantar calcaneonavicular l.
  plantar cuboideonavicular l.
  plantar cuneocuboid l.
  plantar cuneonavicular l.
  plantar intercuneiform l.
  plantar metatarsal l.
  plantar spring l.
  plantar tarsometatarsal l.
  popliteal l.
  posterior cruciate l. (PCL)
  posterior longitudinal l. (PLL)
  posterior meniscofemoral l.
  posterior oblique l. (POL)
  posterior sacroiliac l.
  posterior talofibular l. (PTFL)
  posterior tibiofibular l.
  posterior tibiotalar l.
  Poupart inguinal l.
  quadrate l.
  radial carpal collateral l.
  radial collateral l. (RCL)
  radial metacarpal l.
  radiate carpal l.
  radiate sternocostal l.
  radiocapitate l.
  radiocarpal l.
  radiolunotriquetral l.
  radioscaphocapitate l.
  radioscaphoid l.
  radioscapholunate l.
  radiotriquetral l.
  rearfoot l.
  l. reconstruction
  l. replacement
  retinacular l.
  round l.
  Rouviere l.
  sacroiliac l.
  sacrospinal l.

sacrospinous l.
sacrotuberal l.
sacrotuberous l.
scapholunate interosseous l.
scaphotrapezoid interosseous l.
scapular l.
scapulohumeral l.
l.-scar matrix
sesamoid l.
sesamophalangeal l.
short plantar l. (SPL)
spinal posterior l.
spinal transverse l.
spiral oblique retinacular l.
spring l.
SRL l.
sternoclavicular l.
l. of Struthers
subtalar interosseous l.
superficial medial l.
superficial posterior
  sacrococcygeal l.
superficial transverse l.
superficial TV metacarpal l.
superficial TV metatarsal l.
superior costotransverse l.
superomedial calcaneonavicular l.
  (SMCR)
supraspinal l.
supraspinous l.
syndesmotic l.
talofibular l.
talonavicular l.
l. of tarsus
tectoral l.
tibial collateral l. (TCL)
tibial sesamoid l.
tibiocalcaneal l.
tibiofibular l.
tibionavicular l.
torn meniscotibial l.
transverse acetabular l.
transverse atlantal l.
transverse carpal l.
transverse intertarsal l.
transverse metatarsal l.
transverse retinacular l.
transverse scapular l.
transverse spinal l.
trapezoid l.
traumatized l.
triangular l.

ulnar carpal collateral l.
ulnar collateral l. (UCL)
ulnocarpal l.
ulnolunate l.
ulnotriquetral l.
vaginal hand l.
volar beak l.
volar carpal l.
Weitbrecht l.
l. of Wrisberg
yellow l.
Zenotech biomaterial-synthetic l.

ligamenta
l. carpometacarpalia dorsalia
l. carpometacarpalia palmaria
l. collateralia articulationum
  interphalangealium manus
l. collateralia articulationum
  interphalangealium pedis
l. collateralia articulationum
  metacarpophalangealium
l. collateralia articulationum
  metatarsophalangealium
l. cruciata genus
l. cuneometatarsalia interossea
l. cuneonavicularia dorsalia
l. cuneonavicularia plantaria
l. glenohumeralia
l. intercarpalia interossea
l. intercarpalia palmaria
l. intercuneiformia dorsalia
l. intercuneiformia interossea
l. intercuneiformia plantaria
l. interspinalia
l. intertransversaria
l. metacarpalia dorsalia
l. metacarpalia interossea
l. metacarpalia palmaria
l. metatarsalia dorsalia
l. metatarsalia interossea
l. metatarsalia plantaria
l. palmaria articulationum
  interphalangealium
l. plantaria articulationum
  interphalangealium pedis
l. plantaria articulationum
  metatarsophalangealium
l. sacroiliaca anteriora
l. sacroiliaca interossea
l. sacroiliaca posteriora
l. tarsi
l. tarsi dorsalia

L

NOTES

ligamenta *(continued)*
  l. tarsi interossea
  l. tarsi plantaria
  l. tarsometatarsalia dorsalia
  l. tarsometatarsalia plantaria
ligamentoplasty
ligamentotaxis
  multiplanar l.
ligamentous
  l. ankylosis
  l. attachment
  l. bouncing
  l. box
  l. complex
  l. disruption
  l. injury
  l. insertion
  l. instability test
  l. insufficiency
  l. laxity
  l. luxation
  l. release
  l. repair of the knee for rotatory
    instability
  l. stability
  l. structure
  l. support tissue
  l. thickening
ligamentous-muscular hypertrophy
ligaments
ligamentum
  l. acromioclaviculare
  l. alaria
  l. anulare radii
  l. apicis dentis axis
  l. atlanto-occipitale laterale
  l. bifurcatum
  l. calcaneocuboideum
  l. calcaneocuboideum plantare
  l. calcaneofibulare
  l. calcaneonaviculare
  l. calcaneonaviculare dorsale
  l. calcaneonaviculare plantare
  l. calcaneotibiale
  l. capitis costae intraarticulare
  l. capitis costae radiatum
  l. capitis femoris
  l. capitis fibulae anterius
  l. capitis fibulae posterius
  l. carpi radiatum
  l. carpi transversum
  l. carpi volare
  l. caudale integumenti communis
  l. collaterale carpi radiale
  l. collaterale carpi ulnare
  l. collaterale fibulare
  l. collaterale radiale
  l. collaterale ulnare

  l. collateral tibiale
  l. conoideum
  l. coracoacromiale
  l. coracoclaviculare
  l. coracohumerale
  l. costoclaviculare
  l. costotransversarium
  l. costotransversarium laterale
  l. costotransversarium superius
  l. cruciatum anterius genus
  l. cruciatum cruris
  l. cruciatum posterius genus
  l. cruciforme atlantis
  l. cuboideonaviculare dorsale
  l. cuboideonaviculare plantare
  l. cuneocuboideum dorsale
  l. cuneocuboideum interosseum
  l. cuneocuboideum plantare
  l. flavum
  l. flavum forceps
  l. iliofemorale
  l. iliolumbale
  l. inguinale
  l. intercarpalia dorsalia interossea
  l. interclaviculare
  l. ischiofemorale
  l. laterale articulationis talocruralis
  l. longitudinale anterius
  l. longitudinale posterius
  l. lumbocostale
  l. mediale articulationis talocruralis
  l. meniscofemorale anterius
  l. meniscofemorale posterius
  l. metacarpale transversum
    superficiale
  l. metacarpeum transversum
    profundum
  l. metatarsale transversum
    profundum
  l. metatarsale transversum
    superficiale
  l. mucosum
  l. nuchae
  l. patellae
  l. pisohamatum
  l. pisometacarpeum
  l. plantare longum
  l. popliteum arcuatum
  l. popliteum obliquum
  l. quadratum
  l. radiocarpale dorsale
  l. radiocarpale palmare
  l. sacrococcygeum anterius
  l. sacrococcygeum laterale
  l. sacrococcygeum posterius
    profundum
  l. sacrococcygeum posterius
    superficiale

l. sacrospinalum
l. sacrotuberale
l. supraspinale
l. talocalcaneare laterale
l. talocalcaneare mediale
l. talocalcaneum interosseum
l. talofibulare anterius
l. talonaviculare
l. teres
l. tibiofibulare anterius
l. tibiofibulare posterius
l. transversum acetabuli
l. transversum atlantis
l. transversum cruris
l. transversum genus
l. transversum scapulae inferius
l. transversum scapulae superius
l. trapezoideum
l. ulnocarpale palmare

Ligamentus
L. Ankle ankle orthotic
L. Ankle orthosis

ligand adhesive
ligature (lig)
l. carrier
l. guide
l. passer
stick tie l.

light
l. cast
Cogent l.
l. conductor
l. cross-slot screwdriver
infrared l. (IR)
l. microscopy
l. source
therapeutic l.
l. touch sensation
l. touch test
ultraviolet l. (UV)
L. V sign

lightheadedness
Lightplast athletic tape
LIH
Lars Ingvar Hansson
LIH hook pin

Lilienthal rib spreader
Lima external fixator
limb
l. accurate measurement (LAM)
artificial l.
l. bud

l. girdle
l. gym
hanging of l.
l. holder
ischemic l.
left lower l. (LLL)
left upper l. (LUL)
l. length angulation
l. length discrepancy
l.-length disparity
l. lengthening
plantigrade l.
l. replantation
residual l.
right lower l. (RLL)
right upper l. (RUL)
l. salvage
seal l.
l.-sparing operation
l. synergy
Trowbridge TerraRound sports l.
Utah artificial l.

limb absence
congenital intercalary l. a.
congenital terminal l. a.

Limberg flap
limb-girdle
l.-g. dystrophy
l.-g. lengthening
l.-g.-trunk paresis

limb-salvage
l.-s. procedure
l.-s. surgery

limbus annularis
limit
elastic l.
endurance l.
metal endurance l.
motion l.

limitation
l. of joint motion
motion l.
l. of motion (LOM)
l. of movement

limited
l.-contact dynamic compression
plate
l. fasciectomy
l.-field radiation
l. joint mobility (LJM)
l.-motion metal ankle joint

L

NOTES

347

limited *(continued)*
    l. performance measure
    l. proteoglycan matrix of ligament
limiter
    Becker 655 motion control l.
    motion control l. (MCL)
    Motion Control L. (755 MCL)
limitus
    McKeever arthrodesis for hallux l.
    Regnauld free phalangeal base
      autograft for hallux l.
    Z-slide lengthening in hallux l.
limp
    Trendelenburg l.
LINAC
    linear accelerator
    Boston LINAC
    Siemens LINAC
    University of Florida LINAC
    Varian LINAC
Linberg syndrome
lincomycin
Lindell classification
Lindeman procedure
Linder sign
Lindgren oblique osteotomy
Lindholm
    L. open surgical tendon repair
    L. technique
    L. tendo calcaneus repair
Lindseth osteotomy
Lindsjö method
Lindvall-Stille knife
line
    action l.
    ant ax l. (AAL)
    anterior axillary l. (AAL)
    anterior humeral l.
    antitension l.
    Beau l.'s
    bisector l.
    Blumensaat l.
    cement l.
    Chamberlain l.
    cleavage l.
    coronoid l.
    cyma l.
    l. of demarcation
    divisionary l.
    epiphyseal l.
    Feiss l.
    femoral head l. (FHL)
    fracture l.
    Fränkel white l.
    George l.
    gravitational l.
    l. of gravity
    gravity l.

growth arrest l.
Harris growth arrest l.
Hawkins l.
Hilgenreiner horizontal Y l.
Hilgenreiner-Pauwels l.
Hilgenreiner-Perkins l.
H-P l.
Hueter l.
interteardrop l.
joint l.
Kaplan oblique l.
Köhler l.'s
Langer l.
lateral joint l.
lead l.
Looser l.'s
lumbar gravitational l.
MacNab l.
McGregor l.
medial joint l.
Meyer l.
Meyerding spondylolisthesis
    classification l.
midaxillary l. (MAL)
midheel l.
midmalleolar l.
midsternal l. (MSL)
Moloney l.
Nélaton l.
nipple l.
oblique metacarpal l.
odontoid perpendicular l.
Ombredanne-Perkins l.
parajugular l.
Perkins vertical l.
physeal l.
plumb l.
posterior axillary l. (PAL)
posterior cervical l.
radiocapitellar l.
radiolucent l.
sacral arcuate l.
sacral horizontal plane l. (SHPL)
sclerotic l.
scurvy l.
Shenton l.
spinolaminar l.
Sydney l.
teardrop l.
tibiofibular l.
l.-to-line reaming technique
trapezoid l.
trough l.
Ullman l.
Whitesides l.
Winberger l.
Z l.
l.'s of Zahn

linea
  l. aspera femoris
  l. semilunaris
  l. terminalis
linear
  l. accelerator (LINAC)
  l. fraction
  l. fracture
  l. potentiometer
  l. scar
linear-variable-differential transducer
linebacker's arm
linen suture
liner
  acetabular l.
  acetabular prosthetic l.
  Alpha cushion l.
  Alps ClearLine silicone
    suspension l.
  Alps CustomPro custom l.
  bone l.
  cast l.
  cushion shoe l.
  DePuy acetabular l.
  Duraloc acetabular l.
  elevated rim acetabular l.
  Enduron acetabular l.
  Fillauer prosthesis l.
  Fillauer silicone suspension l.
  Gore-Tex waterproof cast l.
  grommet bone l.
  Hylamer acetabular l.
  Iceross Comfort Plus silicone
    gel l.
  OrthoGel l.
  Plastizote shoe l.
  polyethylene l.
  Polysorb l.
  Reflection l.
  Spenco l.
  splint l.
  TEC l.
Ling cemented hip prosthesis
lingual
  l. artery
  l. dysarthria
  l. vein
lining
  DePuy acetabular l.
link
  L. anatomical hip

  L. custom partial pelvis
    replacement system
  L. Endo-Model rotational knee
    system
  L. MP hip noncemented
    reconstruction prosthesis
  L. MP (microporous) hip stem
  musculotendinous-osseous l.
  L. Saddle Prosthesis Endo-Model
    hip replacement system
  L. Stack Split Splint
  L. toe splint
linkage
  kinematic l.
  rod l.
linked potential
Linton procedure
Linvatec
  L. absorbable screw
  L. arthroscopic infusion pump
  L. driver
**Lionberger-Bishop-Tullos anterior
  arthrodesis**
lion forceps
lion-jaw forceps
Lioresal Intrathecal
lip
  l. of acetabulum
  l. of glenoid
  l. of navicular
  osteophytic bone l.
  posterior l.
  l. of taenia
  l. of tibia
lipid
  l. inclusion cyst
  l. storage disease
  l. tumor
lipoblastomatosis
lipochondrodystrophy
lipofibroma
  intraneural l.
lipofibromatosis
lipofibromatous hamartoma
lipoma
  endovaginal l.
  intraosseous l.
  pleomorphic l.
  spindle-cell l.
lipoprotein
liposarcoma
  myxoid l.

L

NOTES

liposarcoma *(continued)*
    myxoid-type l.
    pleomorphic l.
    round cell l.
    round cell type l.
    well-differentiated myxoid l.
lipoxygenase
lipping
Lippman
    L. hip prosthesis
    L. test
Lipscomb
    L. metatarsophaleangeal arthrodesis
    L. modified McKeever arthrodesis
    L. procedure
    L. technique
Lipscomb-Anderson
    L.-A. drill guide
    L.-A. procedure
liquid
    l. cable
    l. crystal thermography (LCT)
    Lotrimin AF Spray L.
    l. nitrogen cryotherapy
    L. Pred
    Tums Extra Strength L.
Liquiprin
Lisch nodule
Lisfranc
    L. amputation
    L. arthrodesis
    L. articular interline
    L. articular set angle (LASA)
    L. below-knee prosthesis
    L. disarticulation
    L. dislocation
    L. fracture
    L. fracture-dislocation
    L. injury
    L. joint
    L. joint articulation
    L. joint complex
    L. ligament
    L. tubercle
list
    postural l.
Lister
    L. corn
    L. technique
    L. tubercle
listhesis
    anterior-posterior l.
    lateral l.
listing
    dynamic l.
    l. gait
    static l.

Liston
    L. amputating knife
    L. amputation knife
    L. bone-cutting forceps
    L. phalangeal knife
    L. splint
Liston-Key bone-cutting forceps
Liston-Key-Horsley rib shears
Liston-Littauer
    L.-L. bone-cutting forceps
    L.-L. rongeur
Liston-Stille bone-cutting forceps
Lite
    TechCel L.
Lite-Gait partial weight-bearing gait therapy device
lithotomy
    l. legholder
    l. position
litigation reaction
Littauer-Liston bone-cutting forceps
Littauer-West rongeur
litter
    Neal-Robertson l.
little
    L. cargo vest
    l. finger (5th digit)
    l. leaguer's shoulder
    L. release
    L. technique
Littler
    L. opponensplasty
    L. pollicization
    L. technique
    wing excision of L.
Littler-Cooley
    L.-C. abductor digiti quinti transfer
    L.-C. muscle transfer
    L.-C. technique
liver
    l. disease
    l. injury
    l., spleen, kidney (LSK)
Liverpool
    L. elbow prosthesis
    L. knee prosthesis
live splint
living
    activities of daily l. (ADLs)
    instrumental activities of daily l. (IADL)
    Katz index of activities of daily l.
Livingstone therapy
Livingston intramedullary bar
Liviscope scope
Livotrit Plus
Lizzie doll

LJM
    limited joint mobility
LLC
    long leg cast
LLD
    leg length discrepancy
LLE
    left lower extremity
LLI
    leg length inequality
LLL
    left lower limb
    lower fossa active, lateral knee pain, and
      long leg on the side ipsilateral to the
      weak fossa
LLO
    lower limb orthosis
Llorente dissecting forceps
Lloyd
    L. adapter
    L. adapter for Smith-Petersen nail
    L. chiropractic table
    L. nail driver
Lloyd-Roberts
    L.-R. fracture technique
    L.-R. open reduction of Monteggia
      fracture
Lloyd-Roberts-Catteral-Salamon
  classification
LLP
    lower limb prosthesis
LLPS
    low-load prolonged stretch
    low-pressure plasma spray
    LLPS hydroxyapatite
    LLPS hydroxyapatite adhesive
LLS
    long leg splint
LLWBC
    long leg weightbearing cast
LLWC
    long leg walking cast
LMB
    L. finger splint
    L. resting splint
L'Nard
    L. boot
    L. Multi-Podus orthosis
    L. thoracolumbosacral orthosis
LNS
    localized nodular synovitis

LNV
    last normal vertebra
Lo
    L. Bak spinal support
    L. Bak spinal support prosthesis
load
    applied l.
    axial compression l.
    l. beam
    l.-bearing graft
    bending l.
    compression l.
    critical l.
    l.-deflection curve
    l.-deformation curve
    Euler l.
    ramp l.
    rotatory l.
    l. and shift test
    spinal axial l.
    l.-to-grip displacement
    torque l.
    torsional l.
load-displacement
    l.-d. curve
    l.-d. plot
loading
    axial l.
    compression l.
    concentric l.
    cyclic l.
    eccentric l.
    Edwards modular system
      dynamic l.
    fracture callus l.
    functional and anatomic l. (FAL)
    l. mode
    progressive l.
    status l.
    sustained l.
    tension l.
    l. time
    vertical l.
Loban adhesive drape
lobster-claw
    l.-c. deformity
    l.-c. hand
lobster foot
lobster-type clamp
local
    l. adaptation syndrome (LAS)
    l. anesthesia

L

NOTES

351

local *(continued)*
    l. epineurotomy
    l. radical resection
    l. standby anesthesia technique
Localio-Francis-Rossano resection
Localio procedure
localization
    pedicle l.
localized nodular synovitis (LNS)
localizer cast
locating pin
location
    cervical sympathetic chain l.
    pedicle l.
locator
    Berman-Moorhead metal l.
    metal l.
lock
    grip l.
    knee l.
    l. nut
    spring-loaded knee l.
Locke
    L. bone clamp
    L. elevator
locked
    l. knee
    l. nailing
    l. scapula
locking
    anatomic medullary l. (AML)
    l. clamp
    distal l.
    l. hook instrumentation
    l.-hook spinal rod
    l. horizontal mattress suture
    l. of joint
    l. nail
    l. nut
    l. peg
    l.-position test
    l. prosthesis
    proximal l.
    sacroiliac joint l.
    l. screw
lockjaw
locknut wrench
locomotion
locomotor
    l. ataxia
    l. mechanism
    l. pattern
    l. system
Lodine XL
Loeffler-Ballard incision
Lofstrand
    L. brace
    L. crutch

Logan traction
logrolling maneuver
Lok-it screwdriver
Lok-screw double-slot screwdriver
lollipop
LOM
    limitation of motion
London unconstrained elbow prosthesis
long
    l. arm brace
    l. arm cast (LAC)
    l. arm finger cast
    l. arm splint
    l. axial alignment guide
    l. axis
    l. axis of bone
    l. axis ray
    l. bent-knee leg cast
    l. bone
    l. bone deficiency
    l. bone fracture
    l. bone osteomyelitis
    l. coarse bur
    l. curette
    l. deltopectoral approach
    l. extensor
    l. external rotator
    l. finger (3rd digit)
    l. flexor
    l. head
    l. head of biceps
    l. head biceps tendon
    l.-jaw basket forceps
    l.-latency SEP
    l. leg cast (LLC)
    l. leg hinged brace
    l. leg immobilizer
    l. leg orthosis
    l. leg splint (LLS)
    l. leg stockings
    l. leg walking cast (LLWC)
    l. leg weightbearing cast (LLWBC)
    l. nail-mounted drill guide
    l. oblique fracture
    l. opponens orthosis
    l. plantar ligament (LPL)
    l.-radius kyphosis
    l. segment spinal fusion
    l. and short lever rotational
        manipulation
    l.-stemmed powered bur
    l.-term bone-instrumentation
        interface
    l. thoracic nerve injury
    l. thoracic nerve palsy
    l. toe flexor
    l. tract sign
Longevity V-Lign hip prosthesis

longissimus
    l. capitis musculus
    l. cervicis musculus
longitudinal
    l. arch
    l. axis
    l. blood supply
    l. blood supply to ulnar nerve
    l. deficiency
    l. displaced complete tear
    l. distraction
    l. epiphyseal bracket
    l. fracture
    l. incision
    l. incomplete intrameniscal tear
    l. ligament
    l. ligament rupture
    l. member to anchor connector
    l. member to longitudinal member
      connector
    l. meniscal tear
    l. spinal bar
    l. traction
longstanding
longum
    ligamentum plantare l.
    vinculum l.
longus
    adductor hallucis l.
    l. capitis muscle
    l. capitis musculus
    l. cervicis (colli) muscle
    l. colli muscle
    extensor carpi radialis l. (ECRL)
    extensor digitorum l. (EDL)
    extensor hallucis l. (EHL)
    extensor pollicis l. (EPL)
    flexor digitorum l. (FDL)
    flexor hallucis l. (FHL)
    flexor pollicis l. (FPL)
    palmaris l. (PL)
    peroneus l.
loop
    Bunnell finger l.
    l. circumferential wire
    Duncan l.
    figure-of-eight wire l.
    finger l.
    l. fixation
    l. & hook strapping
    l.-lock cock-up splint
    l.-over wrap

    Ransford l.
    l. scissors
    thumb l.
    toe l.
    wire l.
loose
    l. body
    l. body grasper
    l. fracture
    l. fragment
    l. knee procedure
    L. procedure
loosening
    acetabular component l.
    aseptic l.
    Harris criteria for implant l.
    screw l.
    sterile l.
Looser lines
Lo-Por vascular graft prosthesis
Loprox
LOPS
    loss of protective sensation
Lopurin
lorazepam
Lorcet
    L. 10
    L. Plus
Lorcet-HD
Lord
    L. cup
    L. Press-Fit hip prosthesis
lordoscoliosis
lordosis
    cervical l.
    l. creation
    lumbar spine l.
    occipitocervical l.
    l. preservation
    reversal of l.
    reversal of cervical l.
    thoracic spine l.
lordotic curve
lordoticiser
    Posture Pump l.
Lorenz
    L. brace
    L. cast
    L. hip reduction
    L. osteosynthesis system
    L. procedure
    L. sign

L

NOTES

Lorenzo screw
Lore suction tube and tip-holding
forceps
lorry driver's fracture
Lortab ASA
LOS
length of stay
Losee
L. knee instability test
L. modification
L. modification of MacIntosh
technique
L. sling and reef technique
loss
blood l.
bone l.
estimated blood l.
lumbar lordosis iatrogenic l.
l. of motion
motor l.
postmenopausal bone l.
l. of protective sensation (LOPS)
segmental bone l.
sensory l.
Loth-Kirschner drill
lotion
Biotone Polar l.
Criticaid l.
Hydrisinol l.
Lac-Hydrin l.
Lactinol l.
Lotrimin AF L.
Myossage l.
Polysonic ultrasound l.
Restore AF antifungal l.
Senuva l.
Ultra Mide 25 l.
Ureacin-10 l.
Lotrimin
L. AF Cream
L. AF Lotion
L. AF Solution
L. AF Spray Liquid
L. AF Spray Powder
Lotrisone
Lottes
L. nailing
L. pin
L. triflanged medullary nail
lotus position
Lou Gehrig disease
Louisiana
L. ankle wrap technique
L. State University (LSU)
Louis instrumentation
loupe
binocular l.
l. magnification

magnifying l.
surgical l.
Love
L. nerve root retractor
L. splint
Love-Adson periosteal elevator
Love-Gruenwald alligator forceps
Love-Kerrison rongeur forceps
Lovell clubfoot cast
Lovenox Injection
Lovett clinical scale of strength
Lovitt-Uhler modification of Jewett
post-fusion brace
low
l.-air-loss bed
l. back injury
l. back neurosis
l. back pain (LBP)
L. Back Pain Symptom Checklist
l. cervical approach
l.-contact dynamic compression
plate
l. contact stress (LCS)
l.-energy fracture
l.-frequency alternating current
(LFAC)
l.-friction ion treatment (LFIT)
l.-grade central osteogenic sarcoma
l.-impact aerobic dance (LIAD)
l. impedance thermocouple
l.-load prolonged stretch (LLPS)
Low-Contact Stress implant
l. lumbar spine fracture
l. median-low ulnar palsy
l.-neck femoral prosthesis
l.-pressure plasma spray (LLPS)
L. Profile legholder
L. Profile plastic body jacket
l.-purine diet
l. quarter Blucher shoe
l.-riding patella
l. single thoracic curve
l.-surface reactive
l.-temperature plastic
l. T humerus fracture
l. viscosity bone cement
LowDye
L. strapping
L. taping
L. taping technique
Lowe-Breck
L.-B. cartilage knife
L.-B. meniscectomy knife
Lowell
L. reduction
L. view
Lowe-Miller unconstrained elbow
prosthesis

lower
- l. cervical spine
- l. cervical spine fusion
- l. cervical spine posterior stabilization
- l. cervical spine procedure
- l. extremity (LE)
- l. extremity surgery
- l. fossa active, lateral knee pain, and long leg on the side ipsilateral to the weak fossa (LLL)
- l. hand retractor
- l. hook trial
- l. limb orthosis (LLO)
- l. limb prosthesis (LLP)
- l. lumbar spine
- l. motor neuron disease
- l. plexus injury
- l. posterior lumbar spine and sacrum surgery
- l. thoracic pedicle
- l. thoracic spine

lower-extremity amputation (LEA)

Lowman
- L. bone-holding clamp
- L. bone-holding forceps
- L. chisel
- L. hand retractor
- L. shelf procedure

Lowman-Gerster bone clamp

Lowman-Hoglund
- L.-H. chisel
- L.-H. clamp

low-profile
- l.-p. cup
- l.-p. femoral prosthesis
- l.-p. halo traction

LP
lumbar puncture

LPF
leg protection factor

LPL
long plantar ligament

LPPS hydroxyapatite fixation

LRL ligament

L-rod
Luque L-r.

LRS
lateral recess stenosis

LS
lumbosacral
lumbosacral spine

LS⁴ custom spinal jacket

LSE
lifestyle education

L-shaped
- L-s. capsular incision
- L-s. capsulotomy
- L-s. plate
- L-s. rod

LSI
Life Satisfaction Index
LSI Easy Stims self-adhesive electrode
LSI silver self-adhesive disposable electrode

LSK
liver, spleen, kidney

L-spine
lumbar spine

LSU
Louisiana State University
LSU reciprocation-gait orthosis
LSU reciprocation-gait orthosis brace
LSU reciprocator

LT
lactate threshold
lunotriquetral
LT joint
LT ligament

LTC
lateral talocalcaneal ligament

L-tryptophan

Lubinus
- L. acetabular component
- L. AP hip system
- L. knee prosthesis
- L. SP II
- L. SP II anatomically adapted hip system

lubrication

Lucae bone mallet

Lucas
- L. chisel
- L. and Drucker Motor Index
- L. gouge

Lucas-Cottrell osteotomy

Lucas-Murray knee arthrodesis

L

NOTES

lucency
cortical l.
subchondral l.
lucent
Luck
L. bone drill
L. hand procedure
L. hip cup
Luck-Bishop bone saw
Ludington
L. sign
L. test
Ludloff
L. incision
L. medial approach
L. osteotomy
L. sign
L. technique
Ludwig plane
LUE
left upper extremity
Luekens wrinkle test
Luer
L. bone rongeur
L. rongeur forceps
Luer-Friedman bone rongeur
Luer-Hartmann rongeur
Luer-Whiting rongeur forceps
Luhr
L. fixation system
L. Microfixation cranial plate
L. Microfixation System drill bit
L. Microfixation System plate cutter
L. Microfixation System plate-holding forceps
L. Microfixation System pliers
L. microplate
L. miniplate
L. pan plate
L. screw
LUL
left upper limb
Lulu clamp
lumbago-mechanical instability syndrome
lumbar
l. accessory movement technique
l. agenesis
l. anesthesia
l. brace
l. disk
l. disk disorder
l. diskography
l. distraction manipulation
l. epidural endoscopy
l. extension
l. extension test
l. facetal and interbody joint

l. facet injection
l. fascia
l. flat back syndrome
l. gravitational line
l. intersomatic fusion expandable cage (LIFEC)
l. kyphosis
l. lateral flexion
l. lateral flexion test
l. lordosis iatrogenic loss
l. lordosis preservation
l. lordotic curve
l. microtrauma
l. nerve root injection
l. pedicle
l. pedicle fixation
l. pedicle marker
l. pedicle screw
l. plexus injury
l. protective mechanism test
l. puncture (LP)
l. range of motion
l. roll
l. rotation
l. rotation test
l. sagittal mobility
l. scoliosis
l. spine (L-spine)
l. spine biopsy
l. spine burst fracture
l. spine decompression
l. spine fusion
l. spine instability
l. spine instrumentation
l. spine kyphotic deformity
l. spine lordosis
l. spine model
l. spine pedicle diameter
l. spine rotational stability
l. spine segmental fixation
l. spine transpedicular fixation
l. spine trauma
l. spine vertebral osteosynthesis
l. sympathectomy
l. tumor
l. vein
l. vertebra
l. vertebral interbody fusion
lumbocostale
ligamentum l.
lumbocostal ligament
lumbodorsal fascia (LDF)
lumbopelvic
l. complex
l. radiograph
lumbosacral (LS)
l. cartilaginous system
l. corset

l. dislocation
l. flexion
l. fusion
l. fusion elevator
l. joint angle
l. junction
l. junction bone density
l. junction cortical thickness
l. junction fracture
l. kyphosis
l. orthosis
l. plexus
l. series
l. spine (LS)
l. spine transpedicular
  instrumentation
l. spondylolisthesis
l. vertebra

lumbrical

l. bar
l. intrinsic contracture
l. muscle
l. syndrome finger
l. tendon

lumbricalis muscle
lumbrical-plus

l.-p. finger
l.-p. phenomenon

Lumex

L. lightweight wheelchair
L. walker

lunate

l. acrylic cement wrist prosthesis
l. bone
l. dislocation
l. facet dye punch injury
l. fracture
l.-triquetral coalition

lunatomalacia
Lunceford-Pilliar-Engh hip prosthesis
Lunceford total hip replacement
Lundholm

L. plate
L. screw

lunocapitate bone
lunotriquetral (LT)

l. arthrodesis
l. dissociation
l. fusion
l. instability

l. ligament
l. shear test

lunula, pl. lunulae
Luongo hand retractor
lupus

l. anticoagulant
l. erythematosus (LE)
l. erythematosus preparation

Luque

L. cerclage wire
L. fixation device
L. II fixation system
L. II plate
L. II screw
L. II segmental spinal
  instrumentation
L. instrumentation concave
  technique
L. instrumentation convex technique
L. loop fixation
L. L-rod
L. pedicle screw
L. rectangle
L. ring
L. rod
L. rod bender
L. rod fixation
L. rod fixation for kyphosis
L. rod migration
L. segmental fixation
L. semirigid segmental spinal
  instrumentation
L. sublaminar wiring technique
L. wiring

Luque-Galveston

L.-G. fixation
L.-G. post

lurch

abductor l.
gluteal l.
Trendelenburg l.

lurching gait
Luschka

L. bursa
L. joint

Lusskin bone drill
luxans

coxa vara l.

luxated bone
luxatio

l. coxae congenita
l. erecta shoulder dislocation

L

NOTES

luxatio *(continued)*
    l. pedis subtalo
    l. perinealis
luxation
    atlantoaxial l.
    incomplete l.
    ligamentous l.
    palmar l.
Lyden-Lehman technique
Lyden technique
lying
    side l.
Lyman-Smith
    L.-S. toe drop brace
    L.-S. traction
Lyme disease
lymph
    l. vessel
    l. vessel tumor
lymphadenopathy
lymphangiography
lymphangioma
    cavernous l.
lymphangiosarcoma
lymphatic
lymphedema
    familial l.
    l. sling
lymphocyte count
lymphoma
    angiotropic l.

    malignant l.
    non-Hodgkin l.
Lynco
    L. biomechanical orthotic system
    L. foot orthosis
Lynn
    L. technique
    L. tendo calcaneus repair
LYOfoam
    L. C dressing
    L. wound dressing
lyophilization of bone
lyophilized bone graft
Lyphocin
lyre-shaped finger hook
Lysholm
    L. Knee Scale
    L. knee scoring questionnaire
    L. score
Lysholm-Gillquist
    L.-G. knee subjective function
      scale
    L.-G. knee subjective function
      score
lysis
lysosomal absorption
Lyte Fit orthotic
lytic bone lesion
Lytle metacarpal splint

M

    M band
    M wave

3M

    3M fiberglass cast
    3M Maxi Driver blade
    3M prep
    3M skin drape

M/3

    middle third

mA

    milliampere

MAC

    Miami Acute Care
    MAC anesthesia
    MAC cervical collar

MacAusland

    M. lumbar brace
    M. procedure

MacCarthy procedure

maceration

Macewen

    M. classification
    M. drill
    M. sign

Macewen-Shands osteotomy

MacGregor

    M. osteotome
    M. osteotomy

machine

    Accu-Tron microcurrent m.
    ankle exercise m.
    Biodex isokinetic testing m.
    borazone blade cutting m.
    CamStar exercise m.
    continuous passive motion m.
    cooling m.
    CPM m.
    Cybex m.
    elliptical m.
    Griswold distraction m.
    Instron m.
    Isotechnologies B-200 low back m.
    isotonic m.
    KineTec hip CPM m.
    MB-900 AC m.
    MedX functional testing m.
    MedX Mark II lumbar
      extension m.
    MedX stretch m.
    Orthion traction m.
    passive motion m.
    SAM spinal analysis m.
    m. screw
    spinal analysis m. (SAM)

    VersaClimber exercise m.
    Wikco ankle m.

machine-gun-like pain

MacIntosh

    M. extraarticular tenodesis
    M. hip prosthesis
    M. iliotibial band tenodesis
    M. lateral pivot shift test
    M. over-the-top ACL reconstruction
    M. over-the-top repair
    M. technique
    M. tibial plateau prosthesis

MacKentry periosteal

Mackinnon-Dellon

    M.-D. criteria
    M.-D. staging system

MacKinnon nerve injury

Maclaren mobile buggy

MacNab

    M. line
    M. line for facet imbrication
    M. operation
    M. shoulder repair

MacNab-English shoulder prosthesis

MacNichol-Voutsinas classification

macroadhesion

macrocoil

    Gianturco m.

macrodactylia fibrolipomatosis

macrodactyly

macroelectromyography (macro-EMG)

macro-EMG

    macroelectromyography
    macro-EMG needle electrode

Macrofit hip prosthesis

macroglobulinemia

    Waldenstrom m.

**macro motor unit action potential
(MUAP)**

macronychia

macrophage

macroradiograph

macrotrauma

macularis eruptive perstans

Madajet

    M. XL jet-injection anesthesia
      system
    M. XL local anesthesia

Maddacare child bath seat

Maddacrawler Crawler frame

Maddapult Asissto-Seat

Maddox rod test

Madelung deformity

**Madigan-Wissinger-Donaldson proximal
realignment**

M

madreporic hip prosthesis
mafenide
    m. acetate
    m. acetate for burn
MAFO
    molded ankle-foot orthosis
    MAFO cane
Mafucci
    M. disease
    M. syndrome
Magan
Magerl
    M. hook-plate system
    M. plate-screw system
    M. posterior cervical screw fixation
    M. translaminar facet screw
       fixation technique
Magic Wand vibrator
Magilligan
    M. measuring technique
    M. technique for measuring
       anteversion
magna
    arteria radicularis m.
    coxa m.
Magna-FX cannulated screw system
Magnassager massage tool
Magnatherm and Magnatherm SSP
    electromagnetic therapy unit
Magnathotic orthotic
magnesium
    m. deficiency
    m. salicylate
    m. sulfate
magnet
    ankle m.
    Dyonics Golden Retriever m.
    elbow m.
    foot m.
    m. splint
    Tectonic m.
    Tesla m.
    m. therapy
magnetic
    m. motion transducer
    m. resonance arthrography
    m. resonance imaging (MRI)
    m. resonance neurography (MRN)
    m. resonance venography
    m. retriever
    m. source imaging (MSI)
    m. stimulation
    m. therapy
magnification
    loupe m.
    m. view

magnifying
    m. glass
    m. loupe
magnum
    M. 800 bed
    M. chisel
    M. curette
    foramen m.
    M. 101 Plus table
magnus
    adductor m.
    nucleus raphe m. (NRM)
Magnuson
    M. abduction humeral splint
    M. debridement
    M. technique
    M. twist drill
    M. wire
Magnuson-Stack
    M.-S. operation
    M.-S. procedure
    M.-S. shoulder arthrotomy
Ma-Griffith
    M.-G. end-to-end anastomosis
    M.-G. ruptured Achilles tendon
       repair
    M.-G. technique
    M.-G. tendo calcaneus repair
    M.-G. tendon anastomosis
Mahan procedure
MAI
    Movement Assessment of Infants
Maigne test
maintained contraction
Maisel suppression theory
Maisonneuve
    M. fibular fracture
    M. sign
Maitland technique
Majestro-Ruda-Frost
    M.-R.-F. tendon operation
    M.-R.-F. tendon technique
major
    anterosuperior ilium m.
    m. curve
    m. injury vector (MIV)
    posteroinferior ilium m.
MAL
    midaxillary line
malabsorption
maladaptation
    soft-tissue m.
maladjustment
malalignment
    radial m.
    rotational m.
    varus m.
malangulation

Malawer
    M. excision technique
    M. resection
Malcolm-Lynn C-RXF cervical retractor frame
male/female washer
male reamer
malformation
    Arnold-Chiari m.
    arteriovenous m. (AVM)
    medullary venous m. (MVM)
    retromedullary arteriovenous m.
Malgaigne pelvic fracture
Malibu
    M. cervical orthosis
    M. Sandalthotics orthotic
maligna
    lentigo m.
malignancy
    spinal m.
malignant
    m. fasciculation
    m. fibrous histiocytoma
    m. fibrous xanthoma
    m. hyperpyrexia
    m. hyperthermia
    m. lymphoma
    m. melanoma
    m. myeloid sarcoma
    m. schwannoma
Malis
    M. CMC-II bipolar coagulator
    M. curette
    M. elevator
    M. hinge clamp
    M. jeweler bipolar forceps
    M. ligature passer
    M. needle holder
Malis-Jensen microbipolar forceps
Mallamint
malleable
    m. metal finger splint
    structural aluminum m. (SAM)
    m. template
mallei (*pl. of* malleus)
malleolar
    m. fracture
    m. gel sleeve
    m. osteotomy
    m. screw
Malleoloc ankle orthosis
malleolus, pl. malleoli

belly button to medial m. (BB to MM)
    lateral m.
    medial m.
    tip of medial m.
Malleotrain ankle support
mallet
    Acufex m.
    Bergman m.
    bone m.
    boxwood m.
    cervical m.
    Cottle m.
    Crane m.
    Doyen bone m.
    m. finger
    m. finger abouna splint
    m. finger deformity
    m. fracture
    Gerzog bone m.
    Hajek m.
    Heath m.
    Henning m.
    Hibbs m.
    Kirk orthopaedic m.
    Lucae bone m.
    Mead m.
    Meyerding m.
    Ombredanne m.
    polyethylene-faced m.
    Ralks m.
    Richards m.
    Rush m.
    slotted m.
    Steinbach m.
    Surgical No Bounce m.
    Swanson m.
    m. thumb
    m. toe
    m. toe deformity
    Williger bone m.
    Wolfe-Böhler m.
malleus, pl. mallei
    hallux m.
malleus-incus prosthesis
Mallisol
Mallory-Head
    M.-H. hip prosthesis
    M.-H. modular calcar system
    M.-H. porous primary femoral prosthesis
    M.-H. total hip revision

M

NOTES

Mallory technique
Malmö hip splint
malnutrition
    protein m.
malodorous foot
mal perforans
malposed vertebra
malposition
    extension m.
    flexion m.
    lateral flexion m.
    rotational m.
malrotation
Malteno tube implant material
maltracking patella
Maltz
    M. cartilage knife
    M. rasp
malum coxae senilis
malunion
    angulatory m.
    calcaneal m.
    femoral shaft m.
    humeral fracture m.
    talar m.
    varus m.
malunited
    m. acetabulum
    m. calcaneus fracture
    m. forearm fracture
    m. radial fracture
mamillary process
management
    conservative m.
    failure of conservative m.
    neuromechanical spinal
      chiropractic m.
    nonoperative orthopaedic m.
    nonsurgical m.
    preoperative m.
Mandelbaum-Nartolozzi-Carney patellar
  tendon repair
Mandel-Bekhterev sign
mandible
    m. ossification
    osteotomy of m.
mandibular
    m. angle
    m. fracture
    m. nerve
    m. osteotomy
    m. spine
maneuver
    Adson m.
    Allen m.
    Allis m.
    Bárány-Nylen m.
    Barlow m.

    Bigelow m.
    Christiani m.
    circumduction m.
    closed manipulative m.
    costoclavicular m.
    Dandy m.
    Dix-Hallpike m.
    Finkelstein m.
    flexion-extension m.
    flexion-rotation-compression m.
    Foster-Kennedy m.
    Fowler m.
    Gowers m.
    Halsted m.
    Hippocratic m.
    Hubscher m.
    hyperabduction m.
    Jahss m.
    Jendrassik m.
    Kocher m.
    Krackow m.
    Lachman m.
    Leadbetter m.
    logrolling m.
    McKenzie extension m.
    McMurray circumduction m.
    Mendelsohn m.
    Meyn-Quigley m.
    Meyn and Quigley m.
    Ortolani m.
    osteoclasis m.
    Parvin m.
    Phalen m.
    postural fixation back m.
    relative response attributable to
      the m. (RRAM)
    reverse Bigelow m.
    rotation-compression m.
    scalene m.
    Schreiber m.
    Sellick m.
    shear m.
    Slocum m.
    Soto-Hall m.
    Spurling m.
    Steel m.
    Stimson m.
    Valsalva m.
    Walton m.
    Wright m.
Mangled Extremity Severity Score
  (MESS)
manipulate
manipulation
    m. board
    contact m.
    diversified m.
    fine m.

general thrust m.
grading of m.
gross m.
Hippocrates m.
indirect m.
joint m.
Leadbetter hip m.
long and short lever rotational m.
lumbar distraction m.
myofascial m.
noncontact m.
opening wedge m.
osteopathic m.
passive joint m.
specific thrust m.
spinal m.
thrust m.
m. with distraction

manipulative
m. technique
m. therapy

Mankin
M. resection
M. technique

Manktelow
M. pectoralis major transfer
M. transfer procedure

Mann
M. modified McKeever arthrodesis
M. procedure
M. protocol
M. resection arthroplasty
M. technique

Mann-Coughlin
M.-C. arthrodesis
M.-C. procedure

Mann-Coughlin-DuVries cheilectomy
Mann-DuVries arthroplasty
Mann-Thompson-Coughlin arthrodesis
Mann-Whitney
M.-W. analysis
M.-W. U test

MANOVA
multivariate analysis of variance

Manske-McCarroll opponensplasty
Manske-McCarroll-Swanson centralization
Manske technique
M.A.N. Stim. Muscle and Neurological Stimulation
Mantis retrograde forceps

mantle
cement m.
grade A, B, C1, C2, D m.

manual
m. adjustment
m. cavitation
m. contact
m. locking knee prosthesis
m. medicine
m. muscle test
m. muscle testing (MMT)
m. pressure
m. push-pull technique
m. reflex neurotherapy
m. resistance
m. therapy
m. traction
m. treatment
m. wheelchair

manubrium
Manuflex external fixator
manus
ligamenta collateralia articulationum interphalangealium m.

Maolate
MAP
Multiaxial Assessment of Pain

Mapap
MAPF femoral stem prosthesis
mapping
behavioral m.
m. the defect
dermatome m.
MSI m.
paraspinal m.

Maquet
M. advancement
M. anteromedial osteoplasty
M. dome
M. dome osteotomy
M. procedure
M. table extension
M. technique

Maramed
M. Miami fracture brace system
M. ThermoFlex

Maranox
marathon
marathoner's toe
marble
m. bone
m. bone pin

M

NOTES

Marcaine with epinephrine
marcescens
    Serratia m.
marche à petits pas gait
march foot
March fracture
**Marcove-Lewis-Huvos shoulder girdle
  resection**
Marcus-Balourdas-Heiple
    M.-B.-H. ankle fusion
    M.-B.-H. ankle fusion technique
    M.-B.-H. transmalleolar arthrodesis
Marfan syndrome
Margesic H
margin
    anterior m.
marginal
    m. excision
    m. exostosis
    m. fracture
    m. osteophyte
    m. resection
margo, pl. **margines**
Marie-Bamberger disease
Marie-Charcot-Tooth disease
Marie-Foix sign
Marie-Strümpell
    M.-S. arthritis
    M.-S. disease
    M.-S. spondylitis
Marino
    M. transsphenoidal dissector
    M. transsphenoidal enucleator
marinum
    Mycobacterium m.
Marion screw
Mark
    M. II Chandler total knee retractor
    M. II concave total knee retractor
    M. II distal femur distractor
    M. II femoral component extractor
    M. III halo system
    M. II Kodros radiolucent awl
    M. II lateral collateral ligament
      retractor
    M. II modular weight retractor
    M. II Sorrells hip arthroplasty
    M. II Sorrells hip arthroplasty
      retractor system
    M. II "S" total knee retractor
    M. II Stubbs short prong collateral
      ligament retractor
    M. II Stulberg hip positioner
    M. II Stulberg leg positioner
    M. II tibial component extractor
    M. II wide PCL knee retractor
    M. II Wixson hip positioner
    M. II "Z" knee retractor

Markell
    M. brace boot
    M. Mobility Health Clogs
    M. Mobility Shoes
    M. open-toe shoe
    M. tarso medius straight shoe
    M. tarso pronator outflare shoe
marker
    lumbar pedicle m.
    pedicle m.
    retroreflective m.
    skin m.
    tantalum-ball m.
    thoracic pedicle m.
    X-Act podiatric m.
Markham-Meyerding retractor
Markley retention pin
**Marks-Bayne technique for thumb
  duplication**
Markwalder
    M. bone rongeur
    M. rib forceps
Marlex
    M. mesh
    M. methyl methacrylate prosthesis
Marlin
    M. cervical collar
    M. cervical orthosis
Marmor
    M. modular knee prosthesis
    M. replacement
maroon spoon
Maroteaux-Lamy syndrome
Marquardt angulation osteotomy
Marquet fracture table
marrow
    bone m.
    m. cavity
    m. disease
    red m.
    yellow m.
MARS
    Modular Acetabular Revision System
    MARS revision acetabular
      component
Marshall
    M. ligament repair
    M. ligament repair technique
    M. patelloquadriceps tendon
      substitution
Marshall-McIntosh technique
Martel sign
Marthritic
Martin
    M. cartilage chisel
    M. cartilage clamp
    M. cartilage forceps
    M. diamond wire cutter

M. loop circumferential wire
M. meniscal clamp
M. muscular clamp
M. osteotomy
M. patellar wiring technique
M. screw
M. sheet rubber bandage
M. Vigorimeter

Martin-Gruber
M.-G. anastomosis
M.-G. connection

Martini bone curette

Marx osteoradionecrosis protocol

Mary
angle of M.

Maryland
M. Foot Score
M. Foot Score Profile

MAS
milliamperage x seconds

Mason
M. fracture
M. fracture classification system
M. radial head fracture
classification
M. splint

Mason-Allen
M.-A. suture
M.-A. Universal hand splint

mass
bony m.
cellular periosteal
osteocartilaginous m.
center of m.
fat and fat-free m. (FFM)
plantar-hindfoot-midfoot bony m.
soft-tissue m.

massage
Aqua PT water m.
callus m.
connective tissue m. (CTM)
deep friction m.
deep kneading m.
deep stroking and kneading m.
effleurage m.
friction m.
Hoffa m.
ice m.
kneading m.
Shiatsu m.
soft tissue m.
stimulating m.

Swedish m.
m. therapy
M. Time Pro hydroM. table
transverse friction m.

massager
Cryocup ice m.
Jeanie Rub M.
Knobble m.
Morfam M.
Saso Variable Speed M.
The Original Backknobber
muscle m.
Thera Cane m.

massager/percussor
G5 Vibracare m.

Massie
M. driver
M. extractor
M. II nail
M. inserter
M. nail assembly
M. plate
M. screwdriver
M. sliding graft
M. sliding nail

massive
m. herniated disk
m. osteoplysis
m. sliding graft

Masson fasciotome

massotherapy

MAST
military antishock trousers

master
Balance M.
Body M.
m. cement
m. knot of Henry
NeuroCom balance m.
PRO Balance M.
M. screwdriver
SMART Balance M.

Masterson
M. curved clamp
M. pelvic clamp
M. straight clamp

Master-Stim interferential stimulator

Mastin muscular clamp

mastocytosis

mastoid
m. curette

M

NOTES

mastoid *(continued)*
    m. process
    m. rongeur
Mast-Spieghel-Pappas classification
mat
    Airex m.
    air flow m.
    Scoot-Gard m.
    sting m.
Matchett-Brown
    M.-B. cemented hip prosthesis
    M.-B. hip arthroplasty
    M.-B. internal prosthesis
matchstick
    m. graft
    m. test
matchsticked
mater
    dura m.
material
    acrylic implant m.
    Alisoft splinting m.
    allogeneic lyophilized bone graft
      implant m.
    alloplastic m.
    aluminum oxide arthroplasty m.
    Aquaplast splinting m.
    bioceramic implant m.
    bone implant m.
    Bonfiglio bone replacement m.
    Calcitite graft m.
    Carboplast II sheet orthotic m.
    celluloid implant m.
    CHAG bone graft substitute m.
    composite m.
    copolymer orthotic m.
    corundum ceramic implant m.
    Durapatite bone replacement m.
    Duraval Hook & Loop strap m.
    DYNAfabric m.
    Ethrone implant m.
    Evazote cushioning m.
    m. failure break point
    fibrillar absorbable hemostat m.
    Fletching femoral hernia
      implant m.
    gold weight and wire spring
      implant m.
    Graflex m.
    Gypsona cast m.
    homograft implant m.
    hydroxyapatite bone replacement m.
    hydroxyapatite implant m.
    implant m.
    Interpore bone replacement m.
    Iowa implant m.
    Isoloss AC m.
    Keolar implant m.

    Malteno tube implant m.
    methyl methacrylate implant m.
    Ommaya reservoir implant m.
    Ortho-Jel impression m.
    Paladon implant m.
    paraffin implant m.
    PE LITE m.
    Plasti-Pore prosthetic m.
    polyether implant m.
    polyethylene implant m.
    polyurethane implant m.
    polyvinyl alcohol splinting m.
    polyvinyl implant m.
    Porocoat prosthetic m.
    porous prosthetic m.
    ProOsteon bone graft m.
    Proplast I, II porous implant m.
    Proplast prosthetic m.
    purulent m.
    Pyrost bone graft m.
    Schepens hollow silicone
      hemisphere implant m.
    Scutan temporary splint m.
    Shearing posterior chamber
      implant m.
    shell implant m.
    silicone m.
    Silon silicone thermoplastic
      splinting m.
    solid buckling implant m.
    solid silicone exoplant implant m.
    Spitz-Holter valve implant m.
    Stimoceiver implant m.
    synthetic m.
    thermomoldable m.
    tissue mandrel implant m.
    titanium implant m.
    Virtullene brace m.
    viscoelastic m.
    Vitallium implant m.
    Vitox alumina ceramic m.
    zirconium oxide arthroplasty m.
    Zorbacel shock-absorbing m.
maternal serum alpha fetoprotein
   (MSAFP)
Matev sign
Mathews
    M. drill point
    M. hand drill
    M. load drill
    M. olecranon fracture classification
Mathys prosthesis
matricectomy *(var. of* matrixectomy)
matrix, pl. **matrices**
    Collagraft bone graft m.
    demineralized bone m. (DBM)
    germinal m.
    m. Grafton putty

m. injury
ligament-scar m.
nail m.
sterile m.
matrix-bone marrow slurry
matrixectomy, matricectomy
chemical m.
partial m.
phenol m.
Steindler m.
Winograd partial m.
Zadik total m.
Matroc femoral head
Matrol femoral head prosthesis
Matson
M. periosteal elevator
M. procedure
M. rib elevator
Matson-Alexander rib elevator
Matta-Saucedo fixation
matter
gray m.
white m.
Matthew cross-leg clamp
Matthews-Green pin
matting
Dycem roll m.
Matti-Russe
M.-R. bone graft
M.-R. technique
mattress
Akros extended care m.
Akros pressure m.
AkroTech m.
antidecubitus m.
Clinisert m.
Invacare APM m.
Lapidus alternating air-pressure m.
Nirvana m.
OptiMax Supreme pressure
reduction m.
overlay m.
Q Star Voyager pressure
reduction m.
RIK fluid m.
Sofflex m.
Sof Matt pressure relieving m.
m. suture
Tempur-Pedic pressure relieving
Swedish m.
T-Foam m.
Tri-Float pressure reduction m.

Mattrix spinal cord stimulation system
maturation
m. phase
skeletal m.
maturity
Oxford method for scoring
skeletal m.
skeletal m.
Mauch
M. S'n'S
M. Swing and Stance hydraulic
knee
Mauck knee procedure
Mauclaire disease
Mau osteotomy
Max
M. 3 electric handpiece
Thera-Band M.
MaxCast
M. cast
M. casting tape
Maxi-Driver driver
MaxiFloat wheelchair cushion
maxillary
m. fracture
m. spine
maxillectomy
Cocke m.
subtotal m.
maxillofacial bone screw
maxillotomy
extended m.
**Maxima II transcutaneous electrical
nerve stimulator**
maximal
m. oxygen uptake
m. stimulus
m. voluntary contraction (MVC)
m. voluntary ventilation (MVV)
Maxim Modular Knee System
maximum
m. conduction velocity
m. control (MC)
m. eversion velocity
m. inversion velocity
one-repetition m. (1-RM)
m. pressure picture (MPP)
m. radial bow
repetition m. (RM)
M. Strength Desenex Antifungal
Cream
M. Strength Nytol

M

NOTES

Maxon suture
Maxwell body
Maxxus orthopaedic latex surgical glove
May anatomical bone plate
Mayer
    M. orthotic
    M. splint
Mayfield
    M. adapter
    M. fixation frame
    M. forceps
    M. head rest
    M. incision
    M. instrumentation
    M. miniature clip applier
    M. neurosurgical headrest
    M. temporary aneurysm clip
      applier
Mayo
    M. ankle arthroplasty
    M. approach
    M. block anesthesia
    M. bunionectomy
    M. carpal instability classification
    M. clamp
    M. Clinic forefoot scoring system
    M. Clinic hip-scoring system
    M. elbow performance score
    M. hallux valgus modified
      operation
    M. metatarsal head resection
    M. nerve block
    M. resection arthroplasty
    M. scissors
    M. semiconstrained elbow
      prosthesis
    M. total ankle prosthesis
    M. total elbow arthroplasty
Mayo-Collins retractor
Mayo-Hegar needle holder
Mayo-Thomas collar
Mazas totally constrained elbow
  prosthesis
Mazet
    M. disarticulation of knee
    M. technique
Mazur
    M. ankle evaluation
    M. ankle rating system
MB-900 AC machine
MBHI
    Millon Behavioral Health Inventory
MB&J knee positioner
MBS snap-on orthotic
MC
    maximum control
MCA
    motorcycle accident

McAfee approach
McArdle disease
McAtee compression screw device
McAtee-Tharias-Blazina arthroplasty
McBride
    M. bunionectomy
    M. bunion hallux valgus
    M. bunion hallux valgus operation
    M. femoral prosthesis
    M. hallux abductovalgus reduction
    M. hallux valgus reduction
    M. pin
    M. plate
    M. procedure
    M. tripod
    M. tripod pin traction
McBride-Moore prosthesis
McCabe-Farrior rasp
McCain
    M. TMJ arthroscopic system
    M. TMJ cannula
    M. TMJ curette
    M. TMJ forceps
McCarroll-Baker procedure
McCarty hip procedure
McCash
    M. hand procedure
    M. hand surgery
McCauley foot procedure
McClamary elevator
McClintoch brace
McCollough internal tibial torsion brace
McConnell
    M. extensile approach
    M. median and ulnar nerve
      approach
    M. orthopaedic headrest
    M. patellofemoral treatment plan
    M. shoulder positioner
    M. technique
McCormick-Blount procedure
McCullough retractor
McCune-Albright syndrome
McCutchen hip implant
McCutcheon SLT hip prosthesis
McDavid
    M. ankle guard
    M. hinged knee guard
    M. knee brace
McDermott radiological classification
McDonald dissector
McDowell Impairment Index (MII)
McElfresh-Dobyns-O'Brien technique
McElroy
    M. curette
    M. instrumentation

McElvenny
    M. foot procedure
    M. technique
McElvenny-Caldwell procedure
McFarland bone graft
McFarland-Osborne
    M.-O. lateral approach
    M.-O. technique
McFarlane technique
MCF shoulder orthosis
McGee
    M. prosthesis needle
    M. splint
    M. wire-crimping forceps
McGee-Priest wire forceps
McGehee elbow prosthesis
McGill
    M. pain checklist
    M. Pain Questionnaire
McGlamry-Downey procedure
McGlamry elevator
McGregor line
McGuire
    M. pelvic positioner
    M. rating
    M. scoring system
MCI
    midcarpal instability
McIndoe
    M. bone rongeur
    M. rongeur forceps
    M. scissors
McIntire splint
McIver ENT retractor
McKay hip procedure
McKay-Simons
    M.-S. clubfoot operation
    M.-S. CSR
    M.-S. CSR operation
McKee
    M. brace
    M. femoral prosthesis
    M. totally constrained elbow
      prosthesis
    M. tri-fin nail
McKee-Farrar
    M.-F. acetabular cup
    M.-F. total hip arthroplasty
    M.-F. total hip prosthesis
McKeever
    M. arthrodesis for hallux limitus
    M. cartilage knife

M. medullary clavicle fixation
M. metatarsophalangeal arthrodesis
M. metatarsophalangeal fusion
M. open reduction
M. patellar cap prosthesis
M. procedure
M. Vitallium knee prosthesis
McKeever-Buck
    McK.-B. elbow technique
    McK.-B. fragment excision
McKeever-MacIntosh tibial plateau prosthesis
McKenzie
    M. bone drill
    M. cervical roll
    M. enlarging bur
    M. extension exercise
    M. extension maneuver
    M. lumbar roll
    M. night roll
    M. perforating twist drill
McKittrick transmetatarsal amputation
MCL
    medial collateral ligament
    motion control limiter
McLain-Weinstein spinal tumor classification
McLaughlin
    M. acromioplasty
    M. approach
    M. carpal scaphoid screw
    M. modification of Bunnell pull-out suture
    M. nail
    M. operation
    M. osteosynthesis apparatus
    M. osteosynthesis device
    M. plate
    M. procedure
    M. subscapularis transfer
McLaughlin-Hay technique
McLaughlin-Ryder incision
McLeod padded clavicular splint
McLight PCL brace
McMaster bone graft
McMaster-Toronto arthritis patient preference disability questionnaire
McMurray
    M. circumduction maneuver
    M. maneuver for torn knee cartilage

M

NOTES

McMurray *(continued)*
   M. sign
   M. test
McMurry osteotomy
McMurtry
   M. kinematic index
   kinematic indices of M.
McNaught prosthesis
McNutt driver
MCP
   metacarpophalangeal
   mucopolysaccharidosis
   MCP finger joint prosthesis
MCR
   midcarpal radial
   MCR portal
McReynolds
   M. driver
   M. driver-extractor
   M. method
   M. open reduction
   M. open reduction technique
McShane-Leinberry-Fenlin acromioplasty
MCU
   midcarpal ulnar
   MCU portal
McWhorter posterior shoulder approach
MD
   muscular dystrophy
   MD brace
MDCN
   medial dorsal cutaneous nerve
MDI
   multidirectional instability
MDS microdebrider
Mead
   M. bone rongeur
   M. mallet
   M. periosteal elevator
meal
   bone m.
mean value
Mears-Rubash approach
Mears sacroiliac plate
Meary metatarsotalar angle
measure
   emergency closed manipulative m.
   Gross Motor Function M. (GMFM)
   limited performance m.
   outcome m.
   parallel goniometric m.
   reconstructive m.
   standard goniometric m.
measured stress
measurement
   Agliette m.
   arthrometric knee laxity m.
   Blackburn-Peel m.

curve m.
Doppler m.
functional capacity m.
Insall-Salvati m.
limb accurate m. (LAM)
Mehta rib angle m.
motion m.
pedodynographic m.
range-of-motion m.
roof arc m.
Schober m.
skin fluorescence m.
tissue pressure m.
measurer
   Bunnell digital exertion m.
measuring
   m. gauge
   precise lesion m. (PLM)
mechanical
   m. agent
   m. axis
   combined m. (CM)
   m. dermatome
   m. dysfunction
   m. instability
   m. insufficiency
   m. low back pain syndrome
   m. pain threshold (MPTh)
   m. plate design
   m. two-dimensional echo transducer
   m. ventilation
mechanics
   altered intervertebral m.
   altered regional m.
   body m.
mechanism
   abductor m.
   adhesion/cohesion m.
   Adjustable Leg and Ankle
    Repositioning M. (ALARM)
   capsuloligamentous m.
   central extensor m. (CEM)
   clamping m.
   Cook-Gordon m.
   m. of correction
   cranial-sacral respiratory m.
    (CRSM)
   digital extensor m.
   extensor hood m.
   fail-safe m.
   flexor m.
   four-bar linkage prosthetic knee m.
   gliding m.
   Hosmer-Dorrance voluntary control
    four-bar knee m.
   locomotor m.
   MicroStable liner locking m.
   Noiles rotating-hinge knee m.

physiological venous pump m.
post-and-cam m.
primary cranial sacral
    respiratory m.
quadriceps m.
screw-home m.
tendo Achillis m.
terminal extensor m. (TEM)
UHR locking ring m.
Windlass m.

mechanoreceptor
m. activity
joint capsule m.
pacinian m.
Ruffini m.

Meckel cavity
meclofenamate
Meclomen
Mecring acetabluar prosthesis
med
medial
Medak glove
Medarmor puncture-resistant glove
Med-Fit cranial-sacral table
media
Conray contrast m.
contrast m.
Hypaque contrast m.
iohexol contrast m.
meglumine diatrizoate contrast m.
metrizamide contrast m.
Omnipaque contrast m.
Renografin contrast m.

medial (med)
m. antebrachial cutaneous nerve
m. articular nerve
m. aspect
m. aspiration
m. bicortical screw
m. border
m. brachial cutaneous nerve injury
m. brachial nerve
m. capsular imbrication
m. capsular ligament
m. capsule
m. capsulorrhaphy
m. clear space
m. closing wedge phalangeal
    osteotomy
m. collateral ligament (MCL)
m. column calcaneal fracture
m. column instability

m. compartment
m. compartment disruption
m. compartment injury
m. cortical overlap technique
m. disk protrusion
m. displacement
m. displacement osteotomy
m. dorsal cutaneous nerve (MDCN)
m. drainage
m. eminence
m. eminence resection
m. end
m. epicondylar apophysis
m. epicondyle
m. epicondylectomy
m. epicondyle humeral fracture
m. epicondylitis
m. extensor expansion
m. femoral condyle
m. gastrocnemius bursitis
m. geniculate
m. geniculate artery
m. geniculate fascia
m. hamstring
m. head stem offset
m. heel-and-sole wedge
m. heel skive technique
m. heel wedge (MHW)
m. humerus condyle
m. imbrication
m. joint line
m. ligament of ankle
m. malleolar fracture
m. malleolus
m. malleolus cast
m. malleolus fixation
m. malleolus resection
m. meniscus
m. metacarpal bone
m. movement
m. neurovascular bundle
m. opening wedge osteotomy
m. parapatellar arthrotomy
m. parapatellar capsular approach
m. parapatellar incision
m. patellar plica
m. patellofemoral ligament (MPFL)
m. plantar fasciocutaneous flap
m. plantar neurapraxia
m. portal
m. quadruple complex
m. repair

M

NOTES

medial *(continued)*
  m. rotation procedure
  m. shelf
  m. sole wedge
  m. stem pivot
  m. swivel dislocation
  m. talocalcaneal ligament
  m. tennis elbow tendinosis
  m. tibial flare
  m. tibial stress syndrome (MTSS)
  m. tibial syndrome (MTS)
  m. T-strap
  m. tubercle
  m. unicortical screw
  m. V-Y capsulotomy
  m. wall
mediale
  ligamentum talocalcaneare m.
medialis
  m. obliquus imbrication
  vastus m.
medialization
medial/lateral
  m. femoral condyle
  m. meniscus
medial/plantar hinge
median
  m. nerve
  m. nerve block
  m. nerve compression
  m. nerve entrapment
  m. nerve injury
  m. nerve palsy
  m. parapatellar incision
  m. raphe
  m. sagittal plane
Medi-Band bandage
medical
  m. adhesive
  M. Design brace
  m. elastomer X7-2320
  M. Examination and Diagnostic
    Coding System (MEDICS)
  M. Research Council (MRC)
  M. Research Council system
medication
  antiinflammatory m.
  beta blocker m.
  nonsteroidal antiinflammatory m.
  Occlusal-HP wart m.
medicinalis
  Hirudo m.
medicine
  allopathic m.
  American Congress of
    Rehabilitation M. (ACRM)
  American Orthopaedic Society for
    Sports M.

  complimentary alternative m.
    (CAM)
  electrodiagnostic m.
  manual m.
  Native American m.
  occupational and environmental m.
    (OEM)
  sports m.
  vertebral m.
MEDICS
  Medical Examination and Diagnostic
    Coding System
Medicus bed
Mediflow
  M. waterbase pillow
  M. Waterpillow
Mediloy
  M. implant metal
  M. implant metal prosthesis
mediolateral (M/L)
  m. position
  m. rediocarpal angle
  m. stress
  m. tilt
Medipain 5
Medipedic Multicentric knee brace
Mediplast
MEDI Plus compression stockings
Medipore H surgical tape
Medipren
Medi-Quick Topical Ointment
Medi-Rip dressing
Mediskin hemostatic sponge
Medi-Stim stimulator
meditation and mindfulness
medium
  m. callus podi-burr
  m. carbide cone bur
  m. fine bur
  Microfil contrast m.
  m. nail podi-burr
  m. profile femoral prosthesis
Medmetric
  M. knee ligament arthrometer
  M. KT-1000 knee laxity
    arthrometer
Medoff
  M. axial compression screw
  M. sliding plate
Medralone Injection
Medrol
  M. Dosepak
  M. Oral
medroxyprogesterone
  estrogens and m.
Meds eye protector
**Medtronic spinal cord stimulation
  system**

medulla
medullary
    m. bone graft
    m. canal
    m. canal reamer
    m. nail
    m. nail fixation
    m. pin
    m. prosthesis
    m. saw
    m. venous malformation (MVM)
    m. vent tubing
medullostomy
    tarsal m.
MedX
    M. functional testing machine
    M. Mark II lumbar extension
      machine
    M. stretch machine
Meek
    M. clavicular strap
    M. pelvic traction belt
mefenamic acid
Mefoxin
Mega-Air bed
megalodactyly
Mega Tilt and Turn bed
meglumine diatrizoate contrast media
Mehn-Quigley technique
Mehta rib angle measurement
melanoma
    acral lentiginous m.
    Breslow classification of m.
    Clark classification of m.
    lentigo maligna m.
    malignant m.
    metastatic m.
melanosis circumscripta preblastomatosis
  of Dubreuilh
melanotic
    m. panaris
    m. progonoma
    m. Whitlow of Hutchinson
melatonin
Melaware flatware
Meleney
    M. infection
    M. synergistic gangrene
melioidosis
    musculoskeletal m.
melioidotic
Mellaril

mellitus
    diabetes m.
    insulin-dependent diabetes m.
      (IDDM)
    noninsulin-dependent diabetes m.
      (NIDDM)
Melone distal radius fracture
  classification
melorheostosis
melphalan
Melzack Pain Questionnaire
membrane
    anterior atlantooccipital m.
    atlantooccipital anterior m.
    basement m.
    cricothyroid m.
    Golgi m.
    m. instability
    interosseous m. (IOM)
    interposition m.
    intraosseous m.
    mucous m. (mm)
    periprosthetic m.
    Preclude spinal m.
    synovial m.
    m. tectora
    thickened synovial m.
membranous ossification
Memford-Gurd arthroplasty
memory
    m. board
    m. exercise card
    m. splint
men
    meniscectomy
    lat men
      lateral meniscectomy
Menadol
Mendel-Bekhterev
    M.-B. reflex
    M.-B. sign
Mendelsohn maneuver
Menelaus triceps transfer
Menest
meningeal syndrome
meningioma
meningism
meningismus
meningitis
meningocele
meningococcal purpura
meningoencephalomyelitis

M

NOTES

meningomyelitis
meningomyelocele
meniscal
    m. aponeurosis
    m. clamp
    m. curette
    m. cyst
    m. excision
    m. injury
    m. lateral tear
    m. mirror
    m. radial tear
    m. repair
    m. repair needle
    m. scissors
    m. spoon
    m. transverse tear
meniscectomy (men)
    arthroscopic m.
    m. knife
    lateral m. (lat men)
    partial m.
    Patel medial m.
    subtotal m.
    subtotal lateral m.
    total m.
menisci (*pl. of* meniscus)
meniscocapsular
    m. junction
    m. tear
meniscofemoral
    m. capsule
    m. ligament
meniscoid
    m. entrapment
    joint m.
meniscoplasty
meniscorrhexis
meniscosynovial junction
meniscotibial
    m. capsule
    m. ligament
meniscotome
    Bircher m.
    Bowen-Grover m.
    curved m.
    Grover m.
    Storz m.
meniscus, pl. menisci
    bridge of m.
    bucket-handle tear of m.
    clefting of m.
    degenerative m.
    Dickhaut-DeLee classification of
      discoid m.
    discoid lateral m.
    m. forceps
    frayed m.

    m. graft
    m. hook
    m. knife
    lateral m.
    medial m.
    medial/lateral m.
    M. Mender II system
    resection of m.
    torn m.
    trapped m.
    Watanabe classification of
      discoid m.
    Wrisberg ligament type of
      discoid m.
Mennell
    M. sign
    M. test
menopause
MENS
    microamperage electrical nerve
      stimulation
    MENS unit
Mensor-Scheck
    M.-S. hanging-hip operation
    M.-S. technique
mentagrophytes
    Trichophyton m.
Mentax
Mentor
    M. Self-Cath soft catheter
    M. tissue expander
Mepergan
meperidine and promethazine
mepivacaine
MEPP
    miniature end-plate potential
meprobamate
meptazinol
meralgia
    m. paraesthetica
    m. paresthetica
merbromin
Merchant
    M. congruence angle
    M. and Dietz ankle score
    M. radiograph
    M. view
Mercurochrome
mercury
    millimeters of m. (mmHg)
meridian
    M. Intersegmental table
    M. ST femoral implant component
Merit Final Flexion Kit
Merkel cell
Merland classification of perimedullary
    arteriovenous fistulas

Merle
    M. d'Aubigné hip score
    M. d'Aubigné and Postel hip
      rating scale
Merlin arthroscopy blade
meropenem
Merrem I.V.
Merry Walker
Mersilene
    M. Kessler stitch
    M. sling
    M. suture
    M. tape
Mersol
Merthiolate
Meryon sign
mesenchymal
    m. cell
    m. chondrosarcoma
    m. tumor
mesenchyme
mesenchymoma
    pluripotential m.
mesenteric vasculitis
mesh
    chromium-cobalt m.
    m. graft
    Marlex m.
    metal m.
    sintered titanium m.
    stainless steel m.
    tantalum m.
mesher
    Zimmer skin graft m.
mesiodistal plane
mesotendon
MESS
    Mangled Extremity Severity Score
Mestinon
mesylate
    benztropine m.
met
    metatarsal
    met cookie
    met head
metabolic
    m. bone disease
    m. variable
metabolism
    arachidonate m.
    purine m.

metacarpal
    m. base
    m. beak
    m. block
    m. bone
    fifth m.
    first m.
    m. lengthening
    m. ligament
    m. neck
    m. neck fracture
    m. osteotomy
    thumb m.
metacarpocapitate joint
metacarpocarpal joint
metacarpoglenoidal ligament
metacarpohamate joint
metacarpophalangeal (MCP, MP)
    m. articulation
    m. dislocation
    m. implant
    m. joint (MPJ)
    m. joint arthroplasty
    m. ligament
metacarpophalangealium
    ligamenta collateralia
      articulationum m.
metacarpotrapezial joint
metacarpus
metachromatic mucoid substance
metal
    Alivium implant m.
    Biophase implant m.
    Biotex implant m.
    m. clamp
    Coballoy implant m.
    Co-Cr-Mo alloy implant m.
    Co-Cr-W-Ni alloy implant m.
    m. endurance limit
    m. failure
    m. fatigue
    m. femoral head prosthesis
    m. footplate
    HA 65101 implant m.
    Haynes-Stellite 21 implant m.
    m. hemi-toe implant
    m. hybrid orthosis
    implant m.
    m. implant corrosion
    m. locator
    m. measuring triangle
    Mediloy implant m.

M

NOTES

metal *(continued)*
    m. mesh
    Orthochrome implant m.
    m. orthopaedic implant
    m. pin
    PMI-6A1-4V implant m.
    porous m.
    Protasul implant m.
    m. pylon
    Sinterlock implant m.
    m. splint
    Ti-6A1-4V implant m.
    Tivanium implant m.
    Vinertia implant m.
    Vitallium implant m.
    Zimalite implant m.
    Zimaloy implant m.
metal-backed
    m.-b. acetabular component
    m.-b. acetabular component hip
      implant
    m.-b. acetabular cup
    m.-b. patellar implant
    m.-b. prosthesis
    m.-b. socket
metallic
    m. bead
    m. debris
    m. implant
metallograft
metal-on-metal
    m.-o.-m. articulating intervertebral
      disk prosthesis
    m.-o.-m. design
metaphyseal
    m. abscess
    m. artery
    m.-articular nonunion
    m. to diaphyseal width ratio
    m.-epiphyseal angle
    m. head resection with prosthesis
    m. osteotomy
    m. shortening
    m. spike
    m. stapler
    m. tibial fracture
    m. tuberculosis
metaphyseal-diaphyseal
    m.-d. angle
    m.-d. junction
metaphysial-diaphyseal junction
metaphysis, pl. **metaphyses**
    distal m.
    femoral m.
    fibular m.
    funnelization of m.
    tibial m.

metaplasia
    cartilaginous m.
    osteocartilaginous m.
metaplastic
metastasis, pl. **metastases**
    bony m.
    osteoblastic m.
    Picker Magnascanner for bone m.
    spinal m.
metastatic
    m. disease
    m. melanoma
    m. spinal tumor
    m. tumor removal
Metasul
    M. hip joint component
    M. hip system
    M. joint
metatarsal (met, MT)
    angle of declination of m.
    m. artery
    m. axis
    m. bar shoe modification
    m. bone
    m. cookie
    m. cuneiform exostosis
    fifth m.
    first m.
    m. flatfoot bar
    m. fracture
    m. head
    m. head osteotomy
    m. head resection
    m. joint
    lesser m.
    m. neck
    m. neck osteotomy
    m. oblique osteotomy
    osteochondrosis of m.
    m. overload syndrome
    m. pad
    m. parabola
    m.-phalangeal creaking
    m. phalangeal crease
    m. phalangeal fifth angle
    m. proximal dome osteotomy
    m. ray
    m. Reverdin osteotomy
    m. shaft
    m. V-shaped osteotomy
metatarsalgia
    Morton m.
    secondary m.
    transfer m.
metatarsi (*pl. of* metatarsus)
metatarsocalcaneal angle
metatarsocuboid joint
metatarsocuneiform (MTC)

m. arthrodesis
m. articulation
m. joint
m. joint exostosis
m. joint fusion
metatarsophalangeal (MT, MTP)
m.-interphalangeal scale
m. joint (MTPJ)
m. joint arthrodesis
m. joint capsule
m. joint disarticulation
m. joint dislocation
m. joint fusion
m. joint injury
metatarsophalangealium
ligamenta collateralia
articulationum m.
ligamenta plantaria
articulationum m.
metatarsotalar angle
metatarsus, pl. **metatarsi**
m. abductus
m. adductocavus
m. adductovarus
m. adductus (MTA)
m. adductus angle
m. cavus
m. elevatus
m. equinus
m. internus
m. latus
m. primus adductus (MPA)
m. primus angle
m. primus atavicus
m. primus elevatus
m. primus varus (MPV)
m. supinatus
m. valgus
m. varus (MTV)
metaxalone
metazonal region
Metcalf spring drop brace
meter
Fischer pressure threshold m.
pinch m.
methacrylate
antibiotic-impregnated
polymethyl m. (PMMA)
centrifuged methyl m.
methyl m.
polymethyl m. (PMMA)
methadone

methemoglobin
methicillin
methocarbamol and aspirin
method
Abbott m.
antegrade m.
anthropometric m.
biofeedback-assisted m.
Bleck m.
Borggreve m.
Buck m.
Budin-Chandler m.
bundle-nailing m.
Caton m.
Cobb m.
computer-assisted design-controlled
alignment m. (CAD/CAM)
contoured adduction trochanteric-
controlled alignment m. (CAT-
CAM)
cup and cone m.
depth caliper-meter stick m.
disk diffusion m.
dynamic traction m.
Elmslie-Trillat patellar
realignment m.
extension block splinting m.
Fallat-Buckholz m.
Feldenkrais m.
Ferguson scoliosis measuring m.
Fick m.
Gerbert-Mellilo m.
Gohil-Cavolo m.
Hoke triple-section m.
hold-relax m.
hole preparation m.
hydrogen washout m.
Ilizarov m.
immobilization m.
Insall patella alta m.
install m.
Jahss ninety-ninety m.
Kaplan-Meier time-to-event
analysis m.
keyhole m.
Kocher m.
Lindsjö m.
McReynolds m.
Mose m.
Mosley m.
nail length gauge m.
Neufeld dynamic m.

M

NOTES

method *(continued)*
>ninety-ninety m.
>Oil-Red-O m.
>one-inclinometer m.
>Oxford m.
>Palmer m.
>pedicle m.
>m. of perpendiculars
>Pilates exercise m.
>pin-and-plaster m.
>Ponseti m.
>Ranawat-Dorr-Inglis m.
>receptor-tonus m.
>retrograde m.
>Risser m.
>Russe-Gerhardt m.
>Schober m.
>Stimson gravity m.
>Tajima m.
>total mesenteric apron m.
>Trager m.
>two-inclinometer m.
>Wagner limb lengthening m.

methotrexate toxicity
methotrimeprazine
methyl
>m. methacrylate
>m. methacrylate adhesive
>m. methacrylate bead
>m. methacrylate beads implant
>m. methacrylate cement
>m. methacrylate implant material

methylene
>m. bisphenyl diisocyanate
>m. blue
>m. blue dye

methylprednisolone acetate
methyltestosterone
>estrogens and m.
>Premarin With M.

Meticorten
Metrecom
>M. digitizer
>M. spinal analyzer

metrizamide contrast media
MetroGel Topical
metronidazole
metronome
Mettler electrotherapy
metyrosine
Metzenbaum
>M. chisel
>M. gouge
>M. scissors

Meuli arthroplasty
Meurig Williams plate
Meyer
>M. cervical orthosis

>M. dysplasia
>M. line

Meyerding
>M. chisel
>M. curved osteotome
>M. gouge
>M. mallet
>M. retractor
>M. spondylolisthesis classification line
>M. straight osteotome

Meyerding-Van Demark technique
Meyers-McKeever
>M.-M. tibial fracture classification

Meyers quadratus muscle-pedicle bone graft
Meyhoeffer bone curette
Meyn
>M. and Quigley maneuver
>M. reduction of elbow dislocation

Meynet node
Meyn-Quigley maneuver
MFA
>Musculoskeletal Function Assessment
>MFA questionnaire

M-F heel protector
MG
>MG II knee prosthesis
>MG II total knee system

MGH osteotome
MHW
>medial heel wedge

Miacalcin
>M. Injection
>M. nasal spray

Miami
>M. Acute Care (MAC)
>M. acute collar cervical traction
>M. fracture brace
>M. J cervical collar
>M. J collar cervical traction
>M. TLSO scoliosis brace

Micatin Topical
MICA 3x sleeve
mice
>joint m.

Michael Reese articulated prosthesis
Michal deformity
Michel clip
Michele vertebral biopsy
Michelson-Sequoia air drill
miconazole
Micro
>M. Series wire driver

Micro-Aire
>M.-A. debridement of bone surface
>M.-A. drill
>M.-A. osteotome

microamperage
  m. electrical nerve stimulation
    (MENS)
  m. neural stimulation (MNS)
microavulsion
microcellular rubber
microcirculation
microcoil
microcomputer upper limb exerciser
  (MULE)
microcrystalline collagen
microcurrent
  m. electrode
  m. therapy
microdebrider
  MDS m.
microdiskectomy
  arthroscopic m. (AMD)
  uniportal arthroscopic m.
MicroFET2
  M. muscle test
  M. muscle testing device
Microfil contrast medium
Microfoam dressing
microfracture
microgeode
microgeodic syndrome
microinterlock
microirrigating cannula
microirrigator
microknurling
Microloc
  M. knee implant
  M. knee prosthesis
  M. knee system
microlumbar
  m. diskectomy (MLD)
  m. disk excision
  m. diskography
Micro-Mill knee instrument system
micromotion
microneedle holder
microneuroanalysis
  internal m.
microneurography midlatency SEP
microneurosurgical technique
Micro-One dissecting forceps
microoscillating saw
MicroPhor iontophoretic drug delivery
  system
micropin
  Pischel m.

microplate
  Luhr m.
microprocessor
  Intertron therapy m.
microsagittal saw
microscissors
microscope
  double binocular operating m.
  operating m.
microscopy
  light m.
Microsect
  M. curette
  M. shaver
microsis
  avascular m.
MicroStable liner locking mechanism
microstaple
  Barouk m.
microsurgery diskectomy
microsurgical
  m. diskectomy (MSD)
  m. instrument
  m. thoracoscopic vertebrectomy
MicroTeq portable belt
microtiter protein kinase assay
microtrauma
  cervical m.
  lumbar m.
  thoracic m.
Micro-Two forceps
micro-valve
  Hypobaric m.-v.
microvascular
  m. clamp
  m. free flap
  m. osseous transfer
  m. surgical anastomosis
microvasculature
Microvel prosthesis
microwave diathermy (MWD)
micro waveform
Micro-Z neuromuscular stimulator
Midas
  M. Rex acorn
  M. Rex AM1 bone cutter
  M. Rex bur
  M. Rex drill
  M. Rex instrumentation system
  M. Rex knife
  M. Rex pneumatic instrument

M

NOTES

midaxillary
    m. line (MAL)
    m. line incision
midazolam
midcalf
midcarpal
    m. arthrodesis
    m. arthroscopy
    m. injury
    m. instability (MCI)
    m. joint
    m. portal
    m. radial (MCR)
    m. ulnar (MCU)
Middeldorpf
    M. splint
    M. triangle
middle
    m. column injury
    m. finger
    m. glenohumeral ligament
    m. sacral artery
    m. sacral vein
    m. third (M/3, middle/3)
    m. third of shaft
    m. thyroid vein
    m. tibial shaft fracture
middle/3
    middle third
middle-finger
    m.-f. amputation
    m.-f. test
midfacial fracture
midfemur
midfoot
    m. abductus
    m. adductus
    m. fracture
    m. joint
    m. scale
midheel line
Midland tilt table
midlateral
    m. approach
    m. capsule
midline
    m. disk herniation
    M. Hi-Lo Mat Platform
    m. ligament
    m. medial approach
    m. oblique incision
midmalleolar line
midmedial capsule
Midol
    M. IB
    M. PM

midpalmar
    m. abscess
    m. space
midpatellar
    m. portal
    m. tendon
Midrin
midsagittal plane
midshaft fracture
midstance period of gait
midsternal line (MSL)
midsubstance tear
midtarsal
    m. joint
    m. osteoarthritis
midtarsus
midthigh amputation
Midwest Regional Spinal Cord Injury Center
migraine
    basilar artery m.
migrati
    hallux m.
migration
    m. of acetabular cup
    hallux m.
    instrument m.
    Luque rod m.
    rod m.
    trochanteric m.
migratory
    m. arthralgia
    m. arthritis
MII
    McDowell Impairment Index
Mikasa subacromial bursography
Mikhail bone block
Mikulicz
    M. angle
    M. pad
    M. sponge
Milch
    M. classification of humeral fracture
    M. condylar fracture classification
    M. cuff resection
    M. cuff resection of ulna technique
    M. elbow fracture classification
    M. elbow technique
    M. plate
Miles
    M. bone chisel
    M. Nervine Caplets
milestone
    motor m.
Milewski driver
Milford mallet finger technique

military
    m. antishock trousers (MAST)
    m. brace position
    m. posture test
    m. tuck position
milk-alkali
    m.-a. disease
    m.-a. syndrome
milking of vessel
milkmaid's
    m. elbow
    m. elbow dislocation
milkman's
    m. pseudofracture
    m. syndrome
mill
    bone m.
    Lere bone m.
    OrthoBlend powered bone m.
mille
    m. pattes screw
    m. pattes technique
Millender arthroplasty
Millender-Nalebuff wrist arthrodesis
Miller
    M. flatfoot operation
    M. procedure
Miller-Galante
    M.-G. hip prosthesis
    M.-G. I hemiarthroplasty
    M.-G. II knee prosthesis
    M.-G. jig
    M.-G. knee
    M.-G. knee arthroplasty
    M.-G. revision knee system
    M.-G. total knee system
Millesi
    M. modified technique
    M. nerve graft
milliamperage x seconds (MAS)
milliampere (mA)
millimeter (mm)
millimeters of mercury (mmHg)
millimetric rule
milliner's needle
milling cutter
Millon Behavioral Health Inventory (MBHI)
Mills
    M. dressing
    M. test
Milroy disease

Miltex
    M. bone saw
    M. nail nipper
    M. wire twister
Miltner-Wan calcaneus resection
Milwaukee
    M. cervicothoracolumbosacral
      orthosis
    M. scoliosis brace
    M. scoliosis orthosis
    M. shoulder syndrome
mimocausalgia
Minaar
    M. classification of coalition
    M. classification system
    M. coalition classification
mind-body therapy
mindfulness
    meditation and m.
mind language
MindSet toe splint
mineralization
Miner osteotome
Minerva
    M. cast
    M. cervical jacket
    M. fixation
    M. orthosis
mini
    M.-ALIF
    m. AO screw
    m. applier
    m.-core disease
    M.-Flap drain system
    m.-Hoffmann external fixator
    m.-Hohmann retractor
    m.-Lambotte osteotome
    m.-Lexer osteotome
    m.-meniscus blade
    Mini-pad
    m.-Orthofix fixator
    m.-pilon fracture
    m.-Stryker power drill
    m.-Ullrich bone clamp
miniature
    m. end-plate potential (MEPP)
    m. multipurpose clamp
mini-C-arm
    XiScan m.-C.-a.
Minidyne
minifragment plate fixation

M

NOTES

minima
    patella m.
    m. patella
minimal
    m. bactericidal concentration
    m. inhibitory concentration
minimally displaced fracture
MiniMedBall hand exerciser
minimi
    abductor digiti m. (ADM)
    extensor digiti m. (EDM)
    opponens digiti m. (OPM)
minimum incision surgery (MIS)
miniplate
    Luhr m.
ministaple
    Bio-R-Sorb resorbable poly-L-lactic
    acid m.
ministem shaft
Minkoff-Jaffe-Menendez posterior approach
Minkoff-Nicholas procedure
Minneapolis hip prosthesis
Minnesota
    M. Manual Dexterity Test
    M. Multiphasic Personality
    Inventory (MMPI)
    M. Rate of Manipulation test
    M. Spatial Relations Test
minor
    m. curve
    M. sign
Minos air drill
Mira
    M. cautery
    M. drill
    M. reamer
mirabilis
    Proteus m.
Miragel implant
Mirage Spinal System
mirror
    Apfelbaum m.
    dental m.
    m. hand
    meniscal m.
Mirua-Komada release
MIS
    minimum incision surgery
misalignment
mislauxe
misoprostol
    diclofenac sodium and m.
missed fracture
misshapen
missile injury

Mital
    M. elbow release
    M. elbow release technique
Mitchel-Adam multipurpose clamp
Mitchell
    M. bunionectomy
    M. distal osteotomy
    M. hallux valgus procedure
    M. osteotome
    M. osteotomy/bunionectomy
    M. posterior displacement
    osteotomy
    M. step-down osteotomy
Mitek
    M. anchor
    M. anchor system
    M. GII suture anchor system
    M. SuperAnchor instrument
    M. vapor
    M. Vapr tissue removal system
miter technique
Mithracin
mitochondrial
    m. disease
    m. myopathy
mitochondrion, pl. **mitochondria**
mitt
    holding m.
    impact m.
    motion control m.
    paraffin m.
    wash m.
mitten hand
Mittlemeir
    M. broach
    M. ceramic hip prosthesis
    M. noncemented femoral prosthesis
Mitutoyo digital caliper
MIV
    major injury vector
Mivacron
mivacurium
mixed
    m. cord syndrome
    m. headache syndrome
mixer
    MixEvac bone-cement m.
MixEvac bone-cement mixer
Mixter
    M. forceps
    M. ligature-carrier clamp
    M. right-angle clamp
Miyakawa
    M. knee operation
    M. knee procedure
Mize-Bucholz-Grogen approach
Mizuno-Hirohata-Kashiwagi technique
Mizuno technique

MKS II knee brace
M/L
    mediolateral
        M/L lift
MLD
    microlumbar diskectomy
MLSI
    multiple line-scan imaging
mm
    millimeter
    mucous membrane
mmHg
    millimeters of mercury
M-mode transesophageal
  echocardiography
MMPI
    Minnesota Multiphasic Personality
    Inventory
MMT
    manual muscle testing
MNCV
    motor nerve conduction velocity
MNS
    microamperage neural stimulation
moat
Moberg
    M. advancement flap
    M. arthrodesis
    M. deltoid muscle transfer
    M. deltoid-to-triceps transfer
    M. dowel graft
    M. key-grip tenodesis
    M. key-pinch procedure
    M. osteotome
    M. Picking Up Test
    M. screw
    M. splint
Moberg-Gedda
    M.-G. fracture
    M.-G. incision
    M.-G. open reduction
Mobidin
mobile
    m. bearing knee implant
    m. wad
Mobilimb CPM device
mobility
    active m.
    coordinated m.
    fractured bone m.
    hip m.
    intersegmental m.

    joint m.
    limited joint m. (LJM)
    lumbar sagittal m.
    muscle tissue m.
    passive m.
    rotation m.
    sacral m.
    sacroiliac joint m.
    sagittal m.
    segmental m.
    side-bending m.
    symphyseal m.
    m. testing
    translation m.
    unisegmental m.
    vertical symphyseal m.
mobilization
    ASTM augmented soft tissue m.
    grades of m. (grade 1–5)
    joint m.
    Kaltenborn system of joint m.
    lateral band m.
    nonthrust m.
    soft tissue m.
    spinal joint m.
    m. with impulse
mobilize
mobilizer
    Therabite m.
Mobitz type I, II
MOD
    MOD femoral drill guide
    MOD unicompartmental knee
      system
Mod610
    Alps Lock M.
modality
    electrical m.
    Fluidotherapy sterile dry heat m.
mode
    Gruen m.
    loading m.
model
    M. 810 axial closed-loop hydraulic
      mechanical testing
    corpectomy m.
    Currey m.
    Denis Browne three-column m.
    family management m.
    foot m.
    joint m.
    lumbar spine m.

M

NOTES

modeling
cortical bone m.
modification
Bloom-Raney m.
Bonfiglio m.
C-D screw m.
Clark-Southwick-Odgen m.
dietary m.
Duncan-Lovell m.
Fairbanks technique with Sever m.
Harriluque sublaminar wiring m.
Helal m.
Jacobs locking hook spinal rod
instrumentation m.
Kleinert m.
Losee m.
metatarsal bar shoe m.
Neer m.
Seddon m.
Sequeira-Khanuja m.
Stauffer m.
Strickland m.
Youngwhich m.
modified
M. American Shoulder and Elbow
Surgeons Shoulder Patient Self-
Evaluation Form patient
questionnaire
m. Boyd amputation of ankle and
distal tibial physis
m. Boyd ankle arthrodesis
m. Chrisman-Snook ankle
reconstruction
m. Cocklin toe operation
m. Cotrel cast
m. Gait Abnormality Rating Scale
m. Grace plate
m. Harris hip score
m. Hoffmann quadrilateral external
fixator
m. Hoke-Miller flatfoot procedure
m. Keller resection arthroplasty
m. Kessler suture
m. Kessler-Tajima suture
m. Lapidus procedure
m. Mau bunionectomy
m. Mau osteotomy
m. McBride bunionectomy
m. mold and surface replacement
arthroplasty
m. Moore hip locking prosthesis
m. Oppenheimer splint
m. Robert Jones dressing
m. tonsillar prong
m. two-portal endoscopic carpal
tunnel release
m. Wagner classification system
m. Watson-Jones ankle tenodesis

m. Wilson osteotomy
m. Zarins and Rowe
Modny
M. drill
M. pin
modular
M. Acetabular Revision System
(MARS)
m. Austin Moore hip prosthesis
m. implant
m. instrumentation
m. Iowa Precoat total hip
prosthesis
m. large-head component
m. Lenbach hip system
m. Moniflex hip stem
m. S-ROM total hip system
m. temPPThotic kit
m. total hip prosthesis
m. unicompartmental knee
prosthesis
module
Allen Diagnostic M.
Peak gait m.
modulus
m. of elasticity
Young m.
Moe
M. alar hook
M. bone curette
M. bone impactor
M. gouge
M. intertrochanteric plate
M. modified Cotrel cast
M. modified Harrington rod
M. osteotome
M. scoliosis operation
M. scoliosis technique
M. square-end rod
M. system
**Moe-Kettleson distribution of curves in
scoliosis**
Moeltgen flexometer
Mogensen procedure
Mohr finger splint
Moire topographic scoliosis assessment
moist
m. heat
Restore Clean 'N M.
Moisturizer
Betadine First Aid Antibiotics
+ M.
mold
m. acetabular arthroplasty
Aufranc concentric hip m.
Biothotic orthotic m.
caudad anterior m.
cephalad anterior m.

molded
> AFO m.
> m. ankle-foot orthosis (MAFO)
> m. posterior plaster splint
> m. postpartum insole

molding
> compression m.
> elastomer skin m.
> polyethylene compression m.
> m. sock

Mold-In-Place back support
moleskin
> m. padding
> m. traction tape

Molestick padding
Molesworth-Campbell elbow approach
Molesworth osteotomy
molle
> fibroma m.
> heloma m. (HM)

molluscum
> fibroma m.

Moloney line
Molt periosteal elevator
molybdenum
> stainless steel and m. (SMo)

moment
> anterior bending m.
> m. arm
> m. of force
> m. of inertia
> posterior bending m.
> three-point bending m.

momentum
> angular m.

Momma-Too Maternity Support
MOM tractograph
Monarch knee brace
Monark
> M. bicycle
> M. Rehab Trainer

monarthric
monarthritis
> viral m.

monarticular synovitis
Mönckeberg sclerosis
Mondini dysplasia
Moniflex hip stem
Monistat-Derm Topical
monitor
> blood pressure m. (BPM)
> M. Master M. support

> MyoTrac EMG biofeedback m.
> NervePace nerve conduction m.
> Polar Vantage XL heart m.
> Polar wrist m.
> Vantage Performance m. (VPM)

monitored anesthesia control
monitoring
> blood pressure m.
> central venous pressure m.
> evoked external urethral sphincter
>   potential m.
> fluorescein perfusion m.
> screw position perioperative m.
> somatosensory evoked potential m.
> spinal cord function
>   intraoperative m.

MonitorMate monitor arm
monkey paw
Monk hip prosthesis
monoblock femoral component
monocane
Monocid
monoclonal gammopathy
monocyte
monodactyly
monofilament
> nylon m.
> m. pressure test
> Semmes-Weinstein m.
> Softip m.
> m. suture
> m. wire
> m. wire fixation

Monofixateur external fixator
Mono-Gesic
Monogram total knee instrument
monomalleolar ankle fracture
mononeuropathy
> diabetic femoral m.
> embolic m.
> m. multiplex

monophasic
> m. action potential
> m. endplate activity
> m. (high-volt) waveform

monoplace hyperbaric chamber
monoplegia
monopolar
> m. cautery
> m. needle recording electrode

monosodium urate crystal

M

NOTES

monospherical
    m. shoulder arthroplasty
    m. total shoulder arthroplasty
monostotic fibrous dysplasia
monotube
    M. external fixator system
    Howmedica m.
Monteggia
    M. dislocation
    M. equivalent lesion
    M. forearm fracture
    M. fracture-dislocation of ulna
Montenovesi rongeur
Montercaux fracture
Monticelli-Spinelli
    M.-S. circular external fixation
      system
    M.-S. distraction
    M.-S. distraction technique
    M.-S. distractor
    M.-S. fixator
    M.-S. frame
    M.-S. leg fixation
Montreal hip positioner
Moon
    M. boot
    M. Boot brace
    M. Boot shoe
    M. Walker
Mooney
    M. brace
    M. cast
Moon-Robinson
    M.-R. prosthesis inserter
    M.-R. stapes prosthesis
Moore
    M. bone drill
    M. bone elevator
    M. driver
    M. femoral neck prosthesis
    M. fixation pin
    M. fracture
    M. hip endoprosthesis system
    M. hip prosthesis
    J. R. M. procedure
    M. nail
    M. osteotomy-osteoclasis
    M. posterior approach
    M. prosthesis extractor
    M. prosthesis-mortising chisel
    M. sliding nail plate
    M. stem
    M. technique
    M. template
    M. tibial plateau fracture
      classification

Moore-Blount
    M.-B. driver
    M.-B. screwdriver
Moore-Southern approach
mooring
mop-end mid-substance tear
morcellate
morcellation
    Robinson m.
    Robinson-Chung-Farahvar
      clavicular m.
morcellize, morsellize
morcellized
    m. bone
    m. bone graft
Moreira
    M. bolt
    M. plate
Moreland
    M. femoral component extractor
    M. osteotome
    M. total hip revision
      instrumentation
Moreland-Marder-Anspach femoral stem
removal
Morel-Lavele lesion
Morel syndrome
Moretz prosthesis
Morfam Massager
Morgan-Casscells
    M.-C. meniscus suturing
    M.-C. meniscus suturing technique
Moro reflex
morphea-like lesion
morphine sulfate
Morpho Exerciser
morphogenesis
morphogenetic protein
morphologically
morphometry
    pedicle m.
Morquio
    M. disease
    M. sign
    M. syndrome
Morrey-Bryan
    M.-B. total elbow arthroplasty
Morrey elbow arthroplasty rating
system
Morris
    M. biphase screw
    M. retractor
Morris-Hand-Dunn anterior arthrodesis
Morrison
    M. neurovascular free flap
    M. technique

Morrissy
  M. percutaneous fixation of slipped
    epiphysis
  M. percutaneous slipped epiphysis
    fixation
Morscher cervical plate
Morse
  M. taper
  M. tapered prosthetic post
  M. taper lock of modular hip
    implant component
morsellize (*var. of* morcellize)
mortise
  ankle m.
  cuneiform m.
  m. and tenon joint
  m. view
Morton
  M. disease
  M. foot
  M. interdigital neuroma
  M. metatarsalgia
  M. neuroma neurolysis
  M. sign
  M. syndrome
  M. test
  M. toe
  M. toe support
Morton-Horwitz nerve cross-over sign
mosaicplasty technique
mosaic wart
Moseley
  M. bone age graph
  M. fasciotome
  M. glenoid rim prosthesis
  M. straight line graph
Mose method
Mosley method
mosquito
  m. clamp
  m. hemostat
  m.-tip grasping forceps
Moss
  M. cage
  M. fixation system
  M. hook
  M. instrumentation
  M. rod
Mother Jones dressing
Mother-To-Be
  M.-T.-B. abdominal support
  M.-T.-B. Support Maternity Support

motion
  accessory m.
  active ankle joint complex range
    of m. (AAROM)
  active-assisted range of m.
  active-assistive range of m.
  active integral range of m.
    (AIROM)
  active and passive range of m.
  active range of m. (AROM)
  m. activity
  angular m.
  angulation m.
  ankle dorsiflexion range of m.
    (ADROM)
  ankle inversion-eversion range
    of m.
  AP translatory m.
  arc of m.
  axis of rib m.
  back range of m. (BROM)
  m. barrier
  bucket-handle rib m.
  bucket-handle rim m.
  m. concentration
  constant massive m.
  continuous passive m. (CPM)
  m. control
  controlled ankle m. (CAM)
  m. control limiter (MCL)
  M. Control Limiter (755 MCL)
  m. control mitt
  coupled m.
  degrees-of-freedom joint m.
  m. demand
  distractive m.
  double-flexion knee m.
  end range of m.
  frontal m.
  hindfoot m.
  hip extension range of m.
  inherent m.
  intersegmental m.
  m. limit
  limitation of m. (LOM)
  m. limitation
  limitation of joint m.
  loss of m.
  lumbar range of m.
  m. measurement
  osteokinematic m.
  m. palpation

M

NOTES

motion *(continued)*
    passive intervertebral m. (PIVM)
    passive range of m. (PROM)
    pattern of m.
    m. performance
    physiologic m.
    pistoning m.
    plantarflexory m.
    m.-preserving procedure
    protective limitation of range
      of m.
    pump-handle rib m.
    m. quality
    m. range
    range of m. (ROM)
    rectilinear m.
    m. response
    restricted range of m.
    restriction of m.
    m. restriction
    rotary m.
    sacroiliac joint m.
    sagittal m.
    scapulothoracic m.
    m. segment
    m. slack
    sling suspension range of m.
    stable to m.
    subtalar m.
    m. testing
    m. therapy
    total active m. (TAM)
    total eversion range of m.
    total passive m. (TPM)
    translation m.
    translatory m.
    trial range of m.
    triaxial m.
    triplane m.
    uninhibited ankle m.
    valgus knee m.
    m. velocity
    winging m.
Motivator FTR2000 exerciser
motoneuron *(var. of* motor neuron)
motor
    m. activity
    m. branch
    m. deficit
    m. disorder
    m. dysfunction
    m. examination
    m. fascicle
    m. function
    m. function assessment
    m. latency
    m. loss
    m. milestone

    m. nerve conduction velocity
      (MNCV)
    m. neuron
    m. point
    m. point block
    m. reflex
    m. response
    m. strength
    m. unit
    m. unit action potential (MUAP)
    m. unit fraction
    m. unit potential (MUP)
    m. unit territory
    m. vehicle accident (MVA)
    m. weakness
motorcycle accident (MCA)
motorcyclist's knee
motorized
    m. meniscal cutter
    m. meniscal shaver
    m. reamer
    m. shaving system
    m. suction shaver
    m. trimmer
motor neuron, motoneuron
Motricity Index
Motrin
    M. IB
    M. IB Sinus
    Junior Strength M.
mottled
mottling
Mouchet fracture
Mould arthroplasty
Moule screw pin
Mouradian
    M. humeral fixation system
    M. rod
    M. screw
MouseMitt Keyboarders
Mouse Nest mouse rest
move
    push-pull m.
movement
    active hip m.
    active range of m.
    adventitious m.
    anterior-inferior m.
    anterior-posterior m.
    anterosuperior external ilium m.
      (ASEx)
    anterosuperior internal ilium m.
      (ASIn)
    arcuate m.
    m. artifact
    M. Assessment of Infants (MAI)
    atlas-axis m.
    Awareness Through M. (ATM)

caliper rib m.
compensatory m.
dissociation m.
dynamic m.
external ilium m.
freedom of m.
inferior m.
innominate m.
internal m.
intersegmental m.
isokinetic m.
limitation of m.
medial m.
passive m.
m. performance
posteroinferior external m.
posteroinferior internal m.
primary or intentional m.
primary rotation m.
quasi-independent Y-axis m.
sagittal m.
m. science
trick m.
unilateral posterior-anterior m.
universal coronal m.

mover
prime m.
movie sign
Moxa heat therapy
moxalactam
moxibustion heat therapy
Moynihan towel clamp
MP
metacarpophalangeal
MP35N implant metal prosthesis
MPA
metatarsus primus adductus
M-Pact
M-P. cast cutter
M-P. cast spreader
M-P. cast vacuum
M-P. flexible orthotic
MPF
myofascial pain syndrome
MPFL
medial patellofemoral ligament
MPJ
metacarpophalangeal joint
MPM
M. antimicrobial wound cleanser
M. bandage
MPO 2000 Active

MPP
maximum pressure picture
M-Prednisol Injection
MPTh
mechanical pain threshold
MPV
metatarsus primus varus
MRC
Medical Research Council
MRC muscle function classification
MRI
magnetic resonance imaging
MRI-directed surgery
dynamic MRI
flexion-extension MRI
FONAR Stand-Up MRI
Gyroscan superconducting MRI
MRI testing
MRN
magnetic resonance neurography
MS
multiple sclerosis
MS Contin Oral
MSAFP
maternal serum alpha fetoprotein
MSD
microsurgical diskectomy
MSI
magnetic source imaging
MSI mapping
MSIR Oral
MSL
midsternal line
MS/L
MS/S
M.S. splint
MST-6A1-4V implant metal prosthesis
MT
metatarsal
metatarsophalangeal
muscle testing
MT bar
MTA
metatarsus adductus
MTA brace
MTC
metatarsocuneiform
MTE allograft
MTF
Musculoskeletal Transplant Foundation
MTM 2 bur

M

NOTES

MTP
 metatarsophalangeal
  MTP joint
MTPJ
 metatarsophalangeal joint
MTS
 medial tibial syndrome
MTSS
 medial tibial stress syndrome
MTV
 metatarsus varus
MUAP
 macro motor unit action potential
 motor unit action potential
Mubarak-Hargens
 M.-H. decompression
 M.-H. decompression technique
mucate
 isometheptene m.
mucirocin
mucopolysaccharide
 sulfated m.
mucopolysaccharidosis,
 pl. **mucopolysaccharidoses (MCP)**
mucosum
 ligamentum m.
mucous
 m. cyst
 m. membrane (mm)
mucus (noun)
Mudder sign
Mueli wrist prosthesis
Mueller, Müller
 M. anterolateral femorotibial
  ligament tenodesis
 M. arthrodesis
 M. classification of humerus
  fracture
 M. compression apparatus
 M. compression blade plate
 M. cup
 M. distractor
 M. dual-lock hip prosthesis
 M. femoral supracondylar fracture
  classification
 M. fixation device
 M. hip arthroplasty
 M. intertochanteric varus osteotomy
 M. knee procedure
 M. lateral compartment
 M. patellar tendon graft
 M. retractor
 M. technique
 M. template
 M. tibial fracture classification
 M. total hip replacement prosthesis
 M. transposition osteotomy

 M. Ultralite brace
 M. wrench
Mueller-Charnley hip prosthesis
Muir-Torre syndrome
Mulder
 M. click
 M. sign
MULE
 microcomputer upper limb exerciser
 MULE upper limb exerciser
Müller (*var. of* Mueller)
Mulligan Silastic prosthesis
multangular
 greater m.
 lesser m.
 m. ridge fracture
Multi
 M. Axis Ankle
 M. Podus Foot System
multiaction pin cutter
multiaxial
 M. Assessment of Pain (MAP)
 m. screw
multiaxis foot
multicentric
 m. osteogenic sarcoma
 m. reticulohistiocytosis
multidirectional instability (MDI)
multidisciplinary
multielectrode
multifidi musculi
multifidus syndrome
Multiflex prosthesis
Multiflora-ABS
multilead electrode
Multileaf Collimator
multilevel
 m. fracture
 m. fusion
 m. laminectomy
Multi-Lock
 M.-L. hand operating table
 M.-L. hip prosthesis
 M.-L. knee brace
multipartite
 m. fracture
 m. patella
multiplace hyperbaric chamber
multiplanar
 m. computed tomography scan
 m. CT scan
 m. deformity
 m. gradient recall image
 m. ligamentotaxis
multiplane echo probe
multiple
 m. action cutter
 m. axis knee joint

m. cancellous chip graft
m. digits
m. discharge
m. enchondroma
m. enchondromatosis
m. epiphyseal dysplasia
m. finger
m. flexible medullary nail
m. fracture
m. hook assembly
m. hook assembly C-D
  instrumentation
m. injury
m. line-scan imaging (MLSI)
m. myeloma
m. neurofibroma
m. osteochondromatosis
m. pinhole occluder
m.-point sacral fixation
m. pterygium syndrome
m. ray
m.-ray amputation
m. sclerosis (MS)
m. trauma
m. trauma victim

multiplex
mononeuropathy m.

multipotential cell
Multipulse 1000 compression pump
multipurpose
m. angled clamp
m. curved clamp

multiray fracture
multisegmental
m. spinal distortion
m. spinal stenosis

multisensory ballpit
multisided blade handle
multisized reamer
multispan fracture hook
multistaged carrier flap
multitrauma patient
multivariate analysis of variance
  (MANOVA)
multocida
Pasteurella m.
Mumford
M. procedure
M. resection

Mumford-Gurd
M.-G. acromioclavicular operation
M.-G. arthroplasty

Munchausen syndrome
Munchmeyer disease
MUP
motor unit potential

mupirocin
Murphy
M. Achilles tendon advancement
M. brace
M. gouge
M. heel cord advancement
M. osteotome
M. punch test
M. skid
M. sling
M. splint

Murphy-Lane bone skid
Murray-Jones arm splint
Murray knee prosthesis
Murray-Thomas arm splint
muscle
abdominal m.
abductor digiti minimi m.
abductor digiti quinti m.
abductor hallucis m.
abductor pollicis brevis m.
abductor pollicis longus m.
adductor pollicis m.
agonist m.
agonistic m.
m. analysis
antagonist m.
antagonistic m.
anterior scalene m.
anterior serratus m.
anterior tibial m.
m.-balancing procedure
BBC m.'s
m. belly
biceps brachii m.
biceps femoris m.
m. biopsy clamp
brachialis m.
brachioradialis m.
buccinator m.
m. contractility
m. contracture
cricopharyngeal sphincter m.
cucullaris m.
deepithelialized rectus abdominis m.
  (DRAM)
deltoid m.
digastric m.

M

NOTES

muscle *(continued)*

m. disorder
dorsal interosseous m.
ECRB m.
ECRL m.
EDB m.
m. energy
m. energy technique
extensor carpi radialis brevis m.
extensor carpi radialis longus m.
extensor carpi ulnaris m.
extensor comminicus m.
extensor digiti minimi m.
extensor digiti quinti m.
extensor digitorum brevis m.
extensor digitorum communis m.
extensor digitorum longus m.
extensor hallucis brevis m.
extensor hallucis longus m.
extensor indicis proprius m.
extensor pollicis brevis m.
extensor pollicis longus m.
external intercostal m.
external oblique m.
m. fascicle
m. fiber action potential
m. fiber conduction velocity
finger flexor m.
m. flap
flexor carpi radialis m.
flexor carpi ulnaris m.
flexor digiti quinti m.
flexor digitorum longus m.
flexor digitorum profundus m.
flexor digitorum sublimis m.
flexor digitorum superficialis m.
flexor hallucis brevis m.
flexor hallucis longus m.
flexor pollicis brevis m.
flexor pollicis longus m.
gastrocnemius m.
gastroc-soleus m.
gluteus maximus m.
gluteus medius m.
gluteus minimus m.
gracilis m.
greater rhomboid m.
m. guarding
hamstring m.
handbag m.
m. hernia
hypothenar m.
iliacus m.
iliococcygeus m.
iliocostal m.
iliopsoas m.
m. imbalance
infraspinatus m.

m. insufficiency
internal oblique m.
interosseous m.
intervening m.
intraspinous m.
intrinsic m.
m. ischemia
Langer m.
latissimus dorsi m.
levator scapulae m.
longus capitis m.
longus cervicis (colli) m.
longus colli m.
lumbrical m.
lumbricalis m.
m. and neurological stimulation
   electrotherapy device
oblique m.
obturator internus m.
omohyoid m.
opponens digiti quinti m.
opponens pollicis m. (OP)
palmar interosseous m.
palmaris longus m.
paraspinal m.
paravertebral m.
m. patterning sequence
pectoralis major m.
m. pedicle bone graft
peroneal m.
peroneus brevis m.
peroneus longus m.
peroneus tertius m.
plantaris m.
platysma m.
m. play
pollicis longus m.
popliteus m.
posterior deltoid m.
postural m.
profundus m.
pronator quadratus m.
pronator teres m.
psoas m.
quadratus femoris m.
quadratus lumborum m.
quadratus plantae m.
quadriceps femoris m.
rectus abdominis m.
rectus femoris m.
m. relaxant
released ulnar intrinsic m.
sartorius m.
scalene m.
scalenus anticus m.
scapulohumeral m.
scapulothoracic m.
semimembranosus m.

semitendinosus m.
serratus anterior m.
m.-setting exercise
m. sheath
shunt m.
skeletal m.
m. slide
m. sliding operation
m. spasm
m. spindle
m.-splitting incision
spurt m.
sternocleidomastoid m.
sternohyoid m.
sternomastoid m.
sternothyroid m.
m. strain
strap m.
m. stretch reflex
subscapularis m.
supinator m.
supraspinatus m.
synergistic m.
teres major m.
m. testing (MT)
thenar m.
tibial m.
tibialis anterior m.
tibialis posterior m.
m. tissue mobility
toe extensor m.
toe flexor m.
m. tone
m. transfer
transversus abdominis m.
trapezius m.
triceps surae m.
vastus lateralis m.
vastus medialis m.
vastus medialis obliquus m.
muscle-plasty
Speed V-Y m.-p.
muscle-tendon
m.-t. injury
m.-t. transplantation
muscular
m. atrophy
m. attachment
m. clamp
m. contraction
m. coordination
m. cramp

m. dystrophy (MD)
m. lesion
m. neurofibromatosis
m. reeducation
m. tissue
m. torticollis
muscularis
kyphosis m.
musculature
axial m.
left erector spinae m.
paraspinal m.
paravertebral m.
peroneal m.
right erector spinae m.
musculi (*pl. of* musculus)
musculocutaneous
m. free flap
m. nerve
m. nerve block
m. nerve injury
musculofascial
musculoskeletal
M. Function Assessment (MFA)
m. infection
m. melioidosis
M. Transplant Foundation (MTF)
m. trauma
M. Tumor Society
musculotendinous
m. cuff
m. flap
m. junction
m.-osseous link
m. system
m. unit
musculus, pl. **musculi**
abductor digiti minimi magnus m.
abductor digiti minimi pedis m.
extensor indicis proprius m.
intertransversarii laterales musculi
intertransversarii mediales lumborum
musculi
longissimus capitis m.
longissimus cervicis m.
longus capitis m.
multifidi musculi
obliquus capitis inferior m.
obliquus capitis superior m.
rhomboideus major m.
rotatores breves musculi
rotatores longi musculi

M

NOTES

musculus *(continued)*
　　rotatores thoracis musculi
　　sacrospinalis m.
Musgrave
　　M. footprint pedobarograph
　　M. Footprint System
mushroom
　　m. impactor
　　m. walker glide
mushy edema
musician's plight
Mustard iliopsoas transfer
mutilans rheumatoid arthritis
Mutilation
　　Amniotic Deformity, Adhesion, M.
　　　(ADAM)
MVA
　　motor vehicle accident
MVC
　　maximal voluntary contraction
MVM
　　medullary venous malformation
MV1, MV2 receptor
MVP
　　Biodex Multi-Joint System 3 M.
MVR blade
MVV
　　maximal voluntary ventilation
MWD
　　microwave diathermy
myalgia
myasthenia gravis
myatrophy
Mycelex
Mycelex-7
Mycelex-G
mycetoma
Mycifradin Sulfate Topical
Mycitracin Topical
mycobacterial
　　m. arthritis
　　m. infection
Mycobacterium
　　M. avium
　　M. avium-intracellulare
　　M. bovis
　　M. chelonei
　　M. fortuitum
　　M. gordonae
　　M. intracellulare
　　M. kansasii
　　M. marinum
　　M. terrae
　　M. tuberculosis
Mycocide NS
mycological
mycopolysaccharidosis

mycosis
　　cutaneous m.
　　m. fungoides
　　systemic m.
mycotic
　　m. aneurysm
　　m. club nail
　　m. infection
myelalgia
myelanalosis
myelasthenia
myelatelia
myelatrophy
myeleterosis
myelinated
myelitis
　　acute transverse m.
myeloblastoma
myelocele
myelocystocele
myelocystomeningocele
myelodiastasis
myelodysplasia
myelodysplastic kyphosis
myelofibrosis
myelogram
myelographic
myelography
　　bar-like ventral defect on m.
myelolipoma
myeloma
　　multiple m.
　　plasma cell m.
　　solitary m.
　　urine protein m.
myelomalacia
myelomeningocele
myelomere
myeloneuritis
myeloparalysis
myelopathy
　　cervical spondylotic m.
　　m. incidence
　　laminaplasty with extended
　　　foraminoplasty for cervical m.
　　noncompressive m.
　　progressive subacute m.
　　spinal stenotic m.
　　transverse m.
　　vacuolar m.
myelophthisis
myeloplegia
myeloradiculitis
myeloradiculopathy
myelorrhaphy .
　　commissural m.
myelotomy
Myers knee retractor

mylohyoid
myoasthenia
myoblast
myoblastoma
    granular cell m.
Myobock artificial hand
myobradia
myocardial
    m. bridging
    m. infarction
    m. perfusion scan
myocele
myocelialgia
myocelitis
myocerosis
myocervical collar
Myochrysine
myoclasis
myoclonia
myoclonic
    m. epilepsy
    m. epilepsy with ragged-red fibers
myoclonus
MyoComp
myocutaneous flap
myocytoma
MyoDac 2
myodegeneration
myodemia
myodesis
myodysneuria
myodystonia
myoedema
myoelectrical
myoelectrically silent
myoelectric prosthesis
myoencephalopathy
myofascia
myofascial
    m. closure
    m. manipulation
    m. pain
    m. pain syndrome (MPF)
    m. release
    m. tenderness
    m. trigger point
    m. unit
myofasciitis
    interstitial m.
myofibril
myofibroma
myofibrosis

myofibrositis
Myoflex
MyoForce test
myofusio-periostitis
myogelosis
myogenic tonus
myography
    acoustic m.
myohypertrophia
myoinositol level
myo-inositol uptake
myoischemia
myokerosis
myokymia
myokymic discharge
myolipoma
myolysis
myoma
myomalacia
myomatosis
myomectomy, myomatectomy
myomelanosis
myonecrosis
    clostridial m.
myoneural ischemia
myoneurasthenia
myoneurectomy
myoneuroma
myoneurosis
myopachynsis
myopalmus
myoparalysis
myoparesis
myopathic
    m. arthrogryposis
    m. motor unit potential
    m. recruitment
myopathophysiology
myopathy
    acquired m.
    benign congenital m.
    centronuclear m.
    exercise m.
    idiopathic polymyositis m.
    mitochondrial m.
    myotubular m.
    nemaline rod-body m.
    polymyositis m.
    postinfectious m.
    rheumatoid arthritis m.
    sarcotubular m.
    steroid m.

M

NOTES

myopathy *(continued)*
    structural congenital m.
    zebra body m.
    zidovudine-induced m.
myophagism
myoplastic muscle stabilization
myopsychopathy
myosarcoma
Myoscan sensor
myosclerosis
myoseism
myositides myositis
myositis
    cervical tension m. (CTM)
    clostridial m.
    m. fibrosa
    focal nodular m.
    granulomatous m.
    inclusion body m. (IBM)
    inflammatory m.
    ischemic m.
    myositides m.
    m. ossificans
    m. ossificans progressiva
    proliferative m.
    streptococcal m.
    tension m.
    viral m.
myospasia
myospasm
Myossage lotion
myosteoma
myosynizesis

myotatic unit
myotendinous junction
myotenontoplasty
myotomal pain
myotome
myotonia
    chondroplastic m.
    m. congenita
    congenital m.
    drug-induced m.
    m. intermittens
myotonic
    m. discharge
    m. muscular dystrophy
    m. potential
MyoTrac
    M. 2, C device
    M. device
    M. EMG biofeedback monitor
myotube
myotubular myopathy
mytenositis
myxofibroma
myxoid
    m. chondrosarcoma
    m. liposarcoma
    m.-type liposarcoma
myxoma
    soft tissue m.
myxomatous cell
myxosarcoma
M-Zole 7 Dual Pack

NA
  neuropathic arthropathy
Na
  Tui Na
nabumetone
Nada-Chair Back-Up portable back sling
Naden-Rieth prosthesis
NADPH
  nicotinamide-adenine dinucleotide phosphate
Nafcil Injection
nafcillin
Naffziger
  N. syndrome
  N. test
naftifine
Naftin
nail
  adjustable n.
  Ainsworth modification of Massie n.
  Alta tibial n.
  anteroposterior n.
  AO slotted medullary n.
  n. assembly
  Augustine boat n.
  n. avulsion
  Bailey-Dubow n.
  Barr bolt n.
  beak n.
  n. bed
  n. bed graft
  n. bed hematoma evacuation
  n.-bending device
  bent n.
  Bickel intramedullary n.
  blind medullary n.
  boat n.
  Brooker double-locking unreamed tibial n.
  Brooker femoral n.
  Brooker-Wills n.
  cannulated n.
  centromedullary n.
  Chandler unreamed interlocking tibial n.
  Chick n.
  Christensen interlocking n.
  closed Küntscher n.
  cloverleaf Küntscher n.
  clubbed n.
  condylocephalic n.
  crutch and belt femoral closed n.
  Curry hip n.

Delitala T-nail n.
delta femoral n.
Delta Recon n.
delta tibial n.
Derby n.
Diamond n.
diamond-shaped medullary n.
digital n.
n. disorder
Dooley n.
double-ended n.
n. drill
n. driver
n.-driving guide
n. dust
dynamic locking n.
dystrophic n.
elastic stable intramedullary n. (ESIN)
Ender flexible medullary n.
Engel-May n.
n. extender
flexible intramedullary n. (FIN)
flexible medullary n.
fluted Sampson n.
fluted titanium n.
n. fold
n. fold removal
four-flanged n.
gamma locking n.
n. groove
Grosse-Kempf interlocking medullary n.
Grosse-Kempf locking n.
Hackethal n.
Hagie pin n.
Hahn bone n.
Halder locking n.
half-and-half n.
Hall-Pankovich medullary n.
hallux n.
Hansen-Street n.
Harris condylocephalic n.
Harris hip n.
Harris medullary n.
Holt n.
hooked intramedullary n.
hooked medullary n.
Huckstep n.
IMSC five-hole n.
IMSC multihole n.
interlocking medullary n.
intramedullary supracondylar multihole n.
Inyo n.

N

nail *(continued)*
  Jewett n.
  Johannson hip n.
  Kaessmann n.
  Ken sliding n.
  Klemm-Schellman n.
  Knowles pin n.
  Küntscher n.
  left-sided n.
  n. length gauge method
  Lewis n.
  Lloyd adapter for Smith-Petersen n.
  locking n.
  Lottes triflanged medullary n.
  Massie II n.
  Massie sliding n.
  n. matrix
  McKee tri-fin n.
  McLaughlin n.
  medullary n.
  Moore n.
  multiple flexible medullary n.
  mycotic club n.
  nested n.
  Neufeld n.
  No-Lok self-locking n.
  noncannulated n.
  nonreamed n.
  onychocryptosis n.
  Ony-Clear N.
  open-section n.
  OrthoSorb pin n.
  Palmer bone n.
  n.-patella syndrome
  PGP n.
  pincer n.
  Pitcock n.
  n. plate
  n. plate apparatus
  n. plate device
  n. plate fixation
  n. plate removal
  prebent n.
  Pugh sliding n.
  n.-pulling forceps
  reamed n.
  Recon n.
  ReVision n.
  Richards reconstruction n.
  right-sided n.
  n. root
  n. rotational guide
  Rush flexible medullary n.
  Russell-Taylor delta tibial n.
  Russell-Taylor interlocking
    medullary n.
  Rydell n.
  Sage forearm n.

  Sage radial n.
  Sage triangular n.
  Sampson medullary n.
  Sarmiento n.
  Schneider medullary n.
  n.-screw sideplate assembly
  Seidel n.
  self-broaching n.
  self-locking n.
  n. set
  sliding n.
  Slocum n.
  slotted n.
  Smillie n.
  Smith-Petersen femoral neck n.
  Smith-Petersen transarticular n.
  specialized n.
  spring-loaded n.
  standard medullary n.
  n. starter
  static locking n.
  Steinmann extension n.
  Street forearm n.
  supracondylar medullary n.
  n. suture
  Sven-Johansson femoral neck n.
  telescoping n.
  Temple University n.
  Terry n.
  Thatcher n.
  Thornton n.
  Tiemann n.
  triangular medullary n.
  triflanged Lottes n.
  triflanged medullary n.
  TRUE/FLEX Intramedullary n.
  Uniflex humeral n.
  Universal n.
  Venable-Stuck n.
  Vesely-Street split n.
  Vitallium Küntscher n.
  V-medullary n.
  Watson-Jones n.
  Webb bolt n.
  Winograd technique for ingrown n.
  Z fixation n.
  Zickel subcondylar n.
  Zickel subtrochanteric n.
  Zickel supracondylar medullary n.
  Zimmer telescoping n.

nailing
  antegrade n.
  blind medullary n.
  centromedullary n.
  closed Küntscher n.
  closed medullary n.
  condylocephalic n.
  crutch and belt femoral closed n.

elastic stable intramedullary n. (ESIN)
Ender n.
femoral n.
Grosse-Kempf interlocking medullary n.
Harris condylocephalic n.
interlocking n.
intermedullary n.
intramedullary n. (IMN)
Küntscher medullary n.
locked n.
Lottes n.
open medullary n.
retrograde n.
static lock n.
tibiocalcaneal medullary n.
Vertstreken closed medullary n.
Zickel n.

nail plate
sliding n. p.

Nakamura brace
Nakayama staple
nalbuphine
Nalebuff arthrodesis
Nalebuff-Millender lateral band mobilization technique
Nalfon
Nallpen Injection
naloxone hydrochloride
Namaqualand hip dysplasia
NAMES
National Association of Medical Equipment Suppliers

NAP
nerve action potential

napkin
n. ring calcar allograft
n. ring compression

Napoleon hat sign
Naprelan
Naprosyn
naproxen sodium
Naraghi-DeCoster reduction clamp
Narcan
narcissistic personality disorder
Naropin
narrow
n. AO dynamic compression plate
n.-base gait
n.-blade retractor

n.-neck mini-Hohmann retractor
n. toebox shoe

narrowing
intervertebral disk n.

nasal
n. elevator
n. insulin
n. spine

nascent motor unit potential
natatory
n. cord
n. ligament

Nathan-Trung modification of Krukenberg hand reconstruction
National
N. Association of Medical Equipment Suppliers (NAMES)
N. Board of Chiropractic Examiners (NBCE)
N. Football Head and Neck Injury Registry

Native American medicine
Natural-Hip
N.-H. prosthesis
N.-H. titanium hip stem

natural history
Natural-Knee
N.-K. II system

Natural-Lok acetabular cup prosthesis
naturopathy
Naughton-Dunn triple arthrodesis
Nauth
N. traction apparatus
N. traction device

navicular
accessory n.
n. bone
n. cookie in shoe
cornuate n.
n. drop test
n. to first metatarsal angle
n. fracture
Kidner procedure for accessory n.
lip of n.
protrusion of the n.
n. shoe cookie
n. shoe pad
tarsal n.

naviculectomy
naviculocapitate
n. fracture
n. fracture syndrome

NOTES

N

naviculocuneiform
    n. fusion
    n. joint
    n. joint arthrodesis
    n. ligament
NBCE
    National Board of Chiropractic
    Examiners
NC
    neurogenic claudication
NCS
    nerve conduction study
NCT
    nerve compression test
    nerve conduction test
NCV
    nerve conduction velocity
Neal-Robertson litter
near-constant frequency trains
near-far fashion
near-field potential
near-infrared interaction
NEB
    New England Baptist
    NEB acetabular cup
    NEB arthroplasty
    NEB hip arthroplasty
    NEB total hip prosthesis
Necelon surgical glove
necessity
    fracture of n.
neck
    basal n.
    n. diameter
    femoral n.
    n. fracture
    glenoid n.
    N.-Hugger cervical support pillow
    humeral n.
    metacarpal n.
    metatarsal n.
    Neck-Roll aromatherapy hot/cold
      pack
    phalangeal n.
    radial n.
    n. reflex
    n.-righting reflex
    n. roll
    n. shaft
    n.-shaft angle
    supple n.
    surgical n.
    talar n.
    n. wrap
Neckcare pillow
Necktrac
    N. traction
    N. traction device

Nec Loc cervical collar
necrosis
    aseptic n.
    atraumatic n.
    avascular n. (AVN)
    avascular n. of the femoral head
      (AVNFH)
    bone n.
    corticosteroid-induced avascular n.
    epiphyseal ischemic n.
    gangrenous n.
    idiopathic avascular n.
    radiographic avascular n.
    Ratliff avascular n. classification
    septic n.
    skin n.
    steroid-induced avascular n.
necroticans
    osteochondritis n.
necrotic tissue
necrotizing fasciitis
NEECHAM Confusion Scale
needle
    Astralac n.
    atraumatic n.
    Beath n.
    Bergstrom n.
    n. biopsy
    bone biopsy n.
    bore n.
    bouge n.
    Bunnell tendon n.
    cutting n.
    Deschamps n.
    diskogram n.
    n. electrode
    Framer tendon-passing n.
    Gallie n.
    Hawkeye suture n.
    n. holder
    hubbed n.
    Intracath n.
    Jamshidi n.
    Keith n.
    McGee prosthesis n.
    meniscal repair n.
    milliner's n.
    n. placement
    Quincke n.
    retrobulbar prosthesis n.
    Seirin acupuncture n.
    Sklar ligature n.
    spinal n.
    Stimuplex block n.
    tendon n.
    Thomas n.
    Tuohy n.
    Verbrugge n.

Veress n.
Wangensteen n.
Webster n.
needle-nose vise-grip pliers
needling
Neer
N. acromioplasty
N. acromioplasty for rotator cuff
tear
N. capsular shift procedure
N. femur fracture classification
N. hemiarthroplasty
N. humeral replacement prosthesis
N. humerus fracture classification
N. II humeral component
N. II shoulder system
N. II total knee system
N. II total shoulder system implant
N. impingement test
N. modification
N. open reduction
N. posterior shoulder reconstruction
N. shoulder fracture classification
N. shoulder prosthesis (I, II)
N. umbrella prosthesis
N. unconstrained shoulder
arthroplasty
Neer-Horowitz
N.-H. classification
N.-H. classification of humeral
fracture
Neer-Vitallium humeral prosthesis
Neff
N. femorotibial nail system
N. meniscus knife
negative
n. casting
coagulase n.
n. congruence angle
n. ulnar variance (NUV)
n. work
neglect
visual n.
neglected rupture
Neibauer-Cutter prosthesis
Neil-Moore perforator drill
Neisseria
N. gonorrhoeae
N. sicca
Neivert osteotome
Nélaton
N. ankle dislocation

N. dislocation of ankle
N. line
N. rubber tube drain
Nelson
N. finger exerciser
N. rib retractor
N. rib spreader
N. scissors
N. sign
nemaline rod-body myopathy
Nembutal
neoadjuvant chemotherapy
Neo-Cortef
neocortex
NeoDecadron Topical
neoformans
Cryptococcus n.
neolimbus
Neomixin Topical
neomycin
n. and dexamethasone
n. and hydrocortisone
n. and polymyxin B
n., polymyxin B, and
hydrocortisone
neonatal
n. flatfoot
n. sandbag
n. trach tube holder
Neopap
neoplasm
extensive n.
interdigital n.
neoplastic
n. disorder
n. disorder disease
n. fracture
Neoplush foam
neoprene
n. ankle support
n. back support
n. dressing
n. elbow sleeve
n. fabric
n. hinged-knee brace
n. knee sleeve
n. Osgood-Schlatter knee brace
n. wrist brace
n. wrist orthosis
n. wrist strap
Neoral Oral
Neosar Injection

N

NOTES

Neosporin
- N. Cream
- N. Topical Ointment

neotendon

neovascularization

Nephro-Calci

nerve
- abductor digiti minimi n.
- accessory n.
- n. action potential (NAP)
- antebrachial cutaneous n.
- anterior thoracic n.
- articular n.
- axillary n.
- n. cap
- common peroneal n.
- n. compression test (NCT)
- n. conduction study (NCS)
- n. conduction test (NCT)
- n. conduction velocity (NCV)
- n. conduction velocity test
- n. crossing
- cutaneous n.
- deep peroneal n.
- digital n.
- dorsal scapular n.
- n. ending
- n. entrapment syndrome
- femoral cutaneous n.
- n. fiber action potential
- genitofemoral n.
- gluteal n.
- n. graft
- n. hook
- hypoglossal n.
- iliohypogastric n.
- ilioinguinal n.
- inferior laryngeal n.
- n. injury
- intercostal n.
- intercostobrachial n.
- interdigital n.
- n. interference
- intermediate dorsal cutaneous n. (IDCN)
- intermetatarsal n.
- interosseous n.
- n. involvement testing
- n. of Kunzel
- lateral antebrachial cutaneous n.
- lateral anterior thoracic n.
- lateral femoral cutaneous n.
- lateral plantar n.
- longitudinal blood supply to ulnar n.
- mandibular n.
- medial antebrachial cutaneous n.
- medial articular n.
- medial brachial n.
- medial dorsal cutaneous n. (MDCN)
- median n.
- musculocutaneous n.
- obturator n.
- n. palsy
- pectoral n.
- peripheral n.
- peroneal n.
- phrenic n.
- plantar n.
- posterior interosseous n.
- posterior tibial n. (PTN)
- radial digital n.
- radial sensory n.
- recurrent laryngeal n.
- recurrent meningeal n.
- regeneration of n.
- n. root
- n. root block
- n. root compression
- n. root decompression
- n. root entrapment
- n. root injection
- n. root irritability
- n. root irritation
- n. root lesion
- n. rootlet ablation
- sacral n.
- saphenous n.
- scapular n.
- sciatic n.
- sensory n.
- n. separator
- n. sheath tumor
- sinuvertebral n.
- spinal accessory n.
- n. stretching
- superficial peroneal n.
- superficial radial n.
- superior gluteal n.
- superior laryngeal n.
- suprascapular n.
- sural n.
- sympathetic n.
- thoracic n.
- tibial n.
- n. tracing
- n. transmission
- n. trunk action potential
- ulnar n. (UN)
- vagus n.
- n. wrapping

NervePace nerve conduction monitor

Nervocaine

nervorum
- vasa n.

Nervoscope
nervous system
Nesacaine
Nesacaine-MPF
nested
    n. nail
    n. step stool
netting
    splint pan n.
network
    achilleo-calcaneal vascular n.
Neubeiser adjustable forearm splint
Neufeld
    N. apparatus
    N. cast
    N. device
    N. driver
    N. dynamic method
    N. nail
    N. pin
    N. plate
    N. screw
    N. traction
Neurain drill
Neurairtome
    N. drill
    Hall N.
neural
    n. arch resection technique
    n. crest
    n. element
    n. foramen
    n. foraminotomy
    n. injury
    n. nevus
    n. tension
    n. tissue
    n. tumor
neuralgia
    genicular n.
    geniculate n.
    glossopharyngeal n.
    intercostal n.
    traumatic prepatellar n.
    trigeminal n.
    vagoglossopharyngeal n.
    vidian n.
neurapraxia
    medial plantar n.
neurasthenia
neuraxial compression

neurectomy
    adductor tenotomy and obturator n.
    (ATON)
    Eggers n.
    obturator n.
    Phelps n.
    ulnar motor n.
neurilemmoma
neuritis
    axial n.
    obturator nerve n.
    pudendal n.
    suprascapular n.
neuroablative
Neuro-Aide testing device
neuroarthropathic foot
neuroarthropathy
    atrophic n.
neuroarticular
    n. dysfunction
    n. subluxation
    n. syndrome
neuroblastoma
neurocentral synchondrosis
neurocirculation
NeuroCom balance master
neurocutaneous hand flap
neurodevelopmental
    n. approach
    n. training
    n. treatment
NeuroDrape surgical drape
neurodystrophic
neuroectodermal tumor
neurofibroma
    multiple n.
    nonplexiform cutaneous n.
    plexiform n.
neurofibromatosis
    n. kyphoscoliosis
    kyphoscoliosis secondary to n.
    muscular n.
neuroforamen
neurofunctional subluxation
neurogenic
    n. arthrogryposis
    n. claudication (NC)
    n. disease
    n. disorder
    n. fracture
    n. motor-evoked potential (NMEP)

N

NOTES

neurogenic *(continued)*
    n. shock
    n. syndrome
neurography
    magnetic resonance n. (MRN)
neuroleptanalgesia
neurologic
    n. assessment
    n. complication
    n. deficit
    n. disease
    n. pain
neurological
    n. nerve conduction velocity exam
    n. testing
neurologically intact
neurolysis
    distal n.
    external n.
    internal n.
    Morton neuroma n.
neurolytic block
neuroma
    amputation stump n.
    bulb n.
    dorsal n.
    incisional n.
    interdigital n.
    Morton interdigital n.
    refractory n.
    n. sign
    spindle n.
    sural n.
    traumatic n.
neuroma-in-continuity
neuromechanical
    n. correction
    n. lesion
    n. spinal chiropractic management
neuromeningeal pathway
Neurometer
neuromuscular
    n. component
    n. disease
    n. electrical stimulation (NMES)
    n. facilitation
    n. gait pattern change
    n. III stimulator
    n. reflex treatment
    n. scoliosis
    n. scoliosis orthotic treatment
    n. transfer
neuromusculoskeletal
neuromyotonia
neuromyotonic discharge
neuron
    fusimotor n.

    motor n.
    serotonergic n.
neuronal degenerative disease
neuronitis
    Parsonage-Turner n.
neuropathic
    n. ankle
    n. arthropathy (NA)
    n. collapse
    n. foot
    n. forefoot ulceration
    n. fracture
    n. hereditary disease
    n. hyperkyphoscoliosis
    n. knee
    n. midfoot deformity
    n. motor unit potential
    n. osteoarthropathy
    n. recruitment
    n. tarsal-metatarsal joint
    n. ulcer
neuropathogenic
neuropathophysiology
    normalization of n.
neuropathy
    compressive n.
    epineurial n.
    epineurial-perineurial n.
    epiperineurial n.
    fascicular n.
    hereditary sensory motor n.
    hereditary sensory motor n., type III (HSMN III)
    periepineurial n.
    peripheral n.
    peroneal n.
    porphyritic n.
    spontaneous median n.
    sural n.
    ulnar n.
neurophysiologic effect
neurophysiology
neuroplasty
neuroprosthesis
neuropsychologic test
neuroreflexive
neurorrhaphy
    epineurial n.
    perineurial n.
neurosis, pl. neuroses
    low back n.
neurostimulator
    Biotens n.
    Grass n.
    Staodyne EMS+2 n.
neurotherapeutic
neurotherapy
    manual reflex n.

N. hip prosthesis
N. implant
N. wheelchair seating system

N. Stretch night splint
N. Stretch night splint suspension
 system with Sealed Ice
as
N. five-in-one reconstruction
N. five-in-one reconstruction
 technique
N. ligament technique
N. manual muscle tester
plast blank

N. forceps
N. incision
N. shoulder procedure
oni suture
 Compass EMG instrument

N. bone
N. cancellous bone graft
N. cancellous insert graft
N. classification
N. extractor
N. fracture operation
N. fracture repair procedure
N. plate
N. tendon prosthesis
mide-adenine dinucleotide
hate (NADPH)

nsulin-dependent diabetes mellitus

diolucent n.

. finger-joint replacement
prosthesis
. implant
. metacarpophalangeal joint
Silastic prosthesis
 trapeziometacarpal arthroplasty
 trapezium replacement prosthesis
-Cutter implant
-King technique
-Pick disease
t-Pearlman syndrome
e

ergillus n.

 brace
 splint
 splinting
 carpal tunnel support
 fracture

nigricans
 acanthosis n.
Nikon SMZ 2T magnifying lens
Nimmo receptor-tonus technique
ninety-ninety
 n.-n. method
 n.-n. traction
Ninhydrin print test
nipper
 English anvil nail n.
 House-Dieter malleus n.
 Miltex nail n.
 n.'s nail drill
nipple line
Niro
 N. bone-cutting forceps
 N. wire-twisting forceps
Nirschl
 N. operation
 N. technique
Nirvana mattress
Nitalloy
2-nite
 Sleepwell 2-nite
nitinol
nitrate
 silver n.
nitrofurantoin
nitrofurazone
nitrogen
 compressed n.
nitroglycerin
Nitroprusside
Nitro wheelchair
Nizoral
NK 665
NMEP
 neurogenic motor-evoked potential
NMES
 neuromuscular electrical stimulation
NMR
 nuclear magnetic resonance
nociception
nociceptive
 n. receptor
 n. transmission
nociceptor
 n. agent
 bombardment by n.
node
 Bouchard n.
 gouty n.
 Haygarth n.
 Heberden n.
 Meynet n.
 Osler n.
 Parrot n.
 Schmorl n.

NOTES

nodosa
    polyarteritis n.
nodular fasciitis
nodularity
    tendon n.
nodule
    Lisch n.
    rheumatoid n.
    synovial n.
    tendon n.
NOF
    nonossifying fibroma
NoHands Mouse-Foot-Operated Computer Mouse System
Noiles
    N. fully constrained tricompartmental knee prosthesis
    N. hinge
    N. posterior stabilized knee
    N. rotating hinge knee
    N. rotating-hinge knee mechanism
noise
    endplate n.
Nolan system collimator mounted contact shield
No-Lok
    N.-L. bolt
    N.-L. screw
    N.-L. self-locking nail
no man's land (in hand)
nomenclature
    dynamic listing n.
    static listing n.
nonadherent gauze dressing
nonambulation
nonarticular distal radial fracture
nonbeaded guidepin
nonbeveled
nonbipedal
noncannulated nail
noncemented total hip arthroplasty
noncollared Press-Fit femoral stem implantation
noncompliance
noncompressive myelopathy
noncongruent metatarsophalangeal joint
noncontact manipulation
noncontiguous fracture
noncontractile
nondisplaced fracture
nonenzymatic connective tissue glycation
nonfenestrated stem

nonglabrous skin
nonhinged
    n. knee prosthesis
    n. linked prosthesis
non-Hodgkin lymphoma
nonimpulsed base nerve transmission
noninsulin-dependent diabetes mellitus (NIDDM)
noninvasive technique
nonisometric graft
nonlamellated bone
nonlinear lesion
nonoperative
    n. orthopaedic management
    n. treatment
nonossifying fibroma (NOF)
nonosteoconductive bone-void filler
nonpainful
nonphyseal fracture
nonpitting edema
nonplexiform cutaneous neurofibroma
nonporous-coated endoprosthesis
nonreamed nail
nonreconstructable
nonreplantable amputation
nonrotational burst fracture
non-self-tapping screw
nonspasmodic torticollis
nonstanding lateral oblique view
nonsteroidal antiinflammatory medication
nonstructural curve
nonsubluxated metatarsophalangeal joint
nonsubperiosteal cortical defect
nonsuppurative osteomyelitis
nonsurgical management
nontender
nonthreaded wire
nonthrust mobilization
nontotal-contact disorder
nontraumatic idiopathic osteonecrosis
nontubed
    n. closed distant flap graft
    n. open distant flap graft
nontuberculous mycobacterial infection
nonunion
    n. of acromion
    atrophic n.
    avascular n.
    bayonet n.
    bioelectrical repair of delayed union or n.
    defect n.

N

NOTES

nonunion *(continued)*
    draining infected n.
    dry infected n.
    elephant-foot fracture n.
    fracture n.
    n. of fracture site
    gap n.
    hamate hook n.
    horse-hoof fracture n.
    hypertrophic vital n.
    hypervascular n.
    n. incidence
    infected nondraining n.
    metaphyseal-articular n.
    oligotrophic fracture n.
    n. osteomyelitis
    n. rate
    scaphoid n.
    supracondylar n.
    synovial n.
    talar body n.
    torsion wedge fracture n.
    vascular n.
    wedge n.
nonunited fracture
nonvalgus
nonwalking cast
nonweightbearing
    n. brace
    n. crutch walking
No Pain-HP
Norcet
Norco
NordiCare
    N. Back Therapy System
    N. Enabler exerciser
    N. Strider exerciser
NordicTrack ski exerciser
Nordotrack
    N. motion analyzer
    N. motion EMG
Norflex
norfloxacin
Norgesic Forte
Norian SRS cement
Noritate Cream
normal
    n. anatomic position
    n. last shoe
    n. lordotic curve
    upper limits of n.
normalization of neuropathophysiology
Normalize Press-Fit hip prosthesis
Norman
    N. tibial bolt
    N. tibial pin
Normiflo
normoxia

Norm testing and rehabilitation system
Norotrack Motion Analyzer & EMG
Norpramin
North
    N. American blastomycosis
    N. American Malignant
        Hyperthermia protocol
Northville brace
Northwick Park Index of Independence in ADL index
Norton ball reamer
nortriptyline
Norwood iliotibial band tenodesis
notch
    A-frame n.
    clavicular n.
    coracoid n.
    costal n.
    cotyloid n.
    n. cut
    n. cutting guide
    intercondylar n.
    interpeduncular n.
    intervertebral n.
    scapular n.
    sciatic n.
    sigmoid n.
    spinoglenoid n.
    suprasternal n.
    trochlear n.
    n. view
    n. width index (NWI)
notcher device
notchplasty
    n. blade
    n. procedure
note
    SORE n.
no-tie stretch lace
notochord
    persistent n.
no-touch technique
Nottingham
    N. Extended ADL index
    N. Health Profile
nourished
    well developed, well n. (WD, WN)
Novagel gel sheet
Novocain Injection
Noyes flexion rotation drawer test
NP-27
NRM
    nucleus raphe magnus
NRS
    numeric rating scale
NS
    Mycocide NS
    Stadol NS

N-Terface dressing
Nu
    N. Gauze bandage
    N. Gauze dressing
    N. Gauze packing
Nubain
nubbin
nuchae
    ligamentum n.
nuchal ligament
nuclear
    n. arthrogram
    n. injury
    n. magnetic resonance (NMR)
    n. magnetic resonance scan
nucleatum
    Fusobacterium n.
nuclei (*pl. of* nucleus)
Nucleotome
    N. probe
    N. system for lumbar diskectomy
nucleotomy
    laser n.
nucleus, pl. nuclei
    force n.
    periaqueductal gray n.
    n. pulposus
    n. raphe magnus (NRM)
nudge control on prosthesis
NuKO knee orthosis
numb foot
numbness
numeric rating scale (NRS)
Numorphan
Nuprin
Nurick
    N. classification of spondylosis
    N. spondylosis classification
Nurolon suture
NuStep
    N. exerciser
    N. total body recumbent stepper
nut
    n. alignment guide
    close encounter n.
    Kirschner traction bow n.

    lock n.
    locking n.
    nylon n.
nutation
    counter n.
nutcracker fracture
nutrient
    n. artery
    n. flap
NUTRI-SPEC testing
nutrition
    tissue n.
    total parenteral n. (TPN)
nutritional
    n. osteomalacia
    n. status
NUV
    negative ulnar variance
Nuwave transcutaneous electrical nerve stimulator
NV
    neurovascular
NWI
    notch width index
NX
    Talwin NX
Nylatex
    N. strap
    N. wrap
nylon
    n. monofilament
    n. nut
    n. suture
    n. teaspoon
Nystroem nail driver
Nystroem-Stille driver
Nytol
    Maximum Strength N.
    N. Oral
NYU
    New York University
    NYU orthosis insert
NYU-Hosmer electric elbow and prehension actuator
NZ
    neutral zone

NOTES

N

OA
osteoarthritis
OA knee brace
OAS
Oral Analogue Scale
OASIS
osteotomy analysis simulation software
oath hand
OATS
osteochondral autograft transfer system
OATS technique
OAWO
opening abductory wedge osteotomy
Ober
O. anterior transfer
O. incision
O. posterior drainage
O. release
O. tendon technique
O. test
Ober-Barr
O.-B. procedure for brachioradialis transfer
O.-B. transfer technique
obese
o. bed
o. patient
o. support
o. walker
obesity
obl
oblique
OBLA
onset of blood lactate accumulation
oblique (obl)
o. base-wedge osteotomy
o. closing wedge osteotomy (OCWO)
o. displacement
o. displacement osteotomy
o. facet wiring
o. fracture
o. incision
o. meniscal tear
o. metacarpal line
o. metaphyseal osteotomy
o. metatarsocuneiform joint
o. muscle
o. osteotomy for tibial deformity
o. osteotomy with derotation
o. popliteal ligament
o. retinacular ligament
o. retinacular ligament tightness test

o. screw insertion
o. slide osteotomy
o. view
o. wiring facet
obliquity
pelvic o.
obliquum
ligamentum popliteum o.
obliquus
o. capitis inferior musculus
o. capitis superior musculus
vastus medialis o. (VMO)
obliterans
arteriosclerosis o.
endarteritis o.
oblong polyethylene acetabular cup
O₂Boot
O'Brien
O. capsular shift procedure
O. classification of radial fracture
O. goniometer
O. pelvic halo operation
O. radial fracture classification
O. rib hook
O. staple
obstetrician's hand
obstruction
gastrointestinal o.
urinary o.
obturator
o. artery
o. avulsion fracture
conical o.
core biopsy o.
o. internus muscle
o. internus tendon
Keene o.
o. nerve
o. nerve injury
o. nerve neuritis
o. neurectomy
o. oblique view
o. sleeve
OBUS back support
Obwegeser
O. sagittal mandibular osteotomy
O. sagittal mandibular osteotomy technique
occipital
o.-axis joint
o. condyle
o. condyle fracture
o.-fiber analysis
occipitoatlantal dislocation

O

411

occipitoatlantoaxial
  o. fusion
  o. joint
occipitocervical
  o. angle
  o. arthrodesis
  o. articulation
  o. fixation
  o. fusion
  o. junction
  o. lordosis
  o. plate
  o. stabilization
occiput
occluder
  multiple pinhole o.
Occlusal-HP wart medication
occlusal splint
occlusive dressing
occult
  o. fracture
  o. primary malignant tumor
  o. taiar lesion
occulta
  spina bifida o. (SBO)
occupation
  sedentary o.
occupational
  o. behavior
  o. and environmental medicine
    (OEM)
  o. rating system
  o. risk
  o. role
  O. Safety and Health
    Administration (OSHA)
  o. science
  o. stress syndrome (OSS)
  o. therapy (OT)
OCD
  osteochondritis dissecans
ochronosis
OCL volar splint
O'Connor
  O. finger dexterity test
  O. operating arthroscope
  O. tweezer dexterity test
octagon roll
OCT compound
Octocaine Injection
octopus holder
Ocufen Ophthalmic
ocular
  o. prosthesis
  o. sign
oculoauriculovertebral dysplasia
Ocutricin Topical Ointment

OCWO
  oblique closing wedge osteotomy
**Oden peroneal tendon subluxation
classification**
Odgen plate
Odland ankle prosthesis
O'Donoghue
  O. ACL reconstruction
  O. cotton cast
  O. dressing
  O. facetectomy
  O. knee splint
  O. procedure
  O. stirrup splint
  O. test
  triad of O.
  O. unhappy triad
odontoid
  o.-axial area
  o. condyle
  o. condyle fracture
  o. fracture internal fixation
  o. fracture stabilization
  o. perpendicular line
  o. process
  o. process osteosynthesis
  o. x-ray view
odontoidectomy
odontoideum
  os o.
ODQ
  opponens digiti quinti
OEC
  OEC knee immobilizer
  OEC lag screw component with
    keyway
  OEC popliteal pad
  OEC wrist/forearm support
OEM
  occupational and environmental medicine
Oesch hook
officinalis
  valeriana o.
offset
  o. cane
  o. drill hole
  head-stem o.
  o. hinge
  medial head stem o.
  o. suspension feeder
  o. V-osteotomy
ofloxacin
Ogata technique
Ogden
  O. Anchor soft tissue device
  O. epiphyseal fracture classification
  O. fracture classification system
  O. knee dislocation classification

O. plate system
O. tissue reattachment mini system
Ogee acetabular component
Oh
O. cemented hip prosthesis
O. Press-Fit hip prosthesis
OI
osteogenesis imperfecta
oil
Decubitene oxygenated o.
O.-Red-O method
trypsin, balsam peru, and castor o.
ointment
Cortisporin Topical O.
Elase-Chloromycetin o.
Kerasal o.
Medi-Quick Topical O.
Neosporin Topical O.
Ocutricin Topical O.
Panafil o.
Panafil-White o.
papain-urea-chlorophyllin copper
complex debriding and healing o.
Septa Topical O.
Whitfield's O.
OKC
Oklahoma City cable
Oklahoma
O. ankle joint
O. ankle joint orthosis
O. ankle prosthesis
O. City cable (OKC)
OKU
Orthopaedic Knowledge Update
old
o. fracture
o. smoothie bur
o., unreduced dislocation
Olds pin
olecranization
olecranon
o. bursa
o. bursitis
o. fossa
o. fracture
oleoma
Olerud
O. internal fixator
O. pedicle fixation system
O. PSF fixation system
O. PSF rod

O. PSF screw
O. transpedicular fixation
oligoarthritis
oligoarticular
o. arthritis
o. disease
oligosegmental correction
oligotrophic fracture nonunion
olisthesis
olisthetic vertebra
olisthy
Olivecrona clip-applying and removing forceps
olive wire
Ollier
O. arthrodesis approach
O. disease
O. incision
O. lateral approach
O. rake retractor
O. technique
O. thick split free graft
Ollier-Thiersch skin graft
O'Malley jaw fracture splint
Ombredanne mallet
Ombredanne-Perkins line
Omed vented instrument guard
Omega
O. compression hip screw system
O. Plus compression hip system
omental flap
omentum
Omer-Capen
O.-C. carpectomy
O.-C. technique
Ommaya
O. reservoir device
O. reservoir implant material
Omni
O. knee brace
Omniderm dressing
Omnifit
O. HA hip stem prosthesis
O. HA hip stent
O. knee prosthesis
O. total knee system
Omnifit-C
Osteonics O.-C.
Omniflex hip prosthesis
Omni-Flexor
O.-F. device
O.-F. wrist exerciser

O

NOTES

Omnipaque contrast media
OMNI pretibial buttress
Omnitron exercise testing
omohyoid muscle
omosternum
omovertebral bone
OMS Oral
Oncovin Injection
one-and-one-half spica cast
one-bone forearm
one-half
    o.-h. patellar tendon transplant
    o.-h. spica cast
one-inclinometer method
one-leg
    o.-l. hop for distance test
    o.-l. stance test
one-legged
one-part fracture
one-plane
    o.-p. bilateral external fixator
    o.-p. bilateral frame
    o.-p. deformity
    o.-p. instability
    o.-p. unilateral external fixator
    o.-p. unilateral frame
one-repetition maximum (1-RM)
one-stage amputation
one-time sharp debridement tray
"one wound-one scar" concept
onlay
    o. bone graft
    o. bone graft cast
    o. cancellous iliac graft
onset
    o. of blood lactate accumulation
    (OBLA)
    delayed o.
    o. frequency
    o. latency
Ontario Cohort of Running-Related
  injury
onychectomy
onychocryptosis nail
onychogryphosis
onychomadesis
onychomycosis
onychomycotic toenail
onychotomy
Ony-Clear
    O.-C. Nail
    O.-C. Spray
OP
    opponens pollicis muscle
opaque synovium
open
    o. amputation
    o. base wedge osteotomy

o. base wedge
    osteotomy/bunionectomy
o. biopsy
o. bone graft epiphysiodesis
o.-break fracture
o. C-D hook
o.-chain exercise
o. disk surgery
o. double-decked hook cervical
    system
o. drainage
o.-end wrench
o. exit foramen
o. fracture wound drain
o. kinetic chain
o. kinetic chain exercise
o. medullary nailing
o. palm technique
o. pinning
o. reduction
o. reduction, internal fixation
    (ORIF)
o.-section nail
o.-toe shoe
o. wedge (OW)
o. wound
open-air
    o.-a. splint
open-book
    o.-b. fracture
    o.-b. pelvic injury
opener
    Leveron door o.
opening
    o. abductory wedge osteotomy
    (OAWO)
    anterolateral ventricular o. (ALVO)
    blucher o.
    Sierra 2-load voluntary o.
    voluntary o. (VO)
    o. wedge manipulation
    o. wedge manipulation and
    reapplication of plaster
    o. wedge osteotomy
opera-glass hand
Operand
operating
    o. microscope
    o. room
    o. time
operation
    Abbe o.
    Abbott-Lucas shoulder o.
    Adams hip o.
    Albert knee o.
    Armistead ulnar lengthening o.
    Baker patellar advancement o.
    Baker translocation o.

Bankart o.
Bankart-Putti-Platt o.
Barr tendon transfer o.
Bateman modification of Mayer
  transfer o.
Bateman shoulder o.
Bauer-Tondra-Trusler o.
Bennett quadriceps plastic o.
Bora o.
Bosworth shelf o.
Brackett-Osgood-Putti-Abbott o.
Brahms foot o.
bridle posterior tibial tendon
  transfer o.
Bristow o.
Brockman foot o.
Brooks cervical fusion o.
Brooks-Gallie cervical o.
Brooks-Jenkins cervical o.
Broström-Gould ankle instability o.
Bunnell posterior tibial tendon
  transfer o.
Butler fifth toe o.
Caldwell-Coleman flatfoot o.
Caldwell-Durham tendon o.
Cave-Rowe shoulder dislocation o.
centralization of radius o.
Cocklin toe o.
Colonna shelf o.
Contour DF-80 total hip o.
Copeland-Howard shoulder o.
Cotrel-Dubousset derotation o.
Cracchiolo-Sculco implant o.
Debeyre-Patte-Elmelik rotator
  cuff o.
Diamond-Gould syndactyly o.
Dickson-Diveley foot o.
Dunn hip o.
Durham flatfoot o.
DuVries modified McBride hallux
  valgus o.
Dwyer clawfoot o.
Eaton-Malerich fracture-
  dislocation o.
Ellis Jones peroneal tendon o.
Elmslie-Cholmely foot o.
Elmslie peroneal tendon o.
Elmslie-Trillat patellar o.
Evan ankle joint instability o.
Farmer o.
French supracondylar fracture o.
Fried-Green foot o.

Fried-Hendel tendon o.
Galeazzi patellar o.
Gardner o.
Gill modification of Campbell
  ankle o.
hanging hip o.
hanging toe o.
Herndon-Heyman foot o.
Heyman-Herndon clubfoot o.
Hoffmann metatarsal o.
Hoke Achilles tendon
  lengthening o.
I-beam hip o.
Inclan modification of Campbell
  ankle o.
inside-out Bankart shoulder
  instability o.
intermetatarsal angle-reducing o.
Isseis-Aussies scoliosis o.
Janecki-Nelson shoulder o.
Jones cock-up toe o.
Juvara foot o.
Keller foot o.
Keller hallux valgus o.
Kessler posterior tibial tendon
  transfer o.
Kirk distal thigh o.
Kortzeborn hand o.
Krempen-Silver-Sotelo nonunion o.
Krukenberg hand o.
Lambrinudi drop foot o.
limb-sparing o.
MacNab o.
Magnuson-Stack o.
Majestro-Ruda-Frost tendon o.
Mayo hallux valgus modified o.
McBride bunion hallux valgus o.
McKay-Simons clubfoot o.
McKay-Simons CSR o.
McLaughlin o.
Mensor-Scheck hanging-hip o.
Miller flatfoot o.
Miyakawa knee o.
modified Cocklin toe o.
Moe scoliosis o.
Mumford-Gurd acromioclavicular o.
muscle sliding o.
Neviaser o.
Nicoll fracture o.
Nirschl o.
O'Brien pelvic halo o.

O

NOTES

operation *(continued)*
 Osborne-Cotterill elbow
  dislocation o.
 Paddu knee o.
 resurfacing o.
 Sargent knee o.
 Selig hip o.
 Sofield femoral deficiency o.
 Stener-Gunterberg hip o.
 Stewart arm o.
 Suppan foot o.
 T-plasty modification of Bankart
  shoulder o.
 Vulpius equinus deformity o.
 Weaver-Dunn acromioclavicular o.
 Zadik foot o.
 Zickel subtrochanteric fracture o.
operative
 o. arthroscopy
 o. arthrotomy
 o. legholder
 o. roentgenogram
 o. site
O'Phelan technique
ophthalmic
 o. irrigator
 Ocufen O.
 Voltaren O.
Ophthetic
opiate receptor antagonist
Opiela brace
opioid receptor
opisthotonic position
opium
 o. alkaloid
 belladonna and o.
 o. tincture
OPLL
 ossification of the posterior longitudinal
  ligament
OPM
 opponens digiti minimi
OPMI microscopic drape
Oppenheim
 O. brace
 O. disease
 O. gait
 O. reflex
 O. sign
 O. stroke test
Oppenheimer
 O. knuckle-bender splint
 O. spring wire
 O. spring-wire splint
Oppociser
 O. exercise device
 O. hand exerciser

opponens
 o. bar
 o. digiti minimi (OPM)
 o. digiti quinti (ODQ)
 o. digiti quinti muscle
 o. pollicis muscle (OP)
 o. pollicus
 o. splint
 o. transfer
opponensplasty
 abductor digiti minimi o.
 abductor digiti quinti o.
 Bunnell o.
 Goldmar o.
 Groves o.
 Huber adductor digiti quinti o.
 Littler o.
 Manske-McCarroll o.
 Phalen-Miller o.
 Riordan finger o.
opposers
 digital o.
opposite
 o. foot strike phase of gait
 o. toe-off phase of gait
opposition
 o. contracture
 o. test
 thumb o.
Opraflex
 O. drape
 O. dressing
OpSite wound dressing
opsonic activity
opsonization
Optetrak total knee replacement system
optical trapping
Opti-Fix
 O.-F. femoral prosthesis
 O.-F. hip stem
 O.-F. II acetabular cup
 O.-F. prosthesis
 O.-F. total hip system
OptiMax Supreme pressure reduction
 mattress
optimizing motion palpation
Option Orthotic Series
OptiScan 2000
optoelectric
 o. measuring apparatus
 o. measuring system
 o. signal detection apparatus
Optotrak motion measurement system
OPTP
 Orthopaedic Physical Therapy Products
 OPTP Slant

O'Rahilly
    O. classification of limb deficiency
    O. limb deficiency classification
oral
    AllerMax O.
    O. Analogue Scale (OAS)
    Ansaid O.
    Banophen O.
    Belix O.
    Benadryl O.
    Calciferol O.
    Cataflam O.
    Ceftin O.
    Cipro O.
    Cytoxan O.
    o. defensiveness
    Delta-Cortef O.
    Dormarex 2 O.
    Dormin O.
    Drisdol O.
    Estrace O.
    Genahist O.
    Lamisil O.
    Medrol O.
    MS Contin O.
    MSIR O.
    Neoral O.
    Nytol O.
    OMS O.
    Oramorph SR O.
    Pediapred O.
    Phendry O.
    Prelone O.
    Roxanol SR O.
    Sandimmune O.
    Siladryl O.
    Sleep-eze 3 O.
    Sominex O.
    terbinafine, o.
    Toradol O.
    Twilite O.
    Unipen O.
    Valium O.
    VePesid O.
    Voltaren O.
    Voltaren-XR O.
Oralet
    Fentanyl O.
Oramorph SR Oral
Orasone
Oratek
    O. chisel

    O. device
    O. thermal shrinking probe
orbicularis oris
orbicular ligament
orbit
    angular process of o.
Orbital shoulder stabilizer brace
Orbiter treadmill
order of activation
ordinal classification
Oregon Poly II ankle prosthesis
Oretorp retractable knife
Orfit splint
Orfizip
    O. body jacket
    O. knee cast
organ
    Golgi tendon o.
    Ruffini end o.
Orgaran
orientation
    phalangeal articular o.
    visual o.
ORIF
    open reduction, internal fixation
origin
    adductor o.
    deltoid o.
    fever of undetermined o. (FUO)
    flexor-pronator o.
    tripartite muscle o.
Original
    Doan's, O.
    O. Jacknobber II muscle-massage
      device
oris
    orbicularis o.
    O. pin
Orlando hip-knee-ankle-foot orthosis
ORLAU
    O. swivel walker
    O. swivel walker orthosis
Ormandy screw
Ormco pin
ORN
    osteoradionecrosis
oropharyngeal approach
Orozco plate
orphenadrine
    o., aspirin, and caffeine
    o. citrate
Orphengesic

O

NOTES

417

Orr-Buck traction
Orthairtome II drill
Orthawear
    O. antiembolic stockings
    O. antiembolism stockings
Orth-evac autotransfusion system
Orthex
    O. reliever insole
    O. Relievers shoe insert
Orthion traction machine
Orthoairtome wire driver
Ortho-Arch II orthotic
Ortho-Biotic recliner
OrthoBlend powered bone mill
OrthoBone pillow
Ortho-Cel
    O.-C. pad
    O.-C. padding
Orthochrome
    O. implant metal
    O. implant metal prosthesis
Orthocomp cement
ortho disk
orthodox procedure
orthodromic
Orthodyne Enhancer unit
Orthofix
    O. apparatus
    O. external fixation device
    O. external fixator
    O. fixation
    O. M-100 distractor
    O. monolateral femoral external
      fixator
    O. pin
    O. prosthesis
    O. screw
Orthoflex
    O. dressing
    O. elastic plaster bandage
Ortho-Foam
    O.-F. elbow/heel pad
    O.-F. protector
Orthofuse implantable growth stimulator
OrthoGel liner
OrthoGen
    O. bone growth stimulator
    O. implantable stimulator for
      nonunion of fracture
Ortho-Grip silicone rubber handle
Ortho-Jel impression material
orthokinetic exercise
orthokinetics
    orthopaedic o.
    O. travel chair
Ortho-last splint
Ortholav
    O. irrigation and suction device

    O. jet
    O. jet lavage
Ortholen sheet
Ortholoc
    O. Advantim revision knee system
    O. Advantim total knee system
    O. implant metal prosthesis
Orthomedics
    O. brace
    O. Stretch and Heel splint
Orthomerica UFO
Ortho-mesh
Orthomet
    O. Axiom total knee system
    O. Perfecta total hip system
Orthomite II adhesive
Ortho-Mold
    O.-M. spinal brace
    O.-M. splint
orthomolecular medicine/megavitamin
  therapy
orthopaedic
    o. bed
    o. bone file
    o. broach
    o. bur
    o. cement
    o. chisel
    o. curette
    o. cutting instrument
    o. depth gauge
    o. dynamometer
    o. felt
    o. forceps
    o. goniometer
    o. gouge
    o. hammer
    o. hardware
    o. hemostat
    o. impactor
    o. knife
    O. Knowledge Update (OKU)
    o. orthokinetics
    o. osteotome
    o. oxford shoe
    O. Physical Therapy Products
      (OPTP)
    o. prosthesis
    o. rasp
    o. reamer
    o. retractor
    o. rongeur
    o. scissors
    o. shoulder elevator
    o. stockinette
    o. strap clavicular splint
    o. surgical drill
    o. surgical file

o. surgical pliers
o. surgical stripper
o. table
O. Trauma Association
classification
o. Universal drill
OrthoPak
O. bone growth stimulator system
O. II bone growth stimulator
Ortho-Pal body support
orthopedic
O. Positioning Seat
Soft-Tissue Regional O.'s (STO)
O. Systems Inc. (OSI)
Orthopedics
Orthoplast
O. dressing
O. fracture brace
O. isoprene splint
O. jacket
O. plastic
O. slipper cast
orthoPLUG
orthopod
orthoRAP
Orthoset cement
orthosis, pl. orthoses
abduction hip o.
accommodative o.
Adjustable Advanced Reciprocating
Gait O. (ARGO)
A-frame o.
airplane splint o.
Alden CDI o.
AliCork Foot O.
Aliplast custom-molded foot o.
ambulation training o.
Amfit custom o.
ankle o. (AO)
ankle contracture o.
ankle-foot o. (AFO)
ankle-foot plastic o.
Anti-Shox o.
Atlanta brace o.
Atlanta-Scottish Rite abduction o.
bail-lock knee joint o.
balance padding o.
bar-and-shoe o.
Bauerfeind Malleolic Ankle O.
Beaufort seating o.
Bebax o.
BFO O.

Biothotic foot o.
BODI Dynamic O.
BODI knee extension o.
Boston brace thoracolumbosacral o.
Boston post-op hip o.
cable-twister o.
calcaneal spur cookie o.
Canadian Knee O.
CASH o.
C-bar o.
cervical o. (CO)
cervicothoracic o.
cervicothoracolumbosacral o.
(CTLSO)
chairback o.
cock-up splint o.
Comfy Elbow O.
Comfy Knee O.
Controller Shoulder O.
copolymer ankle-foot o.
corrective o.
Craig-Scott o.
cruciform anterior spinal
hyperextension o.
CTLSO o.
Daytona cervical o.
DDH o.
Denis Browne bar foot o.
dermoplast-plastizote o.
developmental dislocated hip o.
Diabetic D-Sole foot o.
dial-lock o.
o. drop-lock ring
dual-photon electrospinal o.
Dynamic elbow o.
Dynamic knee o.
Dynamic wrist o.
elastic knee cage o.
elastic twister o.
elbow o. (EO)
elbow-wrist-hand o. (EWHO)
Engen palmar finger o.
figure-of-eight thoracic o.
Fillauer bar foot o.
FirmFlex custom o.
Flex Foam o.
flexion-extension control cervical o.
floor-reaction ankle-foot o.
foot o. (FO)
Foot Levelers o.
four-poster cervical o.
Frejka pillow o.

O

NOTES

orthosis *(continued)*

gator plastic o.
Gillette joint o.
Gillette modification of ankle-foot o.
GunSlinger shoulder o.
G/W Heel Lift, Inc. o.
halo cervical o.
halo extension o.
halo traction o.
halo-vest o.
hand o. (HO)
heat-molded petroplastic ankle-foot o.
heat-molder petroplastic ankle-foot o.
hindfoot o.
hip o. (HO)
hip-knee-ankle-foot o. (HKAFO)
Hosmer VC four-bar knee o.
Hyperex thoracic o.
Ilfeld splint o.
ipos heel relief o.
J-24 cervical o.
J-45 contraflexion o.
Jewett-Benjamin cervical o.
Jewett contraflexion o.
Jewett hyperextension o.
Jewett post-fusion o.
Jewett thoracolumbosacral o.
J-35 hyperextension o.
Jousto dropfoot splint, skid o.
J-55 postfusion o.
Kallassy o.
Kid-Dee-Lite o.
Klenzak o.
knee o. (KO)
knee-ankle-foot o. (KAFO)
knee extension o.
Knight-Taylor thoracolumbosacral o.
Knight-Taylor and Williams spinal o.
L.A. cervical o.
leather o.
Legg-Perthes disease o.
Lenox Hill knee o.
Lerman multiligamentous knee control o.
Levy & Rappel foot o.
Ligamentus Ankle o.
L'Nard Multi-Podus o.
L'Nard thoracolumbosacral o.
long leg o.
long opponens o.
lower limb o. (LLO)
LSU reciprocation-gait o.
lumbosacral o.
Lynco foot o.

Malibu cervical o.
Malleoloc ankle o.
Marlin cervical o.
MCF shoulder o.
metal hybrid o.
Meyer cervical o.
Milwaukee cervicothoracolumbosacral o.
Milwaukee scoliosis o.
Minerva o.
molded ankle-foot o. (MAFO)
neoprene wrist o.
Newington o.
Newport MC hip o.
New York Orthopedic front-opening o.
New York University insert for o.
NuKO knee o.
Oklahoma ankle joint o.
Orlando hip-knee-ankle-foot o.
ORLAU swivel walker o.
overlapped uprights in o.
o. overlapped uprights
parapodium o.
patellar tendon-bearing o.
patellar tendon weightbearing brace o.
pediatric pressure relief ankle foot o. (PRAFO)
Phelps o.
plastic ankle-foot o.
plastic floor reaction ankle-foot o.
Plastizote cervical collar o.
polypropylene ankle-foot o.
polypropylene glycol-ankle-foot o.
polypropylene glycol-thoracolumbosacral o.
posterior leaf-spring ankle-foot o.
postoperative lumbosacral o.
prehension o.
Profile Sitting O.
Pro-glide o.
Progressive ankle o.
prostheses and orthoses (P&O)
PSA thermoplastic o.
PTB ankle-foot o.
PTB plastic o.
Pucci pediatrics hand o.
Pucci rehab knee o.
reciprocation gait o. (RGO)
resting o.
rib belt o.
Rochester hip-knee-ankle-foot o.
SACH o.
sacroiliac o. (SIO)
safety pin o.
SAWA shoulder o.
Scottish Rite hip o.

Seattle o.
Select joint o.
semirigid o.
semirigid polypropylene ankle-foot o.
Shaeffer rigid o.
short opponens o.
shoulder-elbow-wrist-hand o. (SEWHO)
single-photon electrospinal o.
Slim Option shoe o.
soft collar cervical o.
SOLEutions custom o.
SOMI o.
spinal o. (SO)
Sport-Stirrup o.
spring-loaded lock o.
spring-wire ankle-foot o.
standing frame o.
supramalleolar o. (SMO)
Swede-O-Universal o.
Swedish knee cage o.
Taylor thoracolumbosacral o.
themoplastic ankle-foot o.
Thera-Pos elbow o.
Therapy Carrot Finger O. (TCFO)
Theratotic firm foot o.
Theratotic soft foot o.
Thomas collar cervical o.
Thomas heel o.
thoracic spine o.
thoracolumbosacral o. (TLSO)
thoracolumbosacral o. - flexion, extension, lateral bending, and transverse rotation (TLSO-FELR)
tone-reducing ankle-foot o. (TRAFO)
Toronto parapodium o.
total contact o. (TCO)
total contact bivalve ankle-foot o.
TPE ankle-foot o.
TPE biomechanical foot o.
TRAFO o.
Transpire wrist o.
trilateral knee-ankle-foot o.
trunk-hip-knee-ankle-foot o. (THKAFO)
turnbuckle wrist o.
two-poster cervical o.
UCB foot o.
underarm o.

Universal Plantar Fasciitis O. (UFO)
universal plantar fasciitis o. (UFO)
upper limb o. (ULO)
VAPC dorsiflexion assist o.
Vari-Duct hip and knee o.
Visclas o.
Viscoheel K, N o.
Viscoheel SofSpot o.
von Rosen splint hip o.
weight-relieving o.
Williams o.
wrist-driven flexor hinge o.
wrist-driven prehension o.
wrist-driven wrist-hand o.
wrist-hand o. (WHO)
XPE foot o.
Zinco ankle o.

Orthosleep Pillow

OrthoSorb
O. absorbable pin
O. pin fixation
O. pin nail

Orthotec pressurized fluid irrigation system

orthotic
Alden CDI o.
Amfit o.
ankle-foot o. (AFO)
Anti-Shox o.
o. attachment implant
Bioflex o.
Biofoot o.
Biothotic o.
Blue Line o.
o. coiled spring twister
DesignLine o.
o. device
Diab-A-Thotics o.
DressFlex o.
DSIS o.
D-Soles o.
Duraleve custom molded foot o.
FirmFlex custom o.
FlexiSport o.
foot o.
Foot Levelers custom o.
functional o.
Golden Comfort o.
Golden Fitness o.
Healthflex o.
Jamaica Sandalthotics o.

O

NOTES

orthotic *(continued)*
  Kinetic Wedge o.
  Ligamentus Ankle ankle o.
  Lyte Fit o.
  Magnathotic o.
  Malibu Sandalthotics o.
  Mayer o.
  MBS snap-on o.
  M-Pact flexible o.
  Ortho-Arch II o.
  o. plate
  Polydor Preforms o.
  PRAFO adjustable o.
  ProLite Plus runner's o.
  Pucci Air o.
  Rediform o.
  Rohadur-Polydor o.
  Rohadur-Schaefer o.
  Rohadur-Whitman o.
  SACH o.
  SAFE o.
  Sandalthotics postural support o.
  shoe o.
  o. shoe insert
  Slimthetics o.
  Soft Super Sport o.
  Soft Support Preforms o.
  SOLEutions o.
  solid ankle, cushioned heel o.
  Sporthotics o.
  Sport Preforms o.
  stationary attachment flexible
    endoskeletal o.
  Stratos o.
  Superfeet Custom Pre-Fabricated O.
  Superform Contours o.
  Supralen cradle o.
  Supralen Schaefer o.
  Swiss Balance o.
  Thermo HK/Rohadur o.
  Thermo HK/Tepefom o.
  Thinline uncovered o.
  UCOheal o.
  Wire-Foam O.
  XO-soft-sole o.
orthotist
  certified o. (CO)
orthotome resector
Ortho-Trac adhesive skin traction
  bandage
Orthotron exerciser
Ortho-Turn transfer aid
Ortho-Vent
  O.-V. bandage
  O.-V. traction
OrthoVise orthopaedic instrument
OrthoWedge healing shoe

Ortho-Yomy facebow
Orthozime instrument cleaner
Ortolani
  O. click
  O. maneuver
  O. sign
  O. test
Orudis KT
Oruvail
os
  o. acromiale
  o. calcis
  o. calcis fracture
  o. calcis osteotomy
  o. carpalia accessoria
  o. intercuneiforme
  o. intermetatarseum
  o. lanula
  o. odontoideum
  o. peroneum
  o. sesamoideum
  o. supranaviculare
  o. supratalare
  o. sustentaculum
  o. talocalcaneus
  o. tibiale externum
  o. trapezium bone
  o. trapezoideum bone
  o. triangulare carpi
  o. trigonum
  o. trigonum syndrome
  o. ulnar styloidium
  o. vesalianum
Osada
  O. portable handpiece system
  O. saw
Osborne
  O. plate
  O. posterior approach
  O. punch
Osborne-Cotterill
  O.-C. elbow dislocation operation
  O.-C. elbow technique
  O.-C. procedure
Os-Cal 500
oscillating
  o. gouge
  o. saw
oscillation
  grade I, II o.
oscillococcinum
Osgood
  O. modified technique
  O. rotational osteotomy
Osgood-Schlatter
  O.-S. disease
  O.-S. lesion

OSHA
Occupational Safety and Health
Administration
Osher irrigating implant hook
OSI
Orthopedic Systems Inc.
OSI Arthroscopic legholder
OSI extremity elevator
OSI laxity tester
OSI modular table system
OSI Well Leg Support
OSI-Schlein shoulder positioner
Osler node
OsmoCyte Island wound-care dressing
Osmond-Clarke
O.-C. foot procedure
O.-C. technique
OS-5/Plus
O. 2 knee brace
OSS
occupational stress syndrome
ossa tarsi
Osseodent surgical drill
osseofascial compartment
osseointegrated
osseointegration
osseous
o. adjustment
o. attachment
o. bridge
o. bridge prevention
o. coalition
congenital o.
o. defect
o. drift
o. dystrophy
o. equinus
o. foraminal encroachment
o. homeostasis
o. instability
o. patellae outgrowth
o. pin
o. ring of Lacroix
o. structure
o. tissue
o. tunnel
ossicle
accessory o.
ossicular chain replacement prosthesis
ossiculum terminale
ossificans
myositis o.

osteitis o.
periostitis o.
ossification
bilateral heterotopic o.
Brooker classification of
heterotopic o. I–IV
o. center
ectopic o.
enchondral o.
endochondral o.
endplate o.
heterotopic o.
iliac crest o.
mandible o.
membranous o.
paraarticular heterotopic o.
pelvitrochanteric heterotopic o.
periarticular heterotopic o.
pisiform o.
o. of the posterior longitudinal
ligament (OPLL)
trapezium o.
trapezoid o.
triquetrum o.
ossifying
o. fibroma
o. fibroma of long bone
ossimeter
Küntscher o.
Ossotome bur
ostectomy
fibular o.
partial o.
osteitis
condensing o.
o. deformans
o. distal phalanx
o. fibrosa cystica
o. fibrosa disseminata
o. fragilitans
o. ossificans
o. pubis
sclerosing nonsuppurative o.
suppurative o.
ostemia
ostempyesis
osteoaneurysm
OsteoArthritic knee brace
osteoarthritis (OA)
arthrodesis for primary
degenerative o.
degenerative o.

NOTES

O

osteoarthritis *(continued)*
    o. disease
    midtarsal o.
    tarsometatarsal o.
osteoarthropathy
    neuropathic o.
osteoarticular
    o. allograft
    o. allograft transplantation
    o. defect
    o. graft
    o. tuberculosis
osteoblast
    o. proliferation fluorometric assay
osteoblastic
    o. bone regeneration
    o. metastasis
    o. osteogenic sarcoma
osteoblastoma
    spinal o.
Osteobond copolymer bone cement
Osteo-B Plus
osteobunionectomy
osteocachexia
Osteocalcin Injection
OsteoCap hip prosthesis
osteocartilaginous
    o. exostosis
    o. graft
    o. lesion
    o. loose body
    o. metaplasia
osteochondral
    o. allograft
    o. autograft transfer system
    (OATS)
    o. defect
    o. fracture of the dome of the
    talus
    o. fragment
    o. graft
    o. injury
    o. lesion
    o. prominence
    o. ridge
osteochondritis
    crushing o.
    o. dissecans (OCD)
    epiphyseal o.
    o. ischiopubica
    o. juvenilis
    o. necroticans
    puncture wound o.
osteochondrodesmodysplasia
osteochondrodystrophy
osteochondrofibroma
osteochondrolysis

osteochondroma
    epiphyseal o.
    excision of o.
    intraarticular o.
osteochondromatosis
    multiple o.
    synovial o.
osteochondropathy
osteochondrophyte
osteochondrosarcoma
osteochondrosis
    o. deformans tibiae
    o. dissecans
    o. of metatarsal
osteochrondral slice fracture
osteoclasis
    Blount technique for o.
    o. maneuver
osteoclast
    o.-mediated osteoporosis
    o. tension staple
osteoclastic
    o. erosion
    o. giant cell
    o. resorption
osteoclastoma
osteoconduction
osteocope
osteocutaneous free flap
osteocystoma
osteocyte
osteodistractor
    Ace/Normed o.
osteodystrophy
    Albright hereditary o.
    azotemic o.
    pulmonary o.
    renal o.
osteoenchondroma
osteofascial compartment
osteofibrochondrosarcoma
osteofibromatosis
osteofibrous dysplasia
OsteoGen
    O. bone growth stimulator
    O. implantable stimulator
    O. resorbable osteogenic bone-
    filling implant
osteogenesis imperfecta (OI)
osteogenic
    o. cell
    o. fibroma
    o. sarcoma
Osteoguide
osteohalisteresis
osteoid
    calcified o.
    o. osteoma

o. seam
unmineralized o.
osteoinduction
osteokinematic motion
osteokinematics
osteolipochondroma
osteolipoma
Osteolock
O. acetabular component
O. HA femoral component
O. hip prosthesis
osteolysis
acetabular o.
debris-incited o.
femoral o.
posttraumatic o.
osteoma
intraarticular osteoid o.
intracapsular osteoid o.
osteoid o.
parosteal o.
osteomalacia
nutritional o.
osteomatosis
Osteomed screw
osteomesopyknosis
osteomusculocutaneous flap
osteomyelitic sinus
osteomyelitis
Ackerman criteria for o.
acute hematogenous o. (AHO)
anaerobic o.
blastomycotic o.
Brucella o.
chloramphenicol o.
chronic pyogenic o.
femoral o.
Gaenslen o.
Garré sclerosing o.
hematogenous o.
iatrogenic o.
long bone o.
nonsuppurative o.
nonunion o.
pedal o.
pin-track o.
postfracture o.
posttraumatic chronic o.
pyogenic vertebral o.
Salmonella o.
sclerosing o.

secondary or acute
hematogenous o.
spinal o.
subacute hematogenous o.
suppurative o.
synovitis-acne-pustulosis-
hyperostosis o. (SAPHO)
tuberculous vertebral o.
vertebral o.
osteomyelodysplasia
osteon
osteonal
o. bone union
o. lamellar bone
Osteone air drill
osteonecrosis
dysbaric o.
Ficat and Arlet classification of
stages of o.
Ficat classification of femoral
head o.
idiopathic o.
nontraumatic idiopathic o.
posttraumatic o.
steroid-induced o.
osteoneuralgia
Osteonics
O. acetabular cup
O. acetabular dome hole plug
O. HA femoral implant
O. hip prosthesis
O. jig
O. Omnifit-C
O. Omnifit-HA component
O. Omnifit-HA hip stem
O. Scorpio insert
osteopathia striata
osteopathic
o. lesion
o. manipulation
osteopathy
osteopenia
osteopenic bone
osteoperiosteal
o. bone graft
o. flap
osteoperiostitis
osteopetrosis
osteophlebitis
osteophyte
bony o.
bridging o.

O

NOTES

osteophyte *(continued)*
    o. elevator
    o. formation
    fringe of o.
    marginal o.
    posterior o.
osteophytic
    o. bone lip
    o. spur
osteophytosis
osteoplastic
    o. flap clamp
    o. laminectomy
    o. reconstruction
osteoplastica
osteoplasty
    Maquet anteromedial o.
osteoplysis
    massive o.
osteopoikilosis
osteoporosis
    dual photon densitometry test
      for o.
    femoral o.
    idiopathic juvenile o.
    idiopathic transient o.
    osteoclast-mediated o.
    o. pseudoglioma syndrome
    Singh index of o.
    transient o.
    o. with vertebral collapse and
      neurologic deficit
osteoporotic
    o. bone
    o. spine
osteoprogenitor cell
osteopsathyrosis idiopathica
osteoradionecrosis (ORN)
osteosarcoma
    conventional o.
    intraosseous o.
    parosteal o.
    periosteal o.
    spinal o.
    telangiectatic o.
osteosclerosis fragilis
OsteoSet
    O. bone filler
    O. bone graft substitute
    O.-T medicated bone graft
      substitute
osteosis
osteospongioma
OsteoStat
    O. disposable power tool
    O. single-use power surgical
      equipment

Osteo-Stim implantable bone growth
    stimulator
osteosynovitis
osteosynthesefragen
    Arbeitsgemeinschaft für o. (AO)
osteosynthesis
    anterior column o.
    lumbar spine vertebral o.
    odontoid process o.
    plate-screw o.
    posterior column o.
    thoracic spine vertebral o.
    thoracolumbar spine vertebral o.
    vertebral o.
osteotabes
osteotelangiectasia
osteothrombophlebitis
osteothrombosis
osteotome
    AcuDriver o.
    Acufex o.
    Albee o.
    Alexander costal o.
    Anderson-Neivert o.
    Andrews o.
    Army o.
    arthroscopic o.
    Aufranc o.
    backcutting o.
    bayonet o.
    Blount o.
    Bowen o.
    box o.
    Campbell o.
    Carroll-Legg o.
    Carroll-Smith-Petersen o.
    Cavin o.
    Cherry o.
    Cinelli o.
    Clayton o.
    Cloward spinal fusion o.
    Cobb o.
    Compere o.
    Cottle o.
    Crane o.
    curved o.
    Dautrey o.
    Dawson-Yuhl o.
    Dingman o.
    Epker o.
    Furnas bayonet o.
    grooving o.
    guarded o.
    Hardt-Delima o.
    Hendel guided o.
    Hibbs curved o.
    Hibbs straight o.
    Hoke o.

Joseph o.
Lambotte o.
Leinbach o.
Lexer o.
MacGregor o.
Meyerding curved o.
Meyerding straight o.
MGH o.
Micro-Aire o.
Miner o.
mini-Lambotte o.
mini-Lexer o.
Mitchell o.
Moberg o.
Moe o.
Moreland o.
Murphy o.
Neivert o.
orthopaedic o.
Padgett o.
Parkes o.
Peck o.
Rhoton o.
Rish o.
rotary o.
Sheehan o.
Silver o.
Simmons o.
Smith-Petersen curved o.
Smith-Petersen straight o.
Stille o.
straight o.
Swanson o.
thin o.
unguarded o.
U.S. Army o.
Weck o.
West o.

osteotomize

osteotomy

Abbott-Gill o.
abduction o.
abductor o.
abductory midfoot o.
abductory wedge o.
adduction o.
Agliette supracondylar o.
Aiken o.
Akin proximal phalangeal o.
Amspacher-Messenbaugh closing
  wedge o.
Amstutz-Wilson o.

o. analysis simulation software
  (OASIS)
Anderson-Fowler calcaneal
  displacement o.
angular o.
angulation o.
anterior calcaneal o.
arcuate o.
Austin o.
Axer lateral opening wedge o.
Axer varus derotational o.
Bailey-Dubow o.
Baker-Hill o.
Balacescu closing wedge o.
ball-and-socket trochanteric o.
Barouk microscrew with
  shortening o.
basal o.
base-of-the-neck o.
base wedge o.
basilar crescentic o.
basilar metatarsal o.
Bellemore-Barrett closing wedge o.
Berman-Gartland metatarsal o.
bicorrectional Austin o.
bifurcation o.
biplane trochanteric o.
biplaning of o.
block o.
Blount displacement o.
Blundell-Jones hip o.
Bonney-Kessel dorsiflexionary tilt-
  up o.
Borden-Spencer-Herman o.
Brackett o.
Brett-Campbell tibial o.
o. bunionectomy
calcaneal L o.
Campbell tibial o.
Canale o.
canal innominate o.
Carstan reverse wedge o.
Cartam-Treander reverse wedge o.
Chambers o.
chevron o.
chevron-Akin double o.
Chiari innominate o.
Chiari-Salter-Steel pelvic o.
closed base wedge o. (CBWO)
closed intramedullary o.
closed-wedge o.

O

NOTES

osteotomy *(continued)*

closing abductory-wedge o. (CAWO)
closing base-wedge o.
closing wedge greenstick dorsal proximal metatarsal o.
Cole o.
compensatory basilar o.
controlled rotational o.
Conventry proximal tibial o.
corrective lengthening o.
countersinking o.
Coventry distal femoral o.
Coventry vagal o.
Coventry vagus o.
Crego femoral o.
crescentic base wedge o.
crescentic calcaneal o.
crescentic shelf o. (CSO)
crescent-shaped o.
cuneiform o.
cup-and-ball o.
curved o.
cutting jig for chevron o.
cylindrical o.
decompressive o.
Dega pelvic o.
delayed femoral o.
Derosa-Graziano step-cut o.
derotational o.
dial pelvic o.
dial periacetabular o.
diaphyseal o.
Dickinson-Coutts-Woodward-Handler o.
Dickson geometric o.
Diebold-Bejjani o.
Dillwyn-Evans o.
Dimon o.
Dimon-Hughston intertrochanteric o.
displacement o.
distal Akin phalangeal o.
distal first metatarsal o.
distal L o.
distal oblique sliding o.
dome o.
dome-shaped o.
dorsal closing wedge o.
dorsal proximal metatarsal o.
dorsal-V o.
dorsiflexory wedge o.
double o.
Dunn o.
Dunn-Hess trochanteric o.
Dwyer calcaneal o.
Elizabethtown o.
Emmon o.
epiphyseal-metaphyseal o.

Eppright dial o.
Estersohn o. for tailor's bunion
Evans anterior calcaneal o.
eversion o.
extension o.
failed femoral o.
femoral derotation o.
Ferguson-Thompson-King two-stage o.
Fernandez o.
fibular o.
Fish cuneiform o.
flexion o.
Fowler o.
free-floating o.
French lateral closing-wedge o.
Fulkerson o.
Gant o.
geometric extension o.
geometric supracondylar extension o.
Gerbert o.
Giannestras metatarsal oblique o.
Giannestras oblique metatarsal o.
Giannestras step-down modified o.
Gibson-Piggott o.
Gigli saw o.
Gleich o.
glenoid o.
Golden closing-wedge o.
Grant-Small-Lehman supracondylar extension o.
Greenfield o.
Green-Laird modification of the Reverdin o.
Green-Reverdin o.
greenstick dorsal proximal metatarsal o.
Green-Watermann o.
Gudas scarf Z-plasty o.
Haas o.
Haber-Kraft o.
Haddad metatarsal o.
Hass o.
Helal o.
Herman-Gartland o.
high tibial o. (HTO)
Hirayma o.
Hohmann o.
horizontal o.
iliac o.
Ingram o.
Ingram-Canle-Beaty epiphyseal-metaphyseal o.
innominate o.
intertrochanteric varus o.
intraarticular o.
intracapsular o.

intraepiphyseal o.
Irwin o.
Japas o.
Johnson chevron o.
Kalish o.
Kaplan o.
Kawamura dome o.
Kawamura pelvic o.
Kech and Kelly o.
Kelikian modified Z o.
Kelly-Keck o.
Kelly and Kelly o.
Kempf-Grosse-Abalo Z-step o.
Kessel-Bonney extension o.
Kitaoka-Leventen medial
  displacement metatarsal o.
Koutsogiannis calcaneal
  displacement o.
Koutsogiannis-Fowler-Anderson o.
Kramer-Craig-Noel basilar femoral
  neck o.
Kramer modification of
  Hohmann o.
Lambrinudi o.
lateral closing wedge o.
lateral displacement o.
lateral opening wedge o.
Leach-Igou step-cut medial o.
Lelièvre o.
Lichtblau o.
Lindgren oblique o.
Lindseth o.
Lucas-Cottrell o.
Ludloff o.
Macewen-Shands o.
MacGregor o.
malleolar o.
o. of mandible
mandibular o.
Maquet dome o.
Marquardt angulation o.
Martin o.
Mau o.
McMurry o.
medial closing wedge phalangeal o.
medial displacement o.
medial opening wedge o.
metacarpal o.
metaphyseal o.
metatarsal head o.
metatarsal neck o.
metatarsal oblique o.

metatarsal proximal dome o.
metatarsal Reverdin o.
metatarsal V-shaped o.
Mitchell distal o.
Mitchell posterior displacement o.
Mitchell step-down o.
modified Mau o.
modified Wilson o.
Molesworth o.
Mueller intertochanteric varus o.
Mueller transposition o.
oblique base-wedge o.
oblique closing wedge o. (OCWO)
oblique displacement o.
oblique metaphyseal o.
oblique slide o.
Obwegeser sagittal mandibular o.
open base wedge o.
opening abductory wedge o.
  (OAWO)
opening wedge o.
os calcis o.
Osgood rotational o.
Pauwels proximal o.
Pauwels valgus o.
Pauwels Y o.
peg-in-hole o.
Peimer reduction o.
pelvic o.
Pemberton pericapsular o.
percutaneous o.
pericapsular o.
phalangeal o.
o. pin
plantarflexory proximal
  metatarsal o.
Platou o.
Pol Le Coueur o.
posterior iliac o.
posterior spinal wedge o.
Potts eversion o.
Potts tibial o.
proximal dome o.
proximal femoral o.
proximal first metatarsal o.
proximal metatarsal o.
proximal phalangeal o.
proximal phalanx o.
proximal tibial o.
radial wedge o.
Ranawat-DeFiore-Straub o.
Rappaport o.

O

NOTES

osteotomy *(continued)*
  reduction o.
  Reverdin o.
  Reverdin-Green o.
  Reverdin-Laird o.
  reverse Dillwyn-Evans calcaneal o.
  reverse wedge o.
  Root-Siegal varus derotational o.
  rotational scarf o.
  sagittal-Z o.
  Sakoff o.
  Salter innominate o.
  Salter pelvic o.
  Samilson crescentic calcaneal o.
  Sarmiento intertrochanteric o.
  Scanz o.
  scarf Z o.
  Schanz angulation o.
  Schanz femoral o.
  Schede hip o.
  Schwartz dorsiflexory o.
  shortening o.
  Siffert intraepiphyseal o.
  Siffert-Storen intraepiphyseal o.
  Simmonds-Menelaus metatarsal o.
  Simmonds-Menelaus proximal
    phalangeal o.
  Simmons o.
  Smith-Petersen o.
  Sofield o.
  Southwick biplane trochanteric o.
  spike o.
  spinal o.
  Sponsel oblique o.
  Stamm metatarsal o.
  Steel triple innominate o.
  step o.
  step-cut o.
  step-down o.
  Stren intraepiphyseal o.
  subcapital o.
  subcondylar o.
  subtraction o.
  subtrochanteric o.
  Sugioka transtrochanteric
    rotational o.
  supracondylar femoral
    derotational o.
  supracondylar varus o.
  supramalleolar derotational o.
  supramalleolar varus derotation o.
  supratubercular wedge o.
  Sutherland-Greenfield o.
  Swanson o.
  talar neck o.
  talocalcaneal o.
  tarsal wedge o.
  Thompson telescoping V o.

  through-and-through V-shaped
    horizontal o.
  tibial tuberosity o.
  translational o.
  transtrochanteric rotational o.
  transverse chevron o.
  transverse diaphyseal o.
  transverse metatarsal o.
  transverse supracondylar o.
  trapezoidal o.
  Trethowan metatarsal o.
  Trillat o.
  triplane o.
  triple innominate o.
  trochanteric o.
  tubercle o.
  U o.
  unplanned valgus o.
  V o.
  valgus extension o.
  valgus high tibial o.
  valgus intertrochanteric-wedge o.
  valgus subtrochanteric o.
  valgus wedge-prop o.
  valgus Y-shaped prop o.
  varus derotational o.
  varus rotational o. (VRO)
  varus rotation shortening o.
  varus supramalleolar o.
  V-shaped o.
  Wagdy double-V o.
  Waterman o.
  Weber humeral o.
  Weber subcapital o.
  wedge o.
  wedge-shaped o.
  Whitman o.
  Wilson double oblique o.
  Wilson oblique displacement o.
  Wiltse ankle o.
  Wiltse varus supramalleolar o.
  Yancey o.
  Yu o.

osteotomy/bunionectomy
  base wedge o./b.
  close wedge o./b.
  crescentic base wedge o./b.
  Kelikian modified Z o./b.
  Mitchell o./b.
  open base wedge o./b.
  rotational scarf o./b.
  scarf Z o./b.
  supertubercular wedge o./b.

osteotomy-osteoclasis
  Moore o.-o.

osteotripsy

Osteotron stimulator for bone union

ostium, pl. **ostia**

Ostrup harvesting technique
Oswestry
O. Disability Score
O. index
Oswestry-O'Brien spinal stapler
OT
occupational therapy
Ottawa ankle rule
Otto
O. Bock 1A30 Greissinger Plus foot
O. Bock 1D25 Dynamic Plus foot
O. Bock dynamic prosthesis
O. Bock modular rotary hydraulic knee
O. Bock 3R65 children's hydraulic knee joint
O. Bock 3R60 EBS knee
O. Bock 3R45 modular knee joint
O. Bock 3R80 modular rotary hydraulic knee
O. Bock Safety constant-friction knee
O. Bock system electric hand
O. pelvis dislocation
Oudard procedure
out
draped o.
step out, turn o. (SOTO)
toeing o.
outcome measure
Outerbridge
O. classification
O. ridge
O. scale
O. scale for joint or articular surface damage in chondromalacia
O. staging of degenerative arthritis
outflow cannula
outgrowth
osseous patellae o.
outlet
supraspinatus o.
o. view
outpatient physical therapy
output
urinary o.
outrigger
o. arm
o. cast
dorsal wrist splint with o.

Harrington distraction o.
o. splint
O. wire
outside-in technique
outside-to-outside arthroscopy technique
out-toeing
outward rotation
Ovadia-Beals
O.-B. classification of tibial plafond fracture
O.-B. tibial plafond fracture classification
oval
o. curved-cup curette
o. washer
ovalis
fossa o.
over-bed table
overcorrection
overdistraction
Overdyke hip prosthesis
overgrowth
bone o.
bony o.
terminal o.
overhead
o. exercise test
o. olecranon traction
overhinge
variable flexion o. (VFO)
Overholt clip-applying forceps
overlap
tibiofibular o.
overlapped uprights in orthosis
overlapping fifth toe
overlay
"Bodyline sleeper" mattress o.
o. drafting
o. mattress
o. plate
Stimulite honeycomb mattress o.
x-ray o.
overload
compression o.
torsional o.
overpronation
overpull
overriding fifth toe
oversewn
overstretch weakness
over-the-door traction unit

O

NOTES

over-the-top
> o.-t.-t. knee procedure
> o.-t.-t. position

Overton dowel graft
over-tying wire
overuse
> o. injury
> o. syndrome

OW
> open wedge

Owen gauze dressing
Owens silk
Owestry staple
oxacillin
oxaprozin
oxazepam
Oxford
> O. fixator
> O. method
> O. method for scoring skeletal
>   maturity
> O. prosthesis
> O. uncompartmental device

oxicam
oxiconazole
oxidation
> carbohydrate o.

oxide
> ethylene o.

oximeter
> pulse o.

Oxistat
> O. cream
> O. Topical

oxychlorosene
oxycodone
> o. and acetaminophen
> o. and aspirin
> o. hydrochloride

OxyContin
oxygen
> dysbaric o.
> epiphyseal o.
> hyperbaric o. (HBO)
> o. seizure
> o. tension
> o. therapy

OxyIR
oxymorphone hydrochloride
oxyphenbutazone
oxytoca
> *Klebsiella o.*

Oyst-Cal 500
Oystercal 500

P
>passive

P/3
>proximal third

PA
>posteroanterior

pace card
pachydysostosis
pacinian
>p. corpuscle
>p. mechanoreceptor

pack
>Arctic Blaze hot/cold p.
>Back-Ease aromatherapy hot/cold p.
>Baxter personal Von-Loc ice p.
>BodyIce cold p.
>Coldhot p.
>Colpacs p.
>cool p.
>CP2 inflatable cold p.
>DynaHeat hot p.
>ErgoForm contoured cold p.
>gel p.
>Glacier P.
>hot p. (HP)
>Hydrocollator steam p.
>ice p.
>I.C.E. Down cold p.
>instant cold p.
>Jack Frost hot/cold p.
>Kool Kit cold therapy p.
>M-Zole 7 Dual P.
>Neck-Roll aromatherapy hot/cold p.
>Polar P.
>Softouch Cold/Hot P.
>P. technique
>TheraBeads microwaveable moist
> heat p.
>Thera-Med cold p.
>Thermal P.
>Thermophore heat p.
>Thermophore hot p.
>vaginal p.
>Whitehall Glacier P.

Package
>Cognitive Behavior Therapy P.
> (CBTP)

packed red cell
Pack-Ehrlich deep iliac dissection
packing
>Adaptic p.
>gauze p.
>Nu Gauze p.
>wound p.

Pacs
>Boo-Boo P.

PACU
>postanesthesia care unit

pad
>ABD p.
>abdominal lap p.
>Achilles heel p.
>Airex balance p.
>AirLITE support p.
>Aliplast p.
>alternating pressure p.
>antidecubitus p.
>Aquaflex gel p.
>Aquatech cast p.
>Aquatherm bed p.
>Arthropor cup p.
>artificial fat p.
>balance p.
>buttocks p.
>"buttress" p.
>calcaneal fat p.
>Charnley foam suture p.
>cloverleaf met foot p.
>cold p.
>dancer p.
>Decubinex p.
>digital p.
>elbow p.
>fat p.
>foveal fat p.
>Hapad longitudinal metatarsal
> arch p.
>Hapad medial arch p.
>heel fat p.
>Hoffa fat p.
>horseshoe heel p.
>horseshoe-shaped felt p.
>Hydrocollator p.
>infrapatellar fat p.
>J p.
>Kerlix cast p.
>knee-control orthosis p.
>knuckle p.
>lamb's wool p.
>metatarsal p.
>Mikulicz p.
>navicular shoe p.
>OEC popliteal p.
>Ortho-Cel p.
>Ortho-Foam elbow/heel p.
>patellar fat p.
>patellar orthosis p.
>Pedi-Cushions p.
>Pedifix hammertoe p.

P

pad *(continued)*
    Pelite p.
    Pen/Alps distal p.
    pubic p.
    Redigrip knee p.
    reticulated polyurethane p.
    retropatellar fat p.
    ROHO heel p.
    scalene fat p.
    scaphoid shoe p.
    Scholl p.
    second skin p.
    sensor p.
    shoe heel p.
    Silipos digital p.
    Sof-Rol cast p.
    Sof Sole Sof Gel heel p.
    spur p.
    Staph-Chek p.
    Sure Sport p.
    TenderCloud pressure p.
    T-Foam bed p.
    Thermapad p.
    Zimfoam p.
padded
    p. aluminum splint
    p. board splint
    p. button
    p. clamp
    p. plywood splint
    p. tongue blade splint
padding
    AliBrite p.
    cast p.
    contoured felt p.
    cotton cast p.
    Delta-Rol cast p.
    felt p.
    foam p.
    Kerlix cast p.
    moleskin p.
    Molestick p.
    Ortho-Cel p.
    pressure relief p.
    Protouch synthetic orthopaedic p.
    QuickStick p.
    Reston p.
    Sifoam p.
    splint p.
    Thero-Skin gel p.
    Webril cotton p.
Paddu knee operation
Padgett
    P. electric dermatome
    P. osteotome
    P. prosthesis
pad/protector
    Decubinex p.

PAG
    periaqueductal gray
Page osteitis deformans
Paget
    P.-associated osteogenic sarcoma
    P. disease
pagetoid bone
Paget-Schrötter syndrome
Pagosid
pain
    aches and p.'s
    Achilles tendon p.
    aching p.
    adolescent back p.
    p. at rest
    back p.
    band-like p.
    Behavioral Assessment of P. (BAP)
    burning p.
    causalgic p.
    chronic low back p. (CLBP)
    contralateral p.
    cross leg p.
    deafferentation p.
    dermatomal p.
    diskogenic neck p.
    p. drawing
    dull aching p.
    p. dysfunction syndrome
    endogenous p.
    epicritic p.
    fibromyalgic p.
    functional back p.
    gate control theory of p.
    glenohumeral p.
    gouty p.
    groin p.
    growing p.'s
    impingement p.
    p. induction
    joint line p.
    kinetic foot p.
    lancinating p.
    low back p. (LBP)
    machine-gun-like p.
    Multiaxial Assessment of P. (MAP)
    myofascial p.
    myotomal p.
    neurologic p.
    patellofemoral p. (PFP)
    perimalleolar p.
    periscapulitis shoulder p.
    phantom p.
    pillar p.
    postherpetic p.
    Pronex pneumatic device for cervical p.
    p. provocation test

radicular p.
recalcitrant p.
referred neuritic p.
referred trigger point p.
Roland index of low back p.
scapulothoracic p.
sclerotomal p.
splint-like p.
static foot p.
p. threshold gauge
ticlike p.
vise-like p.
volleys of p.
p. with weightbearing

painful

p. arc
p. femoral head prosthesis
p. gait
p. heel
p. minor intervertebral dysfunction (PMID)
p. spur
p. stump

Pain-HP

No P.-HP

paint

Betadine p.
Castellani p.
p. gun injury
p. thinner injury

paired

p. discharge
p. response
p. scintigraphy
p. stimulus
p. t-test

pairwise comparison
Pais fracture
Pak

Apollo hot/cold P.

PAL

posterior axillary line
PAL Diasole insole

Palacos

P. cement adhesive
P. radiopaque bone cement

Paladon

P. implant material
P. prosthesis

palatasis
Palex expansion screw
Paley classification

palindromic rheumatism
palliative care
pallor
palm

p. guard
p. space
p.-to-axilla dressing
p.-up test

palmar

p. advancement flap
p. aponeurosis
p. approach
p. arch
p. carpometacarpal ligament
p. clip
p. cock-up splint
p. creaking
p. crease
p. cross-finger flap
p. fascia
p. fasciotomy
p. flexion
p. incision
p. intercarpal deltoid ligament
p. interosseous muscle
p. ligaments of interphalangeal articulations
p. luxation
p. metacarpal ligament
p. pinch
p. plate
p. radiocarpal ligament
p. swab kit
p. synovectomy
p. tilt
p. ulnocarpal ligament

palmare

ligamentum radiocarpale p.
ligamentum ulnocarpale p.

palmaria

ligamenta carpometacarpalia p.
ligamenta intercarpalia p.
ligamenta metacarpalia p.

palmaris

p. longus (PL)
p. longus muscle
p. longus tendon

Palmer

P. bone nail
P. method
P. screw
P. technique

NOTES

Palmer (*continued*)
    P. transscaphoid perilunar dislocation
    P. triangular fibrocartilage complex lesion classification
Palmer-Dobyns-Linscheid ligament repair
Palmer-Gonstead-Firth listing system
Palmer-Widen shoulder technique
palpable band
palpation
    p. of anterior superior iliac spine
    digital p.
    end-feel p.
    flat p.
    p. of iliac crest
    intersegmental range of motion p. (IRMP)
    motion p.
    optimizing motion p.
    pincer p.
    p. of posterior superior iliac spine
    screening p.
    static p.
    p. testing
palpatory
    p. diagnosis
    p. examination
    p. skill
palpitation
palsy
    backpack p.
    Bell p.
    brachial plexus p.
    cerebral p. (CP)
    combined nerve p.
    drummer-boy p.
    Erb-Duchenne p.
    handlebar p.
    high median-high radial p.
    high median-high ulnar p.
    high ulnar-high radial p.
    Hoke procedure for tibial p.
    Klumpke p.
    long thoracic nerve p.
    low median-low ulnar p.
    median nerve p.
    nerve p.
    peripheral nerve p.
    peroneal nerve p.
    posterior interosseous nerve p.
    postnatal cerebral p.
    radial nerve p.
    sciatic p.
    tardy ulnar p.
    thenar p.
    tourniquet p.
    ulnar nerve p.

Paltrinieri-Trentani
    P.-T. resurfacing
    P.-T. resurfacing procedure
Palumbo
    P. ankle stabilizer
    P. dynamic patellar brace
    P. knee brace
    P. patella tracker
    P. stabilizing brace
pamidronate
Panadol
    Junior Strength P.
Panafil ointment
Panafil-White ointment
Panalok absorbable anchor
panaris
    melanotic p.
Panasal 5/500
panastragaloid arthrodesis
pancake hand
panclavicular dislocation
pancreas
pancreatic enzyme therapy
pancreatitis
Pandel
pandemic
Panje prosthesis
panmetatarsal head resection
Panner disease
panniculus
pannus
    p. deformity
    p. of synovium
Panogauze Hydrogel wound dressing
Panoview
    P. arthroscope
    P. arthroscopic system
pan splint
pantalar
    p. arthrodesis
    p. fusion
pantalocrural arthritis
pantaloon
    p. brace
    p. spica cast
    p. walking cast
Pantopaque
Pantopon
pants
    prophylactic abduction p.
pants-over-vest
    p.-o.-v. capsulorrhaphy
    p.-o.-v. technique
panty
    Cadenza p.
PAOD
    peripheral arterial occlusive disease

papain-urea-chlorophyllin copper complex debriding and healing ointment
Papavasiliou olecranon fracture classification
papaverine
paper
    tracing p.
papillary adenoma
Papineau
    P. graft
    P. technique
papule
    Gottron p.
papyrus
    Edwin Smith p.
PAR
    postanesthesia recovery
paraaminosalicylic acid
paraarticular
    p. arthrodesis
    p. calcification
    p. heterotopic ossification
Parabath paraffin heat treatment
parabola
    metatarsal p.
paracervical
paracetamol
parachute
    p. jumper's dislocation
    p. reflex
    p. test
    p. therapy
paradoxical lumbrical-plus finger
paraesthesia (*var. of* paresthesia)
paraesthetica
    meralgia p.
paraffin
    p. bath (PB)
    p. heat therapy
    p. implant material
    p. mitt
Paraflex
Parafon
    P. Forte
    P. Forte DSC
parainfluenzae
    Haemophilus p.
parajugular line
parallel
    p. goniometric measure
    p. pin kit

parallelism
parallelogram electrogoniometer
paralysis
    adductor pollicis p.
    p. agitans
    backpack p.
    brachial plexus p.
    Chaves-Rapp p.
    cruciate p.
    Dewar-Harris p.
    Dickson p.
    familial periodic p.
    flaccid p.
    gluteus medius p.
    Haas p.
    hand p.
    Henry p.
    intrinsic p.
    isolated p.
    serratus anterior p.
    spastic p.
    tourniquet p.
    Vastamäki p.
    Volkmann ischemic p.
    Whitman p.
paralytic
    p. contracture
    p. foot
    p. ileus
    p. kyphosis
paramalleolar artery
ParaMax
    P. ACL guide system
    P. angled driver
paramedial incision
paramedian
    p. approach
    p. sagittal plane
paramethasone acetate
Paramount 3-Way Press Bench
paramyotonia congenita
Paramyxoviridae
paraparesis
parapatellar
    p. arthrotomy
    p. incision
    p. plica
    p. synovitis
paraphysiologic zone
paraplegia
    incomplete p.
    postoperative p.

NOTES

P

paraplegia *(continued)*
    Pott p.
    spastic p.
    traumatic p.
paraplegic patient
parapodium orthosis
pararectus approach
parasagittal
    p. groove
    p. scar
parascapular flap
parasite potential
paraspinal
    p. abscess
    p. approach
    p. mapping
    p. muscle
    p. muscle spasm
    p. musculature
    p. rod application
    p. skin temperature thermocouple instrument
parasternal heave
parasympathetic nervous system (PNS)
parasympatholytic
paratenon
parathenar incision
parathyroid disorder
paratrooper fracture
paravertebral
    p. abscess
    p. muscle
    p. muscle spasm
    p. musculature
    p. sympathetic chain
paraxial hemimelia
paregoric
Pare reduction of elbow dislocation
paresis
    limb-girdle-trunk p.
paresthesia, paraesthesia, pl. **paresthesias**
    intermittent p.
paresthetica
    cheiralgia p.
    meralgia p.
Parham
    P. band
    P. support
Parham-Martin
    P.-M. band
    P.-M. bone-holding clamp
    P.-M. fracture apparatus
    P.-M. fracture device
parietal
    p. pleura
    p. tendon sheath layer
parietooccipitalis
    arcus p.

Paris
    P. manual therapy table
    plaster-of-P. (POP)
Park
    transverse lines of P.
Parkes osteotome
Parkes-Weber syndrome
Parkinson disease
parkinsonian gait
Parona space
paronychia bur
parosteal
    p. chondrosarcoma
    p. osteogenic sarcoma
    p. osteoma
    p. osteosarcoma
parosteitis
parosteosis
PAR-Q
    Physical Activity Readiness Questionnaire
parquetry set
Parrish-Mann hammertoe technique
Parrish procedure
parrot
    p.-beak tear
    P. node
    P. pseudoparalysis
parry fracture
pars
    p. defect
    p. interarticularis
    p. interarticularis fracture
Parsonage-Aldren-Turner syndrome
Parsonage-Turner
    P.-T. neuronitis
    P.-T. syndrome
partial
    p. diskectomy
    p. dislocation
    p. fasciectomy
    p. fibulectomy
    p. matrixectomy
    p. meniscectomy
    p. ossicular reconstruction/replacement prosthesis
    p. ossicular replacement prosthesis (PORP)
    p. ostectomy
    p. patellectomy
    p. thromboplastin time (PTT)
    p. weightbearing
partially
    p. necrotic osseous trabecula
    p. threaded pin

particle
- birefringent p.
- p.'s of bone

particulate
- p. cancellous bone graft
- p. debris
- p. synovitis

Partnership
- P. implant
- P. instrument
- P. system

Partridge band

Partsch
- P. chisel
- P. gouge

Parvin
- P. gravity technique
- P. maneuver
- P. reduction

PASA
- proximal articular set angle

PASG
- pneumatic antishock garment

passage
- adiabatic fast p.
- wire p.

passer
- Batzdorf cervical wire p.
- Brand tendon p.
- Bunnell tendon p.
- Charnley wire p.
- Concept two-pin p.
- curved p.
- DeMayo suture p.
- Framer tendon p.
- Hewson suture p.
- Incavo wire p.
- ligature p.
- Malis ligature p.
- Shuttle-Relay suture p.
- suture p.
- tendon p.
- Wedeen wire p.
- wire p.

passing suture

passive (P)
- p. accessory motion test
- p. gliding technique
- p. insufficiency
- p. intervertebral motion (PIVM)
- p. joint manipulation
- p. mobility

- p. mobility testing
- p. motion device
- p. motion machine
- p. movement
- p. patellar glide test
- p. patellar tilt test
- p. physiological test
- p. plantar flexion
- p. positioning device
- p. range of motion (PROM)
- p. range of motion exercise
- p. restraint
- p. spacer
- p. straight leg raising
- p. stretch

Passow chisel

Passport instrumentation

paste
- bone p.
- Coe-pak p.
- Unna p.

Pasteurella multocida

PAT
- Physical Ability Test

Patau syndrome

patch dressing

patella, pl. **patellae**
- absent p.
- p. alta
- apex of head of p.
- p. baja
- ballottement of p.
- bipartite p.
- p. bone saw
- chondromalacia patellae
- p. cubiti
- debridement p.
- dislocated p.
- high-riding p.
- p. infera
- ligamentum patellae
- low-riding p.
- maltracking p.
- minima p.
- p. minima
- multipartite p.
- plastic p.
- prosthetic p.
- skyline x-ray view of p.
- subluxing p.
- superior pole of p.
- p. tendon-bearing-supracondylar

NOTES

P

patella *(continued)*
    p. tracker
    p. turndown approach
    undersurface of p.
patellapexy
patellaplasty
patellar
    p. advancement
    p. affection
    p. aligner
    p. alignment
    p. apprehension test
    p. band
    P. Band knee protector
    p. bar
    p. bone-tendon-bone autograft
    p. bursitis
    p. button
    p. cement clamp
    p. clonus
    p. clunk syndrome
    p. contour
    p. dislocation cast
    p. drill guide
    p. edge
    p. fat pad
    p. glide
    p. groove
    p. instability
    p. intraarticular dislocation
    p. jerk (PJ)
    p. ligament
    p. malalignment syndrome
    p. orthosis pad
    p. osteochondritis dissecans
    p. pair syndrome
    p. portal
    p. realignment
    p. reamer guide
    p. reamer shaft
    p. reduction clamp
    p. reflex
    p. resection guide
    p. resurfacing
    p. resurfacing implant
    p. retinacula release
    p. retinaculum
    p. retraction test
    p. rotation
    p. shelf
    p. sleeve fracture
    p. subluxation
    p. tap test
    p. tendinitis
    p. tendon
    p. tendon-bearing (PTB)
    p. tendon-bearing below-knee
    prosthesis

    p. tendon-bearing brace
    p. tendon-bearing orthosis
    p. tendon-bearing–supracondylar
    (PTB-SC)
    p. tendon graft
    p. tendon repair
    p. tendon substitution
    p. tendon transfer (PTT)
    p. tendon weightbearing brace
    orthosis
    p. tendon weightbearing cast
    p. tracking
    p. transplant
patellectomy
    partial p.
    total p.
    West-Soto-Hall p.
patelloadductor reflex
patellofemoral
    p. alignment
    p. arthritis
    p. articulation
    p. compartment
    p. congruence
    p. crepitation
    p. disorder
    p. dysarthrosis
    p. dysfunction
    p. dysplasia
    p. groove
    p. groove cartilage
    p. joint
    p. joint radiography
    p. joint reaction force
    p. ligament
    p. pain (PFP)
    p. realignment
patellomeniscal ligament
patelloquadriceps
    p. tendon
    p. tendon substitution
patellotibial ligament
Patel medial meniscectomy
Paterson
    P. procedure
    P. technique
Pathocil
pathogenesis
pathognomonic sign
pathokinesiologic
pathologic
    p. barrier
    p. dislocation
    p. fracture
    p. reflex
    p. spondylolisthesis
pathological plica

pathology
    Armed Forces Institute of P.
    heel pad p.
pathomechanical state
pathomechanics
    gait p.
    juvenile flatfoot p.
    kyphotic deformity p.
    spinal fusion p.
pathomechanism
pathway
    neuromeningeal p.
patient
    adult scoliosis p.
    bedbound p.
    p.-controlled analgesia (PCA)
    p.-controlled anesthesia (PCA)
    diabetic p.
    institutionalized p.
    multitrauma p.
    obese p.
    p.-on-table friction
    paraplegic p.
    polytrauma p.
    p. positioning
    p.-resisted internal rotation
    p.-table interface
    variable screw placement system-
        plated p.
PATRAN modelling program
Patrick
    P. drill
    P. sign
    P. test
Patrick/fabere test
Patten bottom
Patten-Bottom-Perthes brace
pattern
    cloverleaf p.
    Collimator plugging p.
    compression p.
    curve p.
    dermatomal p.
    DISI collapse p.
    double major curve p.
    facilitation p.
    firing p.
    full interference p.
    gait p.
    interference p.
    intermediate interference p.
    lamellar p.

    left thoracolumbar major curve p.
    locomotor p.
    p. matching card
    p. of motion
    plantar pressure p.
    posterior depression p.
    primitive locomotor p.
    recruitment p.
    reduced interference p.
    right thoracic, left lumbar curve p.
    right thoracic, left thoracolumbar
        curve p.
    right thoracic minor curve p.
    single-unit p.
    storiform p.
    stretch p.
    p. of thrust
    two-point step-to gait p.
    type II curve p.
    whorled p.
patterning
    Aston p.
PattStrap knee support
patty
    cement p.
    cottonoid p.
pauciarticular arthritis
Paufique blade
Paulos ligament technique
Paulson knee retractor
Paulus plate
Pauly point
Pauwels
    P. angle
    P. femoral neck fracture
        classification
    P. fracture
    P. proximal osteotomy
    P. technique
    P. valgus osteotomy
    P. Y osteotomy
Pavlick harness
Pavlik
    P. bandage
    P. harness
    P. harness splint
    P. sling
paw
    monkey p.
Paxipam
Payr sign

NOTES

P

PB
paraffin bath
peroneus brevis
PBS
peroneus brevis split
PC
PC Performer knee
PC Performer knee prosthesis
PCA
patient-controlled analgesia
patient-controlled anesthesia
porous-coated anatomic
PCA cutting guide
PCA hip stem
PCA medullary guide
PCA primary total knee system
PCA prosthesis
PCA total hip replacement
PCA unconstrained tricompartmental
prosthesis
PCA unicompartmental knee
prosthesis
PCA Universal total knee
instrument system
PCB
proximal communicating branch
PCE
physical capacity evaluation
Smith physical capacities evaluation
PCL
posterior cruciate ligament
PCL-oriented placement (POP)
PCL-oriented placement marking
hook
PCP
phencyclidine hydrochloride
P.C. Williams brace
PDA
plantar digital artery
PDGF
platelet-derived growth factor
PDLS
physical daily living skills
PDS
polydioxanone suture
PDS knot
PDS suture
pDXA
peripheral dual-energy x-ray
absorptiometry
Peabody
P. procedure
P. splint
Peacock
P. transposing index ray
P. transposing technique
peak
P. gait module

p. latency
P. Motus Motion Measurement
System
p.-pressure analysis
PEAK Fixation System
Pean clamp
pear bur
Pearson
P. attachment to Thomas frame
P. attachment to Thomas splint
P. intramedullary saw
P. splint attachment
Pease bone drill
Pease-Thomson traction
Pebax
P. counter unit
P. fastening strap
PEC
PEC modular total knee system
PEC total hip system
Pec-Dec
Peck osteotome
pectoral
p. girdle
p. nerve
p. reflex
pectoralis
p. major flap
p. major muscle
p. muscle implant
pedal
p. exerciser
p. hyperpigmented lesion
p. hypophalangism
p. osteomyelitis
Pedar
P.-in-shoe measurement system
P. pressure measurement system
pedestal
halo p.
IMP surgical leg p.
shelf p.
surgical leg p.
pedestaled
Pediapred Oral
Pediaprofen
pediatric
p. C-D hook
Cleocin P.
p. Cotrel-Dubousset rod
p. PRAFO brace
p. pressure relief ankle foot
orthosis (PRAFO)
p. system
p. TSRH hook
pedicle
adjoining p.
p. anatomy

p. axis angle
p. bone graft
p. C-D hook
p. clamp
p. connector
contralateral hypoplastic/agenetic p.
p. cortex disruption
p. diameter
p. dimension
p. entrance point
p. evaluation
p. fat graft
p. finder
p. fixation
p. fracture
p. groin flap
p. implant
p. landmark
p. localization
p. location
lower thoracic p.
lumbar p.
p. marker
p. method
p. morphometry
p. plate
p. screw
p. screw breakage
p. screw construct
p. screw cord length
p. screw hardware prominence
p. screw insertion
p. screw linkage design
p. screw path length
p. screw plating
p. screw pull-out strength
p. screw system
p. sounder
p. sounding probe
thoracic p.
pedicled
p. fibular transfer
p. transplant
Pedic sponge
pedicular
p. fixation
p. kinking
Pedi-Cushions pad
Pedi-Dri topical powder
Pedifix hammertoe pad
Pedilen polyurethane foam

Pediplast
P. cushion
P. moldable footcare compound
Pedi-Pro Topical
pedis
dorsalis p. (DP)
ligamenta collateralia articulationum
  interphalangealium p.
ligamenta plantaria articulationum
  interphalangealium p.
tinea p.
pedi sandbag
Pedistal
Body P.
pedobarogram
pedobarograph
Biokinetics p.
BTE Dyamic P.
EMED-SF p.
Musgrave footprint p.
pedobarography
pedodynograph
pedodynographic
p. examination
p. measurement
pedography
Pedors orthopedic shoe
pedorthist
certified p. (CPed)
pedorthotic
Pedrialle template
pedunculated loose body
PEER
pronation-eversion-external rotation
Peet Z-plasty
pefloxacin
peg
anchoring p.
p.-base plate
Beath bone intramedullary p.
p. board lateral positioning device
bone p.
p. bone graft
fiber-metal p.
fibular p.
fixation p.
glenoid alignment p.
Harrison-Nicolle polypropylene p.
Kinemax removable fixation p.
locking p.
stringing p.

NOTES

P

pegboard
Purdue p.
pegged tibial prosthesis
pegging
bone p.
peg-in-hole
p.-i.-h. arthroereisis
p.-i.-h. osteotomy
Peimer reduction osteotomy
PE LITE material
Pelite pad
Pelken sign
Pelligrini-Stieda disease
pelvic
p. abscess
p. angle
p. avulsion fracture
p. band
p. bench
p. block
p. brim
p. C-clamp
p. circumference
p. discontinuity
p. drainage
dual drop p. (DDP)
p.-femoral angle
p. fixation
p. flexion contracture (PFC)
p. girdle
p. hyperextension traction
p. injury
p. instability
p. kinematic chain
p. lateral
p. lateral shift
p. lateral tilt
p. obliquity
p. osteotomy
p. plane
p. reconstruction kit
p. ring
p. ring fracture
p. rock (PR)
p. rotation
p. side-shift
p. sling
p. splint
p. splinting
p. straddle fracture
pelvis
pelvitrochanteric heterotopic ossification
Pemberton
P. acetabuloplasty
P. pericapsular osteotomy
P. spur-crushing clamp
PEMF
pulsed electromagnetic field

pen
STA-Pen writer p.
weighted p.
Pen/Alps distal pad
pencil
p. and cup deformity
electrosurgical p.
skin p.
sterile p.
p.-tip drill
penciled
penciling of ribs on x-ray
Penco Walker Sleds
pendulum exercise
penetrating
p. drill
p. fracture
penetration
anterior cortex p.
Penfield
P. 4 dissector
P. periosteal elevator
penguin gait
penicillamine
penicillin
p. G
p. g benzathine and procaine
combined
Penn
P. finger drill
Pennal classification
Pennig dynamic wrist fixator
Pennsylvania bimanual work sample
Penrose drain
pentazocine
p. compound
p. hydrochloride
pentobarbital
Pentothal Sodium
pentoxifylline
peptic ulcer
peptido-leukotriene
Peptococcus
Peptostreptococcus
P-ER
pronation-external rotation
P-ER injury
per
p. hypodermic (H)
p. primam healing
perception
constant-touch p.
visual p.
perceptual deficit
Percocet
Percodan
Percodan-Demi
Percogesic

Percolone
PercScope
percussion tenderness
percutaneous
    p. autogenous dowel bone graft
    p. bone marrow infection
    p. corticotomy
    p. cryoepiphysiodesis
    p. dorsal column stimulator implant
    p. epiphysiodesis
    p. fixation
    p. heel cord lengthening
    p. lengthening of Achilles tendon
    p. lumbar diskectomy
    p. needle placement
    p. osteotomy
    p. pin
    p. pin insertion
    p. pinning
    p. plantar fasciotomy (PPF)
    p. reduction
    p. stapling
    p. tenotomy
Percy
    P. amputating saw
    P. plate
Perez postoperative pain scale
Perfecta
    P. femoral stem
    P. hip prosthesis
    P. Interseal total hip system
PerFixation
    P. screw
    P. system
perforans
    mal p.
perforating
    p. bur
    p. forceps
    p. fracture
    p. twist drill
perforation
    attritional p.
    cortical p.
    esophageal p.
    femoral cortical p.
perforator
    Boyd p.
    Dodd p.
    p. drill
performance
    p. area

    p. component
    p. context
    functional p.
    isokinetic p.
    P. knee prosthesis
    P. modular total knee system
    motion p.
    movement p.
    safety p.
    Test of Infant Motor P. (TIMP)
    P. unicompartmental knee system
performer ultralight knee brace
perfringens
    Clostridium p.
perfusion
    digital blood p.
Periactin
perianal
    p. sensation
    p. skin
periaqueductal
    p. gray (PAG)
    p. gray nucleus
periarthrosis humeri
periarticular
    p. fibrositis
    p. fracture
    p. heterotopic ossification
    p. tissue
pericapsular osteotomy
pericardium
    glutaraldehyde-prepared bovine p.
    p. graft
pericellular halo
perichondral
    p. circulation
    p. ring
perichondrium
PERI-COMFORT cushion
pericyte
    Zimmerman p.
periepineurial neuropathy
perihamate injury
perilesional bone
perilunar
    p. instability
    p. transscaphoid dislocation
perilunate
    p. carpal dislocation
    p. fracture-dislocation
perimalleolar pain
perimysial

NOTES

P

445

perimysiitis
perimysium
perineal
    p. flap
    p. post
    p. sensation
perinealis
    luxatio p.
perineometer
    Peritron p.
perineum
perineural
    p. fibrosis
    p. tissue
perineurial neurorrhaphy
perineurium
period
    absolute refractory p.
    functional refractory p.
    incubation p.
    latent p.
    refractory p.
    relative refractory p.
    silent p.
perionychium
perioperative
    p. antibiotic therapy
    p. reduction
periosteal
    p. bone collar
    p. cambium layer
    p. chondroma
    p. chondrosarcoma
    p. desmoid
    p. elevator
    p. fibroma
    p. ganglion
    MacKentry p.
    p. osteosarcoma
    round-tapped p.
    p. sleeve
    p. tissue
    p. vessel
periosteotome
    Alexander costal p.
    Alexander-Farabeuf p.
    Ballenger p.
    Brown p.
    costal p.
    Fomon p.
    Joseph p.
periosteotomy
periosteum
periostitis
    florid reactive p.
    p. ossificans
    suppurative p.

peripatellar
    p. retinacular support
    p. tendinitis
peripheral
    p. arterial occlusive disease
    (PAOD)
    p. dual-energy x-ray absorptiometry
    (pDXA)
    p. gangrene
    p. nerve
    p. nerve block
    p. nerve block anesthesia
    p. nerve glove
    p. nerve injury
    p. nerve palsy
    p. nervous system (PNS)
    p. neurocompressive disorder
    p. neuropathy
    p. polyneuritis
    p. pulses symmetrical and intact
    p. vascular disease (PVD)
    p. vascular insufficiency
    p. vascular surgery (PVS)
    p. vascular system (PVS)
peripisiform injury
periprosthetic
    p. fracture
    p. membrane
periscapulitis shoulder pain
peritendinitis
    Achilles p.
    p. crepitans
peritendinous scar
peritoneum
peritrapezial injury
peritrapezoidal injury
peritrochanteric fracture
Peritron perineometer
periungual fibroma
PER-IV fracture
Perkins
    P. test
    P. traction
    P. vertical line
Perlstein brace
Perma-Hand silk suture
Permalock
    Weber P.
Perman cartilage forceps
permanent
    p. disability
    p. implant
permanganate
    potassium p.
peroneal
    p. artery
    p. bupivacaine injection
    p. compartment syndrome

p. dislocation
p. groove
p. muscle
p. muscle spasm
p. musculature
p. nerve
p. nerve injury
p. nerve palsy
p. neuropathy
p. spastic flatfoot
p. subluxation
p. tendinitis
p. tendon
p. tendon displacement
p. tendon sheath injection
p. vein
peroneum
os p.
peroneus
p. brevis (PB)
p. brevis elongation
p. brevis graft
p. brevis muscle
p. brevis split (PBS)
p. brevis tendon
p. brevis transfer
p. longus
p. longus muscle
p. longus tendon
p. tertius muscle
p. tertius tendon
peroxide
p. flush
hydrogen p.
perpendiculars
method of p.
perpendicular strumming
perphenazine
Perry
P. extensile anterior approach
P. sensor
P. technique
PerryMeter sensor
Perry-Nickel
P.-N. cranial halo
P.-N. technique
Perry-O'Brien-Hodgson
P.-O.-H. technique
P.-O.-H. triple tenodesis
Perry-Robinson cervical technique
Persian slipper foot

persistent
p. clonus
p. notochord
p. occiput/atlas disrelationship
p. sciatic artery
Persons
American Association of Retired P.
(AARP)
perstans
macularis eruptive p.
Perthes
P. disease
P. epiphysis
P. lesion
P. procedure
P. reamer
P. test
Perthes-Bankart lesion
pertrochanteric fracture
perverted function
pes
p. anserinus
p. anserinus syndrome
p. anserinus transplant
p. cavovalgus
p. cavovarus
p. cavus
p. equinovarus adductus
p. equinus
p. plano valgus
p. planovalgus abductus
p. planovalgus deformity
p. plantigrade planus
p. planus deformity
p. valgo planus
p. valgoplanus deformity
PET
positron emission tomography
PET electrotherapy
petaling the cast
petechia, pl. **petechiae**
Peterson traction
PET/Eurotech 'Generation 2000" table
Petit triangle
Petren gait
Petrie spica cast
petrissage
petroclinoid ligament
petrolatum gauze
petrous temporal bone
Pettibon chiropractic procedure
Peyronie disease

NOTES

P

PFA
  proximal reference axis
Pfannenstiel transverse approach
PFC
  pelvic flexion contracture
  PFC hip stem
  PFC modular total knee system
  PFC TC3 modular knee system
  PFC total hip replacement system
Pfeiffer syndrome
PFFD
  proximal femoral focal deficiency
PF night splint
PFP
  patellofemoral pain
PFS
  Adriamycin PFS
  Folex PFS
PFT
  postop flexor tendon
  PFT traction brace
P/G
  Fulvicin P/G
PGA
  polyglycolic acid
  PGA rod
  PGA screw
PGP
  PGP flexible nail system
  PGP nail
PGR cemented modular system
PGS-3000 pulsed galvanic stimulator
phagocytosis
phal
  phalanges
  phalanx
phalangeal
  p. articular orientation
  p. clamp
  p. condylectomy
  p. diaphyseal fracture
  p. dislocation
  p. fracture fixation
  p. herniation
  p. hypoplasia
  p. malunion correction
  p. microgeodic syndrome
  p. neck
  p. osteotomy
phalangectomy
  intermediate p.
phalangization
phalanx, pl. phalanges (phal)
  accessory p.
  delta p.
  distal p. (DP)
  osteitis distal p.

  proximal p. (PP)
  waist of the p.
Phalen
  P. maneuver
  P. position
  P. wrist flexion test
Phalen-Miller opponensplasty
phantom
  p. frame
  p. pain
  p. pain phenomenon
  p. sensation
phantosmia
pharmacodynamic
pharmacokinetic
pharyngeal tissue
phase
  fibroblastic p.
  flexor p.
  granulation p.
  inflammatory p.
  maturation p.
  remodeling p.
  reparative p.
  stance p.
  swing p.
Pheasant
  P. discotome
  P. elbow technique
Phelps
  P. brace
  P. neurectomy
  P. orthosis
  P. partial resection
  P. scapulectomy
  P. splint
Phemister
  P. acromioclavicular pin fixation
  P. biopsy trephine
  P. elevator
  P. medial approach to tibia
  P. onlay bone graft
  P. onlay bone graft technique
Phemister-Bonfiglio technique
Phenaphen With Codeine
phencyclidine hydrochloride (PCP)
Phendry Oral
Phenergan
phenobarbital
phenol
  camphor and p.
  p. cauterization
  P. EZ swab
  p. matrixectomy
phenolization
phenomenon
  bioelectric p.
  combined-flexion p.

give-way p.
Gordon knee p.
lumbrical-plus p.
phantom pain p.
pivot-shift p.
Raynaud p.
referred anatomic p.
referred trigger point p.
relaxation p.
release p.
staircase p.
temporary cavity p.
wind-up p.
phenoxybenzamine
phentolamine
phenylbutazone
phenyltoloxamine
acetaminophen and p.
phenytoin
Philadelphia
P. cervical collar
P. collar cervical support
P. collar cervical traction
P. Plastizote cervical brace
Philips
P. Angiodiagnostics 96 apparatus
P. toe force gauge
Phillips
P. head screw
P. head screwdriver
P. recessed-head screw
P. screw head
P. splint
pHisoHex
phlebothrombosis
phlegmasia cerulea dolens
phlogistic agent
phocomelia
distal p.
Phoenix
P. foot system
P. Outrigger splint
P. total hip prosthesis
phonophoresis
hydrocortisone p.
ultrasound p.
Phoresor II iontophoretic drug delivery system
phosphatase
alkaline p.
tartrate resistant acid p. (TRAP)

phosphate
Aralen P.
betamethasone sodium p.
calcium p.
chloroquine p.
Cleocin P.
Decadron P.
Hexadrol P.
Hydrocortone P.
nicotinamide-adenine dinucleotide p. (NADPH)
technetium-99m p.
tetracalcium p.
tricalcium p.
phosphokinase
creatine p.
phospholipid
phosphorus
photogrammetry
x-ray p.
photon densitometry
photopenia
hardware p.
photoplethysmography
digital p.
phrenic nerve
phycomycosis
physeal
p. angle
p. cartilage
p. closure
p. damage
p. distraction
p. fracture
p. growth
p. injury
p. line
p. mamillary process
p. region
p. scar
physes (*pl. of* physis)
physiatric
physiatrist
physiatry
physical
P. Ability Test (PAT)
p. activity
P. Activity Readiness Questionnaire (PAR-Q)
p. agent
p. capacity evaluation (PCE)
p. daily living skills (PDLS)

NOTES

P

physical *(continued)*
    p. impairment
    p. therapy (PT)
    p. training (PT)
    p. work
physiognomy
PhysioGymnic exercise ball
physiologic
    p. barrier
    p. lock of the motion segment
    p. motion
    p. response
    p. saline
    p. valgus
physiological
    p. hyperactivity
    p. venous pump mechanism
PhysioLogics Alpha Lipoic Acid
physiology
    exercise p.
physiolysis
    central p.
Physio-Roll-R-Cise
Physio-Roll VisuaLiser exercise ball
Physio-Stim bone growth stimulator
physiotherapist
physique
    ectomesomorphic p.
    ectomorphic p.
physis, pl. physes
    modified Boyd amputation of ankle
      and distal tibial p.
Phytaidr
phytanic acid storage disease
phytoestrogen
Phytolyn
phytonutrient
PI
    posteroinferior
piano-wire dorsiflexion brace
PICA
    Porch Index of Communicative Ability
    PICA index
pick
    P. chisel
    dental p.
    p.-up forceps
    p.-up test
Picker
    P. Magnascanner for bone
      metastasis
picket
    p. fence guide
    P. Fence leg positioner
pickups
picornavirus
Picot incision

picture
    maximum pressure p. (MPP)
Pidcock pin
piece
    chin-occiput p.
piecemeal
pie-crusting skin graft
Piedmont fracture
Pierrot-Murphy
    P.-M. advancement insertion
    P.-M. tendon technique
PIEx
    posteroinferior external
    PIEx ilium
    PIEx subluxation
piezoelectric
    p. accelerometer
    p. potential
Piezo "electro" needle-less stimulator
piezogenic
Piffard curette
pigeonbreast
pigeon-toeing gait
pigmented
    p. nodular synovitis of tendon
      sheath
    p. villonodular bursitis
    p. villonodular synovitis (PVS)
PIIn
    posteroinferior internal
    PIIn ilium
    PIIn subluxation
Pik Stick Reacher
pilar cyst
Pilates exercise method
pillar
    articular p.
    p. pain
    p. tenderness
Pillet hand prosthesis
Pilliar total hip replacement
Pillo
    Knee P.
Pillo-Pedic
    P.-P. cervical traction pillow
pillow
    abduction p.
    antibacterial p.
    Bio-Gel decubitus p.
    Bodynapper Comfort P.
    Capello slim-line abduction p.
    Carter elevation p.
    cervical sleep p.
    crescent p.
    Crescent memory p.
    Crescent-Pillo p.
    Dream P.
    Flip-Flop p.

foot p.
FossFill Health P.
p. fracture
Frejka p.
IMP-Capello slimline abduction p.
Mediflow waterbase p.
Neckcare p.
Neck-Hugger cervical support p.
OrthoBone p.
Orthosleep P.
Pillo-Pedic cervical traction p.
Pillo-Wedge p.
PRN p.
Pron p.
shoulder abduction p.
silicore foot p.
snooze p.
Softeze water p.
p. splint
Tempur-Pedic pressure relieving
  Swedish p.
T-Foam p.
Theracloud p.
Therapeutica Sleeping P.
Therasleep Cervical P.
Tri-Core cervical support p.
Wal-Pil-O neck p.

Pillo-Wedge pillow
pilomatrixoma
pilomotor

p. dysfunction
p. response

pilon fracture
pilonidal

p. cyst
p. dimple
p. sinus

Pil-O-Splint wrist splint
pilot

p. bur
p. drill
P. point screw

pin

A p.
absorbable polyparadioxanone p.
Ace p.
Acufex distractor p.
alignment p.
Allofix cortical bone p.
Apex p.
Arthrex zebra p.
ARUM Colles fixation p.

ASIF screw p.
Asnis p.
Austin Moore p.
p. ball system
Barr p.
beaded hip p.
Beath p.
Belos compression p.
bevel-point Rush p.
Bilos p.
Biofix system p.
bioresorbable p.
Böhler p.
Böhler-Knowles hip p.
Böhler-Steinmann p.
Bohlman p.
p.-bone interface
breakaway p.
Breck p.
calcaneal p.
calibrated p.
Canakis beaded hip p.
cancellous p.
Charnley p.
p. chuck
clavicle p.
cloverleaf p.
Co-Cr-Mo p.
collapsible p.
Compere threaded p.
Compton clavicle p.
Conley p.
cortical p.
Craig p.
Crego-McCarroll p.
p. crimper
Crowe pilot point on Steinmann p.
Crowe tip p.
Crutchfield p.
p. cutter
Davis p.
Day fixation p.
DCS p.
deluxe FIN p.
Denham p.
DePuy p.
derotational p.
Deyerle II p.
distraction p.
distractor p.
drill p.
Ender p.

NOTES

P

451

pin *(continued)*
p. external fixator
Fahey p.
Fahey-Compere p.
femoral guide p.
Fischer transfixing p.
Fisher half p.
fixation p.
p. fixation
Freebody p.
friction lock p.
Furness-Clute p.
Gouffon hip p.
p. guard
p. guide
Hagie hip p.
halo p.
Hansen-Street p.
Hare p.
Hatcher p.
Haynes p.
p. headrest
Hegge p.
Hessel-Nystrom p.
Hewson breakaway p.
hexhead p.
Hoffmann apex fixation p.
Hoffmann transfixion p.
p. holder
hook p.
hook-end intramedullary p.
p. implant
Intraflex intramedullary p.
intramedullary p.
Jones compression p.
Jurgan p.
Kirschner wire p.
Knowles hip p.
Krankendonk p.
Kronendonk p.
Kronfeld p.
Küntscher p.
LIH hook p.
locating p.
Lottes p.
marble bone p.
Markley retention p.
Matthews-Green p.
McBride p.
medullary p.
metal p.
Modny p.
Moore fixation p.
Moule screw p.
Neufeld p.
Norman tibial p.
Olds p.
Oris p.

Ormco p.
Orthofix p.
OrthoSorb absorbable p.
osseous p.
osteotomy p.
partially threaded p.
percutaneous p.
Pidcock p.
Pritchard Mark II p.
Pugh hip p.
rasp p.
resorbable polydioxanon p.
restorative p.
p. retractor
Rhinelander p.
Riordan p.
Rissler p.
Rissler-Stille p.
Roger Anderson p.
Rush intramedullary fixation p.
Safir p.
Sage p.
Scand p.
Schanz p.
Schneider p.
Schweitzer p.
p.-seating forceps
self-broaching p.
self-tapering p.
Serrato forearm p.
Shriners p.
p. site
skeletal p.
Smillie p.
Smith-Petersen fracture p.
SMo Moore p.
smooth Steinmann p.
socket p.
spring p.
Stader p.
Steinmann fixation p.
Street medullary p.
strut-type p.
p. suture
Tachdjian p.
tapered p.
threaded Steinmann p.
tibial p.
titanium half p.
p.-to-bar clamp
p. track
p.-track osteomyelitis
p. tract infection
traction p.
transarticular p.
transcapitellar p.
transfixing p.
transfixion p.

trochanteric p.
Turner p.
union broach retention p.
Varney p.
Venable-Stuck fracture p.
p. vise
von Saal medullary p.
Walker hollow quill p.
Watanabe p.
Webb p.
p. wheel
wrench p.
Z p.
Zimfoam p.
Zimmer p.

pin-and-plaster
p.-a.-p. fixation
p.-a.-p. method

pincer
p. nail
p. palpation
p. testing

pinch
p. callus
p. gauge
P. Gauge and Jackson Strength
Evaluation System
p. grasp
key p.
lateral squeeze p.
p. meter
palmar p.
p. power
p. restoration
p. skin graft
p. strength
p. tree

pinchometer
Prestop p.

ping-pong fracture

Pinkus
fibroepithelioma of P.

pinning
Asnis p.
closed p.
hip p.
Knowles p.
open p.
percutaneous p.
Sherk-Probst percutaneous p.
Sofield p.
Wagner closed p.

pinprick
p. sensation
p. test

Pinto distractor

pinwheel
Cleanwheel disposable
neurological p.
Safe-T-Wheel p.
P. System
Wartenberg p.

Piotrowski sign

PIP
proximal interphalangeal
PIP articulation
PIP flexion creaking
PIP join

PIP/DIP strap

pipe
p. stemming of ankle-brachial
index
p. tree

piperacillin

piperacillin/tazobactam therapy

PIPJ
proximal interphalangeal joint

Pipkin
P. classification of femoral fracture
P. fracture classification system
P. posterior hip dislocation
classification
P. subclassification of Epstein-
Thomas classification

Pirie
P. bone
talonavicular ossicle of P.

piriformis
p. sign
p. syndrome

piriform sclerosis ilium

Pirogoff amputation

piroxicam

Pischel micropin

pisiform
p. bone
p. bursa
p. metacarpal ligament
p. ossification

pisohamate ligament

pisohamatum
ligamentum p.

pisometacarpal ligament

NOTES

P

pisometacarpeum
    ligamentum p.
pisotriquetral
    p. arthritis
    p. joint
pistol-grip hand drill
piston
    cannulated expulsion p.
    p. prosthesis
    p. sign
pistoning
    p. motion
pitching injury
Pitcock nail
pitting edema
Pittsburgh pelvic frame
pituitary
    p. grasper
    p. rongeur
PIVM
    passive intervertebral motion
    PIVM testing
pivot
    Accu-Line dual p.
    calcar p.
    p. of calcar
    p. joint
    medial stem p.
pivoting and cutting activity
pivot-shift
    p.-s. phenomenon
    p.-s. sign
    p.-s. test
PJ
    patellar jerk
PKA
    PRAFO KAFO attachment
PL
    palmaris longus
placement
    bone graft p.
    hand p.
    Kirschner wire p.
    K-wire p.
    needle p.
    PCL-oriented p. (POP)
    percutaneous needle p.
    plate p.
    portal p.
    posterolateral bone graft p.
    rod p.
    sacral screw p.
    variable screw p. (VSP)
Placidyl
placing reflex
plafond
    p. fracture
    tibial p.

plain
    Citanest P.
    p. gauze
    p. pattern plate
    p. rotary scissors
    p. screwdriver
    p. tissue forceps
Plak-Vac oral suction brush
plan
    McConnell patellofemoral
      treatment p.
    preoperative p.
plana
    coxa p.
plane
    anatomic p.
    axial p.
    coronal p.
    facet p.
    fascial p.
    flexion-extension p.
    frontal p.
    Hensen p.
    Hodge p.
    horizontal p.
    internervous p.
    intertubercular p.
    Ludwig p.
    median sagittal p.
    mesiodistal p.
    midsagittal p.
    paramedian sagittal p.
    pelvic p.
    primary movement p.
    sagittal p.
    spinous p.
    sternoxiphoid p.
    subcostal p.
    suprasternal p.
    thigh-shank p.
    thoracic p.
    transverse p.
    p.-type acromioclavicular articulation
    varus-valgus p.
    vertical p.
planer
    calcar p.
planning
    preoperative p.
Planostretch stockings
planovalgus
    p. deformity
    p. feet
    talipes p.
plantar
    p. angulation
    p. aponeurosis
    p. approach

p. arch
p. arch support
p. artery
p. axial view
p. Babinski response
p. bony prominence
p. bromhidrosis
p. calcaneocuboid ligament
p. calcaneonavicular ligament
p. calcaneonavicular ligament-tibialis posterior tendon advancement
p. capsule
p. capsuloligamentous complex
p. condylectomy
p. corn
p. cuboideonavicular ligament
p. cuneocuboid ligament
p. cuneonavicular ligament
p. digital artery (PDA)
p. ecchymosis sign
p. fascia
p. fascial release
p. fasciitis
p. fasciitis night splint
p. fasciotomy
p. fibromatosis
p. flap
p. flexed
p. flexion
p. flexion-inversion deformity
p. intercuneiform ligament
p. keratosis
p. lateral base
p.-lateral release
p. ligaments of interphalangeal articulations
p. ligaments of MTP articulations
p. ligaments of tarsus
p. longitudinal incision
p.-medial release
p. metatarsal angle
p. metatarsal ligament
p. nerve
p. plate
p. plate release
p. pressure
p. pressure pattern
p. reflex
p. shift
p. spring ligament
p. sweating
p. tarsometatarsal ligament

p. tendopathy
p. wart (PW)
plantar-dorsiflexion
plantare
    ligamentum calcaneocuboideum p.
    ligamentum calcaneonaviculare p.
    ligamentum cuboideonaviculare p.
    ligamentum cuneocuboideum p.
plantarflex
plantarflexed first ray
plantarflexion injury
plantarflexion-inversion test
plantarflexory
    p. motion
    p. proximal metatarsal osteotomy
plantar-hindfoot-midfoot bony mass
plantaria
    ligamenta cuneonavicularia p.
    ligamenta intercuneiformia p.
    ligamenta metatarsalia p.
    ligamenta tarsi p.
    ligamenta tarsometatarsalia p.
plantaris
    arcus p.
    keratosis palmaris et p.
    p. muscle
    p. tendon
    p. tendon graft
    verruca p.
plantarward
plantigrade
    p. foot
    p. limb
    p. platform
planum
planus
    Anderson-Fowler anterior calcaneal osteotomy pes p.
    collapsing pes valgo p.
    flexible pes p.
    Gleich osteotomy for pes valgo p.
    pes plantigrade p.
    pes valgo p.
    rigid pes p.
    Selakovich procedure for pes valgo p.
    talipes p.
Plaquenil
plasma
    p. cell myeloma
    coagulated p.

NOTES

P

plasma *(continued)*
    p. β-endorphin
    p. volume shift
plasmacytoma
    aggressive solitary p.
    extramedullary p.
Plasmanate
plasmapheresis drug
plasmin
Plasmodium falciparum
plast
    Putti bone p.
Plastalume
    P. bulb-ended splint
    P. straight splint
Plastazote
    P. blank
    P. foam
    P. insole
plaster
    Batchelor p.
    p. cast
    p. cast application burn
    closing wedge manipulation and
      reapplication of p.
    opening wedge manipulation and
      reapplication of p.
    p. sore
    p. splint
    p. toe cap
    x-ray in p. (XIP)
    x-ray out of p. (XOP)
    Zoroc p.
plaster-of-Paris (POP)
    p.-o.-P. bandage
    p.-o.-P. cast
    elastic p.-o.-P.
    p.-o.-P. splint
plastic
    p. ankle-foot orthosis
    p. ball implant
    p. body jacket
    p. bowing fracture
    p. cast
    p. collar
    p. deformation
    p. end caps
    p. femoral plug
    p. floor reaction ankle-foot orthosis
    p. heel cup
    Hexalite p.
    p. leaf-spring (PLS)
    p. limited-motion joint
    low-temperature p.
    p. marrow canal restrictor
    Orthoplast p.
    p. patella
    p. repair

    p. strain
    thermolabile p.
    unitary p.
PlastiCast adjustable joint cast system
plasticity
    connective tissue p.
Plasticor prosthesis
Plasti-Pore
    P.-P. ossicular replacement
      prosthesis
    P.-P. prosthetic material
Plastiport
    P. TORP
    P. TORP prosthesis
Plastizote
    P. arch support
    P. cervical collar
    P. cervical collar orthosis
    P. foot bed
    P. orthotic device
    P. shoe liner
Plastizote-Kydex cervical immobilizer
plasty
    Coleman p.
    Durham p.
    rotation p.
    skin p.
    V-Y p.
    Y-V p.
plate
    90-90 p.
    acetabular reconstruction p.
    AcroMed VSP p.
    anchor p.
    anterior cervical p. (ACP)
    anterior sacroiliac joint p.
    antiglide p.
    AO-ASIF compression p.
    AO blade p.
    AO condylar blade p.
    AO contoured T p.
    AO dynamic compression p.
    AO hook p.
    AO reconstruction p.
    AO semitubular p.
    AO small fragment p.
    AO spoon p.
    Armstrong p.
    ASIF broad dynamic compression
      bone p.
    ASIF right-angle blade p.
    ASIF T-p.
    autocompression p.
    avulsion of nail p.
    Badgley p.
    Bagby angled compression p.
    barrel p.
    Batchelor p.

p. bender
biodegradable p.
blade p.
Blair talar body fusion blade p.
Blair tibiotalar arthrodesis blade p.
Blanchard traction device blade p.
Blount blade p.
bone flap fixation p.
Bosworth spine p.
bridge p.
broad AO dynamic compression p.
Burns p.
butterfly-shaped monoblock
  vertebral p.
buttress pie p.
buttress-type p.
Calandruccio side p.
calcaneal Y p.
cap-and-anchor p.
carbon fiber-reinforced p.
cartilaginous growth p.
cervical p.
cloverleaf p.
coaptation p.
cobra-head p.
Collison p.
compression p.
Concise side p.
condylar p.
connecting p.
contoured anterior spinal p.
  (CASP)
contoured T-plate p.
cortical p.
craniocervical p.
crosslink p.
cruciform tibial base p.
C-shaped p.
3D p.
deck p.
DePuy p.
Deyerle p.
double Cobra p.
double-H p.
Driessen hinged p.
dual p.
Duopress p.
Dwyer-Hall p.
dynamic compression p. (DCP)
eccentric dynamic compression p.
  (EDCP)
Eggers bone p.

Elliott femoral condyle blade p.
end p.
epiphyseal growth p.
femoral p.
ferromagnetic metal p.
fibrocartilaginous p.
five-hole p.
p. fixation
fixed-angle blade p.
flexor p.
foot p.
force p.
four-hole side p.
fusion p.
gait p.
Gallannaugh p.
Galveston p.
Geibel blade p.
growth p.
Hagie sliding nail p.
Haid cervical p.
Haid Universal bone p.
half-circle p.
Hansen-Street p.
Harlow p.
Harm posterior cervical p.
Harris p.
heavy-duty femur p.
heavy side p.
Hicks lugged p.
Hoen skull p.
11-hole p.
17-hole p.
10-hole blade p.
Holt nail p.
hook p.
hot p.
H-shaped p.
Hubbard p.
Inner Lip P.
interfragmentary p.
intertrochanteric p.
Jergesen I-beam p.
Jergesen tapered p.
Jewett nail overlay p.
Jones compression p.
Kessel p.
L p.
Laing p.
Lane p.
Lawson-Thornton p.
Letournel p.

NOTES

P

plate *(continued)*

limited-contact dynamic
 compression p.
low-contact dynamic compression p.
L-shaped p.
Luhr Microfixation cranial p.
Luhr pan p.
Lundholm p.
Luque II p.
Massie p.
May anatomical bone p.
McBride p.
McLaughlin p.
Mears sacroiliac p.
Medoff sliding p.
Meurig Williams p.
Milch p.
modified Grace p.
Moe intertrochanteric p.
Moore sliding nail p.
Moreira p.
Morscher cervical p.
Mueller compression blade p.
nail p.
narrow AO dynamic
 compression p.
Neufeld p.
neutralization p.
Newman p.
Nicoll p.
occipitocervical p.
Odgen p.
Orozco p.
orthotic p.
Osborne p.
overlay p.
palmar p.
Paulus p.
pedicle p.
peg-base p.
Percy p.
p. placement
plain pattern p.
plantar p.
precurved p.
pressure p.
protection p.
pterygoid p.
Pugh p.
pylon attachment p.
quadrangular positioning plate p.
reconstruction p.
resorbable p.
Richards-Hirschhorn p.
Rohadur gait p.
round-hole compression p.
Roy-Camille p.
RSDCP p.

Schweitzer spring p.
semitubular blade p.
semitubular compression p.
Senn p.
serpentine p.
seven-hole p.
Sherman bone p.
side p.
six-hole p.
slide p.
slotted femur p.
Smith-Petersen intertrochanteric p.
SMO p.
p. spacer washer
spinous process p.
spoon p.
spring p.
stabilization p.
stainless steel p.
static compression p.
Steffee pedicle p.
Steffee screw p.
stem base p.
subchondral p.
supracondylar p.
symmetrical thoracic vertebral p.
symmetric sacral p.
Synthes pie p.
Syracuse anterior I p.
Tacoma sacral p.
tarsal p.
T buttress p.
Temple University p.
tendon p.
tension band p.
thoracolumbosacral p.
Thornton nail p.
three-hole p.
tibial base p.
titanium p.
titanium hollow screw p. (THSP)
toe p.
Townley tibial plateau p.
Townsend-Gilfillan p.
trial base p.
T-shaped AO p.
TSRH p.
tubular p.
Tupman p.
two-hole p.
UCBL foot p.
UCP compression p.
universal bone p. (UBP)
Uslenghi p.
variable screw p. (VSP)
V blade p.
Venable p.
vertebral end p.

Vitallium p.
V nail p.
volar p.
VSP p.
Wainwright p.
Wenger p.
Whitman p.
Wilson p.
wing p.
Wright p.
Wurzburg p.
X p.
X-shaped p.
Y bone p.
Y-shaped p.
Zimmer femoral condyle blade p.
Zimmer side p.
Zimmer Y p.
Z-shaped p.
Zuelzer hook p.
plateau
bicondylar tibial p.
proximal tibial p.
tibial p.
plate-holding forceps
platelet
p. concentrate
p. count
p.-derived growth factor (PDGF)
plate-like atelectasis
plate-screw
p.-s. fixation
p.-s. osteosynthesis
p.-s. system
platform
Hausmann Velcro-Lock mat p.
Kistler force p.
Midline Hi-Lo Mat P.
plantigrade p.
plating
anterior spinal p.
diaphyseal p.
pedicle screw p.
posterior spinal p.
tension band p.
variable spinal p. (VSP)
Platinol
Platinol-AQ
Platinum stationary table
Platou osteotomy
platybasia
platysma muscle

platyspondylisis
play
end p.
joint p.
muscle p.
pledget
Betadine-soaked p.
p. dressing
p. of gauze
Gelfoam p.
pleomorphic
p. fibrous histiocytoma
p. lipoma
p. liposarcoma
p. rhabdomyosarcoma
plethysmography
digital p.
impedance p.
pleura
parietal p.
pleural
p. effusion
p. injury
Plexidure insole
plexiform neurofibroma
Plexiglas
P. jig
P. spacer
PlexiPulse
P. DVT prophylaxis system
P. intermittent pneumatic
compression device
plexus
p. block
brachial p.
cervical p.
fascial p.
lumbosacral p.
sacral p.
subdermal p.
superior hypogastric p.
plica, pl. **plicae**
bucket-handle p.
infrapatellar p.
medial patellar p.
parapatellar p.
pathological p.
suprapatellar p.
symptomatic synovial p.
p. syndrome
synovial p.
p. test

NOTES

P

plicamycin
plication
    capsular p.
    disk p.
    soft tissue p.
plicectomy
pliers
    extraction p.
    Luhr Microfixation System p.
    needle-nose vise-grip p.
    orthopaedic surgical p.
    slip-joint p.
    Sontec p.
    square-end p.
    wire bending p.
PLIF
    posterior lumbar interbody fusion
    posterolateral interbody fusion
plight
    musician's p.
plinth
PLL
    posterior longitudinal ligament
PLLA
    poly-ʟ-lactic acid
    PLLA implant
PLM
    precise lesion measuring
    PLM device
plot
    load-displacement p.
plotter
    X-Y p.
PLS
    plastic leaf-spring
plug
    bone femoral p.
    Buck p.
    cement p.
    p. cutter
    femoral p.
    Osteonics acetabular dome hole p.
    plastic femoral p.
    polyethylene femoral buck p.
plumb
    p. line
    p.-line analysis
plumbism
Plummer-Vinson syndrome
plunger
    dome p.
    p.-type femoral pressurizer
pluri-cal caliper
pluripotential
    p. mesenchymal tumor
    p. mesenchymoma
Plus
    DHC P.

    Extra Strength Bayer P.
    Livotrit P.
    Lorcet P.
    Nexerciser P.
    Osteo-B P.
    Quinsana P.
    Steri-Cuff P.
Plyoback Rebounder
Plyoball
plyometric
    p. exercise
    p. resistance
plyometrics
plyo-sled exerciser
Plystan prosthesis
PM
    Midol PM
P.M.
    Excedrin P.M.
PMD
    progressive muscular dystrophy
PMI-6A1-4V
    P. implant metal
    P. implant metal prosthesis
PMID
    painful minor intervertebral dysfunction
PMMA
    antibiotic-impregnated polymethyl
      methacrylate
    polymethyl methacrylate
    PMMA bone cement
    PMMA centralizer
    PMMA implant
PMR
    posteromedial release
Pneu Knee brace
pneumatic
    p. ankle tourniquet
    p. antishock garment (PASG)
    p. 4-bar linkage knee
    p. compression boot
    p. compression stockings
    p. drill accessory
    p. external compression device
    p. garment
    p. pedal compression
    p. splint
    p. tourniquet cuff
pneumoarthrogram
pneumoniae
    Diplococcus p.
    Klebsiella p.
    Streptococcus p.
pneumonitis
pneumothorax (px)
Pneu-trac cervical collar
PNF
    proprioceptive neuromuscular facilitation

PNF exercise
PNF technique
PNS
  parasympathetic nervous system
  peripheral nervous system
PO
  postoperatively
P&O
  prostheses and orthoses
podalgia
podi-burr
  large callus p.-b.
  large nail p.-b.
  medium callus p.-b.
  medium nail p.-b.
podogeriatrics
podopediatrics
Podospray
  Darco P.
  P. nail drill system
Pogon chair
Pogrund lateral approach
point
  anchoring p.
  associated myofascial trigger p.
  "Back Shu" paraspinal p.
  bleeding p.
  break p.
  contact p.
  Crowe pilot p.
  Crutchfield drill p.
  dorsal p.
  drill p.
  electrodesiccated bleeding p.
  end p.
  entry p.
  Erb p.
  glenoid p.
  inflexion p.
  isometric p.
  Krackow p.
  material failure break p.
  Mathews drill p.
  motor p.
  myofascial trigger p.
  p.-of-reduction clamp
  Pauly p.
  pedicle entrance p.
  pressure p.
  primary myofascial trigger p.
  Raney-Crutchfield drill p.
  referred p.

  satellite myofascial trigger p.
  secondary myofascial trigger p.
  Steinmann pin with Crowe pilot p.
  tender p. (TeP)
  p. tenderness
  trigger p.
  twist drill p.
  Universal drill p.
pointed
  p. awl
  p. toe shoe
pointer
  hip p.
  shoulder p.
Pointer-Plus
Poirier
  space of P.
poisoning
  lead p.
Poisson ratio
poker spine
POL
  posterior oblique ligament
Poland
  P. classification of physeal injury
  P. epiphyseal fracture classification
  P. syndrome
Polar
  P. Care 500 cryotherapy device
  P. Pack
  P. Vantage XL heart monitor
  P. wrap therapy
  P. wrist monitor
polarization
Polar-Mate
  P.-M. coagulator
Polarus
  P. humeral rod
  P. positional humeral fixation
    system
**Policy and Review Committee for
  Human Research**
polio
poliomyelitis treatment
Polk finger goniometer
poll
  pollicis
Pol Le Coueur osteotomy
pollex abductus
pollicis (poll)
  p. longus muscle

NOTES

P

pollicization
  Buck-Gramcko p.
  Gillies p.
  Littler p.
  Riordan p.
pollicized ray
pollicus
  adductor p.
  opponens p.
polly power grip
Polocaine
polo test
polyacetal resin
polyarteritis nodosa
polyarthritis
  juvenile p.
polyarthropathy
polyarticular
  p. arthritis
  p. symmetric tophaceous joint
    inflammation
polyaxial cervical screw
polybutester suture
Polycel bone composite prosthesis
polycentric
  p. knee prosthesis
  p. rotation
  P. and Wide-Track knee system
polyclonal hypergammaglobulinemia
polydactylous cleft foot
polydactyly
  central p.
  postaxial p.
  preaxial p.
  thumb p.
  Wassel classification of thumb p.
Polydek suture
Poly-Dial
  P.-D. insert
  P.-D. prosthesis
  P.-D. socket
Polydine
polydioxanone suture (PDS)
Polydor Preforms orthotic
polyester suture
polyether implant material
polyethylene
  ArCom processed p.
  p. button
  carbon fiber-reinforced p.
  p. compression molding
  p. debris
  p. drain
  extruded bar p.
  p. femoral buck plug
  p. femoral buck plug procedure
  p. foam

high molecular weight p.
  (HMWPE)
  p. implant material
  p. liner
  p. liner implant component
  p. patellar implant prosthesis
  porous p.
  p. proximal brims in quadrilateral
    contour
  p. sleeve
  p. socket
  p. suture
  p. talar prosthesis
  ultrahigh molecular weight p.
    (UHMWPE)
polyethylene-faced
  p.-f. driver
  p.-f. mallet
Polyform splint
polygalactic acid suture
polyglactin suture
polyglycolic
  p. acid (PGA)
  p. acid suture
polyglycolide implant
polyglyconate suture
polylactic acid
polylactide
  p. implant
  p. screw
poly-L-lactic acid (PLLA)
Poly-Lock bonding
PolyMem wound-care dressing
polymer
  cold-curing p.
  Hylamer orthopaedic bearing p.
  P.Q. viscoelastic p.
  self-curing p.
  viscoelastic p.
polymerase chain reaction test
PolymerFriction total knee
polymeric debris
polymerization of bone cement
polymerized cement
polymetatarsalia
polymethyl
  p. methacrylate (PMMA)
  p. methacrylate bone cement
  p. methacrylate implant
polymorphonuclear leukocyte
polymyalgia rheumatica
polymyositis myopathy
polymyxin
  bacitracin, neomycin, and p. B
polyneuritiformis
  heredopathia atactica p.
polyneuritis
  peripheral p.

polyneuropathy
sensory p.
polyolefin elastomer
polyostotic fibrous dysplasia
polyp
fibroepithelial p.
polyphasic action potential
polypropylene
p. ankle-foot orthosis
p. glycol-ankle-foot orthosis
p. glycol-thoracolumbosacral orthosis
p. insert
p. prosthesis
p. suture
polyradiculopathy
acute inflammatory p.
diabetic` p.
polyserositis
Polyskin dressing
Polysonic ultrasound lotion
Polysorb
P. heel cup
P. liner
P. suture
Polysporin Topical
polystyrene
polytetrafluoroethylene (PTFE)
polytomography
polytrauma patient
polyurethane
p. bandage
p. cast
p. implant material
polyvinyl
p. alcohol
p. alcohol splint
p. alcohol splinting material
p. chloride (PVC)
p. implant material
PolyWic dressing
pommel cushion
POMS
Profile of Mood States
poncho restraint
pond
P. adjustable splint
p. fracture
Ponseti
P. method
P. splint
Ponstel
Pontenza arthrodesis

ponticulus posticus
Pontocaine With Dextrose Injection
pontoon spica cast
pool
Aquaciser p.
AquaMotion p.
Endless Pool physical therapy p.
SwimEx p.
p. therapy
poor
p. alignment
p. bone stock
p. cosmesis
POP
PCL-oriented placement
plaster-of-Paris
Popeye arm
popliteal
p. artery
p. crease
p. flexion creaking
p. fossa
p. fossa entrapment
p. giant synovial cyst
p. hiatus
p. ligament
p. pressure sign
p. pterygium syndrome
p. recess
p. space
p. tendon
p. vein
p. vessel
popliteomeniscal fascicle
popliteus
p. bypass
p. muscle
p. tendon
popoff suture
Poppen
P. forceps
P. Gigli saw guide
P. ridge sensitometer
Porch Index of Communicative Ability (PICA)
porcine
p. prosthesis
p. skin graft
Porocoat
P. AML noncemented prosthesis
P. porous coating
P. prosthetic material

NOTES

P

Porocoat *(continued)*
    Tri-Lock total hip prosthesis
      with P.
Porocool prosthesis
Poro-in-between sole
porokeratosis, pl. **porokeratoses**
    p. plantaris discerta
poroma
    eccrine p.
Porometal noncemented femoral
  prosthesis
Poron
    P. cellular urethane
    P. 400 insole
poroplastic splint
porosity
    interfacial p.
porotic bone
porous
    p. cementless component
    p. coating
    p. ingrowth fixation
    p. metal
    p. polyethylene
    p. polyethylene graft
    p. prosthetic material
    p. surfaced prosthesis
porous-coated
    p.-c. anatomic (PCA)
    p.-c. anatomic prosthesis
    p.-c. anatomic total hip
      replacement
    p.-c. anatomic total knee
    p.-c. component
    p.-c. femur prosthesis
    p.-c. hip prosthesis
PORP
    partial ossicular replacement prosthesis
    Richards hydroxyapatite PORP
porphyritic neuropathy
portable
    p. C-arm image intensifier
      fluoroscopy
    P. Topical Hyperbaric Oxygen
      Extremity Chamber
portal
    1–2 p.
    3–4 p.
    4–5 p.
    p. accessory
    anterior p.
    anterocentral p.
    anteroinferior p.
    anterolateral p.
    anteromedial p.
    arthroscopic entry p.
    Caspari arthroscopic p.
    central transpatellar tendon p.

    direct lateral p.
    inside-out technique for establishing
      ankle p.
    lateral transmalleolar p.
    MCR p.
    MCU p.
    medial p.
    midcarpal p.
    midpatellar p.
    patellar p.
    p. placement
    posterior p.
    posteroinferior p.
    posterolateral p.
    posteromedial p.
    P. Pro 2 treatment chair
    proximal midpatellar medial and
      lateral p.'s
    straight posterior p.
    subacromial p.
    superior p.
    superolateral p.
    superomedial p.
    suprapatellar p.
    Swedish p.
    transmalleolar p.
    transpatellar tendon p.
    transtendo calcaneus p.
    6U p.
Porter-Richardson-Vainio
    P.-R.-V. synovectomy
    P.-R.-V. technique
portion
    accessory p.
    cord p.
    proximal p.
Portmann drill
portmanteau procedure
Portola Valley Scale
port-wine stain
Porzett splint
Posada fracture
Posey
    P. bar kit
    P. bed cradle
    P. below-the-knee castbelt
    P. belt
    P. drop seat
    P. grip
    P. Palm Cone
    P. sling
Positex knee wedge
position
    90-90 p.
    angular p.
    antiembolic p.
    "arch and slouch" p.
    barber chair p.

bayonet fracture p.
beach chair p.
Bonner p.
Brickner p.
cottonloader p.
decubitus p. (decub)
de Kleyn p.
dorsal lithotomy p.
dorsal recumbent p.
dorsiflexion-plantar flexion p.
equinus p.
figure-four p.
flexed p.
Fowler p.
frog-leg p.
full lateral p.
p. of function
Gaynor-Hart p.
horizontal p.
intrinsic minus p.
jackknife p.
James p.
Jones p.
jumper's knee p.
kneeling p.
90-90 kneeling p.
Kraske p.
lateral decubitus p.
lateral park-bench p.
lithotomy p.
lotus p.
mediolateral p.
military brace p.
military tuck p.
neutral hip p.
normal anatomic p.
opisthotonic p.
over-the-top p.
Phalen p.
prayer p.
prone p.
proximal bow p.
quasistatic stressed p.
rectus p.
recumbent p.
resting calcaneal stance p. (RCSP)
reverse Trendelenburg p.
scissor-leg p.
semi-Fowler p.
semisitting p.
p. sense
side-lying p.

side-posture p.
Sims p.
sitting p.
sniffer's p.
p. in space
spinal fusion p.
subtalar joint neutral p. (STNP)
supine p.
three-quarters prone p.
tibial sesamoid p. (TSP)
translational p.
Trendelenburg p.
positional
p. dyskinesia
p. release therapy
positioner
acetabular cup p.
Allen arthroscopic elbow p.
Allen arthroscopic knee p.
Allen arthroscopic wrist p.
arm p.
Assistant Free Stulberg leg p.
Bareskin knee p.
cup p.
Grasshopper p.
Hold-and-Hold p.
IMP Universal knee p.
IMP Universal lateral p.
knee p.
leg p.
Mark II Stulberg hip p.
Mark II Stulberg leg p.
Mark II Wixson hip p.
MB&J knee p.
McConnell shoulder p.
McGuire pelvic p.
Montreal hip p.
OSI-Schlein shoulder p.
Picket Fence leg p.
Prep-Assist p.
Profex arthroscopic leg p.
Schlein shoulder p.
shoulder abduction p.
Stulberg hip p.
Stulberg Mark II leg p.
SurgAssist leg p.
Ther-A-Shapes p.
Universal knee p.
Universal lateral p.
Vac-Pac p.
Wixson hip p.

NOTES

P

positioning
  patient p.
  proper neck p.
positive
  p. ability
  coagulase p.
  p. impingement sign
  p. rim sign
  p. sharp wave
  p. ulnar variance (PUV)
  p. wave
positron
  p. emission tomographic scan
  p. emission tomography (PET)
post
  posterior
    4-p. cervical brace
    extrinsic rearfoot p.
    iliac p.
    Isola spinal implant system iliac p.
    Luque-Galveston p.
    Morse tapered prosthetic p.
    perineal p.
    status p.
    thumb p.
    P. total shoulder arthroplasty
postactivation
  p. depression
  p. exhaustion
  p. facilitation
  p. potentiation
postacute sprain
postage stamp skin graft
Postalume finger splint
post-and-cam mechanism
postanesthesia
  p. care unit (PACU)
  p. recovery (PAR)
postaxial polydactyly
postcalcaneal bursitis
postcast compression reflex
postcasting syndrome
Postel hip status system
posterior (post)
  anterior and p. (AP)
  p. arch
  p. arch fracture
  p. atlantoaxial arthrodesis
  p. atlantoodontoid interval
  p. axillary line (PAL)
  p. bending moment
  p. bone block
  p. bone graft
  p. bow
  p. capsule
  p. capsulorrhaphy
  p. capsulotomy
  p. cervical fixation

p. cervical fusion
p. cervical line
p. cervical spinal instrumentation
p. column fracture
p. column osteosynthesis
p. compartment
p. component
p. construct
p. cord syndrome
p. costotransversectomy approach
p. cruciate
p. cruciate condylar knee system
p. cruciate ligament (PCL)
p. cruciate ligament graft
p. cruciate ligament of knee
p. cruciate ligament tear
p. deltoid muscle
p. deltoid-to-triceps transfer
p. depression pattern
p. distraction instrumentation
p. drainage
p. drawer sign
p. drawer test
p. element
p. element fracture
p. facet
p. fixation system biomechanics
p. flap
p. flap technique
p. fracture-dislocation
p. glenoid labrum
p. glenoplasty
p. glide
p. hip dislocation
p. hook-rod spinal instrumentation
p. horn
p. horn meniscal tear
p. iliac osteotomy
p. iliofemoral technique
p. incision
p.-inferior spine
p. innominate
p. innominate rotation
p. instability
p. interosseous branch
p. interosseous nerve
p. interosseous nerve compression
  syndrome
p. interosseous nerve entrapment
p. interosseous nerve palsy
p. interspinous wiring
p. inverted U approach
p. leaf-spring ankle-foot orthosis
p. ligament of head of fibula
p. ligamentous injury
p. lip
p. longitudinal fiber region
p. longitudinal ligament (PLL)

p. lower cervical spine stabilization
p. lower cervical spine surgery
p. lumbar interbody fusion (PLIF)
p. lumbar interbody fusion surgery
p. lumbar spine and sacrum
  surgery
p. meniscofemoral ligament
p. midline approach
p. nerve decompression
p. oblique fiber region
p. oblique ligament (POL)
p. oblique meniscal tear
p. occipitocervical approach
p. osteophyte
p. pelvic tilt
p. pharyngeal abscess
p. portal
p. radial collateral artery
p. rhizotomy
p. rod system
p. rotation on the left side
p. rotation on the right side
p. sacroiliac ligament
p. sacroiliac spine (PSIS)
p. sag sign
p. screw fixation
p. segmental fixation
p. shoulder dislocation
p. spinal fusion
p. spinal plating
p. spinal wedge osteotomy
p. spine
p. splint
p. stability
p. surgical exposure of sacrum and
  coccyx
p. talar process fracture
p. talofibular ligament (PTFL)
p. thigh bar
p. tibial artery
p. tibial nerve (PTN)
p. tibial pulse (PTP)
p. tibial tendinitis (PTT)
p. tibial tendon (PTT)
p. tibial tendon transfer
p. tibiofibular ligament
p. tibiotalar ligament
p. translation
p. transolecranon approach
p. triangle
p. tuberosity

p. upper cervical spine surgery
p. wall fracture
posteriora
  ligamenta sacroiliaca p.
posterior-anterior
  p.-a. glide
  p.-a. pressure
posteriorly
posterior-superior
  p.-s. endplate
  p.-s. oblique projection
posterius
  ligamentum capitis fibulae p.
  ligamentum longitudinale p.
  ligamentum meniscofemorale p.
  ligamentum tibiofibulare p.
posteroanterior (PA)
posterodistal
posteroinferior (PI)
  p. external (PIEx)
  p. external movement
  p. ilium major
  p. internal (PIIn)
  p. internal movement
  p. portal
posterolateral
  p. approach
  p. aspect
  p. bone graft
  p. bone graft placement
  p. bundle
  p. capsule
  p. compartment
  p. costotransversectomy incision
  p. costotransversectomy technique
  p. decompression
  p. drainage
  p. drawer sign
  p. drawer test
  p. herniation
  p. interbody fusion (PLIF)
  p. lumbosacral fusion
  p. portal
  p. release
  p. rotary instability
  p. structure
posteromedial
  p. approach
  p. capsule
  p. compartment
  p. corner
  p. dislocation

NOTES

P

posteromedial *(continued)*
- p. drainage
- p. drawer sign
- p. pivot-shift test
- p. portal
- p. region
- p. release (PMR)
- p. rotary instability

posteroproximal

posterosuperior iliac spine (PSIS)

postfracture
- p. cyst
- p. lesion
- p. osteomyelitis

postganglionic technique

postherpetic pain

posticus
- ponticulus p.

postinfectious
- p. arthritis
- p. myopathy

posting
- heel p.
- strip p.
- wedge p.

postirradiation
- p. fracture
- p. osteogenic sarcoma

postisometric
- p. relaxation
- p. relaxation traction technique
- p. stretch technique

postlaminectomy
- p. kyphosis
- p. two-level spondylolisthesis

postmenopausal
- p. arthritis
- p. bone loss

postmortem fracture

postnatal
- p. cerebral palsy
- p. gangrene

postop
- postoperatively
- postop flexor tendon (PFT)

postoperative
- p. antibiotic
- p. bracing
- p. casting
- p. complication
- p. corticosteroid
- p. extubation
- p. fracture
- p. immobilization
- p. infection
- p. lumbosacral orthosis
- p. paraplegia
- p. regimen

- p. synovitis
- p. therapy
- p. wound care

postoperatively (PO, postop)

postphlebitis syndrome

postpoliomyelitic contracture

postpyelomyelitis syndrome

postradiation kyphosis

postreduction x-ray

poststatic dyskinesia (PSDK)

poststress ankle-arm Doppler index

posttest likelihood of disease

posttetanic
- p. facilitation
- p. potentiation

posttraumatic
- p. algodystrophic syndrome
- p. angulation
- p. apoplexy
- p. chronic cord syndrome
- p. chronic osteomyelitis
- p. dystrophy
- p. edema
- p. hemarthrosis
- p. kyphosis
- **p. osteolysis**
- **p. osteonecrosis**
- p. sacroiliac dysfunction
- p. spinal deformity
- p. stress disorder (PTSD)
- p. syringomyelia

postural
- p. analysis
- p. balance
- p. complex
- p. component
- p. control
- p. development
- p. exteroceptor
- p. fixation back maneuver
- p. interoceptor
- p. list
- p. muscle
- p. receptor
- p. strain
- p. sway
- p. tremor
- p. variation

posture
- batrachian p.
- benediction p.
- P. Curve lumbar cushion
- decerebrate p.
- decorticate p.
- forward flexion p.
- forward head p.
- P. Pump lordoticiser
- P. Pump Spine Trainer

recumbent p.
P. S'port
P. Wedge seat cushion
potassium
p. permanganate
ticarcillin and clavulanate p.
potassium-40 count
potential
action p. (AP)
auditory evoked p. (AEP)
bioelectric p.
biphasic action p.
bizarre repetitive p.
brainstem auditory evoked p.
(BAEP)
brief, small, abundant p. (BSAP)
brief, small, abundant,
polyphasic p. (BSAPP)
complex motor unit action p.
compound mixed nerve action p.
compound motor nerve action p.
compound muscle action p.
(CMAP)
compound muscle-motor action p.
(CMAP)
compound sensory nerve action p.
denervation p.
dermatosensory evoked p.
electrical p.
electrokinetic p.
endplate p. (EPP)
evoked compound muscle action p.
excitatory postsynaptic p. (EPSP)
far-field p.
fasciculation p.
fibrillation p.
giant motor unit action p.
inhibitory postsynaptic p. (IPSP)
injury p.
irregular p.
kilovoltage p. (kVP)
linked p.
macro motor unit action p.
(MUAP)
miniature end-plate p. (MEPP)
monophasic action p.
motor unit p. (MUP)
motor unit action p. (MUAP)
muscle fiber action p.
myopathic motor unit p.
myotonic p.
nascent motor unit p.

near-field p.
nerve action p. (NAP)
nerve fiber action p.
nerve trunk action p.
neurogenic motor-evoked p.
(NMEP)
neuropathic motor unit p.
parasite p.
piezoelectric p.
polyphasic action p.
pseudopolyphasic action p.
regeneration motor unit p.
resting membrane p.
satellite p.
sensory evoked p.
sensory nerve action p. (SNAP)
serrated action p.
short-latency somatosensory
evoked p. (SSEP)
somatosensory evoked p. (SEP,
SSEP)
spinal evoked p.
streaming p.
tetraphasic action p.
triphasic action p.
visual evoked p. (VEP)
potentiation
postactivation p.
posttetanic p.
potentiometer
linear p.
Pott
P. ankle fracture
P. disease
P. paraplegia
P. spinal curvature
Potter arthrodesis
Potts
P. eversion osteotomy
P. splint
P. tibial osteotomy
Potts-Smith dressing forceps
pouce flottant (floating thumb)
pouch
antibiotic bead p.
bead p.
inflamed synovial p.
suprapatellar p.
p.-type sling
pound
foot p.
poundal

NOTES

P

Poupart inguinal ligament
Pouteau syndrome
povidone-iodine
    p.-i. solution
powder
    Absorbine Antifungal Foot P.
    Ammens foot p.
    p. board
    Cida-Gel p.
    Goody's Headache P.'s
    Lotrimin AF Spray P.
    Pedi-Dri topical p.
    thrombin p.
    Zeasorb-AF P.
powdered bone graft
power
    p. bur
    p. drill
    p.-driven saw
    grasping p.
    p. oscillating saw
    pinch p.
    P. Play knee brace
    P. Pogo stationary exerciser
    p. rasp
    p. reamer
    thumb pinch p.
    P. Trainer cycle
    P. Web hand exerciser
    p. wheelchair
PowerAnthro Shoe
PowerBelt lower back and abdominal support belt
PowerCut drill blade
powered metaphyseal stapler
Powerflex
    P. CMP exerciser
    P. tape
Powermatic table
POWERPoint orthotic shoe insert
PowerStar bipolar scissors
PP
    proximal phalanx
PPF
    percutaneous plantar fasciotomy
PPG-AFO brace
PPG-TLSO brace
PPT
    PPT flat insole
    PPT insole system
    PPT MXL soft moulded insole
    PPT orthotic device
    PPT Plastazote insole
    PPT RX firm moulded insole
    PPT sheet
    PPT soft tissue orthotic system
    PPT temPPThotics kit

PQ
    pronator quadratus
P.Q. viscoelastic polymer
PR
    pelvic rock
    progressive-resistive exercise
PRAFO
    pediatric pressure relief ankle foot orthosis
    PRAFO adjustable orthotic
    PRAFO attachment
    PRAFO KAFO
    PRAFO KAFO attachment (PKA)
Pratt
    P. open reduction
    P. T-clamp
    P. technique
prayer position
PRE
    progressive-resistive exercise
preaxial polydactyly
prebent nail
precautions
    universal p.
precise lesion measuring (PLM)
Precision
    P. hip stem
    P. Osteolock femoral component system
    P. Osteolock femoral prosthesis
    P. Osteolock fixation
    P. Osteolock hip prosthesis
    P. Strata hip system
    P. total hip
Preclude spinal membrane
precoat
    p. hip prosthesis
    p. Plus femoral prosthesis
precompression jig
precontoured unit rod
precurved
    p. ball-tipped guidepin
    p. plate
Pred
    Liquid P.
Predate S
Predcor-TBA Injection
prediction
    Anderson-Green growth p.
    growth p.
predictor of injury
predisposition
    congenital p.
Prednicen-M
prednisolone
Prednisol TBA Injection
prednisone
preemptive blockade technique

preganglionic
- p. sympathectomy
- p. technique

prehallux

prehension
- p. force
- p. orthosis

Preiser disease

preload

Prelone Oral

premanipulative testing

Premarin With Methyltestosterone

premature
- p. closure
- p. consolidation
- p. infant

Premphase

Prempro

prenatal dislocation

Prenyl jacket

preop
- preoperatively

preoperative
- p. antibiotic
- p. drawing
- p. evaluation
- p. management
- p. plan
- p. planning
- p. roentgenography
- p. tomography

preoperatively (preop)

prep
- 3M p.

preparation
- bone-patellar tendon-bone p.
- facet joint p.
- graft p.
- lupus erythematosus p.
- rod contour p.
- skin p.
- Spälteholz p.
- wire contour p.

Prep-Assist
- P.-A. legholder
- P.-A. positioner

prepatellar
- p. bursa
- p. bursa inflammation
- p. bursitis

Prep-IM

Preposition ColorCards

Presbyterian
- P. Hospital staphylorrhaphy elevator
- P. Hospital T-clamp

Prescription
- ACSM Guidelines for Exercise Testing and P.
- P. Strength Desenex

preservation
- lordosis p.
- lumbar lordosis p.

press
- CamStar power leg p.
- p. fit
- leg p.
- p. up

Press-Fit
- P.-F. circumferential grommet
- P.-F. condylar knee arthroplasty
- P.-F. Condylar Total knee
- P.-F. condylar total knee prosthesis
- P.-F. cup
- P.-F. femoral component
- P.-F. fixation
- P.-F. stem
- P.-F. total condylar knee system

press-fit
- p.-f. acetabular implant insertion technique

PresSsion pneumatic garment

pressure
- ankle systolic p.
- blood p.
- bone marrow p. (BMP)
- central posterior-anterior p.
- compartmental p.
- disk p.
- p. dressing
- p. epiphysis
- p. glove
- hydrostatic p.
- intraabdominal p.
- intracompartmental p.
- intradiscal p.
- lateral root p.
- manual p.
- plantar p.
- p. plate
- p. point
- posterior-anterior p.
- p.-relief cushion
- p. relief padding
- p. relief shoe

NOTES

P

pressure *(continued)*
>rolfing p.
>P. Sentinel reamer
>sequential p.
>p. sore
>systolic blood p. (SBP)
>p. threshold
>p.-time integral (PTI)
>tissue p.
>toe p.
>p. tolerance
>p.-tolerant tissue
>tourniquet p.
>p. transducer-monitor system
>p. ulcer

pressure-sensitive
>p.-s. area
>p.-s. tissue

pressurization of cement
pressurizer
>acetabular p.
>plunger-type femoral p.

Preston
>P. ligamentum flavum forceps
>P. overhead pulley
>P. pinch gauge
>P. Traveler CPM exerciser

Prestop pinchometer
pretarget filtration system
pretendinous
>p. band
>p. cord

pretest likelihood of disease
pretibial
>p. bearing (PTB)
>p. edema

prevention
>p. of fracture
>heterotopic ossification p.
>infection p.
>osseous bridge p.
>rod rotation p.

prevertebral space
PRICE
>protection, restricted activity, ice, compression, elevation

Price muscular biopsy clamp
prickling
prickly ash bark
Pridie
>P. ankle arthrodesis
>P. incision

Pridie-Koutsogiannis procedure
prilocaine
>lidocaine and p.

Primaderm dressing
Primapore wound dressing

primary
>p. arthroplasty
>p. bone union
>p. closure
>p. cranial sacral respiratory mechanism
>p. curve
>p. cystic arthrosis
>p. intention
>p. or intentional movement
>p. movement plane
>p. myofascial trigger point
>p. repair
>p. rotation movement
>p. tumor
>p. x-ray beam

Primaxin
prime mover
Primer modified Unna boot
primitive
>p. bone
>p. dislocation
>p. locomotor pattern

principal stress
principle
>anatomic fracture reduction p.
>axial compression p.
>biomechanical p.
>Enneking p.
>gliding p.
>Lambotte p.
>SAID p.
>spherical gliding p.

priori
>anlage a p.

prism
>Fresnel p.

Pritchard
>P. Mark II pin
>P. total elbow prosthesis

Pritchard-Walker
>P.-W. semiconstrained elbow prosthesis
>P.-W. total elbow prosthesis

Pritchett-Mallin-Matthews arthrodesis
Prizm
>P. Electro-Mesh Sock electrode
>P. Electro-Mesh Z-Stim-II stimulator

PRN
>P. bandage
>P. pillow
>P. protector
>P. shoe

Pro-8 ankle brace
ProAdvantage knee
probability
>bone cyst fracture p.

PRO Balance Master
Pro-Banthine
probe
    Acufex p.
    angled p.
    arthroscopic p.
    blunt-tip p.
    Bunnell dissecting p.
    Bunnell forwarding p.
    calibrated p.
    dissecting p.
    free-spinning p.
    gearshift p.
    gold p.
    intraosseous p.
    LASE p.
    laser Doppler p.
    multiplane echo p.
    Nucleotome p.
    Oratek thermal shrinking p.
    pedicle sounding p.
    reverse-cutting meniscal p.
    skin temperature monitoring p.
    spinning p.
    ultrasonic p.
    Woodson p.
probenecid
    colchicine and p.
procaine
    p.-phenol motor point injection
procallus formation
Procardia XL
procedure
    Adams p.
    Akin p.
    Albee-Delbert p.
    Albee shelf p.
    AMBRI p.
    anchovy p.
    Anderson-Fowler p.
    anecdotal p.
    antenna p.
    anterior stabilization p.
    AO p.
    Arbeitsgemeinschaft für
      osteosynthesefragen p.
    articulatory p.
    Auto-Implant p.
    Axer-Clark p.
    Badgley combination p.
    Bandi p.
    Bankart p.

    Barsky p.
    Bartlett p.
    Basic I, II cranial adjusting p.
    Baxter-D'Astous p.
    Bell Tawse p.
    Bennett quadriceps plastic p.
    Berman-Gartland p.
    B.H. Moore p.
    Bickel-Moe p.
    Bilhaut-Cloquet p.
    Blatt p.
    Blatt-Ashworth p.
    bone block p.
    bony p.
    Bose p.
    Bosworth shelf p.
    Boyd-Bosworth p.
    Boyd-McLeod p.
    Boyd-Sisk p.
    Boytchev p.
    Brahms p.
    Brantigan-Voshell p.
    Braun p.
    Bridle p.
    Bristow p.
    Bristow-Helfet p.
    Bristow-May p.
    Brockman p.
    Broström p.
    Bryan p.
    Bunnell-Williams p.
    Calandriello p.
    Campbell-Akbarnia p.
    Campbell ankle p.
    Campbell-Goldthwait p.
    capsular imbrication p.
    capsular shift p.
    Castle p.
    Chambers p.
    Chandler p.
    checkrein p.
    chevron p.
    Chrisman-Snook p.
    Clayton p.
    Cole p.
    Connolly p.
    core drilling p.
    Cracchiolo p.
    Darrach p.
    Das Gupta p.
    debulking p.
    degloving p.

NOTES

P

473

procedure *(continued)*

Dewar posterior cervical fixation p.
Dickson-Diveley p.
Dorrance p.
Downey-McGlamery p.
DuVries p.
Dwyer p.
Eden-Hybbinette p.
Eden-Lange p.
Edwards p.
Elmslie-Cholmely p.
Elmslie peroneal tendon p.
Elmslie-Trillat patellar p.
Evans p.
Eve reconstructive p.
extraarticular p.
failed p.
Fairbanks-Sever p.
femorodistal bypass p.
Ficat p.
Fired-Hendel p.
five-incision p.
forage p.
four-incision p.
Fowler p.
Fox-Blazina knee p.
Fried-Green foot p.
Froimson p.
Froimson-Oh arm p.
Frost foot p.
Fulford p.
Gallie p.
Gartland p.
Gelman foot p.
Gerard resurfacing p.
Ghormley shelf p.
Gill modification of Campbell
  ankle p.
Gillquist p.
Gill shelf p.
Girdlestone hip p.
Girdlestone-Taylor p.
Goldner-Hayes p.
Goldthwait-Hauser p.
Gould p.
gracilis p.
Green p.
Grice p.
Gritti-Stokes distal thigh p.
Gruca lower leg p.
Gurd p.
hallux valgus p.
Hambly p.
Hammon foot p.
Hardinge vastus lateralis p.
Hark foot p.
Harmon p.
Hass p.

Hauser heel cord p.
Hauser patellar tendon p.
Hawkins p.
Hay-Groves shelf p.
Heifetz p.
Herndon-Heyman foot p.
Heyman p.
Heyman-Herndon p.
Hibbs p.
His-Haas p.
Hitchcock arm p.
Hodor-Dobbs p.
Hoffer ankle p.
Hoffmann-Clayton p.
Hoffmann metatarsal p.
Hohmann p.
Hoke-Miller p.
Hoke tibial palsy p.
Hovanian p.
Howorth p.
Howorth-Keillor p.
Hughston p.
Hughston-Hauser p.
Hui-Linscheid p.
iliac buttressing p.
Inclan modification of Campbell
  ankle p.
Inclan-Ober p.
Ingram p.
Insall p.
installation p.
intercalary allograft p.
intermetatarsal angle-reducing p.
intraarticular p.
Jaffe p.
Jahss p.
Jansey p.
Jobe-Glousman capsular shift p.
Johnson p.
Johnson-Spiegl p.
Jones p.
J. R. Moore p.
Juvara p.
Karakousis-Vezeridis p.
Karlsson p.
Kawaii-Yamamoto p.
Kelikian p.
Kelikian-McFarland p.
Keller p.
Keller-Brandes p.
Keller-Lelièvre-Hoffman p.
Kendrick p.
Kessel-Bonney p.
Kidner foot p.
Kiehn-Earle-DesPrez p.
Knobby-Clark p.
Kortzeborn p.
Koutsogiannis p.

Krukenberg p.
Lane p.
Lange p.
Langenskiöld p.
Larmon forefoot p.
Latarjet p.
lateral sling p.
Lauenstein p.
Lee p.
Leeds spinal p.
Lepird p.
L'Episcopo-Zachary p.
limb-salvage p.
Lindeman p.
Linton p.
Lipscomb p.
Lipscomb-Anderson p.
Localio p.
Loose p.
loose knee p.
Lorenz p.
lower cervical spine p.
Lowman shelf p.
Luck hand p.
MacAusland p.
MacCarthy p.
Magnuson-Stack p.
Mahan p.
Manktelow transfer p.
Mann p.
Mann-Coughlin p.
Maquet p.
Matson p.
Mauck knee p.
McBride p.
McCarroll-Baker p.
McCarty hip p.
McCash hand p.
McCauley foot p.
McCormick-Blount p.
McElvenny-Caldwell p.
McElvenny foot p.
McGlamry-Downey p.
McKay hip p.
McKeever p.
McLaughlin p.
medial rotation p.
Miller p.
Minkoff-Nicholas p.
Mitchell hallux valgus p.
Miyakawa knee p.
Moberg key-pinch p.

modified Hoke-Miller flatfoot p.
modified Lapidus p.
Mogensen p.
motion-preserving p.
Mueller knee p.
Mumford p.
muscle-balancing p.
Neer capsular shift p.
Neviaser-Wilson-Gardner p.
Newman-Keuls p.
Nicola shoulder p.
Nicoll fracture repair p.
notchplasty p.
O'Brien capsular shift p.
O'Donoghue p.
orthodox p.
Osborne-Cotterill p.
Osmond-Clarke foot p.
Oudard p.
over-the-top knee p.
Paltrinieri-Trentani resurfacing p.
Parrish p.
Paterson p.
Peabody p.
Perthes p.
Pettibon chiropractic p.
polyethylene femoral buck plug p.
portmanteau p.
Pridie-Koutsogiannis p.
Proxiderm p.
Putti-Platt shoulder p.
realignment p.
reefing p.
Regnauld p.
Reichenheim-King p.
resurfacing p.
Reverdin-Green foot p.
reverse Mauck knee p.
reverse Putti-Platt p.
revision p.
Ridlon p.
Rockwood p.
Rockwood-Matsen capsular shift p.
Rose foot p.
Roux-Goldthwait p.
Ruiz-Mora p.
Ryerson p.
sacroiliac buttressing p.
Saha p.
salvage p.
Samilson p.
sartorial slide p.

NOTES

P

procedure *(continued)*
    Sauvé-Kapandji p.
    Schrock p.
    Scuderi p.
    Selakovich p.
    semitendinosus p.
    Sham p.
    short lever specific contact p.
    Silfverskiöld p.
    Silver p.
    sling p.
    Slocum knee p.
    SLURPIE p.
    Somerville p.
    Souter hip p.
    Southwick slide p.
    spinal locking p.
    Spira p.
    Spittler p.
    SPLATT p.
    split anterior tibial tendon p.
    Stack shoulder p.
    Staheli shelf p.
    Stamm p.
    Steindler p.
    Steytler-Van Der Walt p.
    Stone p.
    Strayer p.
    Sutherland hip p.
    Syme p.
    Tachdjian p.
    Taylor p.
    terminal Syme p.
    Thomas p.
    Thomas-Thompson p.
    Tikhoff-Linberg radical arm p.
    p. time
    Trillat p.
    triple-wire p.
    Tsai-Stillwell p.
    TUBS p.
    upper cervical spine p.
    Valpius-Compere p.
    Van Ness p.
    Vulpius p.
    Vulpius-Stoffel p.
    wafer p.
    Wallenberg p.
    Watson-Cheyne-Burghard p.
    Watson-Jones p.
    Weaver-Dunn p.
    Weber p.
    White slide p.
    Whitman talectomy p.
    Whitman-Thompson p.
    Williams p.
    Woodward p.
    Yoke transposition p.
    Young p.
    Yount p.
    Zancolli-Lasso p.
    Zancolli static lock p.
    Zarins-Rowe p.
    Zoeller-Clancy p.

process
    abnormal posterior talar p.
    absent spinous p.
    articular p.
    cleft spinous p.
    coracoacromial p.
    coracoid p.
    coronoid p.
    deficient spinous p.
    inferior p.
    intact spinous p.
    lateral p.
    mamillary p.
    mastoid p.
    odontoid p.
    physeal mamillary p.
    sacralized transverse p.
    spinous p.
    superior p.
    supracondylar p.
    talar p.
    transverse p.
    xiphoid p.
    Zimmer PMMA precoat p.

processed carbon implant
ProCol bovine bioprosthesis tendon
ProComp
procurvatum deformity
procurvature deformity
ProCyte transparent dressing
Proderm topical spray
product
    cyclooxygenase p.
    Innovative Medical P.'s (IMP)
    Orthopaedic Physical Therapy P.'s
      (OPTP)
    Remifemin herbal p.

production
    bone p.
    torque p.

Profex
    P. arthroscopic leg positioner
    P. arthroscopic tourniquet

Proficiency
    Bruininks-Oseretsky Test of
      Motor P.

profile
    Functional Limitation P. (FLP)
    P. hip prosthesis
    P. hip stem
    Maryland Foot Score P.
    P. of Mood States (POMS)

Nottingham Health P.
risk factor p.
Sickness Impact P. (SIP)
P. Sitting Orthosis
Staheli rotational p.
wrist speed p.

Profix
P. confirming tibial insert
P. metaphyseal tibial stem
P. nonporous tibial base
P. porous femoral component
P. total knee replacement system

ProFlex wrist support
ProFlo vascular compression therapy
Profore
P. Four-Layer bandage system
P. wound dressing

profunda femoris
profundum
ligamentum metacarpeum
transversum p.
ligamentum metatarsale
transversum p.
ligamentum sacrococcygeum
posterius p.

profundus
p. advancement
arcus palmaris p.
arcus plantaris p.
arcus volaris p.
p. artery fracture
flexor digitorum p. (FDP)
p. muscle
p. tendon

prog
prognosis
Pro-glide
P.-g. orthosis
P.-g. splint

prognosis (prog)
progonoma
melanotic p.

program
ABAQUS modeling p.
aquatic stabilization p.
Carpal Care rehabilitative p.
Elderberry Sambu Internal
Cleansing P.
four-star exercise p.
home spinal stabilization p.
independent exercise p.

interdisciplinary vocational
evaluation p.
PATRAN modelling p.
Rothman Institute total hip p.
Total Gym Exercise P.
walking p.
Westcott Pyramid P.
Williams exercise p.
work hardening p.

**programmable VariGrip II prosthetic
control system**
progression
curve p.
p. to full weightbearing

progressiva
fibrous dysplasia ossificans p.
myositis ossificans p.

progressive
P. Ambulation Scale
P. ankle orthosis
p. diaphyseal dysplasia
p. loading
p. muscular dystrophy (PMD)
p. myositis fibrosa
p. neurologic disorder
P. Palm Guard
p. perilunar instability
p.-resistance exercise
p.-resistive exercise (PR, PRE)
p. subacute myelopathy
p. systemic sclerosis

proinflammatory
projection
axial calcaneal p.
axial sesamoid p.
bursal p.
cephaloscapular p.
convergence p.
dorsoplantar p.
Harris-Beath p.
Isherwood p.
lateral p. (LC)
posterior-superior oblique p.
stress dorsiflexion p.

prolapse
disk p.
Prolene suture
proliferation
angiofibroblastic p.
reactive periosteal p.
villous lipomatous p.

NOTES

P

477

proliferative
p. fasciitis
p. myositis
p. synovitis
ProLite Plus runner's orthotic
Prolixin
prolonged insertional activity
prolotherapy
PROM
passive range of motion
promazine
promethazine
meperidine and p.
prominence
bony p.
osteochondral p.
pedicle screw hardware p.
plantar bony p.
rotational p.
tibial tubercle p.
prominent heel
promontorium
promontory
sacral p.
pronate
pronated
p. foot
p. straight flatfoot
pronation
p. contracture
p. control
p. of the foot
p. injury
p. sign
p. spring-control device
subtalar p.
p. and supination
pronation-abduction
p.-a. fracture
p.-a. injury
pronation-eversion
p.-e. fracture
p.-e. injury
pronation-eversion-external
p.-e.-e. rotation (PEER)
p.-e.-e. rotation injury
p.-e.-e. rotation injury of ankle
pronation-external
p.-e. rotation (P-ER)
p.-e. rotation fracture
pronation-supination
pronator
p. drift
p. drill
p. quadratus (PQ)
p. quadratus muscle
p. teres (PT)
p. teres muscle

p. teres release
p. teres syndrome
p. teres tendon
pronatory
prone
p. extension test
p. knee-bend test
p. knee flexion test
p. position
p. rectus test
p. reduction
p. sacral push
Pronex pneumatic device for cervical pain
prong
modified tonsillar p.
Pron pillow
Pronto cement
ProOsteon
P. bone graft material
P. Implant 500
P. implant 500 coralline hydroxyapatite bone void filler
P. Implant 500 granule
Propac
Champ Insulated P. II
Propacet
propagation velocity
proparacaine
Propel cannulated interference screw
proper
p. digital nerve branch
p. neck positioning
properitoneal space
properly seated
property
elastic p.
elongation p.
prophylactic
p. abduction pants
p. antibiotic
p. antibiotic therapy
p. anticoagulation
p. bone graft
p. fasciotomy
p. operative stabilization
p. resection
p. skeletal fixation
prophylaxis
deep venous thrombosis p.
dextran p.
DVT p.
tetanus p.
propiomazine
Proplast
P. HA
P. I, II porous implant material

P. prosthesis
P. prosthetic material
propoxyphene
p. and acetaminophen
p. and aspirin
p. hydrochloride
propranolol
proprioception
gravitational p.
proprioceptive
p. deficit
p. neuromuscular facilitation (PNF)
p. neuromuscular facilitation
approach
p. training
proprioceptor
propriosensory training
proprius
extensor indicis p. (EIP)
p. tendon
Prop'r Toes hammer toe cushion
propulsion
p. biomechanics
p. gait
propulsive
ProROM walker
proscope
ProSom
prostaglandin
PROSTALAC
prosthetic antibiotic-loaded acrylic
cement
PROSTALAC total hip prosthesis
PROSTALAC total joint prosthesis
Prostaphlin
prosthesis, pl. **prostheses**
above-knee p., AK p.
acetabular p.
acrylic bar p.
Aequalis shoulder p.
Aesculap-PM noncemented
femoral p.
AFI total hip replacement p.
AGC femoral p.
AGC knee p.
AGC tibial p.
AHP digital p.
AHSC elbow p.
AHSC-Volz elbow p.
AK p. (*var. of* above-knee p.)
Alivium implant metal p.
Allen-Brown p.

Alumina cemented total hip p.
AMC total wrist p.
American Hand P. (AHP)
American Heyer-Schulte chin p.
American Heyer-Schulte-Hinderer
malar p.
American Heyer-Schulte Radovan
tissue expander p.
AML Tang femoral p.
AML total hip p.
Amstutz cemented hip p.
Anametric total knee p.
Anatomic Precoat hip p.
anatomic surface p.
Anderson acetabular p.
ankle p.
APR acetabular p.
APR femoral p.
APR II p.
APRL hand p.
Arafiles elbow p.
Arizona Health Science Center-Volz
elbow p.
Arthropor cup p.
Arthropor II acetabular p.
Atlas modular humeral p.
Attenborough total knee p.
Aufranc-Cobra hip p.
Aufranc-Turner cemented hip p.
Aufranc-Turner hip p.
Austin Moore femoral head p.
Austin Moore hip p.
Autophor ceramic total hip p.
Autophor femoral p.
Averett hip p.
ball-and-socket ankle p.
Bankart shoulder p.
Bateman femoral neck p.
Bateman finger p.
Bateman UPF II bipolar p.
Bateman UPF II shoulder p.
BDH p.
Bechtol hip p.
Bechtol system p.
Becker hand p.
Beck-Steffee total ankle p.
below-knee p.
Bi-Angular shoulder p.
BIAS p.
bicentric p.
bicompartmental knee implant p.
bicondylar ankle p.

NOTES

P

479

prosthesis *(continued)*
    bicondylar knee p.
    Bi-Metric hip p.
    Bi-Metric Interlok femoral p.
    Bi-Metric porous primary
      femoral p.
    Bio-Chromatic hand p.
    Bioclad with pegs reinforced
      acetabular p.
    BioFit Press-Fit acetabular p.
    Bioglass p.
    Bio-Groove acetabular p.
    Bio-Groove Macrobond HA
      femoral p.
    Biomet AGC knee p.
    Biomet hip p.
    Biometric p.
    Biomet total toe p.
    Biophase implant metal p.
    Biotex implant metal p.
    bipolar femoral head p.
    bipolar hip replacement p.
    Björk p.
    BK p.
    Blauth knee p.
    Blazina p.
    Bock knee p.
    Bograb Universal offset
      ossicular p.
    Bombelli-Mathys-Morscher hip p.
    bone p.
    bovine collagen material p.
    Brigham p.
    Bryan total knee implant p.
    Buchholz p.
    Byars mandibular p.
    CAD/CAM p.
    CAD femoral stem p.
    Caffinière trapeziometacarpal p.
    Calandruccio cemented hip p.
    calcar replacement femoral p.
    Callender technique hip p.
    Calnan-Nicolle finger p.
    camouflage p.
    Canadian hip disarticulation p.
    capitellocondylar unconstrained
      elbow p.
    Carbon Copy II Foot p.
    Carbon Copy II Light p.
    Cardona keratoprosthesis p.
    carpal lunate implant p.
    carpal scaphoid implant p.
    Cathcart Orthocentric hip p.
    CDH Precoat Plus hip p.
    p.-cement interface
    Centralign precoat hip p.
    ceramic ossicular p.
    Ceramion p.

CFS hip p.
Charnley acetabular cup p.
Charnley cemented p.
Charnley-Hastings p.
Charnley low-friction hip p.
Charnley-Mueller hip p.
Charnley total hip p.
Chatzidakis hinged Vitallium
  implant p.
Chopart partial foot p.
Choyce MK II keratoprosthesis p.
Christiansen hip p.
Cintor knee p.
Cirrus foot p.
clamshell p.
Cloutier unconstrained knee p.
Coballoy implant metal p.
cobalt-chromium-alloy p.
Co-Cr-Mo alloy p.
Co-Cr-W-Ni alloy p.
Cofield shoulder p.
cold-mold p.
cold-weld femoral p.
collar-calcar support femoral p.
College Park TruStep foot p.
Compartmental II knee p.
p. component
p. component subsidence
compression-molded p.
computer-assisted design/computer
  assisted manufacturing p.
Conaxial ankle p.
constrained hinged knee p.
constrained nonhinged knee p.
Contour internal p.
Coonrad hinged p.
Coonrad-Morrey elbow p.
Coonrad semiconstrained elbow p.
C-2 OsteoCap hip p.
crimped Dacron p.
cruciate-retaining p.
cruciate-sacrificing p.
CSF p.
CUI tendon p.
p. cup
custom p.
custom-threaded p.
DANA shoulder p.
d'Aubigne femoral p.
Deane unconstrained knee p.
DeBakey p.
Dee totally constrained elbow p.
de La Caffinière
  trapeziometacarpal p.
DeLaura knee p.
DeLaura-Verner knee p.
Deon hip p.
DePalma hip p.

DePuy AML Porocoat stem p.
Deune knee p.
DF80 hip internal p.
digital p.
Dimension-C femoral stem p.
Dimension hip p.
distal radioulnar joint p.
Dorrance hand p.
Dow Corning implant p.
Dow Corning Wright finger
 joint p.
p. driver
DRUJ p.
dual-lock total hip p.
Duocondylar knee p.
Duo-Lock hip p.
Duo-Patellar knee p.
Dupaco knee p.
Duracon p.
Dynaplex knee p.
Eaton trapezium finger joint
 replacement p.
Edwards seamless p.
Eftekhar-Charnley hip p.
Eicher femoral p.
Eicher hip p.
Eilers-Armstrong unicompartmental
 knee p.
elbow p.
ELP femoral p.
Endolite p.
Endo-Model hinged knee p.
Endo-Model rotating knee joint p.
Endo-Model sled p.
Endo rotating knee joint p.
Engh porous metal hip p.
Englehardt femoral p.
English-McNab shoulder p.
EPTFE graft p.
Eriksson knee p.
Evolution hip p.
Ewald unconstrained elbow p.
Exeter cemented hip p.
femoral neck p.
Fett p.
finger joint implant p.
Finney p.
Finney-Flexirod p.
FIRST knee p.
fixed femoral head p.
Flatt finger p.
Flatt finger-joint p.

Flatt finger-thumb p.
Flex-Foot p.
foot p.
forearm lift-assist p.
four-bar linkage on knee p.
Four-Bar Polycentric knee p.
Freeman modular total hip p.
Freeman-Samuelson knee p.
Freeman-Swanson knee p.
F. R. Thompson femoral p.
fully constrained tricompartmental
 knee p.
Gaffney ankle p.
Galante hip p.
Gemini hip system p.
Genesis knee p.
Geomedic total knee p.
Geometric total knee p.
Gerard p.
Gianturco p.
Gilfillan humeral p.
Giliberty acetabular p.
Giliberty femoral neck p.
Giliberty hip p.
Gillette joint p.
Gillies p.
Girard keratoprosthesis p.
Gore-Tex knee p.
great toe implant p.
Greissinger foot p.
Gripper acetabular cup p.
Gritti-Stokes knee p.
Gruppe wire p.
GSB elbow p.
GSB expanded version for knee p.
Gschwind-Scheier-Bahler elbow p.
Guepar hinged knee p.
Guilford-Wright p.
Gunston-Hult knee p.
Gunston polycentric knee p.
Gustilo hip p.
Gustilo knee p.
HA 65101 implant metal p.
Hamas upper limb p.
hand p.
Hanslik patellar p.
Harken p.
Harris-CDH hip p.
Harris cemented hip p.
Harris Design femoral p.
Harris-Galante porous hip p.
Harris Micromini p.

NOTES

P

prosthesis *(continued)*
    Hastings hip p.
    Haynes-Stellite implant metal p.
    HD-2 cemented hip p.
    heat-cured acrylic femoral head p.
    Hedley-Hungerford hip p.
    Henschke-Mauch SNS knee p.
    Henschke-Mauch SNS lower
      limb p.
    Herbert knee p.
    Hexcel knee p.
    Hexcel total condylar p.
    HG multilock hip p.
    Hinderer malar p.
    hinged constrained knee p.
    hinged great toe replacement p.
    hinged implant p.
    hinged total knee p.
    hip disarticulation p.
    Hittenberger p.
    homograft p.
    Hosmer WALK p.
    Howmedica Kinematic II knee p.
    Howorth p.
    Howse-Coventry p.
    HPS II total hip p.
    HSS total condylar knee p.
    Hunter Silastic p.
    Hunter tendon p.
    Hydra-Cadence knee p.
    hydraulic knee unit p.
    Hydroxial hip p.
    I-beam hemiarthroplasty hip p.
    ICLH ankle p.
    ICLH knee p.
    Identifit hip p.
    immediate postoperative p. (IPOP)
    Impact modular porous p.
    Indiana conservative p.
    Indong Oh hip p.
    Infinity modular hip p.
    Inronail finger or toenail p.
    Insall-Burstein semiconstrained
      tricompartmental knee p.
    Integral Interlok femoral p.
    Integrity acetabular cup p.
    p. interface
    Intermedics Natural-Knee knee p.
    Iowa internal p.
    Iowa total hip p.
    ischial weightbearing p. (IWP)
    Ishizuki unconstrained elbow p.
    isoelastic pelvic p.
    Ivalon p.
    Jaffe-Capello-Averill hip p.
    Jewett p.
    Jobst p.
    Jonas p.

    Jonathan Livingston Seagull
      patellar p.
    Joplin toe p.
    Judet Press-Fit hip p.
    Kessler p.
    Kinematic fully constrained
      tricompartmental knee p.
    Kinematic II rotating hinge total
      knee p.
    Kinemax Plus knee p.
    Kirschner Medical Dimension p.
    Kirschner total shoulder p.
    KMC femoral stem p.
    KMP femoral stem p.
    KMW/PC femoral p.
    knee p.
    Koenig MPJ p.
    Krause-Wolfe p.
    Kudo unconstrained elbow p.
    Küntscher humeral p.
    Lacey fully constrained
      tricompartmental knee p.
    Lacey hinged knee p.
    LaGrange-Letoumel hip p.
    Laing hip cup p.
    Lanceford p.
    Landers-Foulks p.
    LAPOC p.
    LaPorte total toe p.
    LCS New Jersey knee p.
    Leake Dacron mandible p.
    Leinbach femoral p.
    Leinbach hip p.
    Lewis expandable adjustable p.
      (LEAP)
    Lewis Trapezio p.
    Ling cemented hip p.
    Link MP hip noncemented
      reconstruction p.
    Lippman hip p.
    Lisfranc below-knee p.
    Liverpool elbow p.
    Liverpool knee p.
    Lo Bak spinal support p.
    locking p.
    London unconstrained elbow p.
    Longevity V-Lign hip p.
    Lo-Por vascular graft p.
    Lord Press-Fit hip p.
    Lowe-Miller unconstrained elbow p.
    lower limb p. (LLP)
    low-neck femoral p.
    low-profile femoral p.
    Lubinus knee p.
    lunate acrylic cement wrist p.
    Lunceford-Pilliar-Engh hip p.
    MacIntosh hip p.
    MacIntosh tibial plateau p.

MacNab-English shoulder p.
Macrofit hip p.
madreporic hip p.
malleus-incus p.
Mallory-Head hip p.
Mallory-Head porous primary
  femoral p.
manual locking knee p.
MAPF femoral stem p.
Marlex methyl methacrylate p.
Marmor modular knee p.
Matchett-Brown cemented hip p.
Matchett-Brown internal p.
Mathys p.
Matrol femoral head p.
Mayo semiconstrained elbow p.
Mayo total ankle p.
Mazas totally constrained elbow p.
McBride femoral p.
McBride-Moore p.
McCutcheon SLT hip p.
McGehee elbow p.
McKee-Farrar total hip p.
McKee femoral p.
McKee totally constrained elbow p.
McKeever-MacIntosh tibial
  plateau p.
McKeever patellar cap p.
McKeever Vitallium knee p.
McNaught p.
MCP finger joint p.
Mecring acetabluar p.
Mediloy implant metal p.
medium profile femoral p.
medullary p.
metal-backed p.
metal femoral head p.
metal-on-metal articulating
  intervertebral disk p.
metaphyseal head resection with p.
MG II knee p.
Michael Reese articulated p.
Microloc knee p.
Microvel p.
Miller-Galante hip p.
Miller-Galante II knee p.
Minneapolis hip p.
Mittlemeir ceramic hip p.
Mittlemeir noncemented femoral p.
modified Moore hip locking p.
modular Austin Moore hip p.
modular Iowa Precoat total hip p.

modular total hip p.
modular unicompartmental knee p.
Monk hip p.
Moon-Robinson stapes p.
Moore femoral neck p.
Moore hip p.
Moretz p.
Moseley glenoid rim p.
MP35N implant metal p.
MST-6A1-4V implant metal p.
Mueli wrist p.
Mueller-Charnley hip p.
Mueller dual-lock hip p.
Mueller total hip replacement p.
Mulligan Silastic p.
Multiflex p.
Multi-Lock hip p.
Murray knee p.
myoelectric p.
Naden-Rieth p.
Natural-Hip p.
Natural-Lok acetabular cup p.
NEB total hip p.
Neer humeral replacement p.
Neer shoulder p. (I, II)
Neer umbrella p.
Neer-Vitallium humeral p.
Neibauer-Cutter p.
New Jersey hemiarthroplasty p.
New Jersey LCS shoulder p.
New Jersey LCS total knee p.
Newton ankle p.
Nexus hip p.
Nicoll tendon p.
Niebauer finger-joint replacement p.
Niebauer metacarpophalangeal joint
  Silastic p.
Niebauer trapezium replacement p.
Noiles fully constrained
  tricompartmental knee p.
nonhinged knee p.
nonhinged linked p.
Normalize Press-Fit hip p.
nudge control on p.
ocular p.
Odland ankle p.
Oh cemented hip p.
Oh Press-Fit hip p.
Oklahoma ankle p.
Omnifit HA hip stem p.
Omnifit knee p.
Omniflex hip p.

NOTES

prosthesis *(continued)*
    Opti-Fix p.
    Opti-Fix femoral p.
    Oregon Poly II ankle p.
    Orthochrome implant metal p.
    Orthofix p.
    Ortholoc implant metal p.
    orthopaedic p.
    prostheses and orthoses (P&O)
    ossicular chain replacement p.
    OsteoCap hip p.
    Osteolock hip p.
    Osteonics hip p.
    Otto Bock dynamic p.
    Overdyke hip p.
    Oxford p.
    Padgett p.
    painful femoral head p.
    Paladon p.
    Panje p.
    partial ossicular
      reconstruction/replacement p.
    partial ossicular replacement p.
      (PORP)
    patellar tendon-bearing below-
      knee p.
    PCA p.
    PCA unconstrained
      tricompartmental p.
    PCA unicompartmental knee p.
    PC Performer knee p.
    pegged tibial p.
    Perfecta hip p.
    Performance knee p.
    Phoenix total hip p.
    Pillet hand p.
    piston p.
    Plasticor p.
    Plasti-Pore ossicular replacement p.
    Plastiport TORP p.
    Plystan p.
    PMI-6A1-4V implant metal p.
    Polycel bone composite p.
    polycentric knee p.
    Poly-Dial p.
    polyethylene patellar implant p.
    polyethylene talar p.
    polypropylene p.
    porcine p.
    Porocoat AML noncemented p.
    Porocool p.
    Porometal noncemented femoral p.
    porous-coated anatomic p.
    porous-coated femur p.
    porous-coated hip p.
    porous surfaced p.
    Precision Osteolock femoral p.
    Precision Osteolock hip p.

precoat hip p.
Precoat Plus femoral p.
Press-Fit condylar total knee p.
Pritchard total elbow p.
Pritchard-Walker semiconstrained
    elbow p.
Pritchard-Walker total elbow p.
Profile hip p.
Proplast p.
PROSTALAC total hip p.
PROSTALAC total joint p.
prosthetic antibiotic-loaded acrylic
    cement total joint p.
Protasul femoral p.
Protasul-10 noncemented femoral p.
Protasul-64 WF Zweymuller
    femoral p.
Protek p.
provisional p.
proximal humeral p.
proximal third femoral p.
PTB-SC-SP p.
PTB supracondylar p.
PTB suprapatellar p.
PTS soft wedge p.
Quantum Foot p.
radial head implant p.
Radovan tissue expander p.
RAM knee p.
Ranawat-Burstein hip p.
Randelli shoulder p.
Rastelli p.
retaining knee p.
Reverdin p.
Richards maximum contact cruciate-
    sparing p.
Richards Spectron metal-backed
    acetabular p.
Richards Zirconia femoral head p.
Ring knee p.
Ring total hip p.
RMC p.
RM isoelastic hip p.
Robert Brigham total knee p.
Rock-Mulligan p.
Rosenfeld hip p.
rotating femoral head p.
rotating-hinge knee p.
Rothman Institute femoral p.
SACH foot p.
    solid ankle, cushioned heel
      prosthesis
sacrificing knee p.
saddle p.
SAF p.
SAFE II p.
Saint George-Buchholz ankle p.
Saint George knee p.

Saint Jude p.
Salzer p.
Sampson p.
Sarmiento hip p.
Sauerbruch p.
Savastano Hemi-Knee p.
Sbarbaro hip p.
Sbarbaro tibial plateau p.
Scarborough p.
Schlein semiconstrained elbow p.
Schlein total elbow p.
Schlein trisurface ankle p.
Schuknecht Gelfoam wire p.
Schuknecht Teflon wire piston p.
Seattle foot p.
Select ankle p.
Select shoulder p.
self-bearing ceramic hip p.
self-centering Universal hip p.
semiconstrained tricompartmental
  knee p.
Sense-of-Feel p.
Sharrard-Trentani p.
Sheehan knee p.
Sherfee p.
Shier knee p.
shoulder p.
Silastic ball spacer p.
Silastic radial head p.
Silastic standard elastometer p.
Silastic thumb p.
Silflex intramedullary p.
silicone trapezium p.
single-axis ankle p.
sintered implant p.
Sinterlock implant metal p.
Sivash hip p.
SKI knee p.
SMA p.
Smith ankle p.
Smith-Petersen hip cup p.
SMo p.
solid ankle, cushioned heel p.
  (SACH foot prosthesis)
Souter unconstrained elbow p.
Spectron hip p.
Speed radius cap p.
spherocentric fully constrained
  tricompartmental knee p.
Spotorno hip p.
Springlite lower limb p.
S-ROM femoral stem p.

stainless steel implant metal p.
Stanmore shoulder p.
Stanmore totally constrained
  elbow p.
STD hip p.
STD+ Titanium total hip p.
stemmed tibial p.
Stenzel rod p.
Stevens-Street elbow p.
STH-2 hip p.
Street-Stevens humeral p.
substituting knee p.
Sulzer p.
SuperCup acetabular cup p.
Surgitek p.
Sutter double-stem silicone
  implant p.
Sutter MCP finger joint p.
Swanson finger joint p.
Swanson flexible hallux valgus p.
Swanson great toe p.
Swanson metacarpal p.
Swanson metatarsal p.
Swanson Silastic elbow p.
Swanson T-shaped great toe
  Silastic p.
Swanson wrist p.
Syme amputation p.
Syme foot p.
Synatomic total knee p.
synthetic p.
Taperloc femoral p.
TARA total hip p.
Tavernetti-Tennant knee p.
TCCK unconstrained knee p.
Teflon tri-leaflet p.
p. template
tendon p.
Thackray hip p.
Tharies hip replacement p.
thermomechanical implant metal p.
T28 hip p.
Thompson femoral neck p.
Thompson hemiarthroplasty hip p.
threaded titanium acetabular p.
  (TTAP)
thrust plate p. (TPP)
Ti-Bac II hip p.
tibial plateau p.
Ti/CoCr hip p.
Ti-Con p.
Tilastin hip p.

NOTES

P

485

prosthesis *(continued)*
    Tillman p.
    Titan cemented hip p.
    titanium implant p.
    Ti-Thread p.
    Titian hip p.
    Tivanium hip p.
    Tivanium implant metal p.
    TK Optimizer knee p.
    TMA p.
    toe p.
    TORP p.
    total articular replacement arthroplasty p.
    total condylar knee p.
    total condylar semiconstrained tricompartmental p.
    total hip replacement p.
    total joint replacement p.
    total knee replacement p.
    Townley TARA p.
    Townley total knee p.
    TPR ankle prosthesis p.
    trapezial p.
    trapeziometacarpal joint replacement p.
    trapezium implant p.
    Trapezoidal-28 hip p.
    Trapezoidal-28 internal p.
    TR-28 hip p.
    Triad p.
    trial p.
    Tri-Axial p.
    triaxial semiconstrained elbow p.
    tricompartmental knee p.
    Tricon-M cruciate-sparing p.
    Tricon-M patellar p.
    trileaflet p.
    Tronzo p.
    trunnion-bearing hip p.
    TTAP p.
    TTAP-ST acetabular p.
    Turner p.
    two-prong stem finger p.
    UCI ankle p.
    UHMWPE p.
    ulnar head implant p.
    unconstrained tricompartmental knee p.
    unicompartmental knee p.
    unicondylar p.
    Universal femoral head p.
    Universal hip p.
    UPF p.
    upper extremity myoelectric p.
    upper limb p. (ULP)
    Valls hip p.
    Vanghetti limb p.

    Varikopf hip p.
    Viladot p.
    Vinertia implant metal p.
    Vitallium humeral replacement p.
    Vitallium-W implant metal p.
    Volz wrist p.
    Wadsworth unconstrained elbow p.
    Wagner p.
    Walldius Vitallium mechanical knee p.
    Warsaw hip p.
    Waugh knee p.
    Waugh total ankle replacement p.
    Wayfarer p.
    Weller total hip joint p.
    well-seated p.
    Whitesides knee p.
    Whitesides Ortholoc II condylar femoral p.
    William Harris hip p.
    Wilson-Burstein hip internal p.
    Wright knee p.
    wrist joint implant p.
    Xenophor femoral p.
    YIS knee p.
    Young hinged knee p.
    Young-Vitallium hinged p.
    Zimalite implant metal p.
    Zimaloy femoral head p.
    Zimaloy implant metal p.
    Zimmer Centralign Precoat hip p.
    Zimmer shoulder p.
    Zimmer tibial p.
    Zirconia femoral head p.
    Zirconia orthopedic p.
    zirconium oxide ceramic p.
    Z stent p.
    Zweymuller hip p.

prosthetic
    p. ambulation
    American Board of Certification of Orthotics and P.'s
    American Hand P.'s (AHP)
    p. antibiotic-loaded acrylic cement (PROSTALAC)
    p. antibiotic-loaded acrylic cement total joint prosthesis
    p. arthroplasty
    Cirrus foot p.
    DawSkin p.
    p. design
    p. femorodistal graft
    p. fitting
    p. foam
    p. gait training
    p. hemiarthroplasty
    p. hook
    p. patella

P. Problem Inventory Scale
P. Problem Inventory Scale
  classification
p. replacement
p. socket
p. spacer
p. stance phase shock
p. support
prosthetist
American Academy of Orthotists
  and P.'s
certified p. (CP)
prosthetist/orthotist
certified p. (CPO)
ProStretch exerciser
Protasul
P. femoral prosthesis
P. implant metal
Protasul-10 noncemented femoral
  prosthesis
Protasul-64 WF Zweymuller femoral
  prosthesis
protection
digital artery p.
p. plate
p., restricted activity, ice,
  compression, elevation (PRICE)
protective limitation of range of motion
protector
Alvarado collateral ligament p.
Ankle Ligament p.
ankle ligament p. (ALP)
Cast Gard cast p.
Decubinex p.
grooved p.
Heelbo decubitus heel/elbow p.
Jurgan Pin Ball pin p.
Meds eye p.
M-F heel p.
Ortho-Foam p.
Patellar Band knee p.
PRN p.
ROHO heel p.
Seal-Tight cast p.
ShowerSafe waterproof cast and
  bandage p.
The Heeler inflatable heel p.
tissue p.
Toes P.
UVEX eye p.
Protecto splint

protein
Bence Jones p.
bone morphogenic p.
C-reactive p.
IGF-binding p.
p. malnutrition
morphogenetic p.
protein-polysaccharide synthesis-
  depolymerization equilibrium
Protek prosthesis
proteoglycan
p. degradation
p. synthesis
Proteus mirabilis
prothelen set
prothrombin time (PT)
protocol
Bruce p.
Duran-Houser p.
Evans-Burkhalter p.
Mann p.
Marx osteoradionecrosis p.
North American Malignant
  Hyperthermia p.
p. of Smidt
Protoplast cement
prototype design
Protouch synthetic orthopaedic padding
ProTrac
P. alignment guide
P. cruciate reconstruction system
P. measurement device
P. system for knee surgery
protraction
protractor
arthroidal p.
Demariniff p.
triplanar p.
Zimmer p.
protruding disk
protrusio
p. acetabulum
p. cage
p. deformity
p. ring
p. shell
protrusion
central disk p.
disk p.
lateral disk p.
medial disk p.
p. of the navicular

NOTES

P

protuberans
dermatofibrosarcoma p.
proud flesh
Providence Scoliosis System
provisional
p. fixation
p. prosthesis
p. stabilization
Proxiderm
P. procedure
P. wound closure system
proximal
p. annular pulley of the thumb
p. articular facet angle
p. articular set angle (PASA)
p. bow position
p. carpal row
p. cement spacer
p. communicating branch (PCB)
p. and distal realignment
p. dome osteotomy
p. drill-guide assembly
p. femoral epiphysiolysis
p. femoral focal deficiency (PFFD)
p. femoral fracture
p. femoral metaphyseal shortening
p. femoral osteotomy
p. femoral resection
p. femur
p. fibula
p. first metatarsal osteotomy
p. humeral fracture
p. humeral prosthesis
p. humerus
p. interlocking
p. interphalangeal (PIP)
p. interphalangeal joint (PIPJ)
p. interphalangeal joint approach
p. intrinsic release
p. latency
p. locking
p. medical brim
p. metatarsal approach
p. metatarsal osteotomy
p. midpatellar medial and lateral portals
p. phalangeal epiphysiodesis
p. phalangeal osteotomy
p. phalanx (PP)
p. phalanx osteotomy
p. portion
p. radioulnar articulation
p. radius
p. reference axis (PFA)
p. row carpectomy
p. tendon rupture
p. third (P/3, proximal/3)
p. third femoral prosthesis
p. third of shaft
p. tibia
p. tibial fracture
p. tibial metaphyseal fracture
p. tibial osteotomy
p. tibial plateau
p. tibiofibular joint
p. tibiofibular joint dislocation
p. tibiofibular subluxation
p. tibiofibular synostosis
p.-to-distal ring
p. ulna
p. Wagner metaphyseal shortening
proximal/3
proximal third
proximally
proximal third (P/3, proximal/3)
proximolateral
Prozac
prune-belly syndrome
PSA thermoplastic orthosis
PSC pronation/spring control
PSDK
poststatic dyskinesia
pseudarthrosis, pseudoarthrosis
closed p.
congenital tibial p.
documented p.
extraarticular p.
failed back syndrome with documented p.
fibular p.
Girdlestone p.
interspinous p.
radial p.
p. rate
p. repair
synovial p.
tibial p.
tibular p.
pseudoacetabulum
pseudoaneurysm
pseudoarthrosis (*var. of* pseudarthrosis)
pseudoarticulation
pseudo-Babinski sign
pseudoboutonnière deformity
pseudoclaudication
pseudoclawing
pseudocortex
pseudodislocation
pseudoephedrine and ibuprofen
pseudoepiphysis
pseudoexostosis
pseudofacilitation
pseudofracture
milkman's p.
pseudogamekeeper's injury
pseudogout

pseudohead
pseudo-Hurler deformity
pseudohypertrophy
pseudohypoparathyroidism
pseudomallei
    Pseudomonas p.
pseudometatarsal head
Pseudomonas
    P. aeruginosa
    P. infection
    P. pseudomallei
pseudomyotonic discharge
pseudoneuroma
pseudoosteomyelitis
pseudoparalysis
    Parrot p.
pseudopodium
pseudopolyphasic action potential
pseudoradicular syndrome
pseudosarcomatous reaction
pseudosubluxation
pseudotendon
pseudothrombophlebitis (PTP)
pseudotumorous mucin deposition
pseudovarus
    cubitus p.
PSIS
    posterior sacroiliac spine
    posterosuperior iliac spine
psoas
    p. abscess
    p. muscle
psoriasis
psoriatic arthritis
psychoextended hand
psychoflexed hand
psychogenic
psychologic testing
psychology
    sports p.
psychomotor
psychosomatic
PT
    physical therapy
    physical training
    pronator teres
    prothrombin time
PTB
    patellar tendon-bearing
    pretibial bearing
      PTB ankle-foot orthosis
      PTB brace

      PTB cast
      PTB plastic orthosis
      PTB supracondylar prosthesis
      PTB suprapatellar prosthesis
PT-ball
PTB-SC
    patellar tendon-bearing–supracondylar
PTB-SC-SP prosthesis
pterygium colli
pterygoid plate
PTFE
    polytetrafluoroethylene
      PTFE graft
PTFL
    posterior talofibular ligament
PTI
    pressure-time integral
PTN
    posterior tibial nerve
PTP
    posterior tibial pulse
    pseudothrombophlebitis
PTS
      PTS knee brace
      PTS soft wedge prosthesis
PTSD
    posttraumatic stress disorder
PTT
    posterior tibial tendinitis
PTT
    partial thromboplastin time
    patellar tendon transfer
    posterior tibial tendon
pubalgia
pubic
    p. diastasis
    p. pad
    p. ramus
    p. symphysis
pubicus
    arcus p.
pubis
    osteitis p.
    symphysis p.
pubococcygeus
puboischial area
puborectalis
Pucci
    P. Air orthotic
    P. pediatrics hand orthosis
    P. rehab knee orthosis
    P. splint

NOTES

P

pucker sign
Puddu
>P. drill guide
>P. tendon technique

pudendal
>p. artery
>p. nerve injury
>p. neuritis

Pudenz flushing chamber
Pugh
>P. driver
>P. hip pin
>P. plate
>P. sliding nail
>P. traction

Pugil stick injury
Puka chisel
Pul-Ez
>P.-E. exerciser
>P.-E. shoulder pulley

pull
>p. screw
>spinous p.

pulldown
>lat p.

pulled elbow
pulley
>A1–A4 annular p.
>C1–C3 cruciate p.
>p. exercise
>fibroosseous p.
>Preston overhead p.
>Pul-Ez shoulder p.
>Range-Master p.
>p. reconstruction
>shoulder p.
>weights and p.'s

pull-out
>p.-o. button
>p.-o. strength
>p.-o. suture

Pulmonair 40 bed
pulmonale
>cor p.

pulmonary
>p. atelectasis
>p. complication
>p. contusion
>p. edema
>p. embolism
>p. function test
>p. osteodystrophy

pulp
>p. approach
>finger p.
>p. flap
>p. traction

pulposus
>herniated nucleus p. (HNP, HPN)
>nucleus p.

pulsatile
>p. hypothermic perfusion with
> University of Wisconsin solution
>p. jet lavage
>p. pneumatic plantar-compression
> device
>p. pressure lavage

pulsating electromagnetic field
pulsation
Pulsavac
>P. III wound debridement system
>P. irrigation
>P. lavage

pulse
>blood volume p. (BVP)
>dorsalis pedis p.
>p. irrigator
>p. oximeter
>posterior tibial p. (PTP)
>p. status-pull test

pulsed
>p. electromagnetic field (PEMF)
>p. galvanic stimulator
>p. lavage
>p. short-wave therapy
>p. ultrasound

pulselessness
pulsing current for nonunion of
** fracture**
Pulvertaft
>P. end-to-end suture
>P. fish-mouth stitch
>P. interweave suture
>P. weave technique

pulvinar region
Pulvules
>Darvon Compound-65 P.

pump
>ALZET continuous infusion
> osmotic p.
>ankle rehab p.
>p. bump
>p. bump exostosis
>continuous wave arthroscopy p.
>extremity p.
>EZ hand p.
>p.-handle rib motion
>intermittent extremity p.
>P. It Up pneumatic socket volume
> management system
>Jobst athrombotic p.
>knee p.
>Linvatec arthroscopic infusion p.
>Multipulse 1000 compression p.

sequential extremity p.
venous foot p.
PumpPals insole
punch
Acufex rotary p.
arthroscopic p.
p. biopsy
bone hole p.
boxer's p.
Caspari suture p.
Casselberry suture p.
cervical laminectomy p.
Charnley femoral prosthesis
neck p.
cruciate p.
p. forceps
Hirsch hypophyseal p.
I-beam cement p.
Kerrison p.
keyhole p.
Osborne p.
Rowe glenoid p.
Schlesinger p.
suction p.
tibial p.
TOP ejector p.
tubular p.
punctata
keratosis p.
puncture
p. fracture
lumbar p. (LP)
p. wound
p. wound osteochondritis
Puno-Winter-Byrd (PWB)
P.-W.-B. system
purchase
bony p.
p. and press the ground
socket's p.
toe-ground p.
Purdue pegboard
pure syndactyly
puric
purine metabolism
purposeful activity
purpura
p. fulminans
meningococcal p.
pursestring suture
purulent material
pus

push
p. cuff
knee-chest p.
P. medical brace
prone sacral p.
spinous p.
Push-Ease
P.-E. Quad Cuff
P.-E. wheelchair glove
pusher
Charnley femoral prosthesis p.
hemispherical p.
hook p.
knot p.
Revo loop handle knot p.
push-off
great toe p.-o.
p.-o. by great toe
p.-o. phase of gait
push-pull
p.-p. activity
p.-p. ankle stress view
p.-p. hip view
p.-p. instability
p.-p. move
push-up
p.-u. block
p.-u. test
**putative segmental instantaneous axis of
rotation**
Puth abduction splint
Put-In Driver
Putti
P. bone plast
P. bone rasp
P. knee arthrodesis
P. posterior approach
P. splint
Putti-Platt
P.-P. arthroplasty
P.-P. instrumentation
P.-P. shoulder procedure
putty
AliMed p.
BeOK hand exercise p.
Blue Brand Therapy P.
color-coded therapy p.
Graphton p.
matrix Grafton p.
Thera-Plast p.
Therapy P.

NOTES

P

PUV
　positive ulnar variance
PVC
　polyvinyl chloride
　　PVC drain
　　PVC tubing
PVD
　peripheral vascular disease
　　PVD dressing
PVS
　peripheral vascular surgery
　peripheral vascular system
　pigmented villonodular synovitis
PW
　plantar wart
PWB
　Puno-Winter-Byrd
　　PWB transpedicular spine fixation
　　system
px
　pneumothorax
pyarthrosis
pyelogram
　　intravenous p.
pyknodysostosis
Pyle
　　bone age according to Greulich
　　and P.

pylon
　　AirStance p.
　　p. attachment plate
　　metal p.
　　Stratus impact reducing p.
　　vertical shock p.
pyoderma gangrenosum
pyogenic
　　p. arthritis
　　p. bursitis
　　p. granuloma
　　p. spinal infection
　　p. vertebral osteomyelitis
pyomyositis
　　staphylococcal p.
Pyramesh cage
pyramidal
　　p. fracture
　　p. tract
pyrazinamide
pyridoxine
Pyrilinks-D urine assay
pyrolytic carbon
pyrophosphate
　　p. arthropathy
　　technetium-99m p.
　　technetium stannous p. (TSPP)
Pyrost bone graft material

Q

Q Star Voyager pressure reduction mattress

Q angle
quadriceps angle
Q angle of the knee

QCT
quantitative computed tomography

QF
quadratus femoris

qigong

Qingyangshen (QYS)

Q-Ray bracelet

QST
quantitative sensory testing

quad
quadriceps
quadrilateral
quadriplegic
quad board
quad cane
quad strengthening exercise

quadpolar IF waveform

Quadracut ACL shaver system

quadrangular
q. cartilage
q. positioning plate plate

quadrant
Q. advanced shoulder brace
q. test

quadraphasic scanning

quadrapod cane

quadrate ligament

quadratum
ligamentum q.

quadratus
q. femoris (QF)
q. femoris fascia
q. femoris muscle
q. lumborum muscle
q. lumborum syndrome
q. plantae muscle
pronator q. (PQ)

quadriceps (quad)
q. angle (Q angle)
q. aponeurosis
q. apron
q. atrophy
q. contraction test
q. contracture
q. femoris muscle
q. femoris muscle cast
q. jerk
q. mechanism
q. muscle group

q. reflex
q.-setting exercise
q. tendon
q. wasting

quadricepsplasty
Coonse-Adams q.
Judet q.
Thompson q.
V-Y q.

Quadriflex

quadrilateral (quad)
q. brim
q. frame
q. socket
q. space syndrome

quadriparesis

quadriplegia
spastic q.

quadriplegic (quad)

quadruple complex

Quadtro
Q. cushion
Q. cushion with Isoflap valve

QualCare knee brace

QualCraft
Q. ankle support
Q. short elastic wrist support
Q. splint
Q. strap

quality
q. of gait
q. of life
motion q.

quantitative
q. computed tomography (QCT)
q. sensory testing (QST)

quantity
scalar q.
vector q.

Quantum
Q. foot
Q. Foot prosthesis

Quartzo device

quasi-independent Y-axis movement

quasistatic stressed position

quazepam

Queckenstedt sign

Quengel
Q. apparatus
Q. cast
Q. device
Q. hinge

Quénu-Küss tarsometatarsal injury classification

Quénu nail plate removal technique

Quest
    Fear Avoidance Beliefs Q. (FABQ)
question
    Enneking q.
questionnaire
    American Academy of Orthopaedic
        Surgeons/Hip Society q.
    Behavioral Assessment of Pain Q.
    Children's Comprehensive Pain Q.
        (CCPQ)
    Cincinnati knee scoring q.
    Clinical Analysis Q. (CAQ)
    Cognitive Error Q.
    Cognitive Strategies Q.
    Functional Status Q. (FSQ)
    Illness Behavior Q.
    Illness Depression Q.
    Jan van Breemen Function Q.
        (JVBF)
    Kenney Self-Care Q.
    Lysholm knee scoring q.
    McGill Pain Q.
    McMaster-Toronto arthritis patient
        preference disability q.
    Melzack Pain Q.
    MFA q.
    Modified American Shoulder and
        Elbow Surgeons Shoulder Patient
        Self-Evaluation Form patient q.
    Physical Activity Readiness Q.
        (PAR-Q)
    Roland-Morris Q. (RMQ)
    Shoulder Pain and Disability Index
        patient q.
    Shoulder Severity Index patient q.
    Simple Shoulder Test patient q.
    Subjective Shoulder Rating Scale
        patient q.
    Varni-Thompson Pediatric Pain Q.

Questus leading edge grasper-cutter
Quetelet index
Quickbox container
QuickCast
    Q. splint
    Q. wrist immobilizer
Quickie
    Q. Carbon wheelchair
    Q. EX wheelchair
    Q. GPS wheelchair
    Q. GP Swing-Away wheelchair
    Q. GPV wheelchair
    Q. Kidz wheelchair
    Q. Recliner wheelchair
    Q. Ti wheelchair
Quick-Sil
    Q.-S. silicone system
    Q.-S. starter kit
QuickStick padding
quick stretch
quiescence
quiescent
Quigley traction
Quik splint splint
Quinby pelvic fracture classification
Quincke needle
Quinine
    Hyland's Leg Cramps with Q.
Quinsana Plus
quinti
        abductor digiti q. (ADQ)
        extensor digiti q. (EDQ)
        Huber transfer of abductor
            digiti q.
        opponens digiti q. (ODQ)
QYS
    Qingyangshen

RA
 rheumatoid arthritis
 RA factor
 RA test
rachialgia
rachicentesis, rachiocentesis
rachiochysis
rachiodynia
rachiokyphosis
rachiomyelitis
rachioparalysis
rachioplegia
rachiotomy, rachitomy
rachitic
 r. cat-back
 r. rosary sign
rack
 Hausmann weight r.
racquet-shaped incision
radial
 r. artery
 r. artery injury
 r.-based flap
 r. bearing
 r. bursa
 r. carpal collateral ligament
 r. clubhand
 r. collateral ligament (RCL)
 r. column
 r. deficiency
 r. deviation
 r. digital nerve
 r. drift
 r. epicondylalgia
 r. forearm flap
 r. fracture reduction
 r. head
 r. head anlage
 r. head dislocation
 r. head fracture
 r. head implant prosthesis
 r. head subluxation
 r. hemimelia
 r. laminectomy
 r. malalignment
 r. meniscal tear
 r. metacarpal ligament
 midcarpal r. (MCR)
 r. neck
 r. neck fracture
 r. nerve glove
 r. nerve injury
 r. nerve palsy
 r. pseudarthrosis
 r. reflex

 r. sensory nerve
 r. sensory nerve entrapment
  syndrome
 r. shaft
 r. slab splint
 r. styloid fracture
 r. trial
 r. tuberosity
 r. tunnel
 r. tunnel syndrome
 r. wedge osteotomy
 r. wrist extensor
 r. wrist extensor tendinitis
radiale
 ligamentum collaterale r.
 ligamentum collaterale carpi r.
radialis
 r. brevis
 flexor carpi r. (FCR)
 r. sign
radialized
radian
radiate
 r. carpal ligament
 r. ligament of head of rib
 r. sternocostal ligament
radiation
 r. exposure
 limited-field r.
radiatum
 ligamentum capitis costae r.
 ligamentum carpi r.
radical
 r. compartmental excision
 r. flexor release
 r. nail bed ablation
 r. palmar fasciectomy
 r. resection
radicotomy
radicular
 r. artery
 r. pain
radiculectomy
radiculitis
 cervical r.
radiculomyelopathy
radiculoneuritis
radiculopathy
 cervical r.
radicurogram
radii (*pl. of* radius)
radioactive
 r. iodine-labeled fibrinogen
 r. xenon clearance
radioallergosorbent testing (RAST)

radiocapitate ligament
radiocapitellar
  r. articulation
  r. joint
  r. line
radiocarpal
  r. angle
  r. arthritis
  r. arthrodesis
  r. arthroscopy
  r. articulation
  r. instability
  r. joint
  r. ligament
radiodiagnostic study
radiogram
radiograph
  anterior drawer stress r.
  cross-table lateral r.
  Judet r.
  lumbopelvic r.
  Merchant r.
  spot r.
  stress r.
  tangential standing r.
  Velpeau axillary r.
  weightbearing tangential r.
  West Point axillary lateral r.
radiographic
  r. avascular necrosis
  r. grid
radiography
  biplanar r.
  Brodén stress r.
  carpometacarpal joint r.
  elbow r.
  flexion-extension r.
  patellofemoral joint r.
  scanogram r.
  serendipity view in shoulder r.
  shoulder r.
  stress r.
radiohumeral
  r. articulation
  r. joint
radioisotope
  r. clearance assay
  r. gallium scan
  r. indium-labeled white blood cell scan
  r. technetium scan
  201 r. thallium
radiolucency
radiolucent
  r. line
  r. nidus
  r. roll

  r. sound
  r. splint
radiolunate
  r. fusion
  r. joint
radiolunotriquetral ligament
radionucleotide imaging
radionuclide
  r. scan
  r. scanning
radioscaphocapitate (RSC)
  r. ligament
  r. ligament laxity
radioscaphoid
  r. articulation
  r. fusion
  r. joint
  r. ligament
radioscapholunate
  r. joint
  r. ligament
radiotherapy
  coxa vara deformity pelvic r.
radiotranslucent rod
radiotriquetral ligament
radioulnar
  r. articulation
  r. dissociation
  r. joint
  r. joint injury
  r. subluxation
  r. synostosis (type I, II)
radius, pl. radii
  absent r.
  r. of angulation
  annular ligament of r.
  r. of curvature
  distal r.
  Kapandji fracture of r.
  ligamentum anulare radii
  proximal r.
  thrombocytopenia-absent r. (TAR)
Radley-Liebig-Brown resection
Radovan tissue expander prosthesis
Raeder paratrigeminal syndrome
ragged-red fibers
Ragnell retractor
Raimiste sign
Raimondi hemostatic forceps
Rainbow cast sandal
raising
  contralateral straight leg r.
  crossed-leg straight leg r.
  crossed straight leg r.
  diurnal variation in straight leg r.
  passive straight leg r.
  straight leg r. (SLR)
  well-leg r.

rake-handle effect
rake retractor
rales and rhonchi
Ralks
    R. bone drill
    R. fingernail drill
    R. mallet
raloxifene
Ralston-Thompson pseudarthrosis
    technique
rami (*pl. of* ramus)
RAM knee prosthesis
ramp load
ramus, pl. **rami**
    dorsal rami
    pubic r.
Ranawat-Burstein
    R.-B. hip prosthesis
    R.-B. porous stem
Ranawat classification
Ranawat-DeFiore-Straub
    R.-D.-S. osteotomy
    R.-D.-S. technique
Ranawat-Dorr-Inglis method
Rancho
    R. ankle foot control device
    R. anklet foot control apparatus
    R. Cube System
    R. external fixation instrument
    R. swivel hinge
Randelli shoulder prosthesis
random pattern flap
Raney
    R. bone drill
    R. flexion jacket brace
    R. perforator drill
    R. saw guide
Raney-Crutchfield
    R.-C. drill point
    R.-C. tongs
    R.-C. tong traction
range
    r. of excursion
    motion r.
    r. of motion (ROM)
    r. of motion brace
    r. of motion exercise
    r. of motion therapy
Range-Master pulley
range-of-motion
    r.-o.-m. measurement

    r.-o.-m. restriction
    r.-o.-m. testing
Ranger
    Home R.
Ransford loop
Ranvier
    groove of R.
    zone of R.
raphe
    anterolateral r.
    median r.
RAP-n-roll
Rappaport osteotomy
rarefaction
rasp, raspatory
    Acufex convex r.
    Alexander r.
    Alexander-Farabeuf r.
    angled r.
    Arthrofile orthopaedic r.
    Aufricht glabellar r.
    Austin Moore r.
    Bacon r.
    Bardeleben r.
    bell r.
    BIAS r.
    Black r.
    Bristow r.
    Brown r.
    carbon-tungsten r.
    Charnley r.
    Coryllos r.
    Cottle r.
    Cottle-MacKenty r.
    custom r.
    DePuy r.
    Doyen costal r.
    Doyen rib r.
    Epstein bone r.
    Farabeuf bone r.
    Farabeuf-Collin r.
    femoral r.
    first rib r.
    Fisher r.
    Fomon r.
    Gallagher r.
    Herczel rib r.
    Hylin r.
    Joseph r.
    Key r.
    Kleinert-Kutz r.
    Koenig r.

R

NOTES

rasp *(continued)*
    Langenbeck r.
    Lewis r.
    Maltz r.
    McCabe-Farrior r.
    orthopaedic r.
    r. pin
    power r.
    Putti bone r.
    triangular r.
    ulnar r.
raspatory
    Farabeuf-Lambotte r.
rasped
RAST
    radioallergosorbent testing
Rastelli prosthesis
ratchet
    r. clamp
    r.-type brace
rate
    erythrocyte sedimentation r. (ESR)
    firing r.
    fusion nonunion r.
    heart r. (HR)
    implant survival r.
    nonunion r.
    pseudarthrosis r.
    sed r.
    vertebral osteosynthesis fusion r.
    Westergren sedimentation r.
rated perceived exertion (RPE)
Rath treatment table
rating
    McGuire r.
    r. of perceived exertion
    r. system
ratio
    AB/AD r.
    abductor/adductor r.
    ankle-brachial pressure r.
    Blackburn-Peel r.
    Brattström condylar height r.
    ER/IR r.
    external/internal rotation r.
    Holdaway r.
    Insall-Salvati r.
    metaphyseal to diaphyseal width r.
    Poisson r.
    vastus medialis obliquus:vastus
     lateralis electromyographic r.
     (VMO:VL EMG ratio)
    VMO:VL r.
Ratliff
    R. avascular necrosis classification
rat-tooth forceps
Rauchfuss sling

rave
    fracture en r.
raw bone
ray
    r. amputation
    border r.
    central r.
    finger r.
    long axis r.
    metatarsal r.
    multiple r.
    Peacock transposing index r.
    plantarflexed first r.
    pollicized r.
    r. resection
    R. screw
    transposing index r.
Ray-Clancy-Lemon technique
Rayhack technique
Raymond shoulder immobilizer
Raynaud
    R. disease
    R. phenomenon
Ray-Parsons-Sunday staphylorrhaphy
  elevator
Rayport muscular biopsy clamp
Ray-Tec sponge
razor
    Credo r.
RB1 suture
RC
    rotator cuff
RCAI
    Restorative Care of America,
     Incorporated
RCL
    radial collateral ligament
RCSP
    resting calcaneal stance position
RDF
    Adriamycin R.
reacher
    Double Duty cane r.
    E-Z R.
    Pik Stick R.
reaction
    compensation r.
    curiosity r.
    epidermophytid r.
    exaggeration r.
    r. force
    giant cell r.
    ground r.
    hunting r.
    id r.
    implant r.
    litigation r.
    pseudosarcomatous r.

R

r. time
vagal r.
reactive
low-surface r.
r. periosteal proliferation
r. synovitis
REACT muscle stimulator
Read gouge
Real-EaSE neck and shoulder relaxer
realign
realignment
distal r.
Elmslie-Trillat r.
Galeazzi r.
Genutrain PE patellar r.
Hauser r.
Hughston r.
Insall proximal r.
Madigan-Wissinger-Donaldson
proximal r.
patellar r.
patellofemoral r.
r. procedure
proximal and distal r.
Roux-Goldthwait r.
Reality Orientation Chart
ream
reamed nail
reamer
acetabular r.
acorn r.
Aequalis r.
Anspach r.
Aufranc r.
Austin Moore r.
ball r.
blunt tapered T-handled r.
bone r.
r. brace
brace-type r.
calcar r.
Campbell r.
cannulated Henderson r.
chamfer r.
Charnley deepening r.
Charnley expanding r.
Charnley taper r.
Charnley trochanter r.
cheese-grater hemispherical r.
Christmas tree r.
r. clamp
concave-surface r.

conical r.
corrugated r.
cup r.
debris-retaining r.
deepening r.
DePuy r.
end-cutting r.
expanding r.
female r.
fenestrated r.
flexible medullary r.
fluted r.
grater r.
r. guide
Hall Versipower r.
handle-type r.
Harris brace-type r.
Harris center-cutting acetabular r.
hollow mill r.
humeral r.
Indiana r.
Intracone intramedullary r.
Küntscher r.
male r.
medullary canal r.
Mira r.
motorized r.
multisized r.
Norton ball r.
orthopaedic r.
Perthes r.
power r.
Pressure Sentinel r.
rigid r.
Rush rod awl r.
Smith-Petersen r.
spiral cortical r.
spiral trochanteric r.
spot-face r.
step-cut r.
straight power r.
tapered hand r.
T-handled r.
triple r.
trochanteric r.
Wagner acetabular r.
reaming
r. awl
closed intramedullary nailing
with r.
reamputation

NOTES

reanastomosis of blood supply to bone graft
rear-entry ACL drill guide
rearfoot
  r. ligament
  r. stability system (RSS)
  r. valgus
  r. varus
reassessment
reattachment
  Amstutz r.
  Doll trochanteric r.
  four-wire trochanter r.
  Harris four-wire trochanter r.
  Volz-Turner r.
rebound
  r. hyperextension
  r. tenderness
Rebounder
  Plyoback R.
recalcitrant
  r. pain
  r. plantar fasciitis
receiver operating characteristic (ROC)
recent dislocation
receptor
  delta r.
  epicritic r.
  epsilon r.
  kappa r.
  MV1, MV2 r.
  nociceptive r.
  opioid r.
  postural r.
  sigma r.
receptor-tonus method
recess
  annular periradial r.
  Flatt r.
  lateral r.
  popliteal r.
recession
  Bleck iliopsoas r.
  gastrocnemius r.
  iliopsoas r.
  Strayer gastrocnemius r.
  Strayer gastroc-soleus r.
  tongue-in-groove r.
  ulnar r.
recipient
  r. site
  r. team
reciprocal
  r. innervation
  r. isokinetic testing
  r. planing instrument
  r. relaxation

reciprocating
  r. motor saw
  r. power handpiece
reciprocation gait orthosis (RGO)
reciprocator
  LSU r.
recliner
  Hydro Soothe r.
  Ortho-Biotic r.
Recon
  R. nail
  R. proximal drill guide bolt
reconstituted depolymerized heparin
reconstruction
  ACL r.
  Allman modification of Evans ankle r.
  Andrews iliotibial band r.
  anterior capsulolabral r. (ACLR)
  arthroscopically assisted anterior cruciate ligament r.
  Bankart r.
  bifurcated vein graft (autologous pedal) for vascular r.
  Brown knee joint r.
  capsular-shift r.
  Cho anterior cruciate ligament r.
  Chrisman-Snook r.
  Clancy-Andrews r.
  Clancy cruciate ligament r.
  complex acetabular r.
  cruciate ligament r.
  d'Aubigne femoral r.
  d'Aubigne resection r.
  Eaton-Littler ligament r.
  Ecker-Lotke-Glazer tendon r.
  Ellison lateral knee r.
  Elmslie r.
  endoscopic anterior cruciate ligament r.
  Eriksson cruciate ligament r.
  Evans lateral ankle r.
  exogenous r.
  extraarticular r.
  five-in-one knee r.
  five-one r.
  Goldner r.
  hand r.
  Harmon hip r.
  House r.
  Hughston-Degenhardt r.
  Hughston-Jacobson lateral compartment r.
  index metacarpophalangeal joint r.
  Insall anterior cruciate ligament r.
  intraarticular r.
  joint r.
  Jones-Ellison ACL r.

juxtacubital r.
Krukenberg hand r.
Kugelberg r.
Lange Achilles tendon r.
Larson ligament r.
lateral compartment r.
Lee r.
L'Episcopo hip r.
ligament r.
MacIntosh over-the-top ACL r.
modified Chrisman-Snook ankle r.
Nathan-Trung modification of
  Krukenberg hand r.
Neer posterior shoulder r.
Nicholas five-in-one r.
O'Donoghue ACL r.
osteoplastic r.
r. plate
pulley r.
Rosenberg endoscopic anterior
  cruciate ligament r.
Silfverskiöld Achilles tendon r.
sternoclavicular joint r.
sural island flap for foot and
  ankle r.
Swanson r.
tenoplastic r.
thumb r.
Torg knee r.
two-stage tendon graft r.
Verdan osteoplastic thumb r.
Vulpius Achilles tendon r.
Watson-Jones r.
Whitman femoral neck r.
Zancolli r.
reconstructive measure
record
computerized patient r. (CPR)
recording
r. electrode
intramuscular r.
recovery
postanesthesia r. (PAR)
r. room (RR)
sagittal fast-short T1 inversion r.
  (STIR)
short tau inversion r. (STIR)
recrudescence
recruitment
r. frequency
r. interval
myopathic r.

neuropathic r.
r. pattern
rectal
r. artery
RMS r.
rectangle
Hartshill r.
Luque r.
rectangular
r. awl
r. frame
rectilinear motion
rectus
r. abdominis flap
r. abdominis muscle
r. femoris
r. femoris contracture
r. femoris flap
r. femoris muscle
r. femoris tendon
r. position
r. sheath
recumbency
recumbent
r. cycle
r. position
r. posture
recurrent
r. disorder
r. hyperextension
r. laryngeal nerve
r. laryngeal nerve injury
r. median nerve block
r. meningeal nerve
r. patellar dislocation
r. synovitis
recurvatum
r. angulation deformity
cubitus r.
genu r.
r. test
red
R. Cross freeze-dried allograft
r. light neon laser
r. marrow
r. response
Reddihough scale
Redi-Around finger splint
Rediform orthotic
Redigrip
R. knee pad
R. pressure bandage

NOTES

Redi head halter
Redi-Trac
    R.-T. traction apparatus
    R.-T. traction device
Redi-Vac cast cutter
reduced
    r. insertion activity
    r. interference pattern
reduction
    Ace bandage r.
    Agee force-couple splint r.
    Allen r.
    Aston cartilage r.
    Barsky macrodactyly r.
    Becton open r.
    Boitzy open r.
    Burwell-Charnley classification of
      fracture r.
    Calandriello hip r.
    calcaneal fracture r.
    closed r. (CR)
    concentric r.
    Cooper r.
    Crego hip r.
    Crosby r.
    Cubbins open r.
    delayed open r.
    Dias-Giegerich open r.
    Eaton closed r.
    Eaton-Malerich r.
    Essex-Lopresti open r.
    femoral neck fracture r.
    Ferguson hip r.
    Flynn femoral neck fracture r.
    force-couple splint r.
    r. forceps
    Fowles open r.
    r. of fracture
    fracture r.
    fracture-dislocation r.
    Hankin r.
    Hastings open r.
    hip r.
    Houghton-Akroyd open r.
    incomplete r.
    indirect r.
    internal fixation, closed r.
    Kaplan open r.
    Kinast indirect r.
    King open r.
    Lange hip r.
    Lavine r.
    Lorenz hip r.
    Lowell r.
    McBride hallux abductovalgus r.
    McBride hallux valgus r.
    McKeever open r.
    McReynolds open r.

    Moberg-Gedda open r.
    Neer open r.
    open r.
    r. osteotomy
    Parvin r.
    percutaneous r.
    perioperative r.
    Pratt open r.
    prone r.
    radial fracture r.
    Ridlon hip r.
    r. ring
    shoulder r.
    side posture r.
    Speed-Boyd open r.
    Speed open r.
    spondylolisthesis r.
    stable r.
    sternoclavicular joint r.
    surgical r.
    swan-neck deformity r.
    r. syndactyly
    r. technique
    trial r.
    Wayne County r.
    Weber-Brunner-Freuler open r.
reduction/fixation
    spondylolisthesis r.
Redutemp
Reebok
    R. shoe
    R. Slide System
    R. Step System
Reece
    R. orthopedic shoe
    R. osteotomy guide
Reed cast belt
reeducation
    muscular r.
reefing
    capsular r.
    r. of the medial retinaculum of
      the knee
    r. procedure
reeling gait
Reese
    R. dermatome
    R. osteotomy guide system
reevaluate
reexploration
reference
    biomechanical frame of r.
    r. electrode
referral
referred
    r. anatomic phenomenon
    r. neuritic pain
    r. point

r. trigger point pain
r. trigger point phenomenon

refill

capillary r.

refixation
reflection

Campbell triceps r.
R. I, V, and FSO acetabular cup
R. liner

reflex

abdominal r.
absent r.
accommodation r.
Achilles tendon r.
adductor r.
anal r.
ankle r.
r. arc
asymmetric incurvatum r.
asymmetric tonic neck r. (ATNR)
axon r.
Babinski r.
Bekhterev-Mendel r.
biceps r.
blink r.
Brain r.
bulbocavernosus r.
consensual light r.
cremasteric r.
crossed extensor r.
cutaneous axon r.
deep tendon r. (DTR)
delayed r.
depressed r.
dorsal r.
elbow r.
r. examination
extensor thrust r.
flexor withdrawal r.
r. function
Gordon r.
R. Gun
r. hammer
Hirschberg r.
Hoffmann r.
hyperactive r.
hypoactive deep tendon r.
incurvatum r.
jaw opening r. (JOR)
knee jerk r.
Mendel-Bekhterev r.

Moro r.
motor r.
muscle stretch r.
r. muscular contraction
neck r.
neck-righting r.
r. neurovascular dystrophy
Oppenheim r.
parachute r.
patellar r.
patelloadductor r.
pathologic r.
pectoral r.
placing r.
plantar r.
postcast compression r.
quadriceps r.
radial r.
Remak r.
righting r.
rooting r.
scapular r.
scapulohumeral r.
slow stretch r.
somatosomatic r.
startle r.
Stookey r.
stretch r.
sudomotor startle r.
suprapatellar r.
r. sympathetic dystrophy (RSD)
tendon r.
r. therapy
r. threshold
toe r.
tonic neck r.
triceps surae r.
ulnar r.
vasomotor startle r.
vertebra prominens r.
vertical suspension r.
viscerosomatic r.
von Bekhterev r.

ReFlexion implant system
reflexogenic
reflexology
Re-Flex VSP artificial foot
Refobacin Palacos cement
refractory

r. neuroma
r. period

R

NOTES

Refsum
R. disease
R. syndrome
Regal Acrylic/Stretch prosthetic sock
regenerated fibroblast
regeneration
r. motor unit potential
r. of nerve
osteoblastic bone r.
tibial bone defect r.
r. torus
Regen flexion exercise
regimen
postoperative r.
region
H r.
Hookian r.
hypochondriac r.
metazonal r.
physeal r.
posterior longitudinal fiber r.
posterior oblique fiber r.
posteromedial r.
pulvinar r.
superomedial r.
true acetabular r.
regional
r. anesthesia
r. block
registration
sensory r.
Registry
National Football Head and Neck
Injury R.
Regitine
Regnauld
R. degeneration of MTP joint
R. enclavement
R. free phalangeal base autograft
for hallux limitus
R. modification of Keller
arthroplasty
R. procedure
Regranex Gel, 0.01%
regular
r. sinus rhythm
r. stem
R. Strength Bayer Enteric 500
Aspirin
Rehab
2+2 R. Collar
Jump Start R.
rehabilitation
aquatic r.
remote locomotor r.
Stage model of industrial r.
Rehability
Reichenheim-King procedure

Reichenheim technique
Reichert-Mundinger stereotactic device
Reimers
R. hip position migration index
R. instability index
reimplantation
Reiner plaster knife
Reinert acetabular extensile approach
reinforcement
Bragard r.
Reintegration to Normal Living index
reinterpretation
hypnotic r.
reirrigation
Reiter
R. disease
R. syndrome
ReJuveness scar treatment
Relafen
relapsing ankle sprain
relation to subadjacent segments
relative
r. refractory period
r. response attributable to the
maneuver (RRAM)
r. risk (RR)
Relax-A-Bac posture support
relaxant
muscle r.
relaxation
r. phenomenon
postisometric r.
reciprocal r.
r. response
relaxer
Real-EaSE neck and shoulder r.
relaxing incision
release
adductor tendon and lateral
capsular r.
anterior hip r.
anterior shoulder r.
anterolateral r.
Baxter nerve r.
Beaty lateral r.
bipolar r.
brevis r.
capsular r.
carpal tunnel r. (CTR)
clubfoot r.
complete subtalar r. (CSR)
distal intrinsic r.
distal soft tissue r. (DSTR)
Dupuytren contracture r.
Eberle contracture r.
endoscopic carpal tunnel r. (ECTR,
ECTRA)

Endotrac endoscopic carpal
tunnel r.
Endotrac system for carpal
tunnel r.
entensile r.
fascial r.
Ferkel bipolar r.
r. of the flexor hallucis longus
tendon
flexor hallucis longus tendon r.
flexor-pronator origin r.
Guyon tunnel r.
hamstring r.
Heyman-Herndon r.
Heyman-Herndon-Strong capsular r.
Inglis-Cooper r.
interleukin-1 beta r.
John Barnes myofascial r.
joint r.
key r.
Kinetix instrument for carpel
tunnel r.
lateral capsular r.
lateral extensor r.
lateral retinaculum r.
leg compartment r.
ligamentous r.
Little r.
Mirua-Komada r.
Mital elbow r.
modified two-portal endoscopic
carpal tunnel r.
myofascial r.
Ober r.
patellar retinacula r.
r. phenomenon
plantar fascial r.
plantar-lateral r.
plantar-medial r.
plantar plate r.
posterolateral r.
posteromedial r. (PMR)
pronator teres r.
proximal intrinsic r.
radical flexor r.
retinacular r.
retrogeniculate hamstring r.
Sengupta quadriceps r.
Siegel hip r.
Snow-Littler r.
soft tissue r.
spinal fascial r.

tarsal tunnel r. (TTR)
tendon r.
triceps surae r.
trigger finger r.
trigger thumb r.
Turco clubfoot r.
Turco posteromedial r.
Ueba r.
ulnar nerve r.
unipolar r.
Williams-Haddad r.
Z-plasty r.
released ulnar intrinsic muscle
Reliance CM femoral implant
component
Relief
Solarcaine Aloe Extra Burn R.
Tylenol Extended R.
Reliever
Arthritis Foundation Pain R.
Cama Arthritis Pain R.
relieving incision
relocation test
Relton-Hall frame
Remak reflex
remediation
biokinetic r.
Remifemin herbal product
remifentanil
remobilization
remodeling
bone r.
cortical bone r.
haversian bone r.
r. phase
remote
r. locomotor rehabilitation
r. pedicle flap
removable cast
removal
Cameron femoral component r.
cast r.
cement r.
Collis-Dubrul femoral stem r.
Harris femoral component r.
implant r.
metastatic tumor r.
Moreland-Marder-Anspach femoral
stem r.
nail fold r.
nail plate r.

NOTES

removal *(continued)*
    stem r.
    Winograd nail plate r.
remover
    Biomet Ultra-Drive cement r.
    Craig pin r.
Remular-S
renal osteodystrophy
Renee creak sign
Renografin contrast media
Renolux convertible car seat
reoperation
repair
    Abraham-Pankovich tendo
     calcaneus r.
    ACL r.
    acromioclavicular joint r.
    all-inside r.
    Atasoy-type flap for nail injury r.
    Bankart shoulder r.
    Barnhart r.
    Becker tendon r.
    Black r.
    bone graft r.
    Bosworth tendo calcaneus r.
    Boyd-Anderson biceps tendon r.
    brachial plexus r.
    Bunnell tendon r.
    Caspari r.
    delayed primary r.
    dog-ear r.
    dural r.
    DuVries hammertoe r.
    dynamic r.
    Ecker-Lotke-Glazer patellar
     tendon r.
    end-to-end tendon r.
    end-to-side r.
    epineural r.
    extensor tendon r.
    fascicular r.
    first-toe Jones r.
    five-in-one knee ligament r.
    five-one knee ligament r.
    flexor tendon r.
    fracture r.
    Froimson-Oh r.
    glenohumeral dislocation r.
    grouped fascicular r.
    group fascicular r.
    inguinal TEPP r.
    Jones first-toe r.
    Kelikian-Riashi-Gleason patellar
     tendon r.
    Kessler r.
    Kleinert r.
    r. of the knee for rotatory
     instability

    Lange tendon lengthening and r.
    Lindholm open surgical tendon r.
    Lindholm tendo calcaneus r.
    Lynn tendo calcaneus r.
    MacIntosh over-the-top r.
    MacNab shoulder r.
    Ma-Griffith ruptured Achilles
     tendon r.
    Ma-Griffith tendo calcaneus r.
    Mandelbaum-Nartolozzi-Carney
     patellar tendon r.
    Marshall ligament r.
    medial r.
    meniscal r.
    Palmer-Dobyns-Linscheid ligament r.
    patellar tendon r.
    plastic r.
    primary r.
    pseudarthrosis r.
    rod fracture r.
    rotator cuff r.
    Scuder r.
    semitendinosus augmentation of
     patellar tendon r.
    Sever-L'Episcopo shoulder r.
    shoulder r.
    Speed sternoclavicular r.
    Staples r.
    Staples-Black-Broström ligament r.
    Strickland tendon r.
    suture r.
    Talesnick scapholunate r.
    tendon r.
    TEPP r.
    Teuffer tendo calcaneus r.
    tissue r.
    triad knee r.
    triple ligamentous r.
    Tsuge tendon r.
    Turco-Spinella tendo calcaneus r.
    volar plate r.
    Watson-Jones fracture r.
reparative
    r. granuloma
    r. phase
REP Bands exercise band
repeated
    r. quick stretch (RQS)
    r. quick stretch from elongation
     (RQS-E)
    r. quick stretch superimposed upon
     an existing contraction (RQS-
     SEC)
reperfusion injury
repetition
    r. maximum (RM)
    r. strain injury (RSI)
    r. time (TR)

repetitive
  r. discharge
  r. exercise
  r. nerve stimulation
  r. stress syndrome (RSS)
  r. trauma disorder (RTD)
replacement
  allograft ligament r.
  alumina bioceramic joint r.
  Amstutz total hip r.
  anatomic porous r. (APR)
  Averill total hip r.
  Biolox ceramic ball head for
    hip r.
  calcar r.
  Capello total hip r.
  Charnley total hip r.
  dynamic double tendon r.
  electrolyte r.
  Engh total hip r.
  Ewald total elbow r.
  facet r.
  failed joint r.
  hip r.
  Howse total hip r.
  hybrid total hip r.
  hypnotic r.
  intercalary segmental r.
  Kirschner Medical Dimension
    hip r.
  ligament r.
  Lunceford total hip r.
  Marmor r.
  PCA total hip r.
  Pilliar total hip r.
  porous-coated anatomic total hip r.
  prosthetic r.
  Ring UPM total hip r.
  Ring UPM total knee r.
  SAF hip r.
    self-articulating femoral hip
      replacement
  Scarborough total hip r.
  self-articulating femoral hip r.
    (SAF hip replacement)
  self-bearing ceramic total hip r.
  Stanmore knee r.
  Stanmore total hip r.
  surface r.
  Tharies hip r.
  tile plate facet r.
  total hip r. (THR)

  total joint r. (TJR)
  total knee r. (TKR)
  total ossicular r. (TORP)
  TPL-6 total hip r.
  TR-28 total hip r.
replantable amputation
replantation
  r. bandage
  limb r.
RepliCare wound dressing
Replica total hip replacement system
repolarization
repositioner
  Wilson-Cook prosthesis r.
reprep and drape
reproducibility
reproducible
Repro head halter
reroute
rerouting
  Blair-Omer r.
  r. insertion
  Zancolli biceps tendon r.
Rescudose
  Roxanol R.
Research
  Agency for Health Care Policy
    and R. (AHCPR)
  Alvarado Orthopedic R.
  Foundation for Chiropractic
    Education and R. (FCER)
resect
resecting fracture
resection
  r. arthrodesis
  r. arthroplasty
  Badgley iliac wing r.
  bar r.
  bone r.
  bony bridge r.
  calcaneal r.
  calcaneonavicular bar r.
  Carrell r.
  caudal lamina r.
  Clayton procedure with
    panmetatarsal head r.
  cuff r.
  Darrach r.
  r. dermodesis
  Dillwyn-Evans r.
  Dwar-Barrington r.
  en bloc r.

R

NOTES

resection (*continued*)
    epiphyseal bar r.
    extraarticular r.
    femoral r.
    first rib r.
    Girdlestone r.
    Guller r.
    Gurd r.
    Henry r.
    Hoffmann panmetatarsal head r.
    iliac wing r.
    Ingram bony bridge r.
    innominate bone r.
    intercalary r.
    intralesional r.
    Janecki-Nelson shoulder girdle r.
    Karakousis-Vezeridis r.
    Kashiwagi r.
    kyphos r.
    Langenskiöld bony bridge r.
    Lewis-Chekofsky r.
    Lewis intercalary r.
    Localio-Francis-Rossano r.
    local radical r.
    Malawer r.
    Mankin r.
    Marcove-Lewis-Huvos shoulder girdle r.
    marginal r.
    Mayo metatarsal head r.
    medial eminence r.
    medial malleolus r.
    r. of meniscus
    metatarsal head r.
    Milch cuff r.
    Miltner-Wan calcaneus r.
    Mumford r.
    panmetatarsal head r.
    Phelps partial r.
    prophylactic r.
    proximal femoral r.
    radical r.
    Radley-Liebig-Brown r.
    ray r.
    r.-realignment
    Rockwood r.
    Stener-Gunterberg r.
    Thompson r.
    Tikhoff-Linberg shoulder girdle r.
    transoral odontoid r.
    tumor r.
    vertebral r.
    Weaver-Dunn r.
    wedge r.
resection-arthrodesis
    Enneking r.-a.
resector
    Accu-Line femoral r.

    Accu-Line tibial r.
    r. blade
    full-radius r.
    orthotome r.
    synovial r.
reserve
    breathing r. (BR)
residence ridge
residual
    r. heel equinus
    r. hindfoot equinus
    r. latency
    r. limb
    r. tension
residuum
resilience
resin
    polyacetal r.
resistance
    growth hormone r.
    isometric r.
    isotonic r.
    manual r.
    plyometric r.
    strength against r.
    Thera-Band System of Progressive R.
resistant clubfoot
resisted
    r. active flexion
    r. dorsiflexion
resistive
    r. chair exercise kit
    r. exercise
    r. exerciser
    r. exercise table
resonance
    nuclear magnetic r. (NMR)
resorbable
    r. ceramic
    r. plate
    r. polydioxanon pin
resorption
    bone r.
    osteoclastic r.
    tuftal r.
respiratory
    r. disorder
    r. exhaust system
Respond II muscle stimulator
response
    average evoked r.
    axon r.
    blink r.
    brainstem auditory evoked r. (BAER)
    decremental r.
    "deh chi" r.

delayed r.
evoked r.
foreign body r.
galvanic skin r.
hyperactive r.
incremental r.
incrementing r.
r. interval
late r.
motion r.
motor r.
paired r.
physiologic r.
pilomotor r.
plantar Babinski r.
red r.
relaxation r.
sensory r.
visual evoked r. (VER)

rest
bed r.
Core Hibak R.
Core Lobak R.
Core Sitback R.
foot r.
r., ice, compression, elevation (RICE)
kidney r.
Mayfield head r.
Mouse Nest mouse r.
pain at r.

Restcue bed
resting
r. ankle-arm Doppler index
r. calcaneal stance position (RCSP)
r. foot sling
r. forefoot supination angle
r. length
r. membrane potential
r. orthosis
r. tremor

restless leg
Reston
R. dressing
R. padding

restoration
R. acetabular system
functional r.
R. GAP acetabular cup
intrinsic r.
pinch r.
R. Secur-Fit X'tra acetabular shell

Restoration-HA hip system
Restorative Care of America, Incorporated (RCAI)
restorative pin
restorator
Restore
R. AF antifungal lotion
R. AF antimicrobial skin cleanser
R. AF antimicrobial solution
R. CalciCare dressing
R. Clean 'N Moist

Restoril
restraint
active r.
passive r.
poncho r.
universal canvas body r.

restricted
r. inversion
r. range of motion

restriction
extension r.
flexion r.
intercostal r.
lateral flexion r.
motion r.
r. of motion
range-of-motion r.
rotational r.
skin r.
soft tissue r.

restrictive bandage
restrictor
Biostop G cement r.
cement r.
plastic marrow canal r.

result
false-negative r.

resurfacing
Amstutz r.
bone r.
island adipofascial flap in Achilles tendon r.
r. operation
Paltrinieri-Trentani r.
patellar r.
r. procedure
Salzer r.

retained
retainer
Thermoskin heat r.

retaining knee prosthesis

R

NOTES

retardation
    growth r.
    healing r.
retention
    r. drill
    r. suture
    urinary r.
reticula (*pl. of* reticulum)
reticular cell sarcoma
reticulated polyurethane pad
reticulin stain
reticulocytosis
    cerebroside r.
reticulohistiocytosis
    multicentric r.
reticulum, pl. reticula
    endoplasmic r.
    sarcoplasmic r.
retinacular
    r. artery
    r. hood
    r. ligament
    r. release
retinaculum, pl. retinacula
    caudal r.
    extensor r.
    flexor r.
    inferior peroneal r.
    patellar r.
    superior peroneal r. (SPR)
    Weitbrecht r.
retinal anlage tumor
retraction
    Schink metatarsal r.
retractor
    Adson cerebellar r.
    Adson hemilaminectomy r.
    Allport r.
    Alm wound r.
    amputation r.
    appendiceal r.
    Army-Navy r.
    Assistant Free long prong collateral
      ligament r.
    Assistant Free Shubbs short prong
      collateral ligament r.
    Assistant Free wide PCL r.
    Aufranc cobra r.
    Badgley laminectomy r.
    Balfour self-retaining r.
    Ballantine hemilaminectomy r.
    Beckman r.
    Bennett r.
    Bertin hip r.
    blade-point r.
    blade-spike r.
    Blount anvil r.
    Blount knee r.

    Bodnar r.
    Boyle-Davis r.
    Busenkell posterior hip r.
    Campbell nerve root r.
    Carroll-Bennett r.
    Carroll hand r.
    Caspar r.
    cerebellar r.
    Chandler knee r.
    Charnley horizontal r.
    Charnley initial incision r.
    Charnley pin r.
    Charnley self-retaining r.
    Cloward blade r.
    cobra r.
    Collis r.
    Collis-Taylor r.
    Cooley rib r.
    crank frame r.
    Crego r.
    curved r.
    Cushing r.
    Darrach r.
    Deaver r.
    deep r.
    D'Errico r.
    Doane knee r.
    double bent Hohmann acetabular r.
    double-ended right-angle r.
    double-hook Lovejoy r.
    Downey hemilaminectomy r.
    Dozier radiolucent Bennett r.
    dual nerve root suction r.
    East-West r.
    Fahey r.
    fat pad r.
    Finochietto rib r.
    five-prong rake blade r.
    flat r.
    Freebody-Steinmann r.
    Fukuda humeral head r.
    Gelpi r.
    Gifford mastoid r.
    handheld r.
    Hayes r.
    Hays hand r.
    heavy-duty two-tooth r.
    Hedblom rib r.
    Heiss soft tissue r.
    Henning meniscal r.
    Hibbs r.
    Hibbs-type r.
    Hoen r.
    Hohmann r.
    Holscher knee r.
    Holscher root r.
    Holzheimer r.
    Homan r.

humeral head r.
Inge r.
Israel r.
Kasdan r.
Kirschenbaum r.
Kleinert-Ragdell r.
Kocher r.
Lange bone r.
Lange-Hohmann bone r.
Langenbeck r.
Love nerve root r.
lower hand r.
Lowman hand r.
Luongo hand r.
Markham-Meyerding r.
Mark II Chandler total knee r.
Mark II concave total knee r.
Mark II lateral collateral
  ligament r.
Mark II modular weight r.
Mark II "S" total knee r.
Mark II Stubbs short prong
  collateral ligament r.
Mark II wide PCL knee r.
Mark II "Z" knee r.
Mayo-Collins r.
McCullough r.
McIver ENT r.
Meyerding r.
mini-Hohmann r.
Morris r.
Mueller r.
Myers knee r.
narrow-blade r.
narrow-neck mini-Hohmann r.
Nelson rib r.
Ollier rake r.
orthopaedic r.
Paulson knee r.
pin r.
Ragnell r.
rake r.
rib r.
Richardson r.
ring r.
Rosenberg r.
Sauerbruch r.
Scholten sternal r.
Scoville r.
self-retaining r.
Senn r.

sharp r.
Sims r.
single-prong broad acetabular r.
skid humeral head r.
Smillie r.
Sofield r.
soft tissue blade r.
Southwick two-tined r.
standard 2-inch blade r.
standard 4-inch blade r.
stiff ribbon r.
Tang r.
Taylor r.
three-prong rake blade r.
two-prong rake r.
upper hand r.
U-shaped r.
Volkmann rake r.
Wagner r.
Watanabe r.
Weit-Arner r.
Weitlaner r.
Wichman r.
Williams self-retaining r.
Wilson gonad r.
Wink r.
Z r.

retriever
  Kleinert-Kutz tendon r.
  magnetic r.
retroacetabular lesion
retrobulbar prosthesis needle
retrocalcaneal
  r. bursa
  r. bursitis
  r. exostosis
retrodisplaced fracture
retroflexion
  tibial r.
retrogeniculate hamstring release
retrograde
  r. Beaver blade
  r.-cutting hook-shaped knife
  r. degeneration
  r. meniscal blade
  r. method
  r. nailing
retrolisthesed fragment
retrolisthesis positional dyskinesia
retromedullary arteriovenous
  malformation

R

NOTES

retropatellar
  r. fat pad
  r. fat pad contracture
retroperitoneal
  r. approach
  r. decompression
  r. fibrosis
  r. hemorrhage
  r. space
retropharyngeal
  r. abscess
  r. approach
  r. fascial cleft
  r. space
retropulsed
  r. bone excision
  r. bony fragment
retropulsion of gait
retroreflective marker
retrosacral fascia
retrosternal
  r. abscess
  r. dislocation
retrotorsion
  femoral r.
  tibial r.
retrovascular cord
retroversion
  r. of acetabular cup
  femoral r.
  tibial r.
retrovirus
Rett syndrome
return of sensation
revascularization
  endosteal r.
  r. of graft
revascularized tissue
Reverdin
  R. bunionectomy
  R. epidermal free graft
  R. osteotomy
  R. prosthesis
Reverdin-Green
  R.-G. foot procedure
  R.-G. osteotomy
Reverdin-Laird
  R.-L. bunionectomy
  R.-L. osteotomy
Reverdin-McBride bunionectomy
reversal
  r. of antagonist (ROA)
  r. of cervical lordosis
  r. of fore-aft shear phase of gait
  isotonic r. (IR)
  r. of lordosis
  stabilizing r. (SR)

reverse
  r. Barton fracture
  r. Bigelow maneuver
  r. Colles fracture
  r. cross-finger flap
  r.-cutting meniscal probe
  r. Dillwyn-Evans calcaneal
    osteotomy
  r. forearm island flap
  r. Hill-Sachs lesion
  r. Hill-Sachs sign
  r. knuckle-bender splint
  r. Lasègue test
  r. last shoe
  r. Mauck knee procedure
  r. Monteggia fracture
  r. pivot shift
  r. pivot shift test
  r. Putti-Platt procedure
  r. tennis elbow
  r. Thomas heel
  r.-threaded screw
  r. Trendelenburg position
  r. undercutting lengthening
  r. wedge osteotomy
  r. wedge technique
  r. wrist curl
Revised
  Symptoms Checklist 90 R. (SCL-
    90R)
ReVision
  R. nail
revision
  exploration and r.
  r. hip arthroplasty
  R. hip stem
  Mallory-Head total hip r.
  r. procedure
  stump r.
  r. of total hip
Revo
  R. knot
  R. loop handle knot pusher
  R. suture anchor
Rezaian
  R. external fixation
  R. external fixation apparatus
  R. external fixation device
  R. interbody device
  R. spinal fixator
R-Gel
RGO
  reciprocation gait orthosis
R-HAB
  Rincoe human action bionic ankle
    R-HAB lighter weight ankle
rhabdomyolysis
rhabdomyoma

rhabdomyosarcoma
    alveolar r.
    embryonal r.
    pleomorphic r.
rhachotomy
    Capener lateral r.
    decompression r.
    lateral r.
rheobase
rheumatica
    polymyalgia r.
rheumatism
    palindromic r.
rheumatoid
    r. arthritis (RA)
    r. arthritis factor
    r. arthritis myopathy
    r. arthritis synovitis
    r. cyst
    r. disease
    r. disorder
    r. foot
    r. nodule
    r. vasculitis
rheumatologist
Rheumatology
    American College of R. (ACR)
Rheumatrex
Rhinelander pin
rhizomelic
rhizomesomelic bone dysplasia
rhizotomy
    intradural dorsal spinal root r.
    posterior r.
    selective posterior r. (SPR)
RHOCS
    right-handed orthogonal coordinate
    system
rhomboideus major musculus
rhomboid flap
rhonchus, pl. **rhonchi**
    rales and rhonchi
Rhoton
    R. elevator
    R. enucleator
    R. needle holder
    R. osteotome
rhythm
    regular sinus r.
    scapulohumeral r.
rhythmic
    r. initiation (RI)

    r. initiation technique
    r. stabilization
RI
    rhythmic initiation
rib
    r. approximator
    r. belt
    r. belt orthosis
    bicipital r.
    bucket-handle r.
    r. cage
    cervical r.
    r. contractor
    r. contusion
    costochondral junction of r.'s
    r. cutter
    r. drill
    r. elevator
    false r.
    floating r.
    r. forceps
    r. fracture
    r. graft
    hypoplastic first r.
    interarticular ligament of head
      of r.
    radiate ligament of head of r.
    r. retractor
    rudimentary r.
    slipping r.
    sternal r.
    true r.
    vertebral r.
ribbed hook
Ribble bandage
ribbon sign
riboflavin
ribonucleoprotein (RNP)
rib-penciling
rib-vertebral angle
Rica
    R. bone drill
    R. wire guidepin
RICE
    rest, ice, compression, elevation
rice
    r. body
    joint r.
Rich
    Rolaids Calcium R.
Richards
    R. angle guide

NOTES

R

Richards *(continued)*
R. arthrodesis
R. bone clamp
R. classic compression hip screw
R. Colles external fixator
R. drill guide
R. fixation staple
R. fixator system
R. hip endoprosthesis system
R. hydroxyapatite PORP
R. lag screw
R. lag screw device
R. locking rod
R. Lovejoy bone drill
R. mallet
R. maximum contact cruciate-sparing prosthesis
R. modular hip system
R. modular stem
R. Phillips screwdriver
R. pistol-grip drill
R. reconstruction nail
R. sideplate
R. Solcotrans orthopaedic drainage-reinfusion system
R. Spectron metal-backed acetabular prosthesis
R. Zirconia femoral head prosthesis

Richards-Hirschhorn plate
Richardson
R. retractor
R. rod
R. subtalar arthrodesis

Riche-Cannieu
R.-C. anastomosis
R.-C. connection

Riches artery forceps
Richet
R. bandage
R. tibio-astragalocalcaneal canal

Richmond
R. bolt
R. subarachnoid screw
R. subarachnoid screw sensor
R. subarachnoid twist drill

Richter
R. bone drill
R. bone screwdriver

rickets
florid r.
vitamin D-dependent r. (VDDR)
vitamin D-resistant r. (VDRR)

rickshaw rehab exerciser
Ridaura
Rideau technique
Ridenol
rider's bone

ridge
epicondylar r.
greater multangular r.
osteochondral r.
Outerbridge r.
residence r.
vastus lateralis r.

Ridlon
R. hip reduction
R. plaster knife
R. procedure

Riecken PQ premium heel cup
rifampin
right
r.-angle dental drill
r.-ankle bur
r. erector spinae musculature
r.-handed orthogonal coordinate system (RHOCS)
r. lateral flexion
r. lower extremity (RLE)
r. lower limb (RLL)
r. posterior innominate
r. rotation
r. side bending
r. thoracic curve
r. thoracic curve scoliosis
r. thoracic curve with hypokyphosis
r. thoracic curve with junctional kyphosis
r. thoracic, left lumbar curve pattern
r. thoracic, left lumbar scoliosis
r. thoracic, left thoracolumbar curve pattern
r. thoracic, left thoracolumbar scoliosis
r. thoracic minor curve pattern
r. upper extremity (RUE)
r. upper limb (RUL)

right-hand
r.-h. dominance
r.-h. dominant

righting
r. reflex
trunk r.

right-left
r.-l. discrimination
r.-l. timing

right-sided
r.-s. nail
r.-s. submandibular transverse incision
r.-s. thoracotomy

rigid
r. below-the-knee cast
r. body
r. curve

R

r. curve scoliosis
r. dressing
r. flatfoot
r. foot
r. gait
r. internal fixation
r. metal pelvic band
r. pedicle screw
r. pes planus
r. postoperative brace
r. reamer
r. rockerbottom (RRB)
r. round back
r. sound

rigidity
C-D instrumentation r.
cogwheel r.
Cotrel pedicle screw r.
spinal fixation r.

rigidus
hallux r.

RIK
R. fluid mattress
R. FootHugger fluid heel boot

Riley-Day syndrome

rim
acetabular r.
alar r.
glenoid r.
sclerotic marginal r.
r. sign
tibial r.

Rimadyl

Rincoe human action bionic ankle (R-HAB)

ring
Ace-Colles half r.
arterial r.
r. block anesthesia
carbon fiber half r.
congenital r.
constriction r.
cricoid r.
r. cushion
doughnut r.
drop-lock r.
epiphyseal r.
r. external fixator
extracapsular arterial r.
r. finger (4th digit)
Fischer r.
foam r.

r. forceps
r. fracture
half r.
halo r.
Ilizarov r.
invalid r.
ischial weightbearing r.
Kayser-Fleischer r.
R. knee prosthesis
Lacroix osseous r.
Luque r.
orthosis drop-lock r.
pelvic r.
perichondral r.
protrusio r.
proximal-to-distal r.
reduction r.
r. retractor
r. structure
r. sublimis apponensplasty
r. syndrome
R. total hip prosthesis
R. UPM total hip replacement
R. UPM total knee replacement
V1 halo r.

Ringer
R. arthroscopy
R. lactate

RingLoc
R. acetabular series
R. instrument

Riordan
R. club hand classification
R. finger flexion
R. finger opponensplasty
R. pin
R. pollicization
R. sign
R. tendon transfer technique

RIPA-2 Assessment

RIPA-G Assessment

Riseborough-Radin
R.-R. fracture classification system
R.-R. intercondylar fracture classification

rise time

Rish osteotome

risk
r. factor profile
occupational r.
relative r. (RR)

NOTES

Risser
 R. frame
 R. grade
 R. localizer scoliosis cast
 R. method
 R. sign
 R. stage
 R. technique
 R. turnbuckle cast
Rissler pin
Rissler-Stille pin
Ritchie
 R. index
 R. nail starter
Rivermead
 R. ADL index
 R. Mobility Index (RMI)
rivet gun
RLE
 right lower extremity
RLL
 right lower limb
RM
 repetition maximum
 RM isoelastic hip prosthesis
1-RM
 one-repetition maximum
RMC
 RMC knee replacement device
 RMC prosthesis
RMI
 Rivermead Mobility Index
RMQ
 Roland-Morris Questionnaire
RMS rectal
RNP
 ribonucleoprotein
R/O
 rule out
ROA
 reversal of antagonist
Robaxin
Robaxisal
Robert
 R. Brigham total knee prosthesis
 R. Jones dressing
 R. Jones splint
 R. view
Roberts
 R. approach
 R. technique
Roberts-Gill periosteal elevator
Robinson
 R. anterior cervical diskectomy
 R. anterior cervical fusion
 R. arthrometer
 R. cervical spine fusion
 R. InRigger splint

 R. morcellation
 R. spinal arthrodesis
Robinson-Chung-Farahvar clavicular morcellation
Robinson-Moon prosthesis inserter
Robinson-Riley cervical arthrodesis
Robinson-Smith spinal arthrodesis
Robinson-Southwick
 R.-S. fusion
 R.-S. fusion technique
Robins-Riley spinal fusion
Robodoc robot
robot
 Robodoc r.
ROC
 receiver operating characteristic
 ROC anchor
 Biothesiometer ROC
Rocabado posture gauge
Rocaltrol
Rocephin
Rochester
 R. bone trephine device
 R. compression system
 R. harvest bone cutter
 R. hip-knee-ankle-foot orthosis
 R. lamina elevator
 R. recipient bone cutter
 R. spinal elevator
Rochester-Carmalt forceps
Rochester-Ochsner forceps
Rochester-Pean forceps
rock
 R. ankle exercise board
 pelvic r. (PR)
 R. & Roller exercise board
rocker
 r. balance square
 r. bar
 r. board
 r. boot
 r. knife
 r. sole
 Uniplane r.
rockerbottom
 r. feet
 r. flatfoot
 r. foot
 r. foot deformity
 rigid r. (RRB)
 r. shoe
rocking
 knee-chest r.
Rock-Mulligan prosthesis
Rockwood
 R. anterior acromioplasty
 R. classification

R

R. classification of
   acromioclavicular injury
R. classification of clavicular
   fracture
R. posterior capsulorrhaphy
R. procedure
R. resection
R. shoulder screw
Rockwood-Green technique
Rockwood-Matsen capsular shift
  procedure
rocky boat exerciser
rod
  alignment r.
  alignment guide r.
  Alta CFX reconstruction r.
  Alta tibial-humeral r.
  aluminum master r.
  Amset R-F r.
  auto-reinforced polyglycolide r.
  Bailey-Dubow r.
  r. bender
  r. bending
  Bickel intramedullary r.
  centralizing r.
  r. clamp
  cold rolled r.
  compression r.
  compressive r.
  concave r.
  r. contour preparation
  convex r.
  Cotrel-Dubousset r.
  Dacron-impregnated silicone r.
  degradable polyglycolide r.
  delta r.
  distraction r.
  r. distraction device
  double-L spinal r.
  dual square-ended Harrington r.
  Edwards-Levine r.
  Edwards modular system
   Universal r.
  Ender r.
  Enneking r.
  Fixateur Interne r.
  flared spinal r.
  fluted medullary r.
  r. fracture repair
  guide r.
  Harrington compression r.
  Harrington distraction r.

Harris condylocephalic r.
hinge r.
r. holder
r.-hook construct
Hunter Silastic r.
impactor r.
impingement r.
intramedullary alignment r.
Isola spinal implant system eye r.
Jacobs distraction r.
Jacobs locking hook spinal r.
Kaneda r.
Knodt r.
Küntscher condylocephalic r.
L r.
r. linkage
locking-hook spinal r.
L-shaped r.
Luque r.
r. migration
Moe modified Harrington r.
Moe square-end r.
Moss r.
Mouradian r.
Olerud PSF r.
pediatric Cotrel-Dubousset r.
PGA r.
r. placement
Polarus humeral r.
precontoured unit r.
radiotranslucent r.
Richards locking r.
Richardson r.
r. rotation prevention
round-ended distraction r.
Rush r.
Russell-Taylor delta r.
Sage r.
Sampson r.
Schneider r.
screw alignment r.
Serrato forearm r.
silicone-dacron tendon r.
r. sleeve fixation
spinal fixation r.
square-ended distraction r.
Stenzel r.
straight threaded r.
R. TAG suture anchor system
telescopic r.
telescoping medullary r.
r. template

NOTES

rod *(continued)*
    tendon r.
    threaded r.
    unit spinal r.
    V-A alignment r.
    Williams r.
    Wiltse system aluminum master r.
    Wiltse system spinal r.
    Wissinger r.
    Zickel r.
    Zielke r.
rod-mounted
    r.-m. targeting apparatus
    r.-m. targeting device
rod sleeve
    Edwards modular system spinal r.
    s.
Roeder manipulative aptitude test device
roentgenogram
    biplane r.
    lateral r.
    operative r.
    templating r.
    two-plane r.
roentgenography
    intraoperative r.
    preoperative r.
    stress r.
roentgenometrics
Roentgen-stereophotogrammatic study
roentgenstereophotogrammetric analysis
Roger
    R. Anderson compression device
    R. Anderson external fixation apparatus
    R. Anderson external fixation device
    R. Anderson external fixator
    R. Anderson pin
    R. Anderson splint
    R. Anderson stabilization device
    R. Anderson system
    R. Anderson table
    R. Anderson traction
Rogers cervical fusion technique
Rogozinski
    R. hook
    R. screw system
    R. spinal fixation
    R. spinal fixation system
    R. spinal rod system
Rohadur gait plate
Rohadur-Polydor orthotic
Rohadur-Schaefer orthotic
Rohadur-Whitman orthotic
ROHO
    R. bed

    R. heel pad
    R. heel protector
    R. Pack-It cushion
    R. pediatric seating system
    R. solid seat insert
Rolaids Calcium Rich
Roland index of low back pain
Roland-Morris Questionnaire (RMQ)
Rolando fracture
Rolator walker
role
    intrinsic transverse connector r.
    occupational r.
rolfing pressure
roll
    cervical r.
    chest r.
    r. control bolster
    cotton r.
    Dutchman's r.
    Feldenkrais foam r.
    FLUFTEX gauze r.
    hip r.
    lumbar r.
    McKenzie cervical r.
    McKenzie lumbar r.
    McKenzie night r.
    neck r.
    octagon r.
    radiolucent r.
    Skillbuilder half r.
    r. stitch
    towel r.
    Tumble Forms r.
Roll-A-Bout
Rollator Nova walker
rolled felt
RollerBack self-massage device
roller injury
rolling
    skin r.
Rollocane
Roll-On
    Biofreeze R.-O.
rollover
Rolyan
    R. AquaForm wrist and thumb spica splint
    R. arm elevator
    R. foot support
    R. Reach N Range Pulley System
    R. tibial fracture brace
Rolz device
ROM
    range of motion
    ROM knee brace
    ROM therapy
Roman arch

Romano curved drilling system
Romberg test
Rome
>R. criteria
>R. criteria for rheumatoid arthritis

rongeur
>Adson r.
>angled jaw r.
>angled pituitary r.
>angular bone r.
>Bacon bone r.
>Baer bone r.
>Bane bone r.
>Bane-Hartmann bone r.
>basket r.
>bayonet r.
>Beyer r.
>Beyer-Stille bone r.
>Blumenthal bone r.
>bone-nibbling r.
>bone punch r.
>Bruening-Citelli r.
>Campbell r.
>cervical r.
>Cicherelli bone r.
>Cleveland bone r.
>Cloward r.
>Cohen r.
>Colclough laminectomy r.
>Corbett bone r.
>curved bone r.
>Cushing r.
>Dale first rib r.
>Decker r.
>Defourmentel bone r.
>disk r.
>double-action r.
>downbiting r.
>duckbill r.
>Echlin duckbill r.
>Ferris Smith r.
>Ferris Smith-Spurling disk r.
>flat-bottomed Kerrison r.
>r. forceps
>Friedman bone r.
>Guleke bone r.
>Hartmann bone r.
>Hein r.
>Hoen r.
>Jackson disk r.
>Jackson intervertebral disk r.
>Kerrison downbiting r.

>Kleinert-Kutz bone r.
>Kleinert-Kutz synovectomy r.
>Lebsche r.
>Leksell r.
>Leksell-Stille thoracic r.
>Lempert bone r.
>Liston-Littauer r.
>Littauer-West r.
>Luer bone r.
>Luer-Friedman bone r.
>Luer-Hartmann r.
>Markwalder bone r.
>mastoid r.
>McIndoe bone r.
>Mead bone r.
>Montenovesi r.
>orthopaedic r.
>pituitary r.
>Ruskin r.
>Schlesinger cervical r.
>single-action r.
>Smith-Petersen r.
>Spurling r.
>Spurling-Kerrison r.
>Stille r.
>Stille-Luer bone r.
>straight bone r.
>straight pituitary r.
>Super Cut laminectomy r.
>synovial r.
>upbiting r.
>upcut r.

rongeured
Rood technique
roof
>acetabular r.
>r. arc measurement
>r. impingement
>intercondylar r.
>r.-reinforcement ring hip
> arthroplasty component
>r. wedge

roofplasty
room
>Allender vertical laminar flow r.
>Charnley laminar flow r.
>operating r.
>recovery r. (RR)
>surgical dressing r. (SDR)

Roos
>R. approach

NOTES

Roos *(continued)*
    R. overhead exercise test
    R. rib cutter
root
    r. anomaly
    r. canal broach
    cervical r.
    r. infiltration
    kava r.
    nail r.
    nerve r.
rooting reflex
Root-Siegal varus derotational osteotomy
ropey
ropiness
ropivacaine
Rorabeck fasciotomy
Rosai-Dorfman disease
Rose foot procedure
Rosen
    R. bur
    R. elevator
    R. splint
Rosenberg
    R. endoscopic anterior cruciate
      ligament reconstruction
    R. retractor
Rosenfeld hip prosthesis
Rosenthal classification of nail injury
rosette
    r. Beaver blade
    R. strain gauge
Rosser Classification of Illness States
Ross Information Processing Assessment
Rotablator rotating bur
Rotaflex exerciser
rotary
    r. ankle instability
    r. basket
    r. basket forceps
    r. bur
    r. deviation
    r. displacement
    r. drawer test
    r. instability test
    r. motion
    r. osteotome
    r. stability
rotated
    externally r.
    internally r.
rotating
    r. femoral head prosthesis
    r. hinge
    r.-hinge knee prosthesis
    r. turner
rotation
    abduction-external r. (AER)

abnormal instantaneous axis of r.
anterior innominate r.
axial r.
r. axis
Borggreve limb r.
center of axial r.
cervical general r.
r.-compression maneuver
r. device
r. drawer test
eccentric axis of ankle r.
r. exercise
external r.
external/internal r. (ER/IR)
flexion in abduction and
  external r. (faber)
flexion in adduction and internal r.
  (fadir)
foot r.
r. fracture
functional axial r.
Hermodsson internal r.
hip r.
horizontal external r.
instantaneous axis of r.
intentional r.
internal r.
internal-external r.
intersegmental r.
inversion-eversion r.
inward r.
knee r.
left r.
lumbar r.
r. mobility
neutral r.
outward r.
patellar r.
patient-resisted internal r.
pelvic r.
r. plasty
polycentric r.
posterior innominate r.
pronation-eversion-external r.
  (PEER)
pronation-external r. (P-ER)
putative segmental instantaneous
  axis of r.
r. recurvatum test
right r.
sagittal r.
spine r.
supination-external r. (SER)
synchronous scapuloclavicular r.
r. testing
vertebral r.
rotational
    r. alignment

r. burst fracture
r. contracture
r. correction
r. deformity
r. flap
r. fracture
r. instability
r. kyphosis
r. malalignment
r. malposition
r. prominence
r. restriction
r. scarf osteotomy
r. scarf osteotomy/bunionectomy
r. scoliosis
rotationplasty
Kotz-Salzer r.
tibial hindfoot
osteomusculocutaneous r.
Van Ness r.
Winkelmann r.
rotator
r. cuff (RC)
r. cuff calcified deposit
r. cuff lesion
r. cuff repair
r. cuff tear
r. cuff-tear arthroplasty
r. cuff tendinitis
external r.
Hosmer above knee r.
Howmedica monotube external r.
internal r.
long external r.
short external r.
r. unit
rotatores
r. breves musculi
r. longi musculi
r. syndrome
r. thoracis musculi
rotatory
r. atlantoaxial subluxation
r. load
r. torque
r.-variable-differential transducer
Rothman
R. Institute femoral prosthesis
R. Institute total hip program
Roto-Rest bed
Rotter-Erb syndrome
rough

roughening
roughen the surface
rouleaux formation
round
r. bur
r. cell liposarcoma
r. cell type liposarcoma
r.-ended distraction rod
r.-hole compression plate
r. ligament
r. shoulder deformity
r.-tapped periosteal
roundback stem
Rousek
R. extender
R. extraction set
Roussy-Levy
R.-L. disease
R.-L. syndrome
Rouviere ligament
Roux-duToit staple capsulorrhaphy
Roux-Goldthwait
R.-G. procedure
R.-G. realignment
Roux sign
row
carpal r.
proximal carpal r.
Rowe
R. blanket
R. calcaneal fracture classification
R. disimpaction forceps
R. fusion
R. glenoid punch
R. glenoid-reaming forceps
R. and Lowell classification system
for fracture-dislocation
R. modified-Harrison forceps
modified Zarins and R.
R. posterior shoulder approach
Rowe-Harrison bone-holding forceps
**Rowe-Lowell hip dislocation
classification**
Rowe-Zarins shoulder immobilization
Rowland-Hughes splint
Roxanol
R. Rescudose
R. SR Oral
Roxicet 5/500
Roxicodone
Roxilox
Roxiprin

NOTES

Royalite body jacket
Roy-Camille
    R.-C. plate
    R.-C. posterior screw plate fixation
Roylan
    R. ergonomic hand exerciser
    R. Gel Shell spica splint
Royle-Thompson transfer technique
RPE
    rated perceived exertion
RQS
    repeated quick stretch
RQS-E
    repeated quick stretch from elongation
RQS-SEC
    repeated quick stretch superimposed upon
      an existing contraction
RR
    recovery room
    relative risk
RRAM
    relative response attributable to the
      maneuver
RRB
    rigid rockerbottom
RSC
    radioscaphocapitate
RSD
    reflex sympathetic dystrophy
RSDCP plate
RSI
    repetition strain injury
RSS
    rearfoot stability system
    repetitive stress syndrome
RTD
    repetitive trauma disorder
Rub
    Jeanie R.
rubber
    r. band traction
    r. bolster
    r. drain
    microcellular r.
    r.-shod
    r.-shod clamp
    r. sling
    r. sole cast walker
    r. spacer
    r. walking heel
    r. wedge walker
Ruben gouge
Rubex
Rubinstein-Taybi syndrome
Rubix-Cube
rubor
rubra vera

rubrum
    Trichophyton r.
rudimentary
    r. bone
    r. rib
RUE
    right upper extremity
Ruedi-Allgower
    R.-A. classification
    R.-A. tibial plafond fracture
Ruedi fracture
Ruffini
    R. ending
    R. end-organ
    R. end organ
    R. mechanoreceptor
Ruiz-Mora
    R.-M. correction
    R.-M. procedure
RUL
    right upper limb
rulangemeter
rule
    millimetric r.
    Ottawa ankle r.
    r. out (R/O)
ruler
    Berndt hip r.
    ulnar r.
Rumel
    R. aluminum bridge splint
    R. myocardial clamp
    R. rubber clamp
    R. thoracic clamp
runner
    r. bump
    heel-toe r.'s
    r. knee
    Sprint R.
    r. toe
running
    r.-related injury
    r. suture
    treadmill r.
rupture
    Achilles tendon r. (ATR)
    adductor longus muscle r.
    anterior talofibular ligament r.
    buttonhole r.
    collateral ligament r.
    crescentic r.
    cruciate ligament r.
    distal biceps brachii tendon r.
    flexor tendon r.
    infrapatellar tendon r.
    longitudinal ligament r.
    neglected r.
    proximal tendon r.

stress r.
tendon r.
transverse ligament r.
ulnar collateral ligament r.
ruptured disk excision
Rush
R. bender
R. bone clamp
R. driver
R. driver-bender-extractor
R. extender
R. flexible medullary nail
R. intramedullary fixation pin
R. mallet
R. pin reamer awl
R. rod
R. rod awl reamer
Ruskin
R. bone-splitting forceps
R. rongeur
R. rongeur forceps
Ruskin-Liston bone-cutting forceps
Ruskin-Rowland bone-cutting forceps
Russe
R. bone graft
R. classification
R. technique

Russe-Gerhardt method
Russell
R. fibular head autograft
R. skeletal traction
R. splint
R. traction for femoral fracture
Russell-Silver dwarfism
Russell-Taylor
R.-T. classification
R.-T. delta rod
R.-T. delta tibial nail
R.-T. femoral interlocking nail system
R.-T. interlocking medullary nail
R.-T. screw
Russian
R. forceps
R. waveform
Rust sign
Rüter classification
Rydell nail
Ryder needle holder
Ryerson
R. bone graft
R. procedure
R. technique
R. triple arthrodesis

NOTES

SAARD
    slow-acting antirheumatic drug
SAB
    short-acting block anesthesia
Sabel cast walker
saber-cut
    s.-c. approach
    s.-c. incision
Sabolich socket system
sabre shin deformity
SAC
    short arm cast
    space available for the cord
sac
    bursal s.
    common dural s.
    thecal s.
SACH
    solid ankle, cushioned heel
    SACH foot
    SACH foot adapter
    SACH foot prosthesis
    SACH orthopaedic heel
    SACH orthosis
    SACH orthotic
Sach nerve separator
saclike cavity
sacral
    s. agenesis
    s. ala
    s. alar screw
    s. approach
    s. arcuate line
    s. artery
    s. bar technique
    s. base angle
    s. base distortion
    s. cyst
    s. fracture
    s. horizontal plane line (SHPL)
    s. inclinaton
    s. mobility
    s. nerve
    s. nerve root sparing
    s. pedicle screw
    s. pedicle screw fixation
    s. plexus
    s. plexus injury
    s. promontory
    s. screw placement
    s. segment
    s. spine
    s. spine decompression
    s. spine fixation
    s. spine fusion

s. spine modular instrumentation
s. spine stabilization
s. spine Universal instrumentation
s. support
s. tilt
s. triangle
sacralization
sacralized transverse process
sacral spine (*var. of* sacrum)
sacrificing knee prosthesis
sacrococcygeal chordoma
Sacro-Eze lumbar support
sacrofemoral angle
sacrohorizontal angle
sacroiliac (SI)
    s. belt
    s. binder
    s. buttressing procedure
    s. disarticulation
    s. dislocation
    s. extension fixation
    s. flexion fixation
    s. fracture
    s. joint
    s. joint arthropathy
    s. joint injury
    s. joint locking
    s. joint mobility
    s. joint motion
    s. ligament
    s. orthosis (SIO)
    s. subluxation
    s. syndrome
sacroiliitis
Sacro Occipital Research Society International (SORSI)
sacrooccipital technique (SOT)
sacrospinalis musculus
sacrospinal ligament
sacrospinalum
    ligamentum s.
sacrospinous ligament
sacrotuberale
    ligamentum s.
sacrotuberal ligament
sacrotuberous ligament
sacrovertebral angle
sacrum, sacral spine
    s. fracture
    s. fusion screw fixation
saddle
    basal block cervical s.
    s.-block anesthesia
    cervical s.
    Cloward surgical s.

S

saddle *(continued)*
    s. cushion
    s. joint
    s. prosthesis
saddlebag
    Seidel s.
SAF
    self-articulating femoral
    SAF hip replacement
    SAF prosthesis
SAFE
    solid-ankle flexible endoskeletal
    stationary attachment flexible
      endoskeletal
    SAFE foot
    SAFE II prosthesis
    SAFE orthotic
Safe spine thoracic-lumbar-sacral
  support
Safe-T-Wheel pinwheel
safety
    s.-bolt suture
    s. performance
    s. pin orthosis
    s. pin splint
Safe·Wrap gauze
SAFHS ultrasound device
Safir pin
SAFK
    single-axis friction knee
sag
    sling seat s.
Sage
    S. driver
    S. driver-extractor
    S. extractor
    S. forearm nail
    S. pin
    S. radial nail
    S. rod
    S. triangular nail
Sage-Clark
    S.-C. cheilectomy
    S.-C. technique
Sage-Salvatore
    S.-S. classification
    S.-S. classification of
      acromioclavicular joint injury
sagittal
    s. anatomic alignment
    s. band
    s. deformity
    s. fast-short T1 inversion recovery
      (STIR)
    s. kyphosis
    s. mobility
    s. motion
    s. movement

    s. pedicle angle
    s. pedicle diameter
    s. plane
    s.-plane imaging
    s. plane instability
    s. roll spondylolisthesis
    s. rotation
    s. spinal canal diameter
    s. surgical saw
    s. T1-weighted spin-echo image
    s.-Z osteotomy
Saha
    S. procedure
    S. shoulder muscle classification
    S. transfer technique
SAI
    Schema Assessment instrument
SAID
    specific adaptation to imposed demand
    SAID principle
Saint
    S. George-Buchholz ankle
      prosthesis
    S. George knee prosthesis
    S. John's Wort
    S. Joseph Adult Chewable Aspirin
    S. Jude prosthesis
    S. Vitus dance
Sakellarides
    S. calcaneal fracture classification
Sakellarides-Deweese technique
Sakoff osteotomy
SAL
    self-aligning knee
Salenius meniscus knife
Saleto-200, -400, -600, -800
Salflex
Salgesic
salicylate
    choline s.
    magnesium s.
    sodium s.
    triethanolamine s.
salicylic
    s. acid and lactic acid
    s. acid and propylene glycol
salicylsalicylic acid
salient angle
saline
    s. acceptance test
    physiologic s.
    s. solution
SALK
    single-axis locking knee
salmon calcitonin
Salmonella
    Salmonella arthritis
    Salmonella osteomyelitis

Salmonine Injection
salsalate
Salsitab
salt
    gold s.
saltans
    coxa s.
Salter
    S. epiphyseal fracture classification
    S. fracture
    S. innominate osteotomy
    S. pelvic osteotomy
    S. technique
Salter-Harris
    S.-H. classification
    S.-H. classification of epiphyseal
      fracture
    S.-H. epiphyseal injury
    S.-H. fracture (type I–VI)
    S.-H. tibial-fibular injury
Salter-Harris-Rang
    S.-H.-R. classification of epiphyseal
      fracture
    S.-H.-R. epiphyseal fracture
      classification
Saltiel brace
salvage
    limb s.
    s. procedure
Salzer
    S. prosthesis
    S. resurfacing
SAM
    spinal analysis machine
    structural aluminum malleable
    SAM spinal analysis machine
    SAM splint
Samilson
    S. crescentic calcaneal osteotomy
    S. procedure
**Sammarco-DiRaimondo modification of
Elmslie technique**
Sammons biplane goniometer
sample
    Pennsylvania bimanual work s.
Sampson
    S. medullary nail
    S. prosthesis
    S. rod
Samuels forceps
SANC
    short arm navicular cast

sandal
    Benefoot & Birkenstock orthotic s.
    Exercise S.
    Rainbow cast s.
Sandalthotics
    S. postural support orthotic
sandbag
    neonatal s.
    pedi s.
Sanders CT Classification
Sandimmune
    S. Injection
    S. Oral
sand toe injury
sandwiched iliac bone graft
Sanfilippo syndrome
sanguineous
Sani-Grinder
Sani Vac
San Joaquin Valley fever
Santa Casa distractor
Santyl
saphenous
    s. flap
    s. nerve
    s. vein
SAPHO
    synovitis-acne-pustulosis-hyperostosis
    osteomyelitis
    SAPHO syndrome
Sapphire
    S. table
    S. View arthroscope
Saratoga cycle
Sarbo sign
sarcoid
    Boeck s.
sarcoidosis
sarcoma
    alveolar soft-part s.
    bicompartmental soft-tissue s.
    botryoid s.
    clear cell s.
    deep intracompartmental soft-
      tissue s.
    epithelioid s.
    Ewing s.
    extracompartmental soft-tissue s.
    femoral s.
    high-grade surface osteogenic s.
    human osteogenic s. (HOS)
    intracortical osteogenic s.

S

NOTES

sarcoma *(continued)*
    Kaposi s.
    low-grade central osteogenic s.
    malignant myeloid s.
    multicentric osteogenic s.
    osteoblastic osteogenic s.
    osteogenic s.
    Paget-associated osteogenic s.
    parosteal osteogenic s.
    postirradiation osteogenic s.
    reticular cell s.
    sclerosa osteoblastic osteogenic s.
    small cell osteogenic s.
    soft tissue s.
    subcutaneous intracompartmental
      soft-tissue s.
    subcutaneous soft-tissue s.
    synovial s.
sarcomatous change
sarcopenia
sarcoplasmic reticulum
sarcotubular myopathy
Sargent knee operation
sargramostim
Sarmiento
    S. fracture brace
    S. hip prosthesis
    S. intertrochanteric osteotomy
    S. nail
    S. short leg patellar tendon-bearing
      cast
    S. trochanteric fracture technique
Sarot needle holder
sartorial slide procedure
sartorius
    s. muscle
    s. tendon
SAS
    short arm splint
    shoulder arm system
    SAS II brace
    SAS shoe
Saso Variable Speed Massager
Sat-A-Lite contoured wedge seat
  cushion
Satalite cushion by Bodyline
sateen knee immobilizer
satellite
    s. myofascial trigger point
    s. potential
Saticon tube camera
Satterlee bone saw
saturation
    arterial oxygen s.
saucerization
Sauerbruch
    S. prosthesis
    S. retractor

    S. rib elevator
    S. rib forceps
    S. rib shears
Saunders
    S. cervical HomeTrac
    S. mobilization wedge
    S. traction
sausage
    s. finger
    s. toe
Sauvé-Kapandji
    S.-K. arthroplasty
    S.-K. procedure
Savastano
    S. hemiknee
    S. Hemi-Knee prosthesis
    S. Hemi-Knee system
saver
    intraoperative Cell S.
    knee s.
saw
    Adams s.
    Aesculap s.
    air-driven oscillating s.
    amputation s.
    Bailey wire s.
    bayonet s.
    Beaver s.
    Bishop s.
    bone s.
    Charriere bone s.
    circular s.
    Cottle s.
    counter rotating s.
    crescentic s.
    crosscut s.
    Delrin-handle bone s.
    electric cast s.
    end-cutting reciprocating s.
    Engel plaster s.
    Gigli s.
    Gigli-Strully s.
    s. guide
    Hall air-driven oscillating s.
    Hall sagittal s.
    Hall Versipower oscillating s.
    Hall Versipower reciprocating s.
    hand s.
    Henschke-Mauch s.
    Herbert s.
    Horsley bone s.
    humeral s.
    intramedullary s.
    Lagenback bone s.
    Langenbeck metacarpal s.
    Lebsche wire s.
    Luck-Bishop bone s.
    medullary s.

microoscillating s.
microsagittal s.
Miltex bone s.
Osada s.
oscillating s.
patella bone s.
Pearson intramedullary s.
Percy amputating s.
power-driven s.
power oscillating s.
reciprocating motor s.
sagittal surgical s.
Satterlee bone s.
single-blade s.
single-sided bone s.
Skil s.
Sklar bone s.
Tuke s.
twin-blade oscillating s.
Zimmer oscillating s.

SAWA

SAWA shoulder brace
SAWA shoulder orthosis

sawblade

Stablecut s.

sawcut

Sayre

S. bandage
S. elevator
S. splint
S. traction

Sbarbaro

S. hip prosthesis
S. spica cast
S. tibial plateau prosthesis

SBO

spina bifida occulta

SBP

systolic blood pressure

SB+ testing and treatment
SB− testing and treatment
SC

sternoclavicular
supracondylar
SC suspension

scaffold

collagen s.

scaffolding
Scaglietti

S. closed reduction technique
S. procedure scale

scalar

s. classification
s. quantity

scale

Abbreviated Injury S. (AIS)
Abnormal Involuntary Movement S.
(AIMS)
Alberta Infant Motor S. (AIMS)
American Musculoskeletal Tumor
Society rating s.
Angus-Cowell s.
ankle-hindfoot s.
Arthritis Impact Measurement S.
(AIMS)
Ashworth s.
balance beam s.
Broberg-Morrey elbow function s.
Charnley pain and function
grading s.
Cinti knee rating s.
S.'s of Cognitive Ability
S.'s of Cognitive Ability for
Traumatic Brain Injury (SCATBI)
S.'s of Cognitive Ability for
Traumatic Brain Injury
Assessment
foot and ankle severity s. (FASS)
French s.
Gait Abnormality Rating S.
(GARS)
GED S.
Geissling rating s.
Glasgow Coma s.
Graphic Rating S. (GRS)
Harris hip s.
Health O Meter S.
Hospital for Special Surgery s.
International Knee Documentation
Committee knee s.
JOA S.
Johnson-Boseker s.
Kenna Knee S.
Kitaoka clinical rating s.
Knirk-Jupiter elbow evaluation s.
Lysholm-Gillquist knee subjective
function s.
Lysholm Knee S.
Merle d'Aubigné and Postel hip
rating s.
metatarsophalangeal-
interphalangeal s.
midfoot s.

S

NOTES

scale *(continued)*
  modified Gait Abnormality
    Rating S.
  NEECHAM Confusion S.
  numeric rating s. (NRS)
  Oral Analogue S. (OAS)
  Outerbridge s.
  Perez postoperative pain s.
  Portola Valley S.
  Progressive Ambulation S.
  Prosthetic Problem Inventory S.
  Reddihough s.
  Scaglietti procedure s.
  Stanford Hypnotic Clinical S.
  Steinberg rating s.
  Tegner activity s.
  The Knee Society clinical-rating s.
  UCLA Shoulder Rating s.
  visual analog s. (VAS)
  Volpicelli functional ambulation s.
scalene
  s. block
  s. fat pad
  s. maneuver
  s. muscle
scalenotomy
scalenus
  s. anticus muscle
  s. anticus syndrome
scalloping
  endosteal s.
  s. of vertebra
scalpel
  Bard-Parker s.
scan
  adenosine thallium s.
  bone s.
  CT s.
  DEXA s.
  gallium-67 s.
  gallium citrate s.
  intrathecally enhanced CT s.
  lead-line s.
  leukocyte s.
  multiplanar computed tomography s.
  multiplanar CT s.
  myocardial perfusion s.
  nuclear magnetic resonance s.
  positron emission tomographic s.
  radioisotope gallium s.
  radioisotope indium-labeled white
    blood cell s.
  radioisotope technetium s.
  radionuclide s.
  technetium-99m diphosphonate s.
  technetium-99m pyrophosphate s.
  technetium-99m sulfur colloid s.
  thallium s.

  three-phase bone s.
  transesophageal echocardiography s.
Scand pin
scanner
  Fonar QUAD MRI s.
  thermographic s.
scanning
  cold phase as in bone s.
  s. EMG
  indium-111-labelled leukocyte
    bone s.
  quadraphasic s.
  radionuclide s.
scanogram radiography
scanography
Scanz osteotomy
scaphocapitate
  s. fusion
  s. interval
  s. joint
  s. syndrome
scaphocapitolunate arthrodesis (SCL)
scaphoid
  bipartite s.
  s. bone
  carpal s.
  s. cookie in shoe
  s. fracture
  s. lift test
  s. nonunion
  s. screw guide
  s. shift test
  s. shoe cookie
  s. shoe pad
  s. tuberosity injury
scaphoiditis
Scaphoid-Microstaple system
scapholunate, scaphoid-lunate (SL)
  s. advanced collapse (SLAC)
  s. angle
  s. dissociation
  s. gap
  s. instability
  s. interosseous ligament
  s. joint
scaphotrapeziotrapezoid arthrodesis
scaphotrapezoid interosseous ligament
scaphotrapezoid-trapezial (STT)
scapula, pl. scapulae
  inferior TV ligament of s.
  locked s.
  snapping s.
  superior TV ligament of s.
  winging of s.
scapular
  s. approximation test
  s. elevation
  s. flap

s. graft
s. ligament
s. nerve
s. notch
s. peroneal atrophy
s. reflex
s. winging

scapulectomy
Das Gupta s.
Phelps s.

scapuloclavicular
s. articulation
s. injury

scapulohumeral
s. ligament
s. muscle
s. reflex
s. rhythm

scapulolateral view
scapulometer
scapuloperoneal
s. muscle atrophy disease
s. syndrome

scapulothoracic
s. arthrodesis
s. dissociation
s. fusion
s. joint
s. motion
s. muscle
s. pain

scapulovertebral border
scar
area s.
s. band
s. formation
linear s.
parasagittal s.
peritendinous s.
physeal s.
s. tissue

Scarborough
S. prosthesis
S. total hip replacement

scarf
s. Z osteotomy
s. Z osteotomy/bunionectomy
s. Z-plasty

Scarpa fascia
scarred
scarring and furrowing

SCATBI
Scales of Cognitive Ability for Traumatic
Brain Injury
SCATBI Assessment

SCD
sequential compression device
SCD stockings

Scerratti goniometer
SCFE
slipped capital femoral epiphysis

Schaberg-Harper-Allen technique
Schaffer squeeze
Schanz, Shantz, Shanz
S. angulation osteotomy
S. collar
S. collar brace
S. dressing
S. femoral osteotomy
S. pin
S. screw

**Schatzker tibial plateau fracture
classification**
Schauwecker
S. patellar tension band wire
S. patellar wiring
S. patellar wiring technique

Schede
S. bone curette
S. hip osteotomy

Schedule
General Well-Being S.

Scheffé
S. interval
S. test

Scheie syndrome
Schema Assessment instrument (SAI)
schenckii
Sporothrix s.

**Schepens hollow silicone hemisphere
implant material**
Schepsis-Leach technique
Scherisorb dressing
Scher nail biopsy
Scheuermann
S. disease
S. dystrophic spondylosis
S. juvenile kyphosis (SJK)

Schink metatarsal retraction
Schirmer test
Schlein
S. elbow arthroplasty
S. semiconstrained elbow prosthesis

S

NOTES

531

Schlein *(continued)*
    S. shoulder positioner
    S. total elbow prosthesis
    S. trisurface ankle prosthesis
Schlesinger
    S. cervical punch forceps
    S. cervical rongeur
    S. punch
    S. rongeur forceps
    S. sign
Schmeisser
    S. spica
    S. spica cast
Schmid metaphyseal dysostosis
Schmidt rod holder
Schmitt fan
Schmorl node
Schneider
    S. driver-extractor
    S. extractor
    S. extractor-driver
    S. fixation
    S. hip arthrodesis
    S. medullary nail
    S. nail driver
    S. pin
    S. rod
Schnute wedge resection technique
Schober
    S. measurement
    S. method
    S. technique
    S. test
    S. test of lumbar flexion
Scholl pad
Scholten sternal retractor
Schreiber maneuver
Schrock procedure
Schuind external fixation
Schuknecht
    S. Gelfoam wire prosthesis
    S. Teflon wire piston prosthesis
Schutte shovelnose basket
Schwachman syndrome
Schwann
    S. cell
    S. tumor
schwannoma
    cellular s.
    collagenous s.
    malignant s.
Schwartz
    S. clip-applying forceps
    S. dorsiflexory osteotomy
    S. temporary clamp-applying
        forceps
Schwartz-Blajwas-Marcinko irrigation
    system

Schwartze chisel
Schwartz-Jampel syndrome
Schwarz finger extension bow
Schweitzer
    S. pin
    S. spring plate
Schwinn Air-Dyne bicycle
SCI
    spinal cord injury
sciatic
    s. foramen
    s. function index (SFI)
    s. leg block
    s. nerve
    s. nerve injury
    s. nerve irritation
    s. nerve palsy hematoma
    s. notch
    s. palsy
    s. tension sign
sciatica
science
    epistemology of s.
    exercise s.
    movement s.
    occupational s.
scintigraphy
    bone s.
    combined s.
    indium-111 s.
    paired s.
    triphase technetium s.
scissor-leg
    s.-l. gait
    s.-l. position
scissors
    Acufex s.
    adventitial s.
    arthroscopic s.
    Aslan endoscopic s.
    Bantam wire-cutting s.
    Beebe wire-cutting s.
    Bellucci alligator s.
    blunt-tip iris s.
    cartilage s.
    Crafoord thoracic s.
    crown and collar s.
    curved Mayo s.
    Dean s.
    dissecting s.
    Fiskars s.
    s. gait
    Giertz-Stille s.
    Halsey nail s.
    Harvey wire-cutting s.
    hook rotary s.
    iris s.
    Jones s.

Koenig nail-splitting s.
Laschal suture s.
loop s.
Mayo s.
McIndoe s.
meniscal s.
Metzenbaum s.
s. nail drill
Nelson s.
orthopaedic s.
plain rotary s.
PowerStar bipolar s.
serrated s.
Sistron s.
Sistrunk s.
Slip-N-Snip s.
Smillie meniscal s.
Smith s.
Stephen s.
straight s.
suture s.
wire-cutting s.

SCIWORA
spinal cord injury without radiographic
abnormality

SCL
scaphocapitolunate arthrodesis

scleroderma
sclerosa osteoblastic osteogenic sarcoma
sclerosing
s. nonsuppurative osteitis
s. osteomyelitis

sclerosis, pl. scleroses
amyotrophic lateral s. (ALS, AML)
anterolateral s. (ALS)
Baló s.
endplate s.
Mönckeberg s.
multiple s. (MS)
progressive systemic s.
systemic s.

sclerotic
s. line
s. marginal rim
s. segment

sclerotomal pain
sclerotome pain chart
SCL-90R
Symptoms Checklist 90 Revised

scoliometer
scoliorachitis

scoliosis
adolescent s.
adolescent idiopathic s. (AIS)
adult s.
Aussies-Isseis unstable s.
s. brace
s. cast
Cobb measurement of s.
Cobb method for measuring s.
compensatory s.
congenital s.
s. correction
s. correction with Dwyer cable
Cotrel s.
curve progression in s.
degenerative lumbar s.
dextrorotary s.
dextroscoliosis s.
double major curve s.
double thoracic curve s.
Dwyer correction of s.
electrical surface stimulation
treatment for s.
Fergusson method for measuring s.
fracture with s.
functional s.
Galen s.
hysterical s.
idiopathic s.
infantile idiopathic s.
juvenile idiopathic s.
King classification of thoracic s.
King-Moe s.
King s. (type I–V)
kyphosing s.
levorotary s.
levoscoliosis s.
lumbar s.
Moe-Kettleson distribution of
curves in s.
neuromuscular s.
s. operating frame
right thoracic curve s.
right thoracic, left lumbar s.
right thoracic, left thoracolumbar s.
rigid curve s.
rotational s.
structural s.
s. surgery
thoracic curve s.
thoracolumbar idiopathic s.
thoracolumbar spine s.

S

NOTES

scoliosis *(continued)*
    treatment for s.
    uncompensated rotary s.
scoliotic
    s. curve
    s. curve fixation
ScoliTron instrument
scoop dish
Scoot-Gard mat
scope
    Doppler s.
    GO s.
    Harris s.
    Liviscope s.
score
    Champion Trauma S. (CTS)
    Charnley hip s.
    duPont Bunion Rating S.
    Fulkerson functional knee s.
    Glasgow Coma S. (GCS)
    Harris hip s.
    Harris-Mayo hip s.
    Hospital for Special Surgery
      knee s.
    Hughston knee s.
    IKDC s.
    Injury Severity S. (ISS)
    Iowa hip s.
    Kurtzke s.
    Lysholm s.
    Lysholm-Gillquist knee subjective
      function s.
    Mangled Extremity Severity S.
      (MESS)
    Maryland Foot S.
    Mayo elbow performance s.
    Merchant and Dietz ankle s.
    Merle d'Aubigné hip s.
    modified Harris hip s.
    Oswestry Disability S.
    Tegner activity s.
    Trauma S.
Scorpio total knee system
Scotchcast
    S. 2 casting tape
    S. length splinting system
scotoma, pl. scotomata
    absolute scotomata
Scott
    S. glenoplasty
    S. glenoplasty technique
    S. humeral splint
    S. posterior glenoplasty
Scottish Rite
    S. R. brace
    S. R. hip orthosis
    S. R. Hospital spinal implant
    S. R. splint

Scott-McCracken periosteal elevator
Scott-RCE osteotomy guide
Scotty
    S. dog sign
    S. stainless ankle joint
scout film
Scoville
    S. curette
    S. retractor
Scranton transmalleolar arthrodesis
scraping toe gait
screen
    Fast Lanex rare earth s.
    homogeneous s.
    Lanex s.
    split s.
screening
    generic s.
    ISIS s.
    s. palpation
screw
    Ace s.
    AcroMed s.
    alar s.
    s. alignment bar
    s. alignment rod
    Alta cancellous s.
    Alta cortical s.
    Alta cross-locking s.
    Alta lag s.
    Alta transverse s.
    AMBI hip s.
    Amset R-F s.
    anchor s.
    s.-and-plate fixation
    s.-and-wire fixation
    s. angle guide
    s. angulation
    AO-ASIF s.
    AO cancellous s.
    AO cortex s.
    AO lag s.
    AO spongiosa s.
    Arthrex sheathed interference s.
    arthrodesis s.
    ASIF cancellous s.
    ASIF cortical s.
    ASIF malleolar s.
    Asnis cannulated cancellous s.
    Aten olecranon s.
    Autogenesis automator for
      Ilizarov s.
    axial compression s.
    s. backout
    Barouk cannulated bone s.
    Basile hip s.
    Bechtol s.
    bicortical s.

S

Bio-Absorbable interference s.
biologically quiet interference s.
Bionix self-reinforced PLLA
  smart s.
bone s.
Bosworth coracoclavicular s.
s. breakage
buttress thread s.
Campbell cannulated s.
cancellous bone s.
cannulated hip s.
CAPIS s.
carpal scaphoid s.
Carrell-Girard s.
s.-in ceramic acetabular cup
Cohort bone s.
Collison s.
compression hip s.
compression lag s.
s. compressor
cortex s.
cortical cancellous s.
Cotrel pedicle s.
Coventry s.
crown drill s.
cruciate head bone s.
cruciform head bone s.
Cubbins s.
DDT s.
DeMuth hip s.
s. depth calibrator
s. depth gauge
DePuy interference s.
s. design
Deyerle s.
DHS hip s.
distal locking s.
distraction s.
double-threaded Herbert s.
Duo-Drive s.
Dwyer spinal s.
Dynamic condylar s. (DCS)
ECT bone s.
Edwards modular system
  spinal/sacral s.
Eggers s.
encased s.
s. epiphysiodesis
expansion s.
Fabian s.
femoral head cork s.
Fixateur Interne s.

s. fixation
flutes of cannulated s.
foreign body s.
four-tap s.
s. fusion
Geckler s.
Glasgow s.
Glass-Bessen transfixion s.
glenoid fixation s.
Guardsman femoral interference s.
Hahn s.
Hall spinal s.
Hamilton s.
s. head
Heck s.
Henderson lag s.
Herbert bone s.
Herbert scaphoid s.
Herbert-Whipple bone s.
hex s.
hexagonal slot-cap s.
hip compression s.
s.-holding forceps
hollow mill Asnis cannulated s.
s.-home mechanism
hook trial set s.
Howmedica ICS s.
iliac s.
iliosacral s.
Ilizarov s.
s. implantation
s. insertion
s. insertion technique
Instrument Makar biodegradable
  interference s.
Integrity acetabular cup s.
interference s.
interfragmentary lag s.
Isola spinal implant system iliac s.
Isola vertebral s.
Jewett pick-up s.
Johannson lag s.
Jones s.
Kaessmann s.
Kostuik s.
Kristiansen eyelet lag s.
Kurosaka interference-fit s.
lag s.
Lane bone s.
lateral s.
Leinbach olecranon s.
Leone expansion s.

NOTES

screw *(continued)*
Linvatec absorbable s.
locking s.
s. loosening
Lorenzo s.
Luhr s.
lumbar pedicle s.
Lundholm s.
Luque II s.
Luque pedicle s.
machine s.
malleolar s.
Marion s.
Martin s.
maxillofacial bone s.
McLaughlin carpal scaphoid s.
medial bicortical s.
medial unicortical s.
Medoff axial compression s.
mille pattes s.
mini AO s.
Moberg s.
Morris biphase s.
Mouradian s.
multiaxial s.
Neufeld s.
No-Lok s.
non-self-tapping s.
Olerud PSF s.
Ormandy s.
Orthofix s.
Osteomed s.
Palex expansion s.
Palmer s.
pedicle s.
PerFixation s.
PGA s.
Phillips head s.
Phillips recessed-head s.
Pilot point s.
s.-plate approach
polyaxial cervical s.
polylactide s.
s. position perioperative monitoring
Propel cannulated interference s.
pull s.
Ray s.
reverse-threaded s.
Richards classic compression hip s.
Richards lag s.
Richmond subarachnoid s.
rigid pedicle s.
Rockwood shoulder s.
Russell-Taylor s.
sacral alar s.
sacral pedicle s.
Schanz s.
Scuderi s.

self-tapping bone s.
set s.
Sharpey s.
Shelton bone s.
Sherman bone s.
Simmons double-hole spinal s.
Simmons-Martin s.
sliding compression hip s.
spherical-headed s.
spongiosa s.
s. stabilization
stainless steel s.
Steffee s.
step s.
s. stripout
Stryker lag s.
superior thoracic pedicle s.
Swiss cancellous s.
syndesmotic s.
Synthes compression hip s.
s. tap
Thatcher s.
thoracolumbar pedicle s.
Thornton s.
threaded cancellous s.
thumb s.
s. tip
titanium s.
Tivanium cancellous bone s.
s.-to-screw compression construct
Townley bone graft s.
Townsend-Gilfillan s.
traction tongs s.
transarticular s.
transfixion s.
transpedicular s.
transverse s.
triangulated pedicle s.
TSRH pedicle s.
tulip pedicle s.
varus-valgus adjustment s.
Venable s.
Venable-Stuck s.
Virgin hip s.
Vitallium s.
VLC compression s.
Wagner-Schanz s.
Weise jack s.
wood s., woodscrew
Woodruff s.
Yuan s.
Zimmer compression hip s.
Zuelzer s.

screwdriver
Allen-headed s.
automatic s.
Becker s.
Bosworth s.

CAPIS s.
Cardan s.
Children's Hospital s.
Collison s.
cross-slot s.
cruciform s.
Cubbins bone s.
DePuy s.
Dorsey screw-holding s.
European-style s.
Flatt self-retaining s.
Hall s.
heavy cross-slot s.
hexhead s.
Johnson s.
Ken s.
Lane s.
light cross-slot s.
Lok-it s.
Lok-screw double-slot s.
Massie s.
Master s.
Moore-Blount s.
Phillips head s.
plain s.
Richards Phillips s.
Richter bone s.
self-retaining s.
Shallcross s.
Sherman s.
Sherman-Pierce s.
single cross-slot s.
single-slot s.
skull plate s.
straight hex s.
Stryker s.
torque s.
Trinkle s.
Universal hex s.
V. Mueller s.
White s.
Williams s.
Woodruff s.
Zimmer s.
Screw-Lok tap
screw-plate
    Calandruccio impaction s.-p.
    Zimmer impaction s.-p.
scrub
    Betadine s.
    Exidine S.
    Hibiclens s.

SCS
    spinal canal stenosis
SCSP
    supracondylar-suprapatellar
SC-SP
    supracondylar-suprapatellar
Scuderi
    S. procedure
    S. screw
    S. technique
Scuder repair
sculp
    Concise cementing s.
    s. knife
scultetus
    s. bandage
    s. binder
scurvy line
Scutan temporary splint material
S-cutting block
SD
    shoulder disarticulation
SDD
    sterile dry dressing
SDR
    surgical dressing room
Seaber forceps
seal limb
Seal-Tight cast protector
seam
    osteoid s.
searching big toe
seat
    antithrust s.
    Backjoy s.
    s. belt
    s. belt injury
    Carrie car s.
    Dream Ride car s.
    ischial-bearing s.
    Maddacare child bath s.
    Orthopedic Positioning S.
    Posey drop s.
    Renolux convertible car s.
    Snug s.
    Special S.
    Spelcast car s.
    Tall-ette toilet s.
    Tubsider Kneeling S.
seated
    S. Cable Row exerciser
    s. hamstring curl

S

NOTES

seated *(continued)*
>   properly s.
>   s. root test

seating
>   s. chisel
>   trial s.
>   s. wedge

Seattle
>   S. foot prosthesis
>   S. LightFoot 2
>   S. orthosis
>   S. splint

sebaceous cyst
Sebileau periosteal elevator
secobarbital
>   amobarbital and s.

Seconal Injection
second
>   s. cervical vertebra
>   cycles per s. (cps, c/sec)
>   s. digit
>   s.-generation cementing technique
>   s. impact syndrome
>   s.-look arthroscopy
>   milliamperage x s.'s (MAS)
>   s. skin pad
>   s. toe

secondarius
>   calcaneus s.

secondary
>   s. or acute hematogenous
>   osteomyelitis
>   s. bone union
>   s. closure
>   s. fracture
>   s. hip-spine syndrome
>   s. metatarsalgia
>   s. myofascial trigger point
>   s. posttraumatic syringomyelia
>   s. stabilizer

section
>   bar s.
>   calcaneonavicular bar s.

sectioning
>   sequential s.

**Secure Yet Gentle surgical dressing
  system**
sed
>   sedimentation
>   sed rate

Sedan goniometer
sedation
Seddon
>   S. classification
>   S. coin test
>   S. dorsal spine costotransversectomy
>   S. modification
>   S. technique

sedentary
>   s. lifestyle
>   s. occupation
>   s. work

Sedillot periosteal elevator
sedimentation (sed)
sedimentation rate
>   erythrocyte s. r. (ESR)

Seeburger implant
segment
>   apical s.
>   central s.
>   motion s.
>   physiologic lock of the motion s.
>   relation to subadjacent s.'s
>   sacral s.
>   sclerotic s.
>   spinal s.
>   vertebral motion s.

segmental
>   s. artery
>   s. bone loss
>   s. compression construct
>   s. deficiency
>   s. dysfunction
>   s. fixation
>   s. fracture
>   s. hyperextension
>   s. level
>   s. mobility
>   s. mobility testing
>   s. spinal correction system (SSCS)
>   s. spinal instrumentation (SSI)
>   s. tendon graft
>   s. vertebral
>   cellulotenoperiosteomyalgic
>   syndrome (SVCPMS)

segmentation
>   s. defect
>   supernumerary lumbar s.

Segond fracture
Seidel
>   S. bone-holding clamp
>   S. intramedullary fixation
>   S. nail
>   S. saddlebag

**Seinsheimer femoral fracture
  classification**
Seipi FAL
Seirin acupuncture needle
seizing forceps
seizure
>   oxygen s.

Selakovich
>   S. procedure
>   S. procedure for pes valgo planus

Selby II hook

Select

S. ankle prosthesis
S. joint
S. joint orthosis
S. shoulder prosthesis
S. shoulder system

selection

bone plate s.
Edwards modular system
construct s.

selective

s. posterior rhizotomy (SPR)
Theraform S.'s
s. thoracic spine fusion

selenium sulfide
self-adhering varus/valgus wedge
self-aligning knee (SAL)
self-articulating

s.-a. femoral (SAF)
s.-a. femoral hip replacement (SAF
hip replacement)

self-bearing

s.-b. ceramic hip prosthesis
s.-b. ceramic total hip replacement

self-broaching

s.-b. nail
s.-b. pin

self-centering Universal hip prosthesis
self-curing polymer
self-induced injury
self-inflicted gunshot wound
self-locking nail
self-mutilation
self-propelling wheelchair
self-retaining

s.-r. bone-holding forceps
s.-r. clamp
s.-r. retractor
s.-r. screwdriver

self-sealing cannula
self-tapering pin
self-tapping bone screw
Selig hip operation
Sell-Frank-Johnson

S.-F.-J. extensor shift
S.-F.-J. extensor shift technique

Sellick maneuver
Sellors rib contractor
Selsun

S. Blue
S. Gold for Women

Selverstone rongeur forceps

Semb

S. bone forceps
S. bone-holding clamp
S. rib forceps

sEMG

surface electromyography

semiconstrained

s. total elbow arthroplasty
s. tricompartmental knee prosthesis

semi-Fowler position
semilunar

s. bone
s. cartilage knife

semilunaris

linea s.

semimembranosus

s. bursitis
s. complex
s. muscle
s. tendinitis
s. tendon

semiopen sliding tenotomy
semirigid

s. fiberglass cast (SRF)
s. orthosis
s. polypropylene ankle-foot orthosis
s. shell

semisitting position
semitendinosus

s. augmentation of patellar tendon
repair
s. muscle
s. procedure
s. technique
s. tendon
s. tendon transfer
s. tenodesis

semitendinosus-gracilis graft
semitendinous graft
semitubular

s. blade plate
s. compression plate

Semmes-Weinstein

S.-W. monofilament
S.-W. monofilament pressure
esthesiometry
S.-W. monofilament pressure test

Senegas

S. approach to hip
S. hip approach

senescence
senescent cell

S

NOTES

Sengupta quadriceps release
senile hallux valgus
senilis
> coxa s.
> malum coxae s.

Senn
> S. plate
> S. retractor

sensation
> altered s.
> catching s.
> circulation, muscle s. (CMS)
> diminished s.
> exteroceptive s.
> light touch s.
> loss of protective s. (LOPS)
> perianal s.
> perineal s.
> phantom s.
> pinprick s.
> return of s.
> sharp s.
> shocklike s.
> touch s.
> vibration s.

sense
> joint position s. (JPS)
> S.-of-Feel prosthesis
> position s.

sensibility recovery sequence
sensitometer
> Poppen ridge s.

sensor
> capacitive s.
> DermaTemp infrared
>   thermographic s.
> Myoscan s.
> s. pad
> Perry s.
> PerryMeter s.
> Richmond subarachnoid screw s.
> Servo Pro force s.

Sensorcaine
Sensorcaine-MPF
sensorimotor (*var. of* sensory motor)
sensorimotor
> s. deficit
> s. stimulation approach

sensorineural, sensory/neural
> s. abnormality

sensory
> s. awareness
> s. component
> s. delay
> s. evoked potential
> s. examination
> s. fascicle
> s. function

> s. impairment
> s. integration
> s. loss
> s. or motor deficit
> s.-motor training
> s. nerve
> s. nerve action potential (SNAP)
> s. nerve conduction velocity
> s. peak latency
> s. polyneuropathy
> s. registration
> s. response
> s. stimulation kit

sensory motor, sensorimotor
sensory/neural (*var. of* sensorineural)
sentinel fracture
Senuva lotion
Seoffert triple arthrodesis
SEP
> somatosensory evoked potential
>   long-latency SEP
>   microneurography midlatency SEP

separation
> AC joint s.
> acromioclavicular s.
> articular mass s.
> degree of s.
> lamellar s.
> transepiphyseal s.

separator
> abduction knee s.
> finger s.
> nerve s.
> Sach nerve s.

sepsis
Septacin implant
septal forceps
Septa Topical Ointment
septic
> s. arthritis
> s. bursitis
> s. finger joint
> s. knee
> s. necrosis

SeptiCare antimicrobial wound cleanser
Septisol solution
Septobal bead
septum
> intermuscular s.
> J s.

Sequeira-Khanuja modification
sequela, pl. **sequelae**
sequence
> Carr-Purcell s.
> Carr-Purcell-Meiboom-Gill s.
> muscle patterning s.
> sensibility recovery s.
> turbo-spin-echo imaging s.

sequencing bead patterns set
sequential
    s. compression device (SCD)
    s. extremity pump
    s. pneumatic compression boot
    s. pressure
    s. sectioning
sequestered disk
sequestra (*pl. of* sequestrum)
sequestrated disk
sequestration
sequestrectomy
sequestrum, pl. **sequestra**
    avascular s.
    s. forceps
    kissing s.
SER
    supination-external rotation
Serafin technique
Serax
**serendipity view in shoulder
  radiography**
serial
    s. casting
    s. wedge cast
series
    Davis s.
    HESSCO 300, 500 s.
    lumbosacral s.
    Option Orthotic S.
    RingLoc acetabular s.
    Valpar component work sample s.
Series-II humeral head
SER-IV fracture
Serola sacroiliac belt
seroma
seronegative
    s. arthritis
    s. arthropathy
seronegativity
seropositive arthritis
serosanguineous
serotonergic neuron
serotonin (5-HT)
serpentine
    s. foam collar
    s. foot
    s. incision
    s. plate
serpiginosum
    angioma s.

serrated
    s. action potential
    s. fine-cutting knife
    s. scissors
Serratia marcescens
serration
Serrato
    S. forearm pin
    S. forearm rod
serratus
    s. anterior flap
    s. anterior muscle
    s. anterior paralysis
sertraline
serum
    s. bactericidal concentration
    s. calcium
    s. urate concentration
Services
    American Red Cross Tissue S.
Servo Pro force sensor
Servox device
sesamoid
    accessory s.
    bipartite tibial s.
    s. bone
    fibular s.
    hallucal s.
    hallux s.
    s. injury
    s. ligament
    tibial s.
sesamoidectomy
    s. dissector
    fibular s.
    lateral s.
sesamoideum
    os s.
sesamoiditis
sesamoidometatarsal joint
sesamophalangeal ligament
sessile
set
    acetabular trial s.
    aluminum contouring template s.
    s. angle
    s. angle of toe
    AO minifragment s.
    Bankart shoulder repair s.
    bone drill s.
    Brown-Mueller T-fastener s.
    Craig vertebral biopsy s.

NOTES

set *(continued)*
>Entrex small joint arthroscopy instrument s.
>grid maze s.
>hand evaluation s.
>Henning instrument s.
>s.-hold adjustment
>Hollywood bed extension hook s.
>LIDO lift and work s.
>nail s.
>parquetry s.
>prothelen s.
>Rousek extraction s.
>s. screw
>sequencing bead patterns s.
>Stille bone drill s.
>Stille-pattern trephine and bone drill s.
>vari-balance board s.
>volumeter s.

Seton hip brace
Setopress dressing
setter
>bone plug s.

setting
>bone s.

seven-hole plate
Sever
>S. disease
>S. modification of Fairbank technique

severance
>severe s.

severe
>s. degenerative disk disease
>s. kyphoscoliosis
>s. rigid thoracic curve
>s. severance

Severin
>anatomical classification system of S.
>S. classification
>S. hip criteria

Sever-L'Episcopo
>S.-L. repair of shoulder
>S.-L. shoulder repair

SEWHO
>shoulder-elbow-wrist-hand orthosis

sex
>s. hormone
>s.-linked muscular dystrophy

SF-36
>Short-Form 36
>SF-36 patient assessment form

SFA
>superficial femoral artery

SFEMG
>single fiber electromyography

SFI
>sciatic function index

S-flap incision
Sgarlato toe implant
shadow
>elliptical overlap s.
>s. shield

Shadow-Line ACF spine retractor system
Shaeffer rigid orthosis
Shaffner orthopaedic inserter
shaft
>Cloward drill s.
>distal third of s.
>femoral s.
>s. fracture
>metatarsal s.
>middle third of s.
>ministem s.
>neck s.
>patellar reamer s.
>proximal third of s.
>radial s.

Shallcross screwdriver
Sham procedure
shank
>Bi-Metric tapered reamer with Zimmer-Hudson s.
>calcar trimmer with Zimmer-Hudson s.
>grater-type reamer with Zimmer-Hudson s.
>steel s.
>taper with Zimmer s.
>Zimmer-Hudson s.

Shannon bur
Shantz *(var. of* Schanz)
Shanz *(var. of* Schanz)
shape
>Erlenmeyer-flask s.
>familial s.

Sharbaro driver
sharing
>Edwards modular system load s.

sharp
>acetabular angle of S.
>S. acetabular angle
>s. dissection
>s. retractor
>s. sensation
>s. trocar
>s. worm hook

Sharpey
>S. fiber
>S. screw

sharp-pointed wire
Sharrard
>S. posterior transfer

S. transfer technique
S.-type kyphectomy
Sharrard-Trentani prosthesis
Shar-Tek foot positioning grid
shave biopsy
shaver
arthroscopic s.
automated s.
cutting s.
Dyonics s.
Grierson meniscal s.
Kuda s.
Microsect s.
5.5-mm s.
motorized meniscal s.
motorized suction s.
sucker s.
synovial s.
shaving
arthroscopic s.
femoral condylar s.
s. system
Shea
S. drill
S. prosthesis placement instrument
shear
anterior s.
s. fracture
lateral s.
s. maneuver
s.-off device
s. strain
s. stress
s. test
s. testing
vertical s. (VS)
ShearGuard low-friction interface
shearing
s. callus
s. injury
S. posterior chamber implant
material
shears
airplane s.
Baer rib s.
Bethune-Coryllos rib s.
Brunner rib s.
Brunn plaster s.
Collins rib s.
Cooley rib s.
Esmarch plaster s.
Felt s.

Giertz rib s.
Giertz-Shoemaker rib s.
Gluck rib s.
Hercules plaster s.
Lefferts rib s.
Liston-Key-Horsley rib s.
Sauerbruch rib s.
Stille plaster s.
sheath
arthroscope s.
arthroscopic s.
carotid s.
digital flexor tendon s.
fascia s.
fibroosseous s.
flexor tendon s.
ganglionic cyst in synovial
tendon s.
muscle s.
pigmented nodular synovitis of
tendon s.
rectus s.
synovial s.
tendon s.
tenosynovial s.
visceral tendon s.
sheathed knife
sheath/liner
Silipos Distal Dip prosthetic s.
Sheehan
S. chisel
S. gouge
S. knee prosthesis
S. osteotome
sheepskin
sheet
Alpha flat s.
Antishear gel s.
Barrier lower extremity s.
s. cork
iodoform-impregnated plastic s.
Korex cork s.
laparotomy s.
Novagel gel s.
Ortholen s.
PPT s.
sterile s.
sheeting
Carboplast II s.
Silastic s.
sterile s.

NOTES

S

Sheffield
    S. hand elevator
    S. support
shelf
    s. acetabuloplasty
    Blumer s.
    s. flexion
    lateral s.
    medial s.
    patellar s.
    s. pedestal
shell
    AFO standard s.
    s. allograft
    calf s.
    s. impactor
    s. implant material
    protrusio s.
    Restoration Secur-Fit X'tra
      acetabular s.
    semirigid s.
    thigh s.
    Unna paste s.
shelling off of cartilage
Shelton
    S. bone screw
    S. femoral fracture classification
shelving
Shenton line
Shepherd fracture
shepherd's crook deformity
Sherfee prosthesis
Sherk-Probst
    S.-P. percutaneous pinning
    S.-P. technique
Sherman
    S. block test
    S. bone plate
    S. bone screw
    S. remote podiatric vacuum system
    S. screwdriver
Sherman-Pierce screwdriver
Sherman-Stille drill
Sherrington law
ShiatsuBACK back support
Shiatsu massage
shield
    arthroscopic s.
    bunion s.
    contact s.
    Nolan system collimator mounted
      contact s.
    shadow s.
    Sportelli system collimator mounted
      contact s.
Shier knee prosthesis
Shifrin wire twister

shift
    anterior cruciate instability with
      pivot s.
    anterior talus s.
    inferior capsular s. (ICS)
    lateral lumbar s.
    lateral pivot s.
    lateral trunk s.
    pelvic lateral s.
    plantar s.
    plasma volume s.
    reverse pivot s.
    Sell-Frank-Johnson extensor s.
    s. sign
    s. test
    trochanteric s.
    trunk s.
Shifter
    AliMed Conductive Patient S.
shifting
    vessel s.
shingling
shin splint
Ship hammertoe implant
SHIP-Shaw rod hammertoe implant
Shirley drain
shish kebab technique
shock
    s. absorption
    s. artifact
    cardiogenic s.
    hypovolemic s.
    neurogenic s.
    prosthetic stance phase s.
    spinal s.
    s. treatment
    vasogenic s.
shocklike sensation
Shockmaster heel cushion
shod
    rubber-s.
shoe
    Acor Quikform I, II s.
    Ambulator s.
    Apex ambulator s.
    arthritic s.
    Asics s.
    balmoral laced s.
    Bebax s.
    Bevin s.
    blucher laced s.
    calcaneal spur pad in s.
    cast s.
    s. cookie
    cut-out s.
    Darco s.
    Darco Wedge s.
    s. dermatitis

diabetic pressure relief s.
extended-counter s.
s. extension
extra-depth s.
s. filler
s.-foot interface
s. gear
healing s.
s. heel pad
high heel s.
Hi-Top s.
infant clown cast s.
s. insert
ipos heel relief s.
J&J postoperative s.
Kunzli orthopaedic sports s.
s. lift
low quarter Blucher s.
Markell Mobility S.'s
Markell open-toe s.
Markell tarso medius straight s.
Markell tarso pronator outflare s.
Moon Boot s.
narrow toebox s.
navicular cookie in s.
normal last s.
open-toe s.
orthopaedic oxford s.
s. orthotic
OrthoWedge healing s.
Pedors orthopedic s.
pointed toe s.
PowerAnthro S.
pressure relief s.
PRN s.
Reebok s.
Reece orthopedic s.
reverse last s.
rockerbottom s.
SAS s.
scaphoid cookie in s.
soft-vamp s.
space s.
straight last s.
s. stretcher
tarsal pronator s.
Thera-Medic s.
torque heel s.
Tru-Fit custom molded s.
Tru-Mold s.
Urban Walkers s.
Vibram rockerbottom s.

Viva s.
WACH orthopaedic s.
s. wear
Weaver rockerbottom s.
wedge adjustable cushioned heel s.
wide toebox s.
wooden s.
wooden-soled s.
Zohar s.

shoe insert
UCB s. i.

short
s.-acting block anesthesia (SAB)
s. arm brace
s. arm cast (SAC)
s. arm fiberglass cast
s. arm gauntlet cast
s. arm navicular cast (SANC)
s. arm splint (SAS)
s. arm sugar-tong splint
s. bone
s. coarse bur
s. curette
s. external rotator
s. fine bur
s. head of biceps
s.-latency somatosensory evoked
  potential (SSEP)
s. leg
s. leg caliper brace
s. leg cast (SLC)
s. leg double-upright brace
s. leg splint
s. leg syndrome
s. leg walker
s. leg walking brace
s. leg walking cast (SLWC)
s. lever accessory movement
  technique
s. lever specific contact procedure
s. oblique fracture
s. opponens orthosis
s. plantar ligament (SPL)
s.-radius kyphosis
s. segment spinal fusion
Short-Form 36 (SF-36)
s. stature
s. tau inversion recovery (STIR)
S. Test of Mental Status (STMS)
s. thumb
s. walking cast (SLWC)
s.-wave diathermy (SWD)

S

NOTES

shortening
  Achilles tendon s.
  Broughton-Olney-Menelaus tibial
    diaphyseal s.
  closed femoral diaphyseal s.
  s. collectomy
  s. contraction
  digital s.
  distal Wagner femoral
    metaphyseal s.
  femoral metaphyseal s.
  Hoffa tendon s.
  leg s.
  metaphyseal s.
  s. osteotomy
  proximal femoral metaphyseal s.
  proximal Wagner metaphyseal s.
  tibial diaphyseal s.
  Wagner femoral metaphyseal s.
  Winquist-Hansen-Pearson closed
    femoral diaphyseal s.
short leg plaster cast
shotgun
  s. injury
  s. wound
shot wadding
shoulder
  s. abduction immobilizer
  s. abduction pillow
  s. abduction positioner
  s. abduction test
  s. amputation
  s. ankylosis
  apprehension s.
  archer's s.
  s. arm system (SAS)
  s. arthrodesis
  s. arthroplasty
  baseball s.
  s. clock
  s. complex
  s. controller
  s. cuff
  s. depression test
  s. disarticulation (SD)
  s. dislocation
  s. dislocation bone bank
  s. dome
  s. dystopia
  S. Ease abduction support
  flail s.
  frozen s.
  s. girdle
  s. holder
  s. immobilizer
  s. instability
  s. ladder
  little leaguer's s.

  Neviaser classification of frozen s.
  S. Pain and Disability Index
    patient questionnaire
  s. pointer
  s. prosthesis
  s. pulley
  s. radiography
  s. reduction
  s. repair
  s. ROM arc
  s. saddle sling
  S. Severity Index patient
    questionnaire
  Sever-L'Episcopo repair of s.
  s. spica cast
  s. spica splint
  s. subluxation inhibitor (SSI)
  s. subluxation inhibitor brace
  s. wheel
**shoulder-elbow-wrist-hand orthosis
  (SEWHO)**
shoulderRAP wrap
ShowerSafe
  S. waterproof cast and bandage
    cover
  S. waterproof cast and bandage
    protector
Show'rbag
SHPL
  sacral horizontal plane line
SH popoff suture
Shriners pin
shrinker
  stump s.
**Shriver-Johnson interphalangeal
  arthrodesis**
shucking
shuck test
shuffling gait
shunt
  s. muscle
  Sundt s.
  ventriculoperitoneal s.
Shur-Band self-closure elastic bandage
shuttle
  S. cardiomuscular conditioner
  Caspari s.
Shuttle-Relay suture passer
Shutt Mantis retrograde forceps
SI
  sacroiliac
    SI belt
    SI joint
sibilant
Sibson fascia
sicca
  Neisseria s.

sickle-cell
  s.-c. anemia
  s.-c. disease
sickle-shape Beaver blade
Sickness Impact Profile (SIP)
SID
  source image distance
side
  s. bending
  s.-bending barrier
  s.-bending mobility
  crest sign s.
  s.-cut pin cutter
  s. cutter
  dollar sign s.
  s.-glide test
  s.-jump test
  s. lying
  s.-opening laminar hook
  s. plate
  posterior rotation on the left s.
  posterior rotation on the right s.
  s.-posture position
  s. posture reduction
side-bent
side-cutting
  s.-c. basket forceps
  s.-c. blade
Sidekick foot support
side-lying
  s.-l. hip abductor
  s.-l. iliac compression test
  s.-l. position
sideplate
  s. barrel
  barreled s.
  compression s.
  Richards s.
  sliding compression screw with s.
side-shift
  pelvic s.-s.
sideswipe
  s. elbow fracture
  s. injury
side-to-side anastomosis
sidewall
Siegel hip release
Sielke instrumentation
Sieman table
Siemens LINAC
Sierra 2-load voluntary opening
Siffert-Forster-Nachamie arthrodesis

Siffert intraepiphyseal osteotomy
Siffert-Storen intraepiphyseal osteotomy
Sifoam padding
sigma receptor
sigmoid notch
sign
  Achilles bulge s.
  Adam s.
  Adson s.
  Allen s.
  Allis s.
  Amoss s.
  Anghelescu s.
  anteater-nose s.
  antecedent s.
  anterior drawer s.
  anterior tibial s.
  anvil s.
  Apley s.
  apprehension s.
  arterial occlusion s.
  Ashhurst s.
  Babinski s.
  Barlow s.
  Bassett s.
  Battle s.
  bayonet s.
  Beevor s.
  bottle s.
  bowstring s.
  bow-tie s.
  Bragard s.
  Brudzinski s.
  Bryant s.
  Burton s.
  camelback s.
  Cantelli s.
  Chaddock s.
  Chinese red line s.
  choppy sea s.
  Chvostek s.
  Chvostek-Weiss s.
  Clark s.
  Cleeman s.
  click s.
  Codman s.
  cogwheel s.
  Collier s.
  commemorative s.
  Comolli s.
  contralateral s.
  Coopernail s.

S

NOTES

sign *(continued)*

crescent s.
crest s.
Darier s.
Dawbarn s.
Déjérine s.
Demianoff s.
Desault s.
Destot s.
dollar s.
double-arc s.
double camelback s.
drawer s.
drivethrough s.
drop-arm s.
Dupuytren s.
Earle s.
Egawa s.
Erichsen s.
eye s.
fabere s.
fadir s.
Fairbanks s.
Fajersztajn crossed sciatic s.
fallen-fragment s.
fallen-leaf s.
fan s.
fat pad s.
fishtail s.
flag s.
Fleck s.
fluid s.
Forestier bowstring s.
Fränkel s.
Friedreich s.
Froment paper s.
Gaenslen s.
Gage s.
Galant s.
Galeazzi s.
Goldthwait s.
Gottron s.
Gowers s.
grab s.
Guilland s.
gun barrel s.
halo s.
Hamman s.
hanging heel s.
Hawkins impingement s.
head-at-risk s.
heel varus s.
Helbing s.
Hill-Sachs s.
Hirschberg s.
Hoffmann s.
Homans s.
Hoover s.

hot-cross-bun skull s.
Hueter s.
Huntington s.
iliac apophysis s.
impingement s.
J s.
Jenet s.
jerk s.
jump s.
Kanavel s.
Kaplan s.
Keen s.
Kehr s.
Kellgren s.
Kernig s.
Kerr s.
Kocher-Cushing s.
Lachman s.
Langoria s.
Lasègue s.
lateral capsular s.
Laugier s.
Leichtenstern s.
Leri s.
Leser-Trelat s.
Lhermitte s.
Light V s.
Linder s.
long tract s.
Lorenz s.
Ludington s.
Ludloff s.
Macewen s.
Maisonneuve s.
Mandel-Bekhterev s.
Marie-Foix s.
Martel s.
Matev s.
McMurray s.
Mendel-Bekhterev s.
Mennell s.
Meryon s.
Minor s.
Morquio s.
Morton s.
Morton-Horwitz nerve cross-over s.
movie s.
Mudder s.
Mulder s.
Napoleon hat s.
Nelson s.
neuroma s.
ocular s.
Oppenheim s.
Ortolani s.
pathognomonic s.
Patrick s.
Payr s.

Pelken s.
Piotrowski s.
piriformis s.
piston s.
pivot-shift s.
plantar ecchymosis s.
popliteal pressure s.
positive impingement s.
positive rim s.
posterior drawer s.
posterior sag s.
posterolateral drawer s.
posteromedial drawer s.
pronation s.
pseudo-Babinski s.
pucker s.
Queckenstedt s.
rachitic rosary s.
radialis s.
Raimiste s.
Renee creak s.
reverse Hill-Sachs s.
ribbon s.
rim s.
Riordan s.
Risser s.
Roux s.
Rust s.
Sarbo s.
Schlesinger s.
sciatic tension s.
Scotty dog s.
shift s.
Soto-Hall s.
Speed s.
spilled cup s.
spine s.
spur s.
stairs s.
stepladder s.
Strümpell s.
Strunsky s.
suction s.
sulcus s.
supinator fat pad s.
Terry Thomas s.
theater s.
thermoregulatory s.
thick patella s.
Thomas s.
Thompson s.
thorn s.

Thurston-Holland flag s.
tibialis s.
Tinel s.
Tinel-Hoffmann s.
toe spread s.
toggle s.
too-many-toes s.
Turyn s.
"V" s.
vacant glenoid s.
Vanzetti s.
Voshell s.
Wartenberg s.
Werenskiold s.
Wilson s.
Winberger s.
windshield wiper s.
wink s.
winking owl s.
Yergason s.

SignaDRESS
S. hydrocolloid dressing
signal
intervertebral disk nucleus s.
s. void
significance
statistical s.
significant displacement
Sigvaris stockings
Siladryl Oral
Silapap
Children's S.
Infants' S.
Silastic
S. ball
S. ball spacer prosthesis
S. button
S. drain
S. finger implant
S. finger joint
S. gel dressing
S. lunate arthroplasty
S. radial head prosthesis
S. sheeting
S. standard elastometer prosthesis
S. thumb prosthesis
S. toe implant
silence
electrical s.
silent
s. fascicle
s. hip stage

NOTES

S

silent *(continued)*
    myoelectrically s.
    s. period
Silesian
    S. bandage
    S. bandage prosthetic support
    S. belt
Silflex intramedullary prosthesis
Silfverskiöld
    S. Achilles tendon lengthening
    S. Achilles tendon reconstruction
    S. procedure
    S. technique
    S. test
Silhouette spinal system
silicone
    s. arthritis
    s. breast implant
    s.-dacron tendon rod
    s. elastomer rubber ball implant
    s. gel
    s. gel socket insert
    s. implant arthroplasty
    s. insole
    s. material
    s. MP implant
    s. rubber arthroplasty
    s. rubber sphere
    s. synovitis
    s. thermoplastic splinting (STS)
    s. trapezium prosthesis
    Wonderflex s.
    s. wrist arthroplasty
silicore foot pillow
Silipos
    S. digital pad
    S. Distal Dip prosthetic sheath/liner
    S. gel
    S. mesh cap
    S. mesh tubing
    S. silicone wonder cup
    S. suspension sleeve
silk
    s. mesh gauze dressing
    Owens s.
    s. suture
**Silon silicone thermoplastic splinting
material**
Silopad
    S. body sleeve
    S. toe sleeve
Silosheath
    S. gel
    S. sock
silver
    S. bunionectomy
    s. dollar technique
    s. fork deformity

    s.-fork fracture
    s. nitrate
    S. osteotome
    S. procedure
    s. sulfadiazine
Silver-Simon lengthening
Silymarin
Similarity Discrimination Card
Simmonds-Menelaus
    S.-M. metatarsal osteotomy
    S.-M. proximal phalangeal
    osteotomy
Simmonds test
Simmons
    S. cervical spine fusion
    S. chisel
    S. crimper
    S. double-hole spinal screw
    S. Multi-Matic orthopaedic bed
    S. osteotome
    S. osteotomy
    S. plating system
    S. and Segil classification system
    S. spinal arthrodesis
    S. Vari-Hite orthopaedic bed
Simmons-Martin screw
Simonart band
simple
    S. Shoulder Test patient
    questionnaire
    s. suture
    s. syndactyly
simplex
    S. cement adhesive
    herpes s.
    hidroacanthoma s.
    S. P bone cement
Simpson sugar-tong splint
Simpulse
    S. pulsing lavage
    S. S/I lavage
Sims
    S. position
    S. retractor
simulator
    Baltimore Therapeutic Equipment
    Work S.
    BTE Work S.
    ERGOS work s.
    LIDO WorkSET work s.
    Spinal Physiotherapy S.
Simultaneous Interview Technique (SIT)
S incision
Sinding-Larsen-Johansson
    S.-L.-J. disease
    S.-L.-J. lesion
    S.-L.-J. syndrome
Sine-Aid IB

Sinequan
Singh
S. index of osteoporosis
S. osteoporosis classification
S. osteoporosis index
trabecular index of S.
single
s.-action rongeur
s. axis
s.-blade saw
s.-cannula system
s.-channel surface EMG
s.-condylar graft
s. cross-slot screwdriver
s. fiber electromyography (SFEMG)
s. fiber EMG
s. fiber needle electrode
s.-heel rise test
s.-incision fasciotomy
s.-leg spica cast
s.-level spinal fusion
s.-limb stance
s.-onlay cortical bone graft
s.-photon electrospinal orthosis
s. photon emission computed
tomography (SPECT)
s.-point cane
s.-prong broad acetabular retractor
s. proximal portal technique
s. reference point instrument (SRP
instrument)
s.-rod construct
s.-sided bone saw
s.-slot screwdriver
s.-unit pattern
single-axis
s.-a. ankle joint
s.-a. ankle prosthesis
s.-a. friction knee (SAFK)
s.-a. knee unit
s.-a. locking knee (SALK)
s.-a. Syme DYCOR foot
single-stage
s.-s. tendon graft
s.-s. tissue transfer
single-stemmed
s.-s. silicone hemiprosthesis
s.-s. toe implant
sink
counter s.
sinogram
sinography

sintered
s. implant prosthesis
s. titanium mesh
sintering
s. of cobalt-chrome powder coating
cobalt-chrome power s.
Sinterlock
S. implant
S. implant metal
S. implant metal prosthesis
sinus
s. histiocytosis
Motrin IB S.
osteomyelitic s.
pilonidal s.
talar s.
s. tarsi
s. tarsi syndrome
s. tract
sinusoidal
sinuvertebral nerve
SIO
sacroiliac orthosis
SIP
Sickness Impact Profile
sisomicin
Sisson fracture reducing elevator
Sistron scissors
Sistrunk scissors
SIT
Simultaneous Interview Technique
sit-and-reach
s.-a.-r. box
s.-a.-r. test
site
donor s.
fracture s.
harvest s.
hook s.
nonunion of fracture s.
operative s.
pin s.
recipient s.
SITElite
SITEprobe
SITEtrac
sit/stand chair
Sit-Straight
S.-S. wheelchair cushion
S.-S. wheelchair cushion with
antidecubitus "Gel"

NOTES

S

sitter
  floor s.
sitting
  s. flexion
  s. flexion test
  s. position
  s. root test
  s. side bend
sit-to-stand
  s.-t.-s. test
sit-up test
Sivash hip prosthesis
six
  s.-degrees-of-freedom
    electrogoniometer
  s.-hole plate
  s.-minute walk test
  "s.-pack hand" exercise
  s.-point knee brace
  s.-portal synovectomy
size
  crosslink plate s.
  S. Discrimination Card
sizer
  Brannock Device shoe s.
SJF
  subtalar joint function
SJK
  Scheuermann juvenile kyphosis
Sjögren syndrome
skate
  arm s.
skateboard
skateboarding accident
Skelaxin
skeletal
  s. age
  s. defect
  s.-extraskeletal angiomatosis
  s. hyperostosis syndrome
  s. hypoplasia
  s. hypoplasia disease
  idiopathic s.
  s. limb deficiency
  s. maturation
  s. maturity
  s. muscle
  s. pin
  s. tissue
  s. traction
  s. tuberculosis
skeleton
  bony s.
skeletonize
Skelid
skewer
skewering
skew flap

skewfoot
skid
  bone s.
  hip s.
  s. humeral head retractor
  Murphy s.
  Murphy-Lane bone s.
skier's
  s. fracture
  s. injury
  s. thumb
skijump view
SKI knee prosthesis
Skil-Care
  S.-C. cushion
  S.-C. cushion grip
  S.-C. reclining wheelchair
skill
  ambulation s.'s
  donning-doffing s.
  palpatory s.
  physical daily living s.'s (PDLS)
Skillbuilder half roll
Skillern fracture
Skil Saw
skin
  s. blood flow determination
  s. bone free graft
  s. breakdown
  S. Care kit
  s. closure
  s.-contact instrumentation
  s. coverage
  s. creaking
  s. crease
  dorsal s.
  s. flap
  s. fluorescence measurement
  s.-gliding test
  s. glue
  s. hook
  s. incision
  s. lesion
  s. marker
  s. necrosis
  nonglabrous s.
  s. pencil
  perianal s.
  s. plasty
  s. preparation
  s. resistance test
  s. restriction
  s. rolling
  s. slough
  s. staple
  s. stroker
  s. tag
  s. tape

s. temperature monitoring probe
s.-tight cast
undermined s.

skinfold

s. caliper
s. caliper

SkinTemp collagen skin dressing
skis

walker s.

skive
skived incision
skiving knife
Sklar

S. bone drill
S. bone saw
S. ligature needle
S. pin cutter
S. wire tightener

Skoog

S. fasciotomy
S. procedure for release of
Dupuytren contracture
S. technique

skull

hot-cross-bun s.
s. plate screwdriver
s. tongs

skull-occiput-mandibular immobilization
orthosis
skyline

s. view
s. x-ray view of patella

Skytron bed
SL

scapholunate
stereolithography
SL cage

SLAC

scapholunate advanced collapse

slack

motion s.
tissue s.
s. wrist

Slam'r wheelchair
slant

foam s.
OPTP S.

SLAP

superior labrum anterior and posterior
lesion

slap

s. foot gait
s. hammer

slapping gait
Slätis pelvic fracture frame
slatted plinth table
Slattery-McGrouther dynamic flexion
splint
SLC

short leg cast

SLE

systemic lupus erythematosus
SLE arthropathy

sleds

Penco Walker S.
walker s.

Sleep-eze 3 Oral
Sleepinal
Sleepwell 2-nite
sleeve

BioCompression Pneumatic S.
circumferential ligamentous s.
cylindrical s.
drill s.
Edwards-Levine s.
Edwards polyethylene s.
elbow s.
Electro-Mesh s.
epX suspension s.
s. fracture
gel suspension s.
heel s.
ICEROSS s.
knee s.
Knit-Rite suspension s.
malleolar gel s.
MICA 3x s.
neoprene elbow s.
neoprene knee s.
obturator s.
periosteal s.
polyethylene s.
Silipos suspension s.
Silopad body s.
Silopad toe s.
Super Grip s.
s. type

slide

flexor pronator s.
Glassman-Engh-Bobyn
trochanteric s.
muscle s.

NOTES

S

slide *(continued)*
    s. plate
    trochanteric s.
sliding
    s. abdominal hernia
    s. AFO
    s. arthrodesis
    s. barrel hook
    s. bone graft
    s. compression hip screw
    s. compression screw with sideplate
    s. fixation device
    s. flap
    s. hammer
    s. inlay bone graft
    s. knot
    s. nail
    s. nail device
    s. nail plate
    s. tenotomy
    s. tibial bone graft
SlimLine cast boot
Slim Option shoe orthosis
Slimrest
    Core S.
Slimthetics orthotic
sling
    Ampoxen s.
    arm elevator s.
    Barton s.
    Böhler-Braun leg s.
    collar-and-cuff s.
    cradle arm s.
    CVA S.
    s. dressing
    envelope arm s.
    envelope-type arm s.
    finger s.
    Fits-All s.
    s. frame
    Glisson s.
    Haacker s.
    hanging cast s.
    Harris Hemi Arm S.
    Harris splint s.
    hemiarm s.
    s. immobilization
    Jacksonville s.
    Kenny-Howard shoulder s.
    Kodel knee s.
    leg s.
    Legg-Perthes s.
    lymphedema s.
    Mersilene s.
    Murphy s.
    Nada-Chair Back-Up portable
      back s.
    Pavlik s.

    pelvic s.
    Posey s.
    pouch-type s.
    s. procedure
    Rauchfuss s.
    s. and reef technique
    resting foot s.
    rubber s.
    s. seat sag
    shoulder saddle s.
    sling-and-swathe s.
    Slingers arm s.
    slinger-style envelope s.
    sling and swathe s.
    soft tissue coaptation s.
    stockinette s.
    s. suspension range of motion
    s. suture
    swathe and s.
    Teare s.
    Thomas Kodel s.
    triangular arm s.
    universal s.
    Uni-Versatil s.
    Velpeau s.
    Vogue arm s.
    Weil pelvic s.
    Westfield-style envelope s.
sling-and-swathe
    s.-a.-s. bandage
    s.-a.-s. sling
sling-dressing
    Velpeau s.-d.
Slingers arm sling
slinger-style envelope sling
slip
    s. angle
    s. angle spondylolisthesis
    central s.
    flexor digitorum s.
    s.-joint pliers
    lateral s.
    s. of tendon
Slip-N-Snip scissors
slipped
    s. capital femoral epiphysis (SCFE)
    s. disk
    s. elbow
    s. vertebral apophysis
slipper
    Kite s.
    s.-type cast
slipping rib
slit catheter technique
sliver of bone
Slocum
    S. ALRI test
    S. anterior rotary drawer test

S. fusion technique
S. knee procedure
S. lateral pivot-shift test
S. maneuver
S. meniscal clamp
S. nail
S. pes anserinus transplant
S. rotary instability test
S. splint
Slo-Mo ball
slope
dorsal radial s.
slot
acetabular s.
S. distraction device
glenoid s.
s.-graft
s. table
slotted
s. acetabular augmentation
s. femur plate
s. mallet
s. nail
slough
skin s.
slow
s.-acting antirheumatic drug
(SAARD)
s. cautery
s. distraction
s. stretch
s. stretch reflex
s. union
SL-Plus stem
SLR
straight leg raising
SLR with Bragard test
SLR with external rotation test
SLR with Kernig test
SLRT
straight leg raising test
SL-Stem
sluggishness
slump test
SLURPIE procedure
slurry
bone s.
matrix-bone marrow s.
SLWC
short leg walking cast
short walking cast
Sly syndrome

SMA
spinal muscular atrophy
SMA prosthesis
small
s.-base quad cane
s. cell osteogenic sarcoma
s. fracture
s.-fragment
s.-joint stiffness
s. nail spicule bur
SMART
S. Balance Master
Smart Screw bioabsorbable implant
SMCR
superomedial calcaneonavicular ligament
Smedberg
S. brace
S. hand drill
S. twist drill
Smedley dynamometer
SMI 3000, 5000 bed
SMIC sternal drill
Smidt
protocol of S.
smile
inverted s.
Smillie
S. cartilage chisel
S. cartilage knife
S. meniscal knife
S. meniscal scissors
S. meniscectomy chisel
S. nail
S. pin
S. retractor
Smillie-Beaver
S.-B. blade
S.-B. knife
Smith
S. ankle prosthesis
S. bone clamp
S. cartilage knife
S. dislocation
S. drill
S. flexor pollicis longus abductor-
plasty
S. fracture
S. & Nephew medium barbed
staple
S. & Nephew reflection acetabular
cup implant component
S. & Nephew small barbed staple

S

NOTES

Smith *(continued)*
    S. physical capacities evaluation (PCE)
    S. scissors
    S. STA-peg
    S. technique
Smith-Davis Converta-Hite orthopaedic bed
Smith-Lemli-Opitz syndrome
Smith-Petersen
    S.-P. approach
    S.-P. cup
    S.-P. cup arthroplasty
    S.-P. curved gouge
    S.-P. curved osteotome
    S.-P. femoral neck nail
    S.-P. fracture pin
    S.-P. hemiarthroplasty
    S.-P. hip cup prosthesis
    S.-P. impactor
    S.-P. intertrochanteric plate
    S.-P. nail with Lloyd adapter
    S.-P. osteotomy
    S.-P. reamer
    S.-P. rongeur
    S.-P. sacroiliac joint fusion
    S.-P. straight gouge
    S.-P. straight osteotome
    S.-P. synovectomy
    S.-P. technique
    S.-P. transarticular nail
Smith-Petersen-Cave-Van Gorder anterolateral approach
Smith-Richards instrumentation
Smith-Robinson
    S.-R. anterior cervical diskectomy
    S.-R. anterior fusion
    S.-R. cervical disk approach
    S.-R. cervical fusion
    S.-R. interbody arthrodesis
    S.-R. interbody fusion
    S.-R. technique
Smithwick clip-applying forceps
SMO
    supramalleolar orthosis
    SMO plate
SMo
    stainless steel and molybdenum
    SMo Moore pin
    SMo prosthesis
smooth
    s. broach
    s. cobalt-chromium
    s. endoprosthesis
    s. Steinmann pin
    s.-tipped jeweler's forceps
    s. transfixion wire

smoother
    Gore s.
smoothie junior bur
SMPS
    sympathetic maintained pain syndrome
SMT
    spinal manipulative therapy
SNAP
    sensory nerve action potential
snap
    s. fit
    s.-lock brace
    S. Lock wire/pin extractor
snap-fit
    s.-f. apparatus
    s.-f. device
snapping
    s. hip
    s. scapula
    s. scapula syndrome
    tendon s.
    s. tendon
    s. thumb flexor
snare
    Zimmer s.
Sneppen talar fracture
sniffer's position
snooze
    S. Fast
    S. pillow
Snow-Littler release
SNS
    sympathetic nervous system
S'n'S
    Mauch S.
snuffbox
    anatomic s.
snug
    S. seat
    s. traction
SO
    spinal orthosis
soak
    Betadine s.
    Epson salt s.
soap
    Betadine s.
Soccer Sporthotic
Society
    American Orthopaedic Foot and Ankle S. (AOFAS)
    International Headache S. (IHS)
    Musculoskeletal Tumor S.
sock
    active s.
    AFO brace s.
    s. aid
    ankle foot orthosis brace s.

arthritis s.
Bio-Wick s.
Carolon AFO s.
cast s.
Dero hole-in-one prosthetic s.
diabetic s.
edema s.
electrode s.
gel stump s.
molding s.
Regal Acrylic/Stretch prosthetic s.
Silosheath s.
Soft Walk gel s.
Spandex Lycra three-ply stump s.
STS molding s.
Venosan support s.

socket

adjustable postoperative protective
  prosthetic s. (APOPPS)
all-polyethylene s.
Alps ClearPro silicone suction s.
AML s.
Arthropor II porous s.
concave loading s.
flexible s.
Flo-Tech prosthetic s.
s. gauge
hard s.
Icecross silicone s.
ICEX s.
ischial containment s.
ischial-gluteal weightbearing s.
metal-backed s.
s. pin
Poly-Dial s.
polyethylene s.
prosthetic s.
s. purchase
quadrilateral s.
standard s.
supracondylar s.
suspension-type s.
total contact s.
universal frame outer s. (UFOS)
University of California cuff
  suspension PTB s.
variable circumference
  suprapatellar s. (VCSPS)
s. wrench

sodium

ardeparin s.
bromfenac s.

butabarbital s.
Butisol S.
cefazolin s.
s. etidronate
s. hyaluronate
s. hypochlorite solution
naproxen s.
s. salicylate
thiopental s.
s. thiosulfate
warfarin s.

Sof

S. Gel HeelCup
S. Matt pressure relieving mattress
S. Sole Sof Gel heel pad

Sofamor spinal device

Sofflex

S. mattress
S. mattress system

Sofield

S. femoral deficiency operation
S. femoral deficiency technique
S. osteotomy
S. pinning
S. retractor

Sof-Rol

S.-R. cast pad
S.-R. dressing

SofStep wheelchair footplate cover

soft

s. bulky dressing
s. callus stage
s. collar
s. collar cervical orthosis
s. corn
s. corset
s. fibroma
S. Silicones Wonderzorb
S. Super Sport orthotic
S. Support Preforms orthotic
s. tissue
s. tissue abnormality
s. tissue ankle injury
s. tissue biomechanics
s. tissue blade retractor
s. tissue coaptation sling
s. tissue contracture
s. tissue envelope
s. tissue flap
s. tissue healing
s. tissue hinge
s. tissue injury

S

NOTES

soft *(continued)*
    s. tissue integrity
    s. tissue interface
    s. tissue interposition
    s. tissue irritability
    s. tissue lesion
    s. tissue massage
    s. tissue mobilization
    s. tissue myxoma
    s. tissue plication
    s. tissue release
    s. tissue restriction
    s. tissue sarcoma
    s. tissue stretching
    s. tissue tumor
    s. touch hand exerciser
    s.-vamp shoe
    S. Walk gel sock
softball sliding injury
Softeze water pillow
Softflex Wrist Wear
Softip monofilament
Softouch Cold/Hot Pack
Softsplint foot splint
soft-tissue
    s.-t. maladaptation
    s.-t. mass
    S.-t. Regional Orthopedics (STO)
software
    Image-I analysis s.
    osteotomy analysis simulation s.
      (OASIS)
    Stat Graphics s.
    Yochum chiropractic s.
Sof-Wick dressing
Sofwire cable system
Solarcaine Aloe Extra Burn Relief
Solcotrans
    S. autotransfusion system
    S. orthopaedic drainage-refusion
      system
sole
    Ambulator Bio-Rocker s.
    s. of foot
    s. insert
    Poro-in-between s.
    rocker s.
    Texon s.
    Vibram s.
soleus
    s. complex
    gastrocnemius s.
SOLEutions
    S. custom orthosis
    S. custom orthotic device
    S. orthotic
    S. Prefab orthotic device
Solganal

solid
    s. ankle, cushioned heel (SACH)
    s. ankle, cushioned heel foot
    s. ankle, cushioned heel orthotic
    s. ankle, cushioned heel prosthesis
      (SACH foot prosthesis)
    s. buckling implant material
    s. hex bolt
    s. silicone exoplant implant
      material
solid-ankle
    s.-a. flexible endoskeletal (SAFE)
    s.-a. joint
solitary
    s. enchondroma
    s. myeloma
Solitens TENS unit
Solu-Cortef
Solu-Medrol Injection
Solurex L.A.
Soluspan
    Celestone S.
solution
    acid-citrate-dextrose s.
    antibiotic and saline s.
    bacitracin s.
    Betadine scrub s.
    Boropak astringent s.
    Bunnell s.
    Burroughs s.
    carbol-fuchsin s.
    colloid s.
    crystalloid s.
    Dakin s.
    dextrose s.
    Duofilm S.
    extravasation irrigation s.
    Fungoid AF Topical S.
    heparinized Ringer lactate s.
    Hibiclens s.
    iodophor s.
    irrigating s.
    irrigation s.
    LazerSporin-C s.
    Lotrimin AF S.
    povidone-iodine s.
    pulsatile hypothermic perfusion with
      University of Wisconsin s.
    Restore AF antimicrobial s.
    saline s.
    Septisol s.
    sodium hypochlorite s.
    sterile saline s.
Soma
    S. Compound
    S. Compound w/Codeine
    S. Gonio system

S. pulley system
S. sacroiliac stabilization belt

somatectomy
subtotal s.

somatic dysfunction
somatization
somatoautonomic
somatomedin-C
somatosensory
s. evoked potential (SEP, SSEP)
s. evoked potential monitoring
s. test

somatosomatic reflex
somatovisceral correction
Somerville ·
S. anterior approach ·
S. procedure
S. technique ·

SOMI
sternal-occipital-mandibular
immobilization
SOMI brace
SOMI orthosis

Sominex Oral
Sommaserene
Factor Six: S.

Songer cable
Sonicator
S. Plus ultrasound
S. 720 ultrasound

Sonocut ultrasonic aspirator
sonographic abnormality
sonography
Sontec pliers
**Sony CCD/RGB DXC-151 color video
camera**
Sorbie calcaneal fracture classification
sorbitol level
Sorbothane
S. heel cushion
S. orthotic device

Sorbsan
Sorbuthane II heel cup
sore
plaster s.
pressure s.

Soren
S. ankle fusion
S. arthrodesis

soreness
delayed-onset muscle s. (DOMS)

SORE note

Sorondo-Ferré hindquarter amputation
**Sorrells hip arthroplasty retractor
system**
SORSI
Sacro Occipital Research Society
International

SOT
sacrooccipital technique

SOTO
step out, turn out
SOTO technique

Soto-Hall
S.-H. bone graft
S.-H. maneuver
S.-H. sign
S.-H. test

Soudre autogéné
sound
flexible s.
radiolucent s.
rigid s.
tearing s.

sounder
pedicle s.

source
fiberoptic light s.
s. image distance (SID)
light s.
Wolf light s.

Souter
S. hip procedure
S. Strathclyde total elbow system
S. unconstrained elbow prosthesis

southern access
Southwick
S. biplane trochanteric osteotomy
S. clamp
S. lateral slip angle
S. pin-holding apparatus
S. pin-holding device
S. screw extractor
S. slide procedure
S. two-tined retractor

**Southwick-Robinson anterior cervical
approach**
Sox
Champion Power S.

SP
suprapatellar

Spa Bed
space
s. available for the cord (SAC)

NOTES

S

space *(continued)*
    costoclavicular s.
    dead s.
    disk s.
    epidural s.
    fascial s.
    first web s.
    hypoplastic disk s.
    increased lateral joint s.
    intercondylar s.
    intercostal s. (ICS)
    intermetatarsal s.
    interpeduncular s.
    lateral joint s.
    medial clear s.
    midpalmar s.
    palm s.
    Parona s.
    s. of Poirier
    popliteal s.
    position in s.
    prevertebral s.
    properitoneal s.
    retroperitoneal s.
    retropharyngeal s.
    s. shoe
    Steel rule of thirds for spinal cord
      free s.
    subacromial s.
    subcoracoid s.
    suprasternal s.
    thenar s.
    tibiofibular clear s.
    web s.
spacer
    acetabular s.
    s. bar
    Barouk s.
    bayonet s.
    bone s.
    Button S.
    ceramic vertebral s.
    s. inserter
    joint s.
    Kinemax s.
    passive s.
    Plexiglas s.
    prosthetic s.
    proximal cement s.
    rubber s.
    s.-tensor jig
    trial s.
    true s.
Spahr metaphyseal dysostosis
Spälteholz
    S. preparation
    S. technique
Spandex Lycra three-ply stump sock

spanner gauge
spanning external fixator
Sparine
sparing
    sacral nerve root s.
Spark handheld dynamometer
Spartan jaw wire cutter
spasm
    arterial s.
    carpal pedal s.
    muscle s.
    paraspinal muscle s.
    paravertebral muscle s.
    peroneal muscle s.
spasmodic torticollis
spastic
    s. cerebral palsy
    s. diparesis
    s. diplegia
    s. disorder
    s. equinovalgus
    s. equinus
    s. flatfoot
    s. hand
    s. hemiplegia
    s. intrinsic contracture
    s. paralysis
    s. paraplegia
    s. quadriplegia
    s. thumb-in-palm deformity
    s. varus hindfoot
spasticity
    Ashworth score of muscle s.
spatula
    cement s.
    s. forceps
spatulate thumb
Spearman rank-order test
spear tackler's spine
special
    s. Colles splint
    Heel Spur S.
    S. Seat
Specialists
    American Board of Physical
      Therapy S. (ABPTS)
specialized
    s. cell
    s. nail
specific
    s. adaptation to imposed demand
      (SAID)
    s. adjustment
    s. curve
    s. thrust manipulation
SPECT
    single photon emission computed
      tomography

Spectazole
spectinomycin
Spectric EF stem
Spectrobid
Spectron
    S. EF total hip system
    S. hip prosthesis
spectroscopy
    Fourier transform infrared s.
Spectrum
    The Early Amnion Rupture S.
    (TEARS)
speed
    S. arthroplasty
    free s.
    s. of gait
    S. hand splint
    s.-lock clamp
    S. open reduction
    S. radial head fracture classification
    S. radius cap prosthesis
    S. sign
    S. sternoclavicular repair
    S. test
    S. V-Y muscle-plasty
Speed-Boyd
    S.-B. open reduction
    S.-B. radial-ulnar technique
Spelcast car seat
Spence rongeur forceps
Spencer tendon lengthening
Spenco
    S. arch support
    S. boot
    S. insole
    S. liner
    S. orthotic device
    S. Second Skin dressing
Spenko shoe insert
Spetzler anterior transoral approach
SpF spinal fusion stimulator
sphenoidal fossa
sphenopalatine ganglion block
sphere
    silicone rubber s.
spherical
    s. bur
    s. gliding principle
    s.-headed screw

spherocentric
    s. fully constrained tricompartmental
    knee prosthesis
    s. knee system
sphygmomanometer
spica
    s. cast
    FREEDOM Thumb S.
    hip s.
    Schmeisser s.
    s. splint
    thumb s.
spicule
spider finger
Spiegleman acromioclavicular splint
Spier elbow arthrodesis
spike
    ball-tip s.
    s. of bone
    endplate s.
    Glissane s.
    metaphyseal s.
    s. osteotomy
spilled cup sign
spina
    s. bifida
    s. bifida occulta (SBO)
spinae
    erector s.
    thoracolumbar erector s.
spinal
    s. abscess
    s. accessory nerve
    s. accessory nerve injury
    s. analysis
    s. analysis machine (SAM)
    s. anesthesia
    s. angulation
    s. artery
    s. arthritis
    s. arthrodesis
    s. axial load
    s. axis
    s. board
    s. brucellosis
    s. canal
    s. canal stenosis (SCS)
    s. column
    s. contour
    s. cord
    s. cord block
    s. cord compression

NOTES

spinal *(continued)*
  s. cord function intraoperative monitoring
  s. cord injury (SCI)
  s. cord injury without radiographic abnormality (SCIWORA)
  s. cord-meningeal complex
  S. Cord Motor Index and Sensory Indices
  s. cord syndrome
  s. coronal plane deformity
  s. deformity/instability
  s. degeneration
  s. distraction
  s. dysarthria
  s. dysraphism
  s. evoked potential
  s. fascial release
  s. fixation
  s. fixation rigidity
  s. fixation rod
  s. fracture
  s. fusion pathomechanics
  s. fusion position
  s. fusion stimulator
  s. fusion technique
  s. hitch
  s. implant design
  s. implant load to failure
  s. infection
  s. infection biopsy
  s. injury operative stabilization
  s. instability
  s. instrumentation
  s. joint mobilization
  s. learning
  s. level
  s. locking procedure
  s. malignancy
  s. manipulation
  s. manipulative therapy (SMT)
  s. manual therapy
  s. metastasis
  s. mobilization technique
  s. muscular atrophy (SMA)
  s. needle
  s. orthosis (SO)
  s. osteoblastoma
  s. osteomyelitis
  s. osteosarcoma
  s. osteotomy
  s. osteotomy stabilization
  S. Physiotherapy Simulator
  s. posterior ligament
  s. process apophysis
  s. rod cross-bracing
  s. segment
  s. shock

  s. stenosis
  s. stenotic myelopathy
  S. Technology bivalve TLSO brace
  "s.-tension-band"
  s. transverse ligament
  s. tuberculosis
  s. tumor
  s. turning frame

spindle
  annulospiral ending of muscle s.
  s. cell
  s.-cell lipoma
  s. effect
  muscle s.
  s. neuroma

spine
  adjustment of cervical s.
  adjustment of lumbar s.
  adjustment of thoracic s.
  anterior inferior iliac s. (AIIS)
  anterior occipitocervical s.
  anterior superior iliac s. (ASIS)
  anterior upper s.
  anterosuperior iliac s. (ASIS)
  axial loading of s.
  bamboo s.
  cervical s. (C-spine)
  Chance fracture thoracolumbar s.
  Charcot s.
  coccygeal s.
  convexity of the s.
  s. deformity
  dorsal s. (D-spine)
  fixation dysfunction of the lumbar s.
  s. flexion
  s. frame
  gibbus deformity of the s.
  iliac s.
  ischial s.
  kissing s.
  laminectomized s.
  lower cervical s.
  lower lumbar s.
  lower thoracic s.
  lumbar s. (L-spine)
  lumbosacral s. (LS)
  mandibular s.
  maxillary s.
  nasal s.
  osteoporotic s.
  palpation of anterior superior iliac s.
  palpation of posterior superior iliac s.
  poker s.
  posterior s.
  posterior-inferior s.

posterior sacroiliac s. (PSIS)
posterosuperior iliac s. (PSIS)
S. Power pelvic stabilizer belt
s. rotation
sacral s.
s. sign
spear tackler's s.
thoracic s. (T-spine)
thoracic s. (T1 to T12)
thoracolumbar s.
thoracolumbosacral s.
three-column s.
trochanteric s.
tumor metastatic to s.
upper thoracic s.
variable screw placement system-
instrumented lumbar s.
spin-echo image
spines
SpineScope
Clarus S.
spinning probe
spinocerebellar
s. ataxia
s. degeneration
s. tract
spinoglenoid notch
spinographic angle
spinography
spinolaminar line
Spinoscope noninvasive imaging system
spinothalamic tract
spinous
s. plane
s. process
s. process fracture
s. process plate
s. process wire
s. process wiring
s. pull
s. push
spiral
s. cord
s. cortical reamer
s. drill
s. groove syndrome
s. humeral groove
s. oblique fracture
s. oblique retinacular ligament
s. oblique retinacular ligament
reconstruction splint
s. technique

s. trochanteric reamer
s. or twist drill
Spira procedure
Spirec drill
spiritual healing
spirometer
Buhl s.
Spittler procedure
Spitz-Holter valve implant material
Spitz nevus
SPL
short plantar ligament
SPLATT
split anterior tibial tendon
split anterior tibial tendon transfer
SPLATT procedure
splayfoot deformity
splaying
forefoot s.
s. of toe
spleen injury
splint
Abbott s.
abduction finger s.
abduction humeral s.
abduction pillow cover s.
abduction thumb s.
abouna s.
acrylic cap s.
acrylic template s.
Adam and Eve rib belt s.
Adams s.
adjustable s.
Adjusta-Wrist s.
aeroplane s.
Agnew s.
Ainslie acrylic s.
air s.
Airfoam s.
airplane s.
air pressure s.
Air-Soft S.
AliMed diabetic night s.
AliMed turnbuckle elbow s.
Alumafoam s.
aluminum bridge s.
aluminum fence s.
aluminum finger cot s.
aluminum foam s.
aluminum hand s.
aluminum wire s.
anchor s.

NOTES

563

splint *(continued)*
Anderson s.
angle s.
ankle-foot orthotic s.
anterior acute flexion elbow s.
any-angle s.
Aquaplast s.
Asch s.
Ashhurst leg s.
s. attachment
balanced s.
Baldan fracture s.
Balkan femoral s.
ball-peen s.
banana finger extension s.
banjo s.
Barlow cruciform infant s.
baseball finger s.
Basswood s.
Bavarian s.
Baylor adjustable cross s.
Baylor metatarsal s.
Bend-A-Boot foot s.
birdcage s.
Bloom s.
Blount s.
board s.
Böhler-Braun s.
Böhler wire s.
Bond arm s.
Bosworth s.
boutonnière s.
Bowlby arm s.
bracketed s.
Brady balanced-suspension s.
Brady leg s.
Brant aluminum s.
Brooke Army Hospital s.
Browne s.
Buck extension s.
Buck traction s.
buddy s.
Budin hammertoe s.
Budin toe s.
Bunnell active hand and finger s.
Bunnell finger extension s.
Bunnell gutter s.
Bunnell knuckle-bender s.
Bunnell outrigger s.
Bunnell reverse knuckle bender s.
Bunnell safety-pin s.
Bunny Boot foot s.
Burnham finger s.
Burnham thumb s.
Cabot leg s.
Cabot posterior s.
calibrated clubfoot s.
Campbell traction s.

cap s.
Capener coil s.
Capener finger s.
Capner s.
Carl P. Jones traction s.
Carpal Lock wrist s.
Carter s.
cartilage elastic pullover kneecap s.
Chandler felt collar s.
Chatfield-Girdlestone s.
clavicular cross s.
Clayton greenstick s.
clubfoot s.
CMC s.
cock-up arm s.
cock-up hand s.
COH hip abduction s.
Colles s.
Comforfoam s.
Comfy elbow s.
composite spring elastic s.
compression sleeve shin s.
Comprifix ankle s.
Cone s.
Converse s.
Cordon-Colles fracture s.
Cosmolon closure for s.
counterrotational s.
countertraction s.
Craig abduction s.
Cramer wire s.
CTS Gripfit s.
cubital tunnel s.
Culley ulnar s.
Curry walking s.
Darco toe alignment s.
Davis metacarpal s.
Delbet s.
Denis Browne s. (DBS)
Denis Browne clubfoot s.
Denis Browne hip s.
Denis Browne talipes hobble s.
DePuy aeroplane s.
DePuy any-angle s.
DePuy coaptation s.
DePuy open-spindle s.
DePuy open-thimble s.
DePuy-Pott s.
DePuy rocking leg s.
DePuy rolled Colles s.
DeRoyal/LMB finger s.
digit s.
Digit-Aide fifth toe s.
DonJoy wrist s.
dorsal extension block s.
dorsiflexion foot s.
Dorsiwedge night s.
double-occlusal s.

drop-foot s.
drop wrist s.
Dupuytren s.
Duran-Houser wrist s.
Dyna knee s.
dynamic s.
Early Fit night s.
Easton cock-up s.
Easy Access foot s.
Eaton s.
Eggers contact s.
elbow extension s.
elbow flexion s.
elephant-ear clavicular s.
Engelmann thigh s.
Engen palmar wrist s.
Erich s.
Extend-It finger s.
extension block s.
Ezeform s.
felt collar s.
fence s.
Ferciot tiptoe s.
Fillauer night s.
finger cot s.
finger extension clockspring s.
finger flexion s.
Finger-Hugger s.
flat s.
flexor hinge s.
fold-over finger s.
foot drop night s.
forearm s.
Formatray mandibular s.
Forrester s.
Foster s.
four-prong finger s.
Fox clavicular s.
Frac-Sur s.
Fractomed s.
fracture s.
Framer s.
FREEDOM Neutral Position S.
FREEDOM Omni Progressive S.
FREEDOM Progressive Resting S.
FREEDOM Sportsfit S.
FREEDOM Ultimate Grip S.
Frejka pillow s.
frog s.
frog-leg s.
Froimson s.
Fruehevald s.

full-hand s.
full-occlusal s.
Funsten supination s.
Futuro s.
Gagnon s.
gait lock s. (GLS)
Gallows s.
Galveston s.
Ganley s.
Gibson s.
Gilchrist s.
Gilmer s.
Gooch s.
Gordon s.
Granberry s.
Gunning s.
gutter s.
half-shell s.
hallux valgus night s.
Hammond s.
hand cock-up s.
Hanna night s.
Hare compact traction s.
Harrington outrigger s.
Harris s.
Hart extension finger s.
Haynes-Griffin mandibular s.
Heel Free s.
Hexcelite sheet s.
hinged cylinder s.
hinged Thomas s.
Hirschtick utility shoulder s.
Hodgen hip s.
Hodgen leg s.
humeral fracture abduction s.
HV NightSplint s.
HVO s.
HV SoftSplint s.
Ilfeld s.
Ilfeld-Gustafson s.
infant abduction s.
inflatable elbow s.
Isoprene plastic s.
Jacoby bunion s.
Jacoby heel s.
James s.
Jelanko s.
Jet-Air s.
Joint-Jack finger s.
Jonell countertraction finger s.
Jonell thumb s.
Jones arm s.

S

NOTES

splint *(continued)*

Jones forearm s.
Jones metacarpal s.
Jones traction s.
Joseph s.
Kanavel cock-up s.
Karfoil s.
Kazanjian s.
Keller-Blake half-ring s.
Keller-Blake leg s.
Kenny-Howard s.
Kerr abduction s.
Keystone s.
kinetic s.
Kleinert s.
Klenzak double-upright s.
knee brace s.
knee immobilizer s.
knuckle-bender s.
Lambrinudi s.
leaf s.
Levis arm s.
Lewin baseball-finger s.
Lewin-Stern finger s.
Lewin-Stern thumb s.
s.-like pain
s. liner
Link Stack Split S.
Link toe s.
Liston s.
live s.
LMB finger s.
LMB resting s.
long arm s.
long leg s. (LLS)
loop-lock cock-up s.
Love s.
Lytle metacarpal s.
magnet s.
Magnuson abduction humeral s.
malleable metal finger s.
mallet finger abouna s.
Malmö hip s.
Mason s.
Mason-Allen Universal hand s.
Mayer s.
McGee s.
McIntire s.
McLeod padded clavicular s.
memory s.
metal s.
Middeldorpf s.
MindSet toe s.
Moberg s.
modified Oppenheimer s.
Mohr finger s.
molded posterior plaster s.
M.S. s.

Murphy s.
Murray-Jones arm s.
Murray-Thomas arm s.
Neubeiser adjustable forearm s.
neutral position s.
New Mind Set toe s.
N'ice Stretch night s.
night s.
occlusal s.
OCL volar s.
O'Donoghue knee s.
O'Donoghue stirrup s.
O'Malley jaw fracture s.
open-air s.
Oppenheimer knuckle-bender s.
Oppenheimer spring-wire s.
opponens s.
Orfit s.
Ortho-last s.
Orthomedics Stretch and Heel s.
Ortho-Mold s.
orthopaedic strap clavicular s.
Orthoplast isoprene s.
outrigger s.
padded aluminum s.
padded board s.
padded plywood s.
padded tongue blade s.
s. padding
palmar cock-up s.
pan s.
s. pan netting
Pavlik harness s.
Peabody s.
Pearson attachment to Thomas s.
pelvic s.
PF night s.
Phelps s.
Phillips s.
Phoenix Outrigger s.
pillow s.
Pil-O-Splint wrist s.
plantar fasciitis night s.
Plastalume bulb-ended s.
Plastalume straight s.
plaster s.
plaster-of-Paris s.
pneumatic s.
Polyform s.
polyvinyl alcohol s.
Pond adjustable s.
Ponseti s.
poroplastic s.
Porzett s.
Postalume finger s.
posterior s.
Potts s.
Pro-glide s.

Protecto s.
Pucci s.
Puth abduction s.
Putti s.
QualCraft s.
QuickCast s.
Quik splint s.
radial slab s.
radiolucent s.
Redi-Around finger s.
reverse knuckle-bender s.
Robert Jones s.
Robinson InRigger s.
Roger Anderson s.
Rolyan AquaForm wrist and thumb
  spica s.
Rosen s.
Rowland-Hughes s.
Roylan Gel Shell spica s.
Rumel aluminum bridge s.
Russell s.
safety pin s.
SAM s.
Sayre s.
Scott humeral s.
Scottish Rite s.
Seattle s.
shin s.
short arm s. (SAS)
short arm sugar-tong s.
short leg s.
shoulder spica s.
Simpson sugar-tong s.
Slattery-McGrouther dynamic
  flexion s.
Slocum s.
Softsplint foot s.
special Colles s.
Speed hand s.
spica s.
Spiegleman acromioclavicular s.
spiral oblique retinacular ligament
  reconstruction s.
spreading hand s.
spring cock-up s.
spring-wire safety pin s.
Stack s.
Stader s.
static s.
Stax finger s.
Stax fingertip s.
stirrup plaster s.

Stock finger s.
Strampelli s.
strap clavicular s.
Stretch and Heel s.
Stromeyer s.
Stuart Gordon hand s.
Stulberg HIPciser abduction s.
sugar-tong plaster s.
Swan Neck s.
Swanson dynamic toe s.
Swanson hand s.
synergistic wrist motion s.
Synergy s.
Tauranga s.
Taylor s.
Teare arm s.
tennis elbow s.
tension night s. (TNS)
T-finger s.
therapeutic s.
Thomas full-ring s.
Thomas hinged s.
Thomas knee s.
Thomas leg s.
Thomas posterior s.
Thomas suspension s.
Thompson s.
Thompson modification of Denis
  Browne s.
thumb web s.
ThumZ'Up thumb s.
Ticonium s.
Titus forearm s.
Titus wrist s.
Toad finger s.
Tobruk s.
Tomberlin-Alemdaroglu s.
Toronto s.
torsion bar s.
traction s.
triangular pillow s.
turnbuckle elbow s.
type 501, 502, 504, 602 finger s.
ulnar gutter s.
Universal acromioclavicular s.
Universal gutter s.
Universal support s.
Urias air s.
Urias pressure s.
U-splint s.
Valentine s.
Van Arsdale triangular s.

S

NOTES

splint *(continued)*
    Van Rosen s.
    Velcro extenders s.
    Vesely-Street s.
    volar plaster s.
    Volkmann s.
    von Rosen abduction s.
    von Rosen cruciform s.
    Wanchik neutral position s.
    Weil s.
    well-leg s.
    Wertheim s.
    Wilson s.
    Winter s.
    wire s.
    wraparound s.
    WristJack wrist s.
    yucca wood s.
    Zimfoam s.
    Zimmer airplane s.
    Zimmer clavicular cross s.
    Zim-Trac traction s.
    Zim-Zip rib belt s.
    Zollinger s.
    Zucker s.
splintage
splinted in position of function
splinter
splinting
    dynamic s.
    night s.
    pelvic s.
    silicone thermoplastic s. (STS)
    Strong dorsal extension block s.
SplintsRite stabilization device
split
    s. anterior tibialis tendon transfer
    s. anterior tibial tendon (SPLATT)
    s. anterior tibial tendon procedure
    s. anterior tibial tendon transfer
      (SPLATT)
    s. calvarial bone graft
    s.-finger hook
    s. fracture
    s.-hand deformity
    s. incision
    Link Stack S. Splint
    s.-nail deformity
    s. patellar approach
    peroneus brevis s. (PBS)
    s. Russell skeletal traction
    s. screen
    s. thickness cranial bone
    s. thin graft
split-heel
    s.-h. approach
    s.-h. fracture
    s.-h. incision

split-thickness
    s.-t. skin excision (STSE)
    s.-t. skin graft (STSG)
splitting fracture
Sponastrine dysplasia
spondylalagia
spondylarthritis
spondylectomy
spondylexarthrosis
spondylitic bar
spondylitis
    ankylosing s.
    Marie-Strümpell s.
    tuberculosis s.
spondylizema
spondyloarthropathy
spondyloarthrosis
spondylo construct
spondylodesis
    ventral derotation s. (VDS)
spondylodiscitis
spondylodynia
spondyloepiphyseal dysplasia
spondylogenic
spondylolisthesis
    anteroinferior s.
    congenital s.
    degenerative s. (type 3)
    doweling s.
    dysplastic s.
    five classifications of s.
    Gill-Manning-White s.
    high-grade s.
    isthmic s.
    lumbosacral s.
    pathologic s.
    postlaminectomy two-level s.
    s. reduction
    s. reduction/fixation
    sagittal roll s.
    slip angle s.
    symptomatic s.
    traumatic s.
    Winter s.
    s. with significant displacement
spondyloloptosis
spondylolysis
    cervical s.
    contralateral s.
spondylometer
spondylophyte
spondyloptosis
spondylosis
    central spine s.
    degenerative s.
    Nurick classification of s.
    Scheuermann dystrophic s.
    thoracolumbar s.

spondylotherapy
spondylotic
    s. bar
    s. spur
spondylotomy
sponge
    Adaptic s.
    bone wax gelatin s.
    gauze s.
    s.-holding forceps
    laparotomy s.
    Mediskin hemostatic s.
    Mikulicz s.
    Pedic s.
    Ray-Tec s.
    s. stick
    s. test
    Vistec x-ray detectable s.
spongiosa screw
spongoide
    couche s.
spongy
    s. appearance
    s. bone
Sponsel oblique osteotomy
spontaneous
    s. activity
    s. fracture
    s. hyperemic dislocation
    s. median neuropathy
spoon
    maroon s.
    meniscal s.
    s. plate
Sporanox
Sporothrix schenckii
sporotrichosis
S'port
    S. Max back support
    Posture S.
Sport
    S. Cord
    S. Preforms orthotic
Sportelli system collimator mounted
   contact shield
Sporthotic
    Soccer S.
Sporthotics orthotic
sports
    S. Brace
    s. injury

    s. medicine
    S. Plus II back belt
    s. psychology
    s. terminal device
Sports-Caster I, II knee brace
Sportscreme
sportstape
    Leukotape P s.
Sport-Stirrup orthosis
SporTX
    S. pulsed direct current stimulator
    S. stimulation device
spot
    café au lait s.
    de Morgan s.
    s.-face reamer
    s. film
    s. radiograph
    s. view
    s. weld
    s.-weld
Spotorno hip prosthesis
SPR
    selective posterior rhizotomy
    superior peroneal retinaculum
Sprague arthroscopic technique
sprain
    s. fracture
    inversion ankle s.
    lateral ankle s.
    postacute s.
    relapsing ankle s.
    syndesmotic s.
    talocrural s.
    talonavicular s.
Spratt
    S. bone curette
    S. mastoid curette
spray
    air plasma s. (APS)
    AliCool splint s.
    Aqua S.
    Fluori-Methane Topical S.
    HandClens ultra antiseptic s.
    L'Aprina topical s.
    low-pressure plasma s. (LLPS)
    Miacalcin nasal s.
    Ony-Clear S.
    Proderm topical s.
    s. and stretch
    s. and stretch technique

S

NOTES

spread
> Fowler s.
> s. hand

spreader
> Assistant Free calibrated femoral tibial s.
> Bailey rib s.
> Beeson cast s.
> Blount bone s.
> Blount laminar s.
> Bobechko s.
> bone s.
> Burford-Finochietto rib s.
> Burford rib s.
> Cloward s.
> Feochetti rib s.
> Haglund-Stille plaster s.
> Haight-Finochietto rib s.
> Harrington s.
> Henning cast s.
> Henning plaster s.
> Hoffer-Daimler cast s.
> Inge s.
> laminar s.
> Lemmon sternal s.
> Lilienthal rib s.
> M-Pact cast s.
> Nelson rib s.
> TSRH eyebolt s.

spreading
> s. forceps
> s. hand splint

Sprengel deformity
spring
> s. cock-up splint
> compression s.
> s. fixation
> Gruca-Weiss s.
> internal fixation s.
> s. ligament
> s.-mounted electromagnet
> s. pin
> s. plate
> s. swivel thumb
> s. test
> Weiss s.

Springer fracture
Springlight footplate
Springlite
> S. G foot component
> S. II foot component
> S. lower limb prosthesis
> S. low profile Symes II
> S. polyolefin BK cover
> S. polyurethane AK, BK conical cover
> S. super low profile Symes II
> S. toe filler

spring-loaded
> s.-l. knee lock
> s.-l. lock orthosis
> s.-l. nail

spring-wire
> s.-w. ankle-foot orthosis
> s.-w. safety pin splint

Sprint
> S. Climber
> S. cross trainer
> S. Runner

sprinter's fracture
Spri Xercise board
sprout
> axon s.

S.P. 100 transcutaneous electrical neural stimulator
spur
> acromial s.
> bone s.
> calcaneal s.
> cartilaginous s.
> chondroosseous s.
> s.-crushing clamp
> fibrous s.
> s. formation
> heel s.
> osteophytic s.
> s. pad
> painful s.
> s. sign
> spondylotic s.
> subacromial s.
> traction s.
> uncovertebral s.

spurious ankylosis
Spurling
> S. maneuver
> S. rongeur
> S. test

Spurling-Kerrison
> S.-K. rongeur
> S.-K. rongeur forceps

spurring
> anterior s.
> bony s.
> inferior s.

spurt muscle
spyrolace shoe lace
squamous cell
square
> s.-end pliers
> s.-hole broach
> s.-hollow chisel
> S. Module Seating System
> rocker balance s.
> s.-shaped awl

square-ended
    s.-e. distraction rod
    s.-e. hook
squat test
squatting
    s. ability
    s. test
squeeze
    s. ball
    s. exerciser
    Schaffer s.
    s. test
SR
    stabilizing reversal
Srb syndrome
SRF
    semirigid fiberglass cast
SRL ligament
S-ROM
    S.-R. femoral stem prosthesis
    S.-R. hip replacement system
    S.-R. modular stem
    S.-R. modular total knee system
    S.-R. Poly-Dial insert
    S.-R. proximally modular total hip
      system
    S.-R. Super Cup
SRP instrument
SSCS
    segmental spinal correction system
SSEP
    short-latency somatosensory evoked
      potential
    somatosensory evoked potential
S-shaped
    S-s. deformity
    S-s. incision
SSI
    segmental spinal instrumentation
    shoulder subluxation inhibitor
      anterior-posterior fusion with SSI
      SSI brace
S-Soles insole
stab
    s. incision
    s. wound
stabilimetry
stability
    elbow s.
    s. of fracture
    glenohumeral joint s.
    knee s.

    Kostuik-Errico classification of
      spinal s.
    lateral s.
    ligamentous s.
    lumbar spine rotational s.
    posterior s.
    rotary s.
    tibiotalar s.
stabilization
    anterior short-segment s.
    s. approach
    atlantoaxial s.
    cervical spine s.
    cervicothoracic junction s.
    definitive s.
    distal radioulnar joint s.
    Dunn-Brittain foot s.
    dynamic lumbar s.
    flexion compression spine injury s.
    fracture s.
    Gruca s.
    iliac crest bone graft s.
    lower cervical spine posterior s.
    myoplastic muscle s.
    occipitocervical s.
    odontoid fracture s.
    s. plate
    posterior lower cervical spine s.
    prophylactic operative s.
    provisional s.
    rhythmic s.
    sacral spine s.
    screw s.
    spinal injury operative s.
    spinal osteotomy s.
    subluxation s.
    thoracolumbar spine s.
    s. training
    TSRH crosslink s.
    wire s.
stabilizer
    ankle s.
    Dynamic foot s.
    foot s.
    FREEDOM Thumb S.
    Heel Hugger therapeutic heel s.
    kneecap s.
    KT1000 foot s.
    Palumbo ankle s.
    secondary s.
    Verteflex arthrotonic s.

S

NOTES

stabilizing
s. bar
s. hinge
s. reversal (SR)
stable
s. burst fracture
s. cervical spine injury
s. gait
s. to motion
s. reduction
s. vertebra
Stablecut sawblade
Stableloc
S. Colles fracture external fixator
S. II external fixator system
Stack
Link S. Split Splint
S. shoulder procedure
S. splint
stacking cones
Stader
S. pin
S. pin guide
S. splint
Stadol NS
stage
Ficat and Arlet disease s.
hard callus s.
implant s.
S. model of industrial rehabilitation
Risser s.
silent hip s.
soft callus s.
staged
Stagesic
staggering gait
Stagnara
S. gouge
S. wake-up test
Staheli
S. rotational profile
S. shelf procedure
S. technique
S. test
Stahl staging system
stain
Gram s.
port-wine s.
reticulin s.
Van Geesen s.
stainless
s. steel
s. steel alloy
s. steel clamp
s. steel equipment
s. steel implant metal prosthesis
s. steel mesh
s. steel and molybdenum (SMo)

s. steel plate
s. steel screw
s. steel wire
staircase phenomenon
StairClimber assist device
stairclimbers foot
stairclimbing
stair-climbing exercise
StairMaster
S. exercise system
stair-running test
stairs
s. hopple test
s. sign
stairstep
cervical s.
s. fracture
stall bar
Stamm
S. metatarsal osteotomy
S. procedure
S. procedure for intra-articular hip fusion
stamp
Gelfoam s.
stance
late s.
s. phase
s. phase of gait
single-limb s.
StanceGuard internal support
stand
Atlas adjustable s.
Cherf cast s.
Grand Stand support s.
heel s.
IMP turnstile casting s.
stork s.
turnstile casting s.
Versa-Helper floor s.
standard
s. deviation
S. E-Z-On Vest
s. goniometric measure
s. 2-inch blade retractor
s. 4-inch blade retractor
s. medullary nail
s. retroperitoneal flank incision
s. socket
s. thoracotomy
standing
s. dorsoplantar view
s. flexion
s. flexion test
s. frame orthosis
s. Gillet test
s. knee bend PSIS-sacrum contact
s. lateral view

s. side bend
s. weightbearing view
Stanford Hypnotic Clinical Scale
Stanisavljevic technique
Stanmore
    S. knee replacement
    S. shoulder arthroplasty
    S. shoulder prosthesis
    S. total hip replacement
    S. totally constrained elbow
      prosthesis
Staodyne EMS+2 neurostimulator
STA-peg
    Smith S.-p.
STA-Pen writer pen
Staph-Chek
    S.-C. pad
    S.-C. Synergy fabric
staphylococcal
    s. arthritis
    s. pyomyositis
Staphylococcus
    S. aureus
    S. epidermidis
staphylorrhaphy elevator
staple
    ASP clip s.
    automatic s.
    barbed s.
    Blount fracture s.
    Bostick s.
    s. capsulorraphy bone bank
    capsulorrhaphy s.
    s. capsulorrhaphy
    Coventry s.
    Day fixation s.
    DePalma s.
    Downing s.
    s. driver
    duToit shoulder s.
    Ellison fixation s.
    epiphyseal s.
    s. extractor
    Fastlok implantable s.
    s. fixation
    GIA s.
    s. gun
    Hernandez-Ros bone s.
    s. holder
    Howmedica Vitallium s.
    s. inserter
    s. introducer

Johannesberg s.
Krackow HTO blade s.
Nakayama s.
O'Brien s.
osteoclast tension s.
Owestry s.
Richards fixation s.
skin s.
Smith & Nephew medium
  barbed s.
Smith & Nephew small barbed s.
Stone four-point s.
Stryker soft tissue s.
s. suture
tabletop Stone s.
TA metallic s.
TA Premium 30, 55, 90 s.
Vitallium s.
Wiberg fracture s.
Zimaloy s.
stapler
    Dwyer spinal mechanical s.
    EEA s.
    Hall double-hole spinal s.
    metaphyseal s.
    Oswestry-O'Brien spinal s.
    powered metaphyseal s.
    Wiberg fracture s.
Staples
    S. elbow arthrodesis
    S. repair
    S. technique
Staples-Black-Broström ligament repair
stapling
    Blount s.
    epiphyseal s.
    percutaneous s.
starch
    s. bandage
    s. test
Stark
    S. arthrodesis
    S. graft
Stark-Moore-Ashworth-Boyes technique
Starrett pin vise
STAR technique
starter
    nail s.
    Ritchie nail s.
startle reflex
stasis ulcer

S

NOTES

Statak
> S. anchor system
> S. soft tissue attachment device

state
> pathomechanical s.
> Profile of Mood S.'s (POMS)
> Rosser Classification of Illness S.'s

Stat Graphics software
static
> s. alignment
> s. compression
> s. compression plate
> s. evaluation
> s. fixation
> s. foot pain
> s. listing
> s. listing nomenclature
> s. locking nail
> s. lock nailing
> s. palpation
> s. splint
> s. stretch
> s. tendon transfer
> s. traction

statically
Staticin Topical
station
> Aquatrend water workout s.
> gait and s.
> s. and gait
> s. test

stationary
> s. angle guide
> s. attachment flexible endoskeletal (SAFE)
> s. attachment flexible endoskeletal orthotic

statistical significance
stature
> short s.

status
> ambulatory s.
> intact neurovascular s.
> s. loading
> neurovascular s.
> nutritional s.
> s. post
> Short Test of Mental S. (STMS)

Stauffer modification
Stax
> S. finger splint
> S. fingertip splint

stay
> length of s. (LOS)

stay-retractor
> Freebody s.-r.

S-T Cort
STC 900-series travel chair

STD hip prosthesis
STD+ Titanium total hip prosthesis
steal
> s. effect
> s. syndrome

Stealth frame
Stedman awl
steel
> S. correction
> S. maneuver
> S. rule of thirds for spinal cord free space
> s. shank
> stainless s.
> S. triple innominate osteotomy

Steffee
> S. instrument
> S. instrumentation technique
> S. pedicle plate
> S. pedicle screw-plate system
> S. plates and screws for lumbar fusion
> S. screw
> S. screw plate
> S. spinal instrumentation
> S. thumb arthroplasty
> S. variable spine plating system

Steffensmeier board
Steichen neurovascular free flap
Steinbach mallet
Steinberg
> S. infiltration block
> S. rating scale

Steinbrocker
> S. classification of rheumatoid arthritis
> S. rheumatoid arthritis classification

Steindler
> S. effect
> S. elbow arthrodesis
> S. flexorplasty
> S. matrixectomy
> S. procedure
> S. stripping

Steinert
> S. classification of epiphyseal fracture
> S. epiphyseal fracture classification

Steinhauser bone clamp
Steinmann
> S. extension nail
> S. fixation pin
> S. pin fixation
> S. pin with ball bearing
> S. pin with Crowe pilot point
> S. pin with pin chuck
> S. tendon forceps

S. test
S. traction
Stelazine
stellate
    s. fracture
    s. laceration
    s. sympathetic ganglion block
Stellbrink fixation device
stem
    Aequalis s.
    APR hip s.
    APR I femoral s.
    Aufranc-Turner s.
    s. base plate
    Biomet revision hip s.
    brain s.
    calcar replacement s.
    collarless s.
    contoured femoral s. (CFS, CSF)
    Corail HA-coated s.
    CRM s.
    s. deformation
    Deon s.
    Engh-Glassman femoral s.
    Extend s.
    s. extractor
    s. failure
    fenestrated s.
    Harris-Galante s.
    HG multilock hip s.
    hydroxyapatite-coated s.
    implant s.
    intramedullary s.
    Iowa s.
    Kirschner s.
    KMP femoral s.
    Link MP (microporous) hip s.
    modular Moniflex hip s.
    Moniflex hip s.
    Moore s.
    Natural-Hip titanium hip s.
    nonfenestrated s.
    Opti-Fix hip s.
    Osteonics Omnifit-HA hip s.
    PCA hip s.
    Perfecta femoral s.
    PFC hip s.
    Precision hip s.
    Press-Fit s.
    Profile hip s.
    Profix metaphyseal tibial s.
    Ranawat-Burstein porous s.

regular s.
s. removal
Revision hip s.
Richards modular s.
roundback s.
SL-Plus s.
Spectric EF s.
S-ROM modular s.
straight femoral s.
Taperloc femoral s.
trial s.
Ultima calcar s.'s
Ultima Fx s.'s
Zimmer bone s.
Stemex
stemmed tibial prosthesis
Stener-Gunterberg
    S.-G. hip operation
    S.-G. resection
Stener lesion
stenosed
stenosing tenosynovitis
stenosis
    ankylosing spinal s.
    aortic s. (AS)
    central canal s.
    foraminal s.
    lateral recess s. (LRS)
    lateral recess spinal s.
    multisegmental spinal s.
    spinal s.
    spinal canal s. (SCS)
stent
    Carcon s.
    Dacron s.
    s. dressing
    Omnifit HA hip s.
    synthetic s.
stenting
Stenzel
    S. rod
    S. rod prosthesis
step
    s. defect
    s. drill
    s. length
    s.-off of fracture
    s. osteotomy
    s. out, turn out (SOTO)
    s. screw
    s. time
    s. width

S

NOTES

step-cut
  s.-c. lengthening
  s.-c. osteotomy
  s.-c. reamer
  s.-c. transection
step-down
  s.-d. drill
  s.-d. osteotomy
Stephen
  S. scissors
  S. spreader bar
stepladder sign
steppage
stepper
  NuStep total body recumbent s.
step-up
  lateral s.-u.
stereognosis
stereolithography (SL)
  s. cage
stereophotogrammetry
stereotaxic anterior capsulotomy
Steri-Clamp
  S.-C. clamp
  IMP S.-C.
  Innovative Medical Products S.-C.
Steri-Cuff
  S.-C. disposable tourniquet cuff
  S.-C. Plus
sterile
  s. condition
  s. dry dressing (SDD)
  s. loosening
  s. matrix
  s. pencil
  s. saline solution
  s. sheet
  s. sheeting
  s. towel
sterilization
  ethylene oxide s.
Steri-Strips
sternal
  s. approximator
  s. rib
sternal-occipital-mandibular immobilization (SOMI)
sternal-occipital-mandibular-immobilizer
sternoclavicular (SC)
  s. joint
  s. joint dislocation
  s. joint injury
  s. joint reconstruction
  s. joint reduction
  s. ligament
sternocleidomastoid
  s. muscle
  s. muscle fibromatosis

sternohyoid muscle
sternomastoid muscle
sternooccipital-mandibular immobilizer brace
sternooccipitomanubrial immobilizer
sternothyroid muscle
sternotomy
sternoxiphoid plane
sternum
  duplicate s.
  s.-splitting approach
steroid
  anabolic s.
  epidural s.
  s. flare
  s. injection
  s. myopathy
  tapering dose s.
  s. therapy
steroid-induced
  s.-i. avascular necrosis
  s.-i. osteonecrosis
Stevens-Johnson syndrome
Stevenson
  S. alligator forceps
  S. grasping forceps
Stevens-Street
  S.-S. elbow prosthesis
  S.-S. elbow prosthesis template
Steward-Milford fracture classification
Stewart
  S. arm operation
  S. distal clavicular excision
  S. styloidectomy
Stewart-Harley transmalleolar ankle arthrodesis
Stewart-Morel syndrome
Steytler-Van Der Walt procedure
STH-2 hip prosthesis
sthenometry
stick
  dressing s.
  FMS Intracell s.
  Intracell Sprinter s.
  sponge s.
  switching s.
  s. tie ligature
  weighted walking s.
Stickler syndrome
Stieda fracture
stiff
  s.-knee gait
  s.-legged gait
  s. ribbon retractor
stiffness
  axial s.
  fusion s.
  joint s.

small-joint s.
torsional s.
stigmatic electrode
Stiles-Bunnell transfer technique
Still disease
Stille
    S. bone biter
    S. bone chisel
    S. bone drill
    S. bone drill set
    S. bone gouge
    S. brace
    S. bur
    S. hand drill
    S. osteotome
    S. plaster shears
    S. rongeur
Stille-Horsley rib forceps
Stille-Liston bone-cutting forceps
Stille-Luer
    S.-L. bone rongeur
    S.-L. rongeur forceps
**Stille-pattern trephine and bone drill
set**
Stille-Sherman bone drill
Stilphostrol
Stimoceiver implant material
Stimprene
    S. electrotherapy brace
    S. wrap
Stimson
    S. anterior shoulder reduction
     technique
    S. dressing
    gravity method of S.
    S. gravity method
    S. maneuver
stimulating
    s. electrode
    s. massage
stimulation
    antidromic s.
    cranial electrical s. (CES)
    direct electrical nerve s. (DENS)
    double simultaneous sensory s.
    electrical nerve s.
    electrical surface s.
    electronic bone s. (EBI)
    electrotherapeutic point s. (ETPS)
    external-coil electrical s.
    functional electrical s. (FES)
    functional neuromuscular s.

galvanic s.
high-voltage pulse galvanic s.
  (HVPGS)
interferential electrical s.
lateral electrical surface s. (LESS)
magnetic s.
M.A.N. Stim. Muscle and
  Neurological S.
microamperage electrical nerve s.
  (MENS)
microamperage neural s. (MNS)
neuromuscular electrical s. (NMES)
repetitive nerve s.
transcutaneous electrical nerve s.
  (TENS)
stimulator
    Acupoint s.
    AME bone growth s.
    AMREX muscle s.
    battery-pack Osteo-Stim bone s.
    bone growth s.
    constant direct current s.
    dorsal column s. (DCS)
    EBI Medical OsteoGen bone
     growth s.
    electrical bone-growth s.
    Electro-Acuscope 85 s.
    EMHI galvanic electrode s.
    EMS 2000 neuromuscular s.
    Endo Multi-Mode s.
    Freedom Micro Pro s.
    galvanic electrode s.
    G5 Porta-Plus muscle s.
    implanted bone growth s.
    Intelect Legend s.
    Intelect 600MP microcurrent s.
    interferential s.
    Master-Stim interferential s.
    Maxima II transcutaneous electrical
     nerve s.
    Medi-Stim s.
    Micro-Z neuromuscular s.
    neuromuscular III s.
    Nuwave transcutaneous electrical
     nerve s.
    Orthofuse implantable growth s.
    OrthoGen bone growth s.
    OrthoPak II bone growth s.
    OsteoGen bone growth s.
    OsteoGen implantable s.
    Osteo-Stim implantable bone
     growth s.

S

NOTES

stimulator *(continued)*
    PGS-3000 pulsed galvanic s.
    Physio-Stim bone growth s.
    Piezo "electro" needle-less s.
    Prizm Electro-Mesh Z-Stim-II s.
    pulsed galvanic s.
    REACT muscle s.
    Respond II muscle s.
    SpF spinal fusion s.
    spinal fusion s.
    SporTX pulsed direct current s.
    S.P. 100 transcutaneous electrical neural s.
    Stimuplex-S nerve s.
    Super Stimm MF s.
    Synchrosonic s.
    SysStim 226 muscle s.
    Theramini 1, 2 electrotherapy s.
    Theratouch 4.7 s.
    Z-Stim s.
Stimulite honeycomb mattress overlay
stimulus
    s. artifact
    conditioned s. (CS)
    conditioning s.
    maximal s.
    paired s.
    submaximal s.
    subthreshold s.
    supramaximal s.
    test s.
    threshold s.
    unconditional s. (US)
Stimuplex block needle
Stimuplex-S nerve stimulator
Stinchfield test
sting mat
stippled epiphysis
stippling
STIR
    sagittal fast-short T1 inversion recovery
    short tau inversion recovery
stirrup
    Böhler s.
    s. brace
    s. plaster splint
    Swivel-Strap ankle s.
    traction s.
stirrups
    Allen s.
stitch
    Allgöwer s.
    Bunnell s.
    Frost s.
    intracuticular s.
    Kessler s.
    Mersilene Kessler s.

    Pulvertaft fish-mouth s.
    roll s.
Stiwer
    S. bone-holding forceps
    S. hand drill
STJ
    subtalar joint
STMS
    Short Test of Mental Status
STNP
    subtalar joint neutral position
STO
    Soft-Tissue Regional Orthopedics
stock
    bone s.
    S. finger splint
    poor bone s.
Stockholm HAVS staging system
stockinette
    s. bandage
    basket s.
    bias-cut s.
    orthopaedic s.
    s. sling
    s. tube
    tubular s.
    Velpeau s.
stockings
    antiembolic s.
    drop-foot redression s.
    elastic s.
    Jobst s.
    long leg s.
    MEDI Plus compression s.
    Orthawear antiembolic s.
    Orthawear antiembolism s.
    Planostretch s.
    pneumatic compression s.'s
    SCD s.
    Sigvaris s.
    TED s.
    Zimmer antiembolism s.
stone
    s. arthrodesis
    s. basket screw mounted handle
    S. bunionectomy
    S. clamp-locking device
    S. four-point staple
    S. procedure
Stookey reflex
stool
    foot s.
    nested step s.
stop
    Elite posterior adjustable s.
stopwatch
storiform pattern

stork
- s. leg
- s. stand

Storz
- S. meniscotome
- S. Microsystems drill bit
- S. Microsystems plate cutter
- S. Microsystems plate-holding forceps
- S. oblique arthroscope

stout-neck curette

straddle
- s. fracture
- s. injury

straight
- s. basket forceps
- s. bone rongeur
- s. curette
- s. femoral stem
- s. gouge
- s. hex screwdriver
- s. incision
- s. last shoe
- s. lateral instability
- s. leg raising (SLR)
- s. leg raising exercise
- s. leg raising test (SLRT)
- s. osteotome
- s. periosteal elevator
- s. pituitary rongeur
- s. posterior portal
- s. power reamer
- s. scissors
- s. threaded rod
- s. walker brace

strain
- acute foot s.
- articular s.
- back s.
- Brunhilde s.
- compression s.
- s.-counterstrain
- elastic s.
- s. energy
- s. fracture
- s. gauge
- muscle s.
- plastic s.
- postural s.
- shear s.
- s.-sprain injury
- s.-stress curve
- tensile s.
- vertebroligamentous sprain s.

strain/counterstrain technique

Strampelli splint

strap
- Band-It tennis elbow s.
- Beta Pile II, III splint s.
- buddy s.
- Butterfly cushion with s.
- capsular s.
- Cho-Pat Achilles tendon s.
- Cho-Pat elbow s.
- Cho-Pat knee s.
- s. clavicular splint
- crotch s.
- D-ring s.
- Eclipse Gel elbow s.
- external elastic s.
- extremity mobilization s.
- Lema s.
- Levine patellar tendon s.
- S. Lok ankle brace
- Meek clavicular s.
- s. muscle
- neoprene wrist s.
- Nylatex s.
- Pebax fastening s.
- PIP/DIP s.
- QualCraft s.
- stretch-out s.
- suspension s.
- Velcro s.

Strap-Pad
- DAW S.-P.

strapping
- adhesive s.
- garter s.
- loop & hook s.
- LowDye s.

strategy
- cuing s.
- diagnostic s.

Stratos orthotic

stratum corneum

Stratus impact reducing pylon

Straub technique

Strayer
- S. gastrocnemius recession
- S. gastroc-soleus recession
- S. lengthening
- S. procedure
- S. tendon technique

S

NOTES

streaming potential
Street
    S. forearm nail
    S. medullary pin
Streeter dysplasia
Street-Stevens humeral prosthesis
strength
    5/5 s.
    s. against resistance
    Aspirin Free Anacin Maximum S.
    axial gripping s.
    Bayer Low Adult S.
    bending s.
    bone-screw interface s.
    C-D instrumentation fixation s.
    cervical extension s.
    Cotrel pedicle screw fixation s.
    s. curve
    s.-duration curve
    Ecotrin Low Adult S.
    Excedrin, Extra S.
    extensor hallucis longus s.
    extrinsic muscle s.
    graft s.
    hand grasp s.
    hand grip s.
    intrinsic muscle s.
    isometric cervical extension s.
    Lovett clinical scale of s.
    motor s.
    pedicle screw pull-out s.
    pinch s.
    pull-out s.
    tensile s.
    s. testing
    torsional gripping s.
    s. training
strengthened
    gas atomized dispersion s. (GADS)
strengthening exerciser
Stren intraepiphyseal osteotomy
streptococcal myositis
Streptococcus
    S. faecalis
    S. pneumoniae
streptokinase
streptomycin
stress
    bending s.
    s.-corrosion cracking
    s. distribution
    s. dorsiflexion projection
    s. examination
    s. film
    s. fracture
    hyperextension s.
    s. injury
    laxity to varus s.

    low contact s. (LCS)
    measured s.
    mediolateral s.
    principal s.
    s. radiograph
    s. radiography
    s. roentgenography
    s. rupture
    shear s.
    s.-strain curve
    tensile s.
    s. test
    s. testing
    s.-testing arthrometer
    torsional s.
    s. transfer
    s.-type fracture
    valgus s.
    s. view
    VonMises s.
stressor
Stress-Ray varus-valgus device
stress-relaxation
    intraoperative s.-r.
stretch
    diagonal s.
    elastic s.
    general capsular s.
    heel cord s.
    S. and Heel splint
    s. injury
    low-load prolonged s. (LLPS)
    s.-out strap
    passive s.
    s. pattern
    quick s.
    s. reflex
    repeated quick s. (RQS)
    slow s.
    spray and s.
    static s.
    s. test
    Vapo coolant spray and s.
stretcher
    shoe s.
stretching
    gastroc-soleus s.
    nerve s.
    soft tissue s.
striata
    osteopathia s.
striatal lesion
Strickland
    S. modification
    S. technique
    S. tendon repair
stride
    S. Analyzer

s. length of gait
s. time
strike
s. phase of gait
string drawing board
stringiness
stringing peg
strip
Fas-Trac s.
gastrocnemius-soleus fascial s.
s. posting
Thera-Band s.
stripout
screw s.
stripper
Acufex microsurgical tendon s.
Brand tendon s.
Bunnell tendon s.
Fischer tendon s.
Furlong tendon s.
Grierson tendon s.
orthopaedic surgical s.
tendon s.
stripping
Steindler s.
stroker
skin s.
stroke test
stroma
fibrovascular connective tissue s.
Stromeyer splint
Stromgren
S. ankle brace
S. support
Stromqvist hook pin system
Strong dorsal extension block splinting
Stronghands hand exerciser
structural
s. aluminum malleable (SAM)
s. bone graft
s. component
s. congenital myopathy
s. curve
s. derangement
s. intersegmental distortion
s. scoliosis
structure
articular s.
contiguous vertebral s.
cordlike s.
extraarticular s.
graft s.

intraarticular s.
keystone s.
ligamentous s.
neurovascular s.
osseous s.
posterolateral s.
ring s.
uniaxial s.
strumming
perpendicular s.
Strümpell sign
Strunsky sign
strut
s. fusion technique
s. graft
s. plate fixation
s.-type pin
Struthers
arcade of S.
ligament of S.
Stryker
S. arthrometer
S. bed
S. camera
S. cartilage knife
S. CPM exerciser
S. dermatome
S. drill
S. fracture frame
S. lag screw
S. leg exerciser
S. power instrumentation
S. screwdriver
S. SE3 drive system
S. soft tissue staple
S. surgical hand table
S. turning frame
S. viewing arthroscope
Stryker-Notch view
STS
silicone thermoplastic splinting
STS molding sock
STSE
split-thickness skin excision
STSG
split-thickness skin graft
STT
scaphotrapezoid-trapezial
STT joint
Stuart Gordon hand splint
Student-Newman-Keuls test
Student's t-test

NOTES

study
    air contrast s.
    anatomopathological s.
    cohort s.
    Doppler s.
    double contrast s.
    evoked potential s.
    fluorescein s.
    injection s.
    kinematic s.
    nerve conduction s. (NCS)
    radiodiagnostic s.
    Roentgen-stereophotogrammatic s.
    sudomotor s.
    in vivo s.
Stulberg
    S. HIPciser abduction splint
    S. hip positioner
    S. Mark II leg positioner
stump
    amputation s.
    s. edema
    painful s.
    s. revision
    s. shrinker
    s. wrapping
Sturge-Weber syndrome
stuttering of gait
STx
    S. lumbar traction device
    S. Saunders lumbar disc device
stylet
    blunt s.
stylohyoid
styloidectomy
    Stewart s.
styloidium
    os ulnar s.
stylus
    tibial s.
Styrofoam filler block
subacromial
    s. bursa
    s. bursal adhesion
    s. bursography
    s. decompression
    s. impingement syndrome
    s. portal
    s. space
    s. spur
subacute hematogenous osteomyelitis
subaponeurotic abscess
subarachnoid block
subarticular cyst
subastragalar
    s. dislocation
    s. fusion

subaxial
    s. posterior cervical spinal fusion
    s. subluxation
subcapital
    s. fracture
    s. osteotomy
subchondral
    s. bone
    s. bone cyst
    s. lesion
    s. lucency
    s. plate
subclavian
    s. artery
    s. artery injury
    s. steal syndrome
    s. vein
    s. vein injury
subclavicular approach
subclavius tendon graft
subcondylar
    s. deformity
    s. osteotomy
subcoracoid
    s. bone
    s. shoulder dislocation
    s. space
subcortical defect
subcostal plane
subcutaneous
    s. abscess
    s. anterior transposition
    s. drain
    s. fracture
    s. granuloma annulare
    s. intracompartmental soft-tissue sarcoma
    s. palmar fasciotomy
    s. pseudosarcomatous fibromatosis
    s. soft-tissue sarcoma
    s. tibialis posterior tenotomy
    s. tissue
subcuticular suture
subdeltoid
    s. bursa
    s. bursal adhesion
    s. bursitis
subdermal plexus
subfascial
    s. incision
    s. transposition
subglenoid shoulder dislocation
subgluteal
    s. bursitis
    s. hematoma
subjacent
Subjective Shoulder Rating Scale patient questionnaire

sublaminar
    s. fixation
    s. wire
    s. wiring
sublesional ulceration
subligamentous dissection
Sublimaze Injection
sublimis
    flexor digitorum s. (FDS)
    s. tendon
    s. tenodesis
subluxated metatarsophalangeal joint
subluxation
    AS s.
    ASEx s.
    ASIn s.
    atlantoaxial s. (AAS)
    atlantoaxial rotatory s.
    atlantooccipital s.
    calcaneocuboid s.
    compensatory structural s.
    congenital hip s.
    Crowe s.
    facilitated s.
    fixation s.
    foraminal encroachment s.
    functional s.
    glenohumeral joint s.
    hip s.
    neuroarticular s.
    neurofunctional s.
    patellar s.
    peroneal s.
    PIEx s.
    PIIn s.
    proximal tibiofibular s.
    radial head s.
    radioulnar s.
    rotatory atlantoaxial s.
    sacroiliac s.
    s. stabilization
    subaxial s.
    tibiofibular s.
    unilateral interfacetal dislocation
        or s. (UID/S)
    vertebral s.
    Yergason test of shoulder s.
subluxing patella
submandibular
submaximal stimulus
subperiosteal
    s. abscess

    s. cortical defect
    s. dissection
    s. exposure
    s. fracture
    s. new bone
subphrenic abscess
subplatysmal abscess
subsartorial tunnel
subscapular
    s. artery injury
    s. nerve injury
    s. tendinitis
subscapularis
    s. bursitis
    s. muscle
    s. tendon
    s. tendon transfer
subscapularis-capsular lengthening
subsidence
    component s.
    prosthesis component s.
    vertical s.
subspinous dislocation
substance
    bone s.
    metachromatic mucoid s.
    s. P
substantia gelatinosa
substitute
    OsteoSet bone graft s.
    OsteoSet-T medicated bone graft s.
substituting knee prosthesis
substitution
    arthroscopy-assisted patellar
        tendon s.
    Carrell fibular s.
    creeping s.
    extensor s.
    Marshall patelloquadriceps tendon s.
    patellar tendon s.
    patelloquadriceps tendon s.
    tendon s.
subtalar
    s. arthralgia
    s. arthrodesis
    s. arthroereisis
    s. arthrosis
    s. arthrotomy
    s. articulation
    s. axis
    s. capsulotomy
    s. dislocation

S

NOTES

subtalar *(continued)*
    s. distraction bone block fusion
    s. instability
    s. interosseous ligament
    s. joint (STJ)
    s. joint function (SJF)
    s. joint neutral position (STNP)
    s. motion
    s. pronation
    s. supination
    s. tilt
subtalo
    luxatio pedis s.
subthreshold
    s. force
    s. stimulus
subtotal
    s. lateral meniscectomy
    s. maxillectomy
    s. meniscectomy
    s. somatectomy
subtraction osteotomy
subtrochanteric
    s. femoral fracture
    s. osteotomy
subungual
    s. abscess
    s. exostosis
    s. fibroma
    s. granuloma
    s. hematoma
sucker
    KAM Super S.
    s. shaver
suction
    autotransfusion s.
    s. biter
    s. drainage
    irrigation s.
    s. irrigation system
    s. punch
    s. sign
    SureTran s.
    s. suspension
    s. tube
suction-irrigation
    s.-i. system
    s.-i. technique
Sudeck
    S. atrophy
    S. disease
sudomotor
    s. activity
    s. activity test
    s. function
    s. startle reflex
    s. study
Sufenta Injection

sufentanil citrate
sugar-tong
    s.-t. cast
    s.-t. plaster splint
    s.-t. traction
suggestion
    indirect hypnotic s.
Sugioka transtrochanteric rotational osteotomy
suit
    body-exhaust s.
    G s.
Sukhtian-Hughes fixation device
sulbactam
    ampicillin and s.
sulconazole
sulcus
    s. angle
    condylopatellar s.
    s. sign
sulfadiazine
    silver s.
sulfamethoxazole
    trimethoprim s.
Sulfamylon
sulfate
    ferrous s. ($FeSO_4$)
    glucosamine s.
    magnesium s.
    morphine s.
sulfated mucopolysaccharide
sulfide
    selenium s.
sulfinpyrazone
Sulfix-6 cement
sulfoxide
    dimethyl s. (DMSO)
sulindac
Sully shoulder stabilizer brace
Sulzer prosthesis
summary
    discharge s.
Sunday staphylorrhaphy elevator
Sunderland classification of nerve injury
Sundt shunt
sunrise view
sunset view
sup
    superior
super
    S. Cut laminectomy rongeur
    S. Grip sleeve
    S. Stimm MF stimulator
    Valorin S.
    s. wedge
    s. wrap
Superblade blade

SuperCup acetabular cup prosthesis
Superfeet Custom Pre-Fabricated
  Orthotic
superficial
  s. circumflex iliac artery
  s. femoral artery (SFA)
  s. infection
  s. medial ligament
  s. palmar arch
  s. peroneal nerve
  s. posterior compartment
  s. posterior sacrococcygeal ligament
  s. radial nerve
  s. temporal artery
  s. temporal vein
  s. transverse ligament
  s. TV metacarpal ligament
  s. TV metatarsal ligament
  s. varicosity
superficiale
  ligamentum metacarpale
    transversum s.
  ligamentum metatarsale
    transversum s.
  ligamentum sacrococcygeum
    posterius s.
superficialis
  s. arcade
  arcus palmaris s.
  arcus volaris s.
  flexor digitorum s. (FDS)
  s. tendon
Superform Contours orthotic
Superglue adhesive
superincumbent
superior (sup)
  s. border
  s. costotransverse ligament
  s. dislocation
  s. extensor retinaculum of foot
  s. glide
  s. gluteal nerve
  s. gluteal neurovascular bundle
  s. hypogastric plexus
  s. labrum anterior and posterior
    lesion (SLAP)
  s. laryngeal artery
  s. laryngeal nerve
  s. laryngeal nerve external branch
  s. leaf
  s. mesenteric artery syndrome

  s. peroneal retinaculum (SPR)
  s. pole of patella
  s. portal
  s. process
  S. Sleeprite Hi-Lo orthopaedic bed
  s. sulcus tumor
  s. thoracic pedicle screw
  s. thyroid artery
  s. thyroid vein
  s. TV ligament of scapula
  s. vena cava
superius
  ligamentum costotransversarium s.
  ligamentum transversum scapulae s.
supermarket elbow
supernumerary
  s. bone
  s. digit
  s. lumbar segmentation
  s. thumb
  s. toe
superoinferior tilt
superolateral portal
superomedial
  s. calcaneonavicular ligament
    (SMCR)
  s. portal
  s. region
supersensitivity
  Cannon Law of Denervation S.
  denervation s.
Super-Seven exercise
SuperSkin thin film dressing
Superstabilizer
  S. cemented stem extender
  S. press-fit stem extender
supertubercular wedge
  osteotomy/bunionectomy
supinated
supination
  s. contracture
  s. deformity
  s. of the foot
  s. injury
  s.-outward rotation injury
  s.-plantarflexion injury
  pronation and s.
  subtalar s.
supination-adduction
  s.-a. fracture
  s.-a. injury

NOTES

supination-eversion
s.-e. fracture
s.-e. injury
supination-external
s.-e. rotation (SER)
s.-e. rotation injury
s.-e. rotation IV fracture (SER-IV
fracture)
supination-inversion
s.-i. injury
s.-i. rotation injury
supinator
s. fat pad sign
s. jerk
s. muscle
supinatus
metatarsus s.
supine
s. C-Trax traction
s. C-Trax traction system
s. iliac gapping test
s. long sitting test
s. position
s. position driver
s. straight leg raising test
Suppan foot operation
supple neck
Suppliers
National Association of Medical
Equipment S. (NAMES)
supply
blood s.
longitudinal blood s.
support
Accommodator arch s.
Accu-Back back s.
Achillotrain active Achilles
tendon s.
Act joint s.
AliMed-Freedom arthritis s.
AliMed wrist/thumb s.
ANNA-DOTE Positioning S.
arch s.
Arizona leg s.
Assistant Free foot/ankle s.
back s.
Back-Hugger lumbar s.
BackThing lumbar s.
base of s.
BIOflex Magnet Back S.
BioSkin s.
Birkenstock Blue Footbed arch s.
Body Gard neoprene s.
Carabelt lower back s.
Castech extremity s.
Cavus foot s.
cervical s.
ChinUpps cervicofacial s.

cock-up wrist s.
Comprifix active ankle s.
Conve back s.
Corfit System 7000 Series
Lumbosacral S.
DayTimer Carpal Tunnel S.
Deltoid-Aid arm s.
DePuy s.
Desk-rest arm s.
Dr. Kho's CMC S.
Epitrain active elbow s.
Ergo Cush back s.
Ergoflex Premiere back s.
external s.
Ezy Wrap lumbosacral s.
FlexLite hinged knee s.
Foot Hugger foot s.
fork strap prosthetic s.
FREEDOM Arthritis S.
FREEDOM Back S.
FREEDOM Elastic Long Wrist S.
Friedman s.
Futuro wrist s.
Genutrain P3 knee s.
geriatric chair trunk s.
Houston halo cervical s.
Kallassy ankle s.
Kerr-Lagen abdominal s.
Lo Bak spinal s.
Malleotrain ankle s.
Mold-In-Place back s.
Momma-Too Maternity S.
Monitor Master monitor s.
Morton toe s.
Mother-To-Be abdominal s.
Mother-To-Be Support Maternity S.
neoprene ankle s.
neoprene back s.
Nightimer carpal tunnel s.
obese s.
OBUS back s.
OEC wrist/forearm s.
Ortho-Pal body s.
OSI Well Leg S.
Parham s.
PattStrap knee s.
peripatellar retinacular s.
Philadelphia collar cervical s.
Plastizote arch s.
ProFlex wrist s.
prosthetic s.
QualCraft ankle s.
QualCraft short elastic wrist s.
Relax-A-Bac posture s.
Rolyan foot s.
sacral s.
Sacro-Eze lumbar s.
Safe spine thoracic-lumbar-sacral s.

Sheffield s.
ShiatsuBACK back s.
Shoulder Ease abduction s.
Sidekick foot s.
Silesian bandage prosthetic s.
Spenco arch s.
S'port Max back s.
StanceGuard internal s.
Stromgren s.
Taylor clavicle s.
tibial fracture brace proximal s.
  (TFB-PS)
Valeo back s.
well-leg s.
wrist hand extension
  compression s. (WHECS)
supported extension exercise
Supprettes
Aquachloral S.
B&O S.
suppurative
s. arthritis
s. flexor tenosynovitis
s. joint infection
s. osteitis
s. osteomyelitis
s. periostitis
supraclavicular
s. approach
s. brachial block anesthesia
s. fossa artery
supracollicular spike of cortical bone
supracondylar (SC)
s. amputation
s. femoral derotational osteotomy
s. humeral fracture
intramedullary s. (IMSC)
s. medullary nail
s. nonunion
patellar tendon-bearing–s. (PTB-SC)
s. plate
s. process
s. process syndrome
s. socket
s. suspension (SC suspension)
s. varus osteotomy
s. Y-shaped fracture
supracondylar-suprapatellar (SC-SP, SCSP)
supraganglionic injury
suprahyoid

Supralen
S. cradle orthotic
S. Schaefer orthotic
supramalleolar
s. derotational osteotomy
s. flap
s. open amputation
s. orthosis (SMO)
s. varus derotation osteotomy
s. venous ulcer
supramaximal stimulus
supranaviculare
os s.
suprapatellar (SP)
s. cannula
s. plica
s. portal
s. pouch
s. reflex
suprapubic
suprascapular
s. nerve
s. nerve entrapment test
s. nerve injury
s. neuritis
suprasellar capsule
supraspinale
ligamentum s.
supraspinal ligament
supraspinatus
s. implant
s. muscle
s. outlet
s. syndrome
s. tendinitis
s. tendon
s. test
supraspinous ligament
suprasternal
s. notch
s. plane
s. space
suprasyndesmotic
s. fixation
s. fracture
s. screw fixation
supratalare
os s.
supratubercular wedge osteotomy
suprofen
sural
s. island flap

S

NOTES

sural *(continued)*
    s. island flap for foot and ankle reconstruction
    s. nerve
    s. neuroma
    s. neuropathy
Surbaugh legholder
Sureclosure closure
Sure-Closure skin stretching system
Sure-Flex III prosthetic foot
Sure Sport pad
SureStep ankle support system
Suretac
    S. bioabsorbable shoulder fixation device
    S. shoulder fixation
SureTran suction
surface
    apposing articular s.
    articular s.
    Bazooka support s.
    cancellous s.
    concave articular s.
    contiguous articular s.
    distal concave articular s.
    s. electrode
    s. electromyography (sEMG)
    endosteal s.
    erosion of articular s.
    freshen the s.
    Micro-Aire debridement of bone s.
    s. replacement
    s. replacement hip arthroplasty
    roughen the s.
    volar s.
    weightbearing s.
surfer's knot
Surfit adhesive
Surgairtome air drill
SurgAssist
    S. leg positioner
    S. surgical legholder
surgeon's
    S. tarsal joint
    s. thumb
surgery
    ablative s.
    adult scoliosis s.
    anterior cervical spine s.
    anterior cervicothoracic junction s.
    anterior lower cervical spine s.
    arthroscopic laser s.
    bypass s.
    cervical disk s.
    cervicothoracic junction s.
    Elite Farley retractor for spinal s.
    failed s.
    first ray s.

    hypotensive s.
    intradural tumor s.
    limb-salvage s.
    lower extremity s.
    lower posterior lumbar spine and sacrum s.
    McCash hand s.
    minimum incision s. (MIS)
    MRI-directed s.
    open disk s.
    peripheral vascular s. (PVS)
    posterior lower cervical spine s.
    posterior lumbar interbody fusion s.
    posterior lumbar spine and sacrum s.
    posterior upper cervical spine s.
    ProTrac system for knee s.
    scoliosis s.
    thoracic and thoracolumbar spine s.
    Unilink system for hand s.
    vascular s.
Surgibone
    Boplant S.
    S. implant
    Unilab S.
surgical
    s. ablation
    s. approach
    s. autoimmunization
    s. dressing room (SDR)
    s. exposure
    s. glove
    s. knife handle
    s. leg pedestal
    s. loupe
    s. neck
    s. neck fracture
    S. No Bounce mallet
    s.-orthopaedic drill
    s. pin driver
    s. reduction
    S. Simplex P bone cement
    S. Simplex P radiopaque cement
    s. staple applier
    s. technique
Surgicel
    S. fibrillar hemostat
    S. implant
    S. Nu-Knit absorbable hemostat
Surgilase CO$_2$ laser
Surgilast tubular elastic dressing
Surgi-Med clamp
Surgitek prosthesis
Surgitube tubular gauze
Surgivac drain
Surmontil
survivorship
    Kaplan-Meier s.

susceptibility testing
suspension
    Children's Advil Oral S.
    Children's Motrin Oral S.
    corset s.
    cuff s.
    s. feeder
    fingertrap s.
    flexible hinge s.
    SC s.
        supracondylar suspension
    s. strap
    suction s.
    supracondylar s. (SC suspension)
    s. traction
    s.-type socket
sustained
    s. ankle clonus
    s. loading
    s. pressure technique
sustentacular fragment
sustentaculum
    os s.
    s. tali
    s. tali fracture
Sutherland
    S. hip procedure
    S. lateral transfer
Sutherland-Greenfield osteotomy
Sutherland-Rowe incision
Sutter
    S. double-stem silicone implant
      prosthesis
    S. implant
    S. MCP finger joint prosthesis
Sutter-CPM
    S.-C. knee apparatus
    S.-C. knee device
suture
    s. abscess
    s. anchor
    s. anchor technique
    Bell s.
    Bondek s.
    braided s.
    bregmatomastoid s.
    bulb s.
    Bunnell crisscross s.
    Bunnell figure-eight s.
    Bunnell wire pull-out s.
    button s.
    Caprolactam s.

    Chinese fingertrap s.
    core s.
    cotton s.
    Cottony Dacron s.
    CT1 s.
    Dacron s.
    Dexon s.
    Donati s.
    double right-angle s.
    end-to-end s.
    epitenon s.
    Ethibond s.
    Ethiflex s.
    Ethilon s.
    fascial s.
    figure-of-eight s.
    fingertrap s.
    fishmouth end-to-end s.
    s. fixation
    Gillis s.
    Gore-Tex nonabsorbable s.
    grasping s.
    guy s.
    s. hole drill
    horizontal mattress s.
    interrupted s.
    intradermal s.
    jugal s.
    Kessler grasping s.
    Kessler-Tajima s.
    s. of Krause
    lamboid s.
    lashing s.
    lateral trap s.
    Le Dentu s.
    linen s.
    locking horizontal mattress s.
    Mason-Allen s.
    mattress s.
    Maxon s.
    McLaughlin modification of
      Bunnell pull-out s.
    Mersilene s.
    modified Kessler s.
    modified Kessler-Tajima s.
    monofilament s.
    nail s.
    Nicoladoni s.
    Nurolon s.
    nylon s.
    s. passer
    passing s.

S

NOTES

suture *(continued)*
    PDS s.
    Perma-Hand silk s.
    pin s.
    polybutester s.
    Polydek s.
    polydioxanone s. (PDS)
    polyester s.
    polyethylene s.
    polygalactic acid s.
    polyglactin s.
    polyglycolic acid s.
    polyglyconate s.
    polypropylene s.
    Polysorb s.
    popoff s.
    Prolene s.
    pull-out s.
    Pulvertaft end-to-end s.
    Pulvertaft interweave s.
    pursestring s.
    RB1 s.
    s. repair
    retention s.
    running s.
    safety-bolt s.
    s. scissors
    SH popoff s.
    silk s.
    simple s.
    sling s.
    staple s.
    subcuticular s.
    Tajima modified Kessler s.
    Tevdek s.
    transosseus s.
    Tycron s.
    undyed s.
    USP#2 s.
    vertical mattress s.
    Vicryl s.
    wire s.
suturing
    Johnson medial meniscal s.
    Morgan-Casscells meniscus s.
SVCPMS
    segmental vertebral
    cellulotenoperiosteomyalgic syndrome
Sven-Johansson
    S.-J. driver
    S.-J. extender
    S.-J. femoral neck nail
swab
    Phenol EZ s.
Swafford-Lichtman division
swager
swan-neck
    s.-n. chisel

    s.-n. deformity reduction
    s.-n. facies
    s.-n. finger deformity
    s.-n. gouge
Swan Neck splint
Swann-Morton surgical blade
Swanson
    S. carpal lunate implant
    S. carpal scaphoid implant
    S. classification
    S. Convex condylar arthroplasty
    S. dynamic toe splint
    S. elevator
    S. finger joint
    S. finger joint implant
    S. finger joint prosthesis
    S. flexible hallux valgus prosthesis
    S. great toe implant
    S. great toe prosthesis
    S. Grip-X hand exerciser
    S. hand splint
    S. interpositional wrist arthroplasty
    S. mallet
    S. metacarpal prosthesis
    S. metacarpophalangeal implant
    S. metatarsal broach
    S. metatarsal prosthesis
    S. metatarsophalangeal joint
    arthroplasty
    S. osteotome
    S. osteotomy
    S. PIP joint arthroplasty
    S. radial head implant
    S. radial head implant arthroplasty
    S. radiocarpal implant
    S. reconstruction
    S. scaphoid awl
    S. Silastic elbow prosthesis
    S. silicone wrist arthroplasty
    S. small joint implant
    S. technique
    S. trapezium implant
    S. T-shaped great toe Silastic
    prosthesis
    S. ulnar head implant
    S. wrist joint implant
    S. wrist prosthesis
swathe, swath
    arm s.
    s. and sling
sway
    anteroposterior s.
    anteroposterior/lateral s.
    body s.
    lateral s.
    postural s.
swaying gait

SWD
> short-wave diathermy

sweating
> plantar s.

sweat test

Swede-O
> S.-O. ankle brace
> S.-O. Arch-lok

Swede-O-Universal
> S.-O.-U. brace
> S.-O.-U. orthosis

Swedish
> S. approach
> S. Helparm
> S. knee cage
> S. knee cage orthosis
> S. massage
> S. portal

swelling
> boggy s.
> joint s.

SwimEx
> S. hydrotherapy system
> S. pool

swimmer's view

swimming pool granuloma

swing
> s.-to gait
> s. phase
> s.-phase acceleration
> s.-phase control
> s. phase of gait
> s.-through gait
> s. time

Swinger car bed

Swiss
> S. Balance orthotic
> S. ball
> S. cancellous screw
> S. MP joint implant

switching stick

swivel
> s. dislocation
> s. utensil
> s. walker

Swivel-Strap
> Aircast S.-S.
> S.-S. ankle brace
> S.-S. ankle stirrup

swollen disk

sx
> symptom

Sydney line

Syed-Neblett implant

Syed template implant

symbrachydactyly

symbrachytactylous hand

Syme
> S. amputation prosthesis
> S. ankle disarticulation amputation
> S. Dycor prosthetic foot
> S. foot prosthesis
> S. procedure

symmetric
> s. sacral plate
> s. thumb duplication
> s. vertebral fusion

symmetrically

symmetrical thoracic vertebral plate

symmetry
> weightbearing s.

sympathectomy
> cervical s.
> chemical s.
> lumbar s.
> preganglionic s.

sympathetic
> s. block
> s. chain
> s. component
> s. dystrophy
> s. maintained pain syndrome
> (SMPS)
> s. nerve
> s. nervous system (SNS)
> s. reflex dystrophy
> s. trunk

sympathetically maintained pain syndrome

symphalangism

symphyseal mobility

symphysis
> pubic s.
> s. pubis
> s. pubis diastasis

sympt
> symptom

symptom (sx, sympt)
> functionally debilitating s.
> irritable s.
> s. magnification syndrome

symptomatic
> s. spondylolisthesis
> s. synovial plica

S

NOTES

symptomatology
Symptoms Checklist 90 Revised (SCL-90R)
Syms traction
Synalgos-DC
Synaptic 2000 pain management system
synarthrosis
Synatomic total knee prosthesis
synchondrosis
    neurocentral s.
    tibiofibular s.
synchondrotomy
synchronized fibrillation
synchronous scapuloclavicular rotation
synchrony
    arm heel-strike s.
Synchrosonic stimulator
syndactylization
syndactylized finger
syndactyly
    burn s.
    complete s.
    complex s.
    complicated complex s.
    Diamond-Gould reduction s.
    incomplete s.
    Kelikian-Clayton-Loseff surgical s.
    pure s.
    reduction s.
    simple s.
syndesmectomy
syndesmophyte
syndesmosis, pl. syndesmoses
    s. sprain of ankle
    tibiofibular s.
syndesmotic
    s. avulsion
    s. ligament
    s. screw
    s. sprain
syndrome
    abdominal s.
    acetabular rim s.
    acquired immunodeficiency s. (AIDS)
    acute low-back s.
    adrenogenital s.
    adult respiratory distress s. (ARDS)
    Aicardi s.
    Albright s.
    Albright-McCune-Sternberg s.
    alcohol fat embolism s.
    algodystrophy s.
    amniotic band s. (ABS)
    annular constricting band s.
    anterior cervical cord s.
    anterior compartment s. (ACS)
    anterior impingement s.

    anterior interosseous nerve s.
    anterior tarsal tunnel s.
    anterior tibial s.
    anteversion s.
    Apert s.
    Arnold-Chiari s.
    arthroonychodysplasia s.
    Baastrupi s.
    Babinski-Fröhlich s.
    Barre-Lieou s.
    Bart-Phumphery s.
    battered child s.
    Behcet s.
    Behr s.
    bicipital s.
    bilateral acute radicular s.
    bilateral chronic radicular s.
    bio-energy imbalance s. (BIS)
    BK mole s.
    black heel s.
    Block-Sulzberger s.
    blue rubber bleb nevus s.
    blue toe s.
    broad thumb-big toe s.
    Brown-Séquard s.
    burning-feet s.
    Cacchione s.
    calcaneal spur s.
    carpal tunnel s. (CTS)
    Carpenter s.
    cast s.
    cauda equina s.
    central cord s.
    central heel pad s.
    cervical acceleration/deceleration s.
    cervical dorsal outlet s.
    cervicoencephalic s.
    cervicogenic s.
    Chédiak-Higashi s.
    Chiari-Foix-Nicolesco s.
    chronic compartment s. (CCS)
    chronic heel pain s. (CHPS)
    chronic intractable benign pain s. (CIBPS)
    chronic musculoskeletal pain s. (CMPS)
    clenched-fist s.
    Cobb s.
    common peroneal nerve s.
    compartment s.
    congenital band s.
    congenital ring s.
    constriction band s.
    conus medullaris s.
    copper deficiency s.
    coracoid impingement s.
    cord-traction s.
    Cornelia de Lange s.

Costen s.
costoclavicular s.
Cotton-Berg s.
CREST s.
Crouzon s.
cubital tunnel s.
cuboid s.
Cushing s.
dancing bear s.
dead-arm s.
de Barsy s.
deconditioned s.
deconditioning s.
Déjérine-Sottas s.
de Lange s.
diffuse idiopathic skeletal
  hyperostosis s.
DiGeorge s.
DISH s.
DOOR s.
dorsi jam s.
double crush s.
Down s.
droopy shoulder s.
Dyke-Davidoff-Masson s.
dysplastic nevus s.
Eagle s.
Eagle-Barrett s.
Eaton-Lambert s.
Edwards s.
Ehlers-Danlos s. (EDS)
Ekbom restless leg s.
empty can s.
entrapment s.
eosinophilia-myalgia s.
exertional anterior compartment s.
  (EACS)
exertional compartment s.
exertional deep posterior
  compartment s. (EDPCS)
extraarticular pain s.
facet joint s.
failed back s. (FBS)
failed back surgery s. (FBSS)
failed surgery s.
Fanconi s.
far-out s.
fat embolism s.
Fazio-Londe s.
Felty s.
fetal alcohol s.
fibromyalgia s. (FMS)

filum terminale s.
flat back s.
flexor carpi ulnaris s.
flexor origin s.
forearm compartment s.
Freeman-Sheldon s.
Frey s.
Funston s.
Gardner s.
General Adaption S. (GAS)
Gillespie s.
Goldenhar s.
Goodpasture s.
Gorlin s.
Grisel s.
Guillain-Barré s.
Haglund s.
hammer digit s.
hand-foot s.
heart-and-hand s.
heel spur s.
heel spur/plantar fasciitis s.
Heerfort s.
hip joint s.
Hoffa s.
Hoffmann s.
Horner s.
Hunter s.
Hurler s.
hyperostosis s.
hypothenar hammer s.
idiopathic skeletal hyperostosis s.
iliocostalis lumborum s.
ilioinguinal s.
iliotibial band friction s.
impingement s.
infrapatellar contracture s. (IPCS)
inguinal ligament s.
interosseous s.
intersection s.
Isaacs s.
Jaccoud s.
Jackson s.
Jackson-Gorham s.
Jackson-Weiss s.
Jaddassohn-Lewandowsky s.
Jarcho-Levin s.
Kasabach-Merritt s.
Kast-Maffucci s.
Kearns-Sayre s.
Kinsbourne s.
Kleine-Levin s.

S

NOTES

syndrome *(continued)*
  Klinefelter s.
  Klippel-Feil s. (KFS)
  Klippel-Trenaunay s.
  Klippel-Trenaunay-Weber s.
  Kocher-Debré-Semelaigne s.
  Kretschmer s.
  Lambert-Eaton myasthenic s.
   (LEMS)
  Larsen s.
  Larson s.
  lateral hyperpressure s.
  lateral patellar compression s.
  leopard s.
  Leriche s.
  levator scapulae s.
  Linberg s.
  local adaptation s. (LAS)
  lumbago-mechanical instability s.
  lumbar flat back s.
  Mafucci s.
  Marfan s.
  Maroteaux-Lamy s.
  McCune-Albright s.
  mechanical low back pain s.
  medial tibial s. (MTS)
  medial tibial stress s. (MTSS)
  meningeal s.
  metatarsal overload s.
  microgeodic s.
  milk-alkali s.
  milkman's s.
  Milwaukee shoulder s.
  mixed cord s.
  mixed headache s.
  Morel s.
  Morquio s.
  Morton s.
  Muir-Torre s.
  multifidus s.
  multiple pterygium s.
  Munchausen s.
  myofascial pain s. (MPF)
  Naffziger s.
  nail-patella s.
  naviculocapitate fracture s.
  nerve entrapment s.
  neuroarticular s.
  neurogenic s.
  Nievergelt-Pearlman s.
  occupational stress s. (OSS)
  osteoporosis pseudoglioma s.
  os trigonum s.
  overuse s.
  Paget-Schrötter s.
  pain dysfunction s.
  Parkes-Weber s.
  Parsonage-Aldren-Turner s.

  Parsonage-Turner s.
  Patau s.
  patellar clunk s.
  patellar malalignment s.
  patellar pair s.
  peroneal compartment s.
  pes anserinus s.
  Pfeiffer s.
  phalangeal microgeodic s.
  piriformis s.
  plica s.
  Plummer-Vinson s.
  Poland s.
  popliteal pterygium s.
  postcasting s.
  posterior cord s.
  posterior interosseous nerve
   compression s.
  postphlebitis s.
  postpyelomyelitis s.
  posttraumatic algodystrophic s.
  posttraumatic chronic cord s.
  Pouteau s.
  pronator teres s.
  prune-belly s.
  pseudoradicular s.
  quadratus lumborum s.
  quadrilateral space s.
  radial sensory nerve entrapment s.
  radial tunnel s.
  Raeder paratrigeminal s.
  Refsum s.
  Reiter s.
  repetitive stress s. (RSS)
  Rett s.
  Riley-Day s.
  ring s.
  rotatores s.
  Rotter-Erb s.
  Roussy-Levy s.
  Rubinstein-Taybi s.
  sacroiliac s.
  Sanfilippo s.
  SAPHO s.
  scalenus anticus s.
  scaphocapitate s.
  scapuloperoneal s.
  Scheie s.
  Schwachman s.
  Schwartz-Jampel s.
  secondary hip-spine s.
  second impact s.
  segmental vertebral
   cellulotenoperiosteomyalgic s.
   (SVCPMS)
  short leg s.
  Sinding-Larsen-Johansson s.
  sinus tarsi s.

Sjögren s.
skeletal hyperostosis s.
Sly s.
Smith-Lemli-Opitz s.
snapping scapula s.
spinal cord s.
spiral groove s.
Srb s.
steal s.
Stevens-Johnson s.
Stewart-Morel s.
Stickler s.
Sturge-Weber s.
subacromial impingement s.
subclavian steal s.
superior mesenteric artery s.
supracondylar process s.
supraspinatus s.
sympathetically maintained pain s.
sympathetic maintained pain s.
 (SMPS)
symptom magnification s.
synovial plica s.
TAR s.
tarsal tunnel s. (TTS)
temporomandibular joint s.
tensor fascia lata s.
tethered cord s.
thoracic inlet s.
thoracic outlet s. (TOS)
thrombocytopenia-absent radius s.
Tietze s.
Torres s.
transversospinalis s.
traumatic compartment s.
Turner s.
ulnar cubital tunnel s.
ulnar impaction s.
ulnar nerve entrapment s.
ulnocarpal abutment s.
unilateral acute radicular s.
unilateral chronic radicular s.
valgus extension overload s.
VATER s.
vertebral subluxation s.
vibrator hand s.
volar compartment s.
von Hippel-Lindau s.
Wallenberg s.
washboard s.
Weber s.
whiplash-shaken infant s.

Wilkie s.
windblown hand, whistling face s.
wrist pain s.
yellow nail s.
synergist
synergistic
 s. muscle
 s. wrist motion splint
synergy
 limb s.
 S. splint
 S. Therapeutic System
syngraft
synostosis
 cervical s.
 congenital radioulnar s.
 fibula protibial s.
 proximal tibiofibular s.
 radioulnar s. (type I, II)
 tibial-profibular s.
 tibiofibular s.
Synovator arthroscopic blade
synovectomy
 Albright s.
 arthroscopic s.
 s. blade
 carpal s.
 dorsal s.
 Inglis-Ranawat-Straub elbow s.
 palmar s.
 Porter-Richardson-Vainio s.
 six-portal s.
 Smith-Petersen s.
 volar s.
 Wilkinson s.
synovia (*pl. of* synovium)
synovial
 s. biopsy
 s. cavity
 s. chondromatosis
 s. cyst
 s. disease
 s. fistula
 s. fluid
 s. fold
 s. fringe
 s. frond
 s. herniation
 s. joint
 s. membrane
 s. nodule
 s. nonunion

S

NOTES

synovial *(continued)*
   s. osteochondromatosis
   s. plica
   s. plica syndrome
   s. pseudarthrosis
   s. resector
   s. rongeur
   s. sarcoma
   s. shaver
   s. sheath
   s. tag
   s. tap
   s. tumor
synoviochondromatosis
synoviocyte
synoviogram
synoviorthesis
synovitis
   boggy s.
   crystal-induced s.
   disseminated pigmented
    villonodular s.
   extraarticular pigmented
    villonodular s.
   Finkelstein sign for s.
   Finkelstein test for s.
   florid s.
   focal pigmented villanodular s.
   hypertrophic s.
   lead s.
   localized nodular s. (LNS)
   monarticular s.
   parapatellar s.
   particulate s.
   pigmented villonodular s. (PVS)
   postoperative s.
   proliferative s.
   reactive s.
   recurrent s.
   rheumatoid arthritis s.
   silicone s.
   villonodular s.
   villous s.
synovitis-acne-pustulosis-hyperostosis
  osteomyelitis (SAPHO)
synovium, pl. **synovia**
   exuberant s.
   opaque s.
   pannus of s.
synpolydactyly
Synthaderm dressing
Synthes
   S. compression hip screw
   S. drill
   S. guidepin
   S. ligament washer
   S. Microsystem drill bit
   S. Microsystem plate cutter

   S. Microsystems plate-holding
    forceps
   S. pie plate
   S. system
   S. wire guide
synthesis
   activity s.
   proteoglycan s.
synthetic
   s. augmentation
   s. bone
   s. graft bypass to ankle
   s. material
   s. prosthesis
   s. stent
Synvisc injection therapy
syovector
   arthroscopic s.
syphilis
Syracuse anterior I plate
syringe
   cement s.
   s. grip
   Terumo s.
syringohydromyelia
syringoma
   chondroid s.
syringometaplasia
syringomyelia
   posttraumatic s.
   secondary posttraumatic s.
SysStim 226 muscle stimulator
Systec irrigation
system
   ABG cement-free hip s.
   above-knee suction enhancement s.
   Accu-Flo ultrafiltration s.
   Acculength arthroplasty
    measuring s.
   Accusway balance measurement s.
   Ace intramedullary femoral nail s.
   ACET s.
   achilleo-calcaneal-plantar s.
   AcroMed VSP fixation s.
   Action traction s.
   Acufex microsurgical rear-entry to
    front-entry femoral guide s.
   Acutrak small bone fixation s.
   Adjustaback wheelchair backrest s.
   Advantim knee s.
   Aequalis s.
   AGC Biomet total knee s.
   Agee carpal tunnel release s.
   Agee-WristJack fracture reduction s.
   AIM femoral nail s.
   Air-Back spinal s.
   Aircast Knee S.
   air inflation s.

AITA modular trauma s.
Alcon Closure S.
Allen shoulder/wrist arthroscopy traction s.
Alliance rehabilitation s.
S. Alloclassic hip system
Allo-Pro hip s.
Alta modular trauma s.
AMBI compression hip screw s.
American shoulder and elbow s. (ASES)
American Society of Anesthesiologists physical status classification s.
AMK fixed bearing knee s.
AMK total knee s.
AML total hip s.
Amplatz anchor s.
Amset ALPS anterior locking plate s.
Amset R-F fixation s.
Anametric total knee s.
anatomic medullary locking hip s.
Anchorlok soft tissue suture anchor s.
Anderson s.
Andersson hip status s.
AnkleTough ankle rehabilitation s.
AnkleTough Rehab S.
Anspach 65K Universal instrument s.
anterior Kostuik-Harrington distraction s.
anterior locking plate s. (ALPS)
anterior plate s. (APS)
antimigration s. (AMS)
Apex Universal Drive and Irrigation S.
Apollo total knee s.
APR II hip s.
APR total hip s.
Aqua-Cel heating pad s.
Aquaciser hydrodynamic measurement s.
Aquaciser 100R underwater treadmill s.
Aquanex hydrodynamic measurement s.
AquaSens fluid monitoring s.
Ariel computerized exercise s.
Arthro-Flo arthroscopic irrigation s.
ArthroProbe laser s.

articular-ligamentous s.
Artisan cement s.
Ashhurst fracture classification s.
ASIF s.
Asnis 2 guided-screw s.
Assistant Free self-retaining hip surgery retractor s.
Association Research Circulation Osseous classification s.
Atlantis cervical plate s.
Atlas cable s.
autonomic nervous s. (ANS)
A-V Impulse s.
axial spinal s.
Axiom modular knee s.
Axis fixation s.
BacFix S.
Back Bull lumbar support s.
BAPS Ankle S.
Bassett electrical stimulation s.
Bateman UPF II bipolar knee s.
Becker orthopaedic spinal s. (BOSS)
Becker orthopedic thermoformable ankle s.
BIAS total hip s.
bilateral variable screw placement s.
Biodynamic Molding S.
Biofix absorbable fixation s.
Bio Flote air flotation s.
Biomechanical Ankle Platform S. (BAPS)
Biomet revision knee s.
Biomet Ultra-Drive ultrasonic revision s.
Bio-Modular total shoulder s.
bioresorbable drug delivery s.
BIOWARE software for Biodex isokinetic exercise s.
BioZone nutrition s.
Blajwas-Schwartz-Marcinko irrigation drainage s.
BMP cabling and plating s.
body logic rehabilitation s.
Body Masters MD 510 hi-lo pulley s.
Body Response s.
Bolin wedge filter s.
Boston Classification S.
Boston elbow s.
Bottoms-Up posture s.

NOTES

S

system *(continued)*

Bowden cable suspension s.
Boyer degenerative joint disease
  grading s.
Bremer halo s.
Bridge hip s.
Brighton electrical stimulation s.
BTM hip s.
cable suspension s.
cannula s.
cannulated guided hip screw s.
Cannulated Plus screw s.
CAPIS bone plate s.
capsuloligamentous s.
Carbon Monotube long bone
  fracture external fixation s.
Cascade Up and About s.
CC Rider closed-chain
  rehabilitation s.
central nervous s. (CNS)
Ceraver Osteal knee replacement s.
Charnley-Maerle D'Aubigné
  disability grading s.
Charnley total hip s.
Chiba spinal s.
C-2 hip s.
Chirotech x-ray s.
Cincinnati Knee Rating S.
CircPlus bandage/wrap s.
Circul'Air shoe process s.
Circulator boot s.
CKS knee s.
closed drainage s.
CLS hip s.
Codman ACP s.
Codman anterior cervical plate s.
Codman anterior cervical plating s.
Codman Ti-frame posterior
  fixation s.
Cofield total shoulder s.
Cohort anterior plate s.
Combi Multi-Traction S.
Command hip instrumentation s.
Compass stereotactic s.
Concept arthroscopy power s.
Concept beach chair shoulder
  positioning s.
Concept Precise ACL guide s.
Concept rotator cuff repair s.
Concept self-compressing cannulated
  screw s.
Concept Sterling arthroscopy
  blade s.
concurrent force s.
Constant and Murley shoulder
  scoring s.
ConstaVac autoreinfusion s.
contact laser delivery s.

Contact SPH cups s.
Continuum knee s. (CKS)
Coombs bone biopsy s.
Coordinate complete revision
  knee s.
Corail hip s.
Counter Rotation S. (CRS)
CPT hip s.
CRM s.
Crowe congenital hip dysplasia
  classification s.
CRS Tibial Torsion S.
cruciate condylar knee s.
Cryo/Cuff Knee Compression
  Dressing S.
curved Küntscher nail s.
Cybex I, II+ exercise s.
Cybex 340 isokinetic rehabilitation
  and testing s.
Cybex training s.
Dall-Miles cable/crimp cerclage s.
Dall-Miles cable grip s.
DataHand s.
d'Aubigne hip status s.
DawSkin flexible protective skin s.
deep bonding s. (DBS)
Deknatel orthopedic
  autotransfusion s.
Diab-A-Foot protection s.
Digi-Flex exercise s.
Digital Biofeedback S.
Dimension hip s.
double-cannula s.
double inflow cannula s.
DTT s.
Dual Range Limiter S.
Dupont distal humeral plate s.
Duracon total knee replacement s.
Duraloc acetabular cup s.
Dwyer-Wickham electrical
  stimulation s.
DynaFix external fixation s.
Dyna-Flex multilayer
  compression s.
Dyna-Lok pedicle screw s.
Dyna-Lok plate s.
Dyna-Lok plating s.
dynamic stabilizing innersole s.
EBI Medical Systems bone
  healing s.
EBI Medical Systems Orthofix
  fixation s.
ECTRA s.
EDG s.
Edwards modular s.
ElastaTrac home lumbar traction s.
Electri-Cool cold therapy s.
electrotherapy s. (ES)

Elite hip s.
Emerald implantation s.
Endoprothetik CSL-Plus cemented-hip s.
Endoprothetik CS-Plus cemented-hip s.
endoscopic carpal tunnel release s.
endoskeletal alignment s. (EAS)
Endotrac blade s.
EPIC functional evaluation s.
E-Series hip s.
Estraderm estradiol transdermal s.
Ewald elbow arthroplasty rating s.
Exact-Fit ATH hip replacement s.
facet screw s.
Facial Grading S. (FGS)
facilitated spinal s.
felt apron Bowden cable suspension s.
Fenlin total shoulder s.
Fernandez point-score wrist assessment s.
Fernandez scale posttraumatic wrist assessment s.
Ferno AquaCiser underwater treadmill s.
Ficat-Marcus grading s.
Fillauer endoskeletal alignment s.
filtration s.
FIN s.
Finn knee s.
Fitnet joint testing s.
Fixateur Interne fixation s.
FlexiTherm Thermographic S.
Flowtron pneumatic compression system BioCryo s.
FOAMART Foot Impression S.
Foot-Station 3-D foot imaging s.
Fowler knee s.
FP5000 pump s.
Freeman-Swanson knee s.
F-Scan foot force and gait analysis s.
fusimotor s.
GDLH posterior spinal s.
GD Regainer S.
Genesis II total knee s.
genital s.
Genucom ACL laxity analysis s.
Genucom knee flexion analysis s.
Geomedic s.

Gillette double-flexure ankle joint s.
Global total shoulder arthroplasty s.
Golden mean testing s.
Golf Exercise S.
Gonstead pelvic marking s.
Graf stabilization s.
Granberg cervical traction s.
gravity extension locking s. (GELS)
Gray revision instrument s.
Green-O'Brien evaluation s.
Guldmann Overhead Trac S.
Gustilo fracture classification s.
Haid UBP s.
Hall mandibular implant s.
Hall modular acetabular reamer s.
halo cervical traction s.
Hands Free Knee Retractor S.
Harrington rod and hook s.
Harris hip status s.
Hausmann Work-Well work hardening s.
haversian s.
HCMI Chiropractic S.
Herbert and Fisher fracture classification s.
Heritage hip s.
Hermes Evolution tricompartmental knee s.
Hermes total knee s.
Herndon hip classification s.
Hexcel total condylar knee s.
Heyman hip classification s.
hipGRIP pelvic positioning s.
Hipokrat bimodular shoulder s.
Histofreezer cryosurgical s.
HJD total hip s.
Hoek-Bowen cement removal s.
Hoffmann external fixation s.
Hohl fracture classification s.
Hot/Ice S. III
Howmedica knee s.
Howmedica total ankle s.
HybridFit total hip s.
HybridFit total knee s.
hydraulic test s.
Hypobaric transfemoral s.
Hypobaric transtibial s.
Ilizarov limb-lengthening s.
immune s.
Impact modular total hip s.

S

NOTES

system *(continued)*

Impingement-Free Tibial Guide S.
Indiana tome carpal tunnel
syndrome release s.
Infinity hip s.
Inglis-Pellicci elbow arthroplasty
rating s.
Innomed arthroplasty measuring s.
Insall-Burstein II modular knee s.
Insight knee positioning and
alignment s.
instrumentation s.
Integral hip s.
integrated shape and imaging s.
(ISIS)
InteliJet fluid management s.
Inteq small joint suturing s.
Intermedics natural hip s.
internal fixation plate-screw s.
International 10-20 s.
International Listing S.
Iowa hip status s.
ipos arch support s.
irrigation s.
Isola fixation s.
Isola spinal implant s.
Isola spinal instrumentation s.
Itrel II, III spinal cord
stimulation s.
Jacobson s.
joint activated s. (JAS)
Judet hip status s.
Jurgan pin-ball s.
J-Vac closed drainage s.
Kaplan-Meier survivorship
analysis s.
Kellgren-Lawrence grading s.
Kendall A-V impulse s.
K-Fix Fixator s.
Kinamed Exact-Fit ATH s.
Kin-Con isokinetic exercise s.
Kinematic II condylar and
stabilizer total knee s.
Kinematic II rotating hinge knee s.
Kinemax modular condylar and
stabilizer total knee s.
Kinemax Plus total knee s.
Kinemetric guide s.
Kirschner II-C shoulder s.
Kirschner integrated shoulder s.
KMC hip s.
KMW hip s.
knee signature s.
Kofoed scoring s.
Kostuik-Harrington distraction s.
Kyle fracture classification s.
Langenskiöld grading s.
Larson hip status s.

LCS mobile bearing knee s.
Leibinger Profyle hand s.
Liberty spinal s.
Lichtman staging s.
Lido Active Multijoint S.
Lidoback isokinetic dynamometry s.
Lido Passive Multijoint S.
Link custom partial pelvis
replacement s.
Link Endo-Model rotational knee s.
Link Saddle Prosthesis Endo-Model
hip replacement s.
locomotor s.
Lorenz osteosynthesis s.
Lubinus AP hip s.
Lubinus SP II anatomically adapted
hip s.
Luhr fixation s.
lumbosacral cartilaginous s.
Luque II fixation s.
Lynco biomechanical orthotic s.
Mackinnon-Dellon staging s.
Madajet XL jet-injection
anesthesia s.
Magerl hook-plate s.
Magerl plate-screw s.
Magna-FX cannulated screw s.
Mallory-Head modular calcar s.
Maramed Miami fracture brace s.
Mark III halo s.
Mark II Sorrells hip arthroplasty
retractor s.
Mason fracture classification s.
Mattrix spinal cord stimulation s.
Maxim Modular Knee S.
Mayo Clinic forefoot scoring s.
Mayo Clinic hip-scoring s.
Mazur ankle rating s.
McCain TMJ arthroscopic s.
McGuire scoring s.
Medical Examination and
Diagnostic Coding S. (MEDICS)
Medical Research Council s.
Medtronic spinal cord
stimulation s.
Meniscus Mender II s.
Metasul hip s.
MG II total knee s.
Microloc knee s.
Micro-Mill knee instrument s.
MicroPhor iontophoretic drug
delivery s.
Midas Rex instrumentation s.
Miller-Galante revision knee s.
Miller-Galante total knee s.
Minaar classification s.
Mini-Flap drain s.
Mirage Spinal S.

Mitek anchor s.
Mitek GII suture anchor s.
Mitek Vapr tissue removal s.
modified Wagner classification s.
Modular Acetabular Revision S.
  (MARS)
modular Lenbach hip s.
modular S-ROM total hip s.
MOD unicompartmental knee s.
Moe s.
Monotube external fixator s.
Monticelli-Spinelli circular external
  fixation s.
Moore hip endoprosthesis s.
Morrey elbow arthroplasty rating s.
Moss fixation s.
motorized shaving s.
Mouradian humeral fixation s.
Multi Podus Foot S.
musculotendinous s.
Musgrave Footprint S.
Natural-Knee II s.
Neer II shoulder s.
Neer II total knee s.
Neff femorotibial nail s.
nervous s.
Newport hip s.
NexGen complete knee s.
Nexus wheelchair seating s.
NoHands Mouse-Foot-Operated
  Computer Mouse S.
NordiCare Back Therapy S.
Norm testing and rehabilitation s.
occupational rating s.
Ogden fracture classification s.
Ogden plate s.
Ogden tissue reattachment mini s.
Olerud pedicle fixation s.
Olerud PSF fixation s.
Omega compression hip screw s.
Omega Plus compression hip s.
Omnifit total knee s.
open double-decked hook
  cervical s.
Optetrak total knee replacement s.
Opti-Fix total hip s.
optoelectric measuring s.
Optotrak motion measurement s.
Orth-evac autotransfusion s.
Ortholoc Advantim revision knee s.
Ortholoc Advantim total knee s.
Orthomet Axiom total knee s.

Orthomet Perfecta total hip s.
OrthoPak bone growth stimulator s.
Orthotec pressurized fluid
  irrigation s.
Osada portable handpiece s.
OSI modular table s.
osteochondral autograft transfer s.
  (OATS)
Palmer-Gonstead-Firth listing s.
Panoview arthroscopic s.
ParaMax ACL guide s.
parasympathetic nervous s. (PNS)
Partnership s.
PCA primary total knee s.
PCA Universal total knee
  instrument s.
PEAK Fixation S.
Peak Motus Motion
  Measurement S.
PEC modular total knee s.
PEC total hip s.
Pedar-in-shoe measurement s.
Pedar pressure measurement s.
pediatric s.
pedicle screw s.
Perfecta Interseal total hip s.
PerFixation s.
Performance modular total knee s.
Performance unicompartmental
  knee s.
peripheral nervous s. (PNS)
peripheral vascular s. (PVS)
PFC modular total knee s.
PFC TC3 modular knee s.
PFC total hip replacement s.
PGP flexible nail s.
PGR cemented modular s.
Phoenix foot s.
Phoresor II iontophoretic drug
  delivery s.
pin ball s.
Pinch Gauge and Jackson Strength
  Evaluation S.
Pinwheel S.
Pipkin fracture classification s.
PlastiCast adjustable joint cast s.
plate-screw s.
PlexiPulse DVT prophylaxis s.
Podospray nail drill s.
Polarus positional humeral
  fixation s.
Polycentric and Wide-Track knee s.

S

NOTES

system *(continued)*
4 in 1 positioning block s.
Postel hip status s.
posterior cruciate condylar knee s.
posterior rod s.
PPT insole s.
PPT soft tissue orthotic s.
Precision Osteolock femoral
component s.
Precision Strata hip s.
Press-Fit total condylar knee s.
pressure transducer-monitor s.
pretarget filtration s.
Profix total knee replacement s.
Profore Four-Layer bandage s.
programmable VariGrip II
prosthetic control s.
ProTrac cruciate reconstruction s.
Providence Scoliosis S.
Proxiderm wound closure s.
Pulsavac III wound debridement s.
Pump It Up pneumatic socket
volume management s.
Puno-Winter-Byrd s.
PWB transpedicular spine
fixation s.
Quadracut ACL shaver s.
Quick-Sil silicone s.
Rancho Cube S.
rating s.
rearfoot stability s. (RSS)
Reebok Slide S.
Reebok Step S.
Reese osteotomy guide s.
ReFlexion implant s.
Replica total hip replacement s.
respiratory exhaust s.
Restoration acetabular s.
Restoration-HA hip s.
Richards fixator s.
Richards hip endoprosthesis s.
Richards modular hip s.
Richards Solcotrans orthopaedic
drainage-reinfusion s.
right-handed orthogonal
coordinate s. (RHOCS)
Riseborough-Radin fracture
classification s.
Rochester compression s.
Rod TAG suture anchor s.
Roger Anderson s.
Rogozinski screw s.
Rogozinski spinal fixation s.
Rogozinski spinal rod s.
ROHO pediatric seating s.
Rolyan Reach N Range Pulley S.
Romano curved drilling s.

Russell-Taylor femoral interlocking
nail s.
Sabolich socket s.
Savastano Hemi-Knee s.
Scaphoid-Microstaple s.
Schwartz-Blajwas-Marcinko
irrigation s.
Scorpio total knee s.
Scotchcast length splinting s.
Secure Yet Gentle surgical
dressing s.
segmental spinal correction s.
(SSCS)
Select shoulder s.
Shadow-Line ACF spine
retractor s.
shaving s.
Sherman remote podiatric
vacuum s.
shoulder arm s. (SAS)
Silhouette spinal s.
Simmons plating s.
Simmons and Segil classification s.
single-cannula s.
Sofflex mattress s.
Sofwire cable s.
Solcotrans autotransfusion s.
Solcotrans orthopaedic drainage-
refusion s.
Soma Gonio s.
Soma pulley s.
Sorrells hip arthroplasty retractor s.
Souter Strathclyde total elbow s.
Spectron EF total hip s.
spherocentric knee s.
Spinoscope noninvasive imaging s.
Square Module Seating S.
S-ROM hip replacement s.
S-ROM modular total knee s.
S-ROM proximally modular total
hip s.
Stableloc II external fixator s.
Stahl staging s.
StairMaster exercise s.
Statak anchor s.
Steffee pedicle screw-plate s.
Steffee variable spine plating s.
Stockholm HAVS staging s.
Stromqvist hook pin s.
Stryker SE3 drive s.
suction-irrigation s.
suction irrigation s.
supine C-Trax traction s.
Sure-Closure skin stretching s.
SureStep ankle support s.
SwimEx hydrotherapy s.
sympathetic nervous s. (SNS)
Synaptic 2000 pain management s.

Synergy Therapeutic S.
Synthes s.
System Alloclassic hip s.
TAB tibial augmentation block s.
TAG anchor s.
Tamarack flexure joint s.
TCIV knee s.
TCPM pneumatic tourniquet s.
TEC interface s.
The Healthy Back S.
Thera-Band resistive therapy s.
Therabath paraffin heat therapy s.
Therabite jaw motion
  rehabilitation s.
Thera-Ciser light exercise s.
Thera-Ciser therapeutic exercise s.
Thompson hip endoprosthesis s.
Thompson leg check s.
three-point pressure s.
THSP s.
tibial torsion s.
Ti-Fit total hip s.
titanium hollow screw plate s.
Townley anatomic knee s.
TPL-6 hip s.
Trilogy acetabular cup s.
Tri-Motion Knee S.
triple envelope s.
Tri-Wedge total hip s.
Trunkey fracture classification s.
TSRH crosslink s.
TSRH spinal implant s.
TSRH Universal spinal
  instrumentation s.
TurnAide therapeutic s.
Turning Board Exercise S.
Tylok high-tension cable s.
UBP s.
UCO Quick-Sil silicone s.
UE Tech Weight Well Exercise S.
Ulson fixator s.
Ultima hip replacement s.
Ultima total hip s.
Ultra-Drive bone cement
  removal s.
Ultra-Drive ultrasonic revision s.
UltraFix RC suture anchor s.
Ultra-Guard FS hip bracing s.
Ultra-Guard hip orthosis s.
UltraPower drill s.
Ultra-X external fixation s.

Unicondylar Geomedic hemi-knee s.
Uniflex nailing s.
unilateral variable screw
  placement s.
Universal bone plate s.
Universal Spine S. (USS)
Up and About s.
variable axis knee s.
variable screw placement s.
Vector low back analysis s.
Vermont pedicle fixation s.
Verruca-Freeze freezing s.
Versalok low back fixation s.
Versa-Trac lumbar spine
  retractor s.
VerSys hip s.
Vertetrac ambulatory traction s.
Vilex cannulated screw s.
VSP s.
Wagner revision hip s.
WalkAide s.
Warm-Up active wound therapy s.
WATSMART stereography s.
Weber fracture classification s.
Wedge TAG suture anchor s.
West Point Ankle Grading S.
Wiltse pedicle screw fixation s.
Winquist-Hansen fracture
  comminution classification s.
Wisconsin Compression s. (WCS)
Wit portable TENS s.
Wrightlock posterior fixation s.
Wrightlock spinal fixation s.
X-Y sensor s.
Y-knot tying s.
Zickel fracture classification s.
Zimmer Anatomic hip prosthesis s.
Zimmer crossover instrumentation s.
Zimmer-Hall drive s.
Zimmer hip implant s.
Zimmer Pulsavac wound
  debridement s.
ZMS intramedullary fixation s.
Zuni exercise s.
Zweymuller hip s.

systemic
  s. lupus erythematosus (SLE)
  s. mycosis
  s. sclerosis
Systems 2000 TENS unit
systolic blood pressure (SBP)

S

NOTES

T

T buttress plate
T fracture
T handle elevator
T wave

T28

Trapezoidal-28
T28 hip prosthesis

T1-weighted image
T2-weighted image
TA

TA metallic staple
TA Premium 30, 55, 90 staple

Tab

T. Grabber

tabes dorsalis
tabetic

t. foot
t. gait

table

Adapta physical therapy t.
Albee-Compere fracture t.
Albee orthopaedic t.
Allen arm/hand surgery t.
AM-MI orthopedic t.
Andrews SST-3000 spinal
surgery t.
Apollo TM electric flexion t.
Back Specialist electric t.
Back Specialist manual t.
Bell t.
Berstein cast t.
cast t.
Chick fracture t.
Chick-Langren orthopaedic t.
circumductor t.
Cobb attachment for Albee-
Compere fracture t.
crank t.
cutout t.
DDP t.
Diamond biomechanical t.
Ergo style flexion t.
Eurotech t.
flexion-distraction t.
fluoroscopic t.
fracture t.
friction-reduced examination t.
friction-reduced segmented t.
Galaxy McManis hylo t.
Green-Anderson growth t.
Hercules TM drop-adjusting t.
Hill Air-Drop HA90C t.
hi-lo t.
hydromassage t.

inner t.
Intersegmental t.
Jackson spinal surgery and
imaging t.
knavel t.
knee-chest t.
Leander chiropractic t.
Leander motorized flexion t.
Leander 79- Series distraction t.
Lloyd chiropractic t.
Magnum 101 Plus t.
Marquet fracture t.
Massage Time Pro hydromassage t.
Med-Fit cranial-sacral t.
Meridian Intersegmental t.
Midland tilt t.
Multi-Lock hand operating t.
orthopaedic t.
over-bed t.
Paris manual therapy t.
PET/Eurotech 'Generation 2000" t.
Platinum stationary t.
Powermatic t.
Rath treatment t.
resistive exercise t.
Roger Anderson t.
Sapphire t.
t. short leg
Sieman t.
slatted plinth t.
slot t.
Stryker surgical hand t.
Telos fracture t.
t. tie
tilt t. (TT)
Titan Apollo electric flexion t.
Titan Meridian Intersegmental
Traction t.
Titan Nova manual flexion-
extension multi flex t.
Topaz flexion t.
Tri W-G t.
TX-1, TX-7 traction t.
VAX-D therapy t.
Verteflex Intersegmental Traction T.
Williams Advantage t.
Williams Model 170 t.
Winco Folding Treatment T.
Zenith ACS t.
Zenith-Cox flexion/distraction t.
Zenith Hylos t.
Zenith stationary t.
Zenith Thompson t.
Zenith Verti-Lift t.

T

table *(continued)*
    Zodiac TM Manual Flexion-
       Distraction t.
tablet
    bonemeal t.
    Tums E-X Extra Strength T.
tabletop Stone staple
taboparesis
Tab-Strap knee immobilizer
TAB tibial augmentation block system
Tac-3
Tac-40
TACE
Tachdjian
    T. classification
    T. fractional lengthening
    T. hamstring lengthening
    T. pin
    T. procedure
Tacit threaded anchor
tack
    t.-and-pin forceps
    biodegradable surgical t.
    t. breakage
tackler's
    t. arm
    t. exostosis
Tacoma sacral plate
tacrine HCl
Tacticon
    T. peripheral neuropathy kit
    T. peripheral neuropathy screening
      device
    T. quantitative sensory testing
tactile
    t. anesthesia
    t. defensiveness
taenia
    lip of t.
tag
    skin t.
    synovial t.
TAG anchor system
t'ai chi
Tai Chi Chuan exercise
tailbone
tailored
tailor's
    t. ankle
    t. bunion
    t. bunionectomy
Tait
    T. flap
    T. graft
Tajima
    T. metacarpal lengthening
    T. method

    T. modified Kessler suture
    T. suture technique
Takahashi forceps
Takakura index
Takayasu arteritis
Take-apart forceps
takeoff
Take-Out Extractor
TAL
    tendo Achilles lengthening
Talacen
talanavicular capsule
talar
    t. avulsion fracture
    t. axis-first MT base angle
      (TAMBA)
    t. beak
    t. beaking
    t. body
    t. body nonunion
    t. canal
    t. dislocation
    t. dome
    t. malunion
    t. neck
    t. neck exostosis
    t. neck fracture
    t. neck osteotomy
    t. osteochondral fracture
    t. osteochondritis dissecans
    t. process
    t. sinus
    t. tilt
    t.-tilt angle
    t. triple arthrodesis
talectomy
    Trumble t.
Talesnick scapholunate repair
tali
    sustentaculum t.
talipes
    t. calcaneocavus
    t. calcaneovalgus
    t. calcaneus
    t. cavovalgus
    t. cavovarus
    t. cavus deformity
    t. convex pes valgus
    t. equinovalgus
    t. equinovarus (TEV)
    flexible t.
    t. planovalgus
    t. planus
Tall-ette toilet seat
talocalcaneal
    t. angle
    t. coalition
    t. fusion

t. index
t. joint
t. osteotomy
talocalcaneonavicular
t. complex
t. joint
t. ligament articulation
talocalcaneus
os t.
talocrural
t. alignment
t. angle
t. fusion
t. joint
t. sprain
talocruralis
ligamentum laterale articulationis t.
ligamentum mediale articulationis t.
talofibular
t. joint
t. ligament
talometatarsal angle
talonavicular
t. angle
t. arthrodesis
t. bone
t. capsulotomy
t.-cuneiform complex
t. dislocation
t. fusion
t. joint
t. ligament
t. ossicle of Pirie
t. sprain
talonaviculare
ligamentum t.
talotibial exostosis
talus
t. accessorius
beaking of head of t.
congenital vertical t. (CVT)
flattop t.
osteochondral fracture of the dome of the t.
Tricodur T. compression dressing
truncated-wedge tarsometatarsal arthrodesis vertical t.
vertical t.
Talwin
T. Compound
T. NX

TAM
total active motion
Tamae harvesting
Tamarack
T. flexure joint
T. flexure joint system
TAMBA
talar axis-first MT base angle
tamp
bone t.
Kiene bone t.
tension band wire t.
Tandearil
tandem
t. connector
t. gait
t. gait test
tangential
t. hand
t. incision
t. standing radiograph
t. x-ray view
Tang retractor
Tanita Professional Body Composition Analyzer
tank
Hubbard t. (HT)
Hubbard physical therapy t.
tantalum
t.-ball marker
t. mesh
tap
AO t.
t. drill
dynamic condylar screw t.
screw t.
Screw-Lok t.
synovial t.
tape
anthropometric measuring t.
benzoin adherent t.
bias-cut t.
cast t.
Delta-Lite casting t.
Elastikon t.
Expandover athletic t.
foam t.
graded Gore-Tex t.
Gulick Anthropometric T.
Lightplast athletic t.
MaxCast casting t.
Medipore H surgical t.

NOTES

tape *(continued)*
Mersilene t.
moleskin traction t.
Powerflex t.
Scotchcast 2 casting t.
skin t.
t. traction
TufStuf II cast t.
Ultra-Light athletic t.
umbilical t.
Zonas porous t.
taper
collarless polished t. (CPT)
t.-jaw forceps
Morse t.
t. with Zimmer shank
tapered
t. hand reamer
t. pin
tapering dose steroid
Taperloc
T. femoral component
T. femoral prosthesis
T. femoral stem
taping
buddy t.
Gibney t.
LowDye t.
tapir
bouche de t.
tapotement
tapper
TAR
thrombocytopenia-absent radius
TAR syndrome
TARA
total articular replacement arthroplasty
total articular resurfacing arthroplasty
TARA total hip prosthesis
Taractan
taratologic dislocation
Taratynov disease
tardy ulnar palsy
targeter
bone screw t.
IMP bone screw t.
targeting
t. bead
distal t.
t. drill guide
tarsal
t. amputation
t. arthrodesis
t. bone
t. bone fracture
t. canal
t. coalition
t. dislocation

t. joint
t. joint infection
t. medullostomy
t. navicular
t. navicular bursitis
t. plate
t. pronator shoe
t. sinus artery
t. tunnel
t. tunnel release (TTR)
t. tunnel syndrome (TTS)
t. wedge osteotomy
tarsalmetatarsal fracture-dislocation
tarsi (*pl. of* tarsus)
tarsometatarsal (TMT)
t. amputation
t. angle
t. articulation
t. dislocation
t. fracture-dislocation
t. joint
t. joint arthrodesis
t. joint injury
t. junction
t. osteoarthritis
t. truncated-wedge arthrodesis
tarsonavicular
tarsus, pl. **tarsi**
dorsal ligaments of t.
interosseous ligaments of t.
ligament of t.
ligamenta tarsi
ossa tarsi
plantar ligaments of t.
sinus tarsi
tartrate
levorphanol t.
t. resistant acid phosphatase (TRAP)
Task Force on Standards of Physical Therapy
Tauranga splint
taut band
Tavernetti-Tennant knee prosthesis
Taylor
T. back brace
T. clavicle support
T. percussion hammer
T. procedure
T. retractor
T. spinal frame
T. spinal retractor blade
T. spine brace
T. splint
T. technique
T. thoracolumbosacral orthosis
Taylor-Daniel-Weiland technique
Taylor-Knight brace

Taylor-Townsend-Corlett iliac crest bone graft
Tazicef
Tazidime
tazobactam
T-bar guide
T broach
T-C
> T-C pin cutter
> T-C ring-handle pin and wire extractor

Tc
> T. 99m sestamibi myocardial perfusion imaging

^{99m}Tc (*var. of* Tc 99m)
TCA
> transcondylar axis

TCAT
> Toglia Category Assessment Test

TCC
> total contact cast
> total contact casting

TCCK unconstrained knee prosthesis
TCFO
> Therapy Carrot Finger Orthosis
> > TCFO placement wand

TCIV knee system
TCL
> tibial collateral ligament

T-clamp
> Pratt T.-c.
> Presbyterian Hospital T.-c.

Tc 99m, ^{99m}Tc
> technetium-99m

TCO
> total contact orthosis

T-condylar fracture
TCPM
> T. pneumatic tourniquet
> T. pneumatic tourniquet system

T-Cube
TD
> temperature differential
> terminal device

TE
> echo time

tea
> t.-and-toast diet
> Chiro-Klenx t.

teacup fracture

team
> donor t.
> recipient t.

tear
> anterior horn meniscal t.
> anterior oblique meniscal t.
> bowstring t.
> bucket-handle t.
> cleavage t.
> complex meniscal t.
> degenerative t.
> deltoid ligament t.
> flap meniscal t.
> full-thickness cuff t.
> horizontal meniscal t.
> iatrogenic dural t.
> incomplete t.
> interstitial meniscal t.
> intraoperative dural t.
> Johnson-Jahss classification of posterior tibial tendon t.
> labral t.
> lateral t.
> longitudinal displaced complete t.
> longitudinal incomplete intrameniscal t.
> longitudinal meniscal t.
> meniscal lateral t.
> meniscal radial t.
> meniscal transverse t.
> meniscocapsular t.
> midsubstance t.
> mop-end mid-substance t.
> Neer acromioplasty for rotator cuff t.
> oblique meniscal t.
> parrot-beak t.
> posterior cruciate ligament t.
> posterior horn meniscal t.
> posterior oblique meniscal t.
> radial meniscal t.
> rotator cuff t.
> TFC t.
> through-and-through t.
> transverse t.
> triangular fibrocartilage complex t.
> vertical longitudinal t.

teardrop
> t. fracture
> t. line
> t.-shaped flexion-compression fracture

T

NOTES

Teare
  T. arm splint
  T. sling
tearing sound
TEARS
  The Early Amnion Rupture Spectrum
teaspoon
  nylon t.
TEC
  TEC interface system
  TEC liner
TechCel Lite
Techmedica implant
technetium
  t. labeled methylene diphosphonate
  t. stannous pyrophosphate (TSPP)
technetium-99 methylene diphosphonate
technetium-99m (Tc 99m, ^{99m}Tc)
  t. diphosphonate scan
  t. phosphate
  t. pyrophosphate
  t. pyrophosphate scan
  t. sulfur colloid scan
technique
  abduction traction t.
  accessory movement t.
  Ace-Colles frame t.
  active-release t. (ART)
  adduction traction t.
  Alexander t.
  Allgöwer suture t.
  Amspacher-Messenbaugh t.
  Amstutz resurfacing t.
  Anderson-Hutchins t.
  Anderson screw placement t.
  Andrews t.
  anterior iliofemoral t.
  anterior quadriceps
    musculocutaneous flap t.
  AO t.
  AO-ASIF compression t.
  Armistead t.
  Aronson-Prager t.
  arthrographic capsular distension
    and rupture t.
  Asher physical build assessment t.
  ASIF screw fixation t.
  Asnis t.
  Atasoy V-Y t.
  Avila t.
  avulsion t.
  axial pin t.
  Badgley t.
  bag-of-bones t.
  Bailey-Badgley t.
  Bailey-Dubow t.
  Baker t.
  Balacescu-Golden t.

Bandi t.
Banks-Laufman t.
Barbour t.
Barsky t.
basic t.
Basmajian t.
Batch-Spittler-McFaddin t.
Bauer-Tondra-Trusler t.
Baumgard-Schwartz tennis elbow t.
Beall-Webel-Bailey t.
Beckenbaugh t.
Becker t.
Becton t.
Bellemore-Barrett-Middleton-Scougall-
  Whiteway t.
Bell-Tawse open reduction t.
Bevin-Aurglass t.
biframed distraction t.
Bircher-Weber t.
Black t.
Black-Broström staple t.
Blackburn t.
Blair t.
Bleck recession t.
Bloom-Raney modification of
  Smith-Robinson t.
Blount tracing t.
Blundell-Jones t.
Bobrath t.
Bohlman cervical fusion t.
Bohlman triple-wire t.
bone t.
Bonfiglio-Bardenstein t.
Bonfiglio modification of
  Phemister t.
Bonola t.
Bora t.
Borggreve-Hall t.
Bosworth t.
Bowers t.
Boyd-Anderson t.
Boyd-McLeod tennis elbow t.
Boyes brachioradialis transfer t.
Brackett-Osgood-Putti-Abbott t.
Brady-Jewett t.
Brand tendon transfer t.
Brannon-Wickström t.
Brooks t.
Brooks-Jenkins atlantoaxial fusion t.
Brooks-Seddon transfer t.
Broström injection t.
Brown t.
Bruser t.
Bryan-Morrey t.
Buck-Gramcko t.
Bugg-Boyd t.
Buncke t.
Bunnell atraumatic t.

Bunnell tendon suturing t.
Bunnell tendon transfer t.
bur-down t.
Burgess t.
Burkhalter modification of Stiles-Bunnell t.
Burkhalter transfer t.
Burow skin flap t.
Burrows t.
Caldwell-Coleman flatfoot t.
Callahan fusion t.
Camino catheter t.
Camitz t.
Campbell t.
Canale t.
cannulated reaming t.
Capello t.
Carnesale t.
Carrell fibular substitution t.
Cave-Rowe shoulder dislocation t.
CBP t.
cement t.
cementless t.
central slip sparing t.
cervical screw insertion t.
cervical spondylotic myelopathy fusion t.
Chaves-Rapp muscle transfer t.
chevron t.
Chiari t.
Childress ankle fixation t.
chiropractic manipulative reflex t. (CMRT)
Cho tendon t.
Chow t.
Chrisman-Snook ankle t.
Cierny-Mader t.
Cincinnati t.
Clancy ligament t.
Clark transfer t.
Clayton-Fowler t.
Cleveland-Bosworth-Thompson t.
Cloward t.
t. of Cobb
Cobb scoliosis measuring t.
Codivilla tendon lengthening t.
Cofield t.
Cole t.
Coleman flatfoot t.
Collis broken femoral stem t.
Coltart fracture t.
combination of isotonics t.

compression t.
Connolly t.
contoured anterior spinal plate t.
contract-relax t.
conventional t.
Conyers t.
Coonse-Adams t.
coracoclavicular t.
costotransversectomy t.
cotyloplasty t.
Cox flexion-distraction t.
Cozen-Brockway t.
craniosacral therapy t.
Crawford-Marxen-Osterfeld t.
Crego tendon transfer t.
Cubbins shoulder dislocation t.
Cuniard and Campell t.
Curtis t.
Curtis-Fisher knee t.
Cyriax t.
Darrach-McLaughlin shoulder t.
Davey-Rorabeck-Fowler decompression t.
Davis drainage t.
DeBastiani t.
Debeyre-Patte-Elmelik rotator cuff t.
decompression t.
decortication t.
DePalma modified patellar t.
Dewar-Barrington clavicular dislocation t.
Dewar-Harris shoulder t.
Dewar posterior cervical fusion t.
Deyerle femoral fracture t.
Dias-Giegerich fracture t.
Dickinson calcaneal bursitis t.
Dickson transplant t.
Dimon-Hughston t.
distraction t.
Doll trochanteric reattachment t.
Doppler t.
double-looped semitendinous and gracilis hamstring graft knee reconstruction t.
double portal t.
double-rod t.
dowel graft t.
doweling spondylolisthesis t.
DREZ modification of Eriksson t.
drilling t.
Drummond spinous wiring t.
Drummond wire t.

T

NOTES

technique *(continued)*

Dunn t.
Dunn-Brittain foot stabilization t.
DuVries deltoid ligament
  reconstruction t.
Eastwood t.
Eaton-Littler t.
Eaton-Malerich fracture-dislocation t.
Eberle contracture release t.
Ecker-Lotke-Glazer tendon
  reconstruction t.
Eftekhar broken femoral stem t.
Eggers tendon transfer t.
Ellis-Jones peroneal tendon t.
Ellison t.
Ellis skin traction t.
Ender femoral fracture t.
Erickson-Leider-Brown t.
Eriksson brachial block t.
Eriksson ligament t.
Essex-Lopresti axial fixation t.
Essex-Lopresti calcaneal fracture t.
European compression t. (ECT)
Evans ankle reconstruction t.
excision-curettage t.
extraarticular t.
extremity mobilization t.
facet excision t.
facilitatory t.
Fahey t.
Fahey-O'Brien t.
Fairbanks t.
Farmer t.
Ferkel torticollis t.
Fielding modification of Gallie t.
Fish cuneiform osteotomy t.
fixation t.
Flatt t.
Flick-Gould t.
Flynn t.
Forbes modification of Phemister
  graft t.
Ford triangulation t.
Forest-Hastings t.
Fowler t.
Fowles dislocation t.
Freebody-Bendall-Taylor fusion t.
freehand suturing t.
French fracture t.
Fried-Hendel tendon t.
Froimson t.
Frost posterior tibialis t.
functional t.
Furnas-Haq-Somers t.
fusion t.
Gaenslen split-heel t.
Gallie atlantoaxial fusion t.
Gallie wiring t.

Galveston t.
Ganley t.
Garceau tendon t.
Ger t.
Getty decompression t.
Giannestras modification of
  Lapidus t.
Gilbert-Tamai-Weiland t.
Gillies-Millard cocked-hat t.
Gill-Manning-White
  spondylolisthesis t.
Gill sliding graft t.
Gledhill t.
gliding-hole-first t.
Glynn-Neibauer t.
Goldberg t.
Goldner-Clippinger t.
Goldstein spinal fusion t.
Gonstead t.
Gordon-Broström t.
Gordon joint injection t.
Gordon-Taylor t.
great toe arthroplasty implant t.
  (GAIT)
Green-Banks t.
Greulich-Pyle t.
Grice-Green t.
Grosse-Kempf tibial t.
Groves-Goldner t.
Guhl t.
Guttmann t.
Hackethal stacked nailing t.
Hall t.
Hamas t.
Hardinge t.
Harmon transfer t.
Harriluque t.
Hassmann-Brunn-Neer elbow t.
Hauser patellar realignment t.
Hendler unitunnel t.
Henning inside-to-outside t.
Henry acromioclavicular t.
Hermodsson internal rotation t.
Hey-Groves fascia lata t.
Hey-Groves-Kirk t.
Hey-Groves ligament
  reconstruction t.
Heyman-Herndon-Strong t.
Hill-Nahai-Vasconez-Mathes t.
HIO t.
Hirschhorn compression t.
Hitchcock tendon t.
Hodgson t.
Hohl-Moore t.
Hoke-Kite t.
hold-relax t.
hole-in-one t.
Hoppenfeld-Deboer t.

Hori t.
hot dog t.
Houghton-Akroyd fracture t.
Hovanian transfer t.
Howard t.
Hughston-Jacobson t.
Hungerford t.
Huntington tibial t.
Ilizarov limb-lengthening t.
Inglis-Cooper t.
Inglis-Ranawat-Straub t.
injection t.
Insall-Hood reconstruction t.
Insall ligament reconstruction t.
inside-to-outside t.
interference screw t.
interspinous segmental spinal
  instrumentation t. (ISSI)
inverting knot t.
ischemic tourniquet t.
isometric t.
Jacobs locking hook spinal rod t.
Jansey t.
Jeffery t.
Johnson pelvic fracture t.
Johnson staple t.
Jones-Brackett t.
Kapandji t.
Kapel elbow dislocation t.
Kaplan t.
Kashiwagi t.
Kates-Kessel-Kay t.
Kaufer tendon t.
Kaufmann t.
Kelikian-Clayton-Loseff t.
Kelikian-Riashi-Gleason t.
Kellogg-Speed fusion t.
Kendrick-Sharma-Hassler-Herndon t.
Kennedy ligament t.
Kessler suture t.
keyhole tenodesis t.
King t.
King-Richards dislocation t.
King-Steelquist t.
Kjolbe t.
Klagsbrun harvesting t.
Klein t.
Klisic-Jankovic t.
Kloehn craniofacial remodeling t.
Krackow-Cohn t.
Krackow-Thomas-Jones t.

Krempen-Craig-Sotelo tibial
  nonunion t.
Kumar-Cowell-Ramsey t.
Kumar spica cast t.
Küntscher t.
Lamb-Marks-Bayne t.
Lambrinudi t.
Lapidus hammertoe t.
Larson t.
Leadbetter t.
Lee t.
Lehman t.
Leibolt t.
Lenart-Kullman t.
Lewit stretch t.
Lichtman t.
Liebolt radioulnar t.
Lindholm t.
line-to-line reaming t.
Lipscomb t.
Lister t.
Little t.
Littler t.
Littler-Cooley t.
Lloyd-Roberts fracture t.
local standby anesthesia t.
Losee modification of MacIntosh t.
Losee sling and reef t.
Louisiana ankle wrap t.
LowDye taping t.
Ludloff t.
lumbar accessory movement t.
Luque instrumentation concave t.
Luque instrumentation convex t.
Luque sublaminar wiring t.
Lyden t.
Lyden-Lehman t.
Lynn t.
MacIntosh t.
Magerl translaminar facet screw
  fixation t.
Magilligan measuring t.
Magnuson t.
Ma-Griffith t.
Maitland t.
Majestro-Ruda-Frost tendon t.
Malawer excision t.
Mallory t.
manipulative t.
Mankin t.
Mann t.
Manske t.

T

NOTES

technique *(continued)*

manual push-pull t.
Maquet t.
Marcus-Balourdas-Heiple ankle fusion t.
Marshall ligament repair t.
Marshall-McIntosh t.
Martin patellar wiring t.
Matti-Russe t.
Mazet t.
McConnell t.
McElfresh-Dobyns-O'Brien t.
McElvenny t.
McFarland-Osborne t.
McFarlane t.
McKeever-Buck elbow t.
McLaughlin-Hay t.
McReynolds open reduction t.
medial cortical overlap t.
medial heel skive t.
Mehn-Quigley t.
Mensor-Scheck t.
Meyerding-Van Demark t.
microneurosurgical t.
Milch cuff resection of ulna t.
Milch elbow t.
Milford mallet finger t.
mille pattes t.
Millesi modified t.
Mital elbow release t.
miter t.
Mizuno t.
Mizuno-Hirohata-Kashiwagi t.
Moe scoliosis t.
Monticelli-Spinelli distraction t.
Moore t.
Morgan-Casscells meniscus suturing t.
Morrison t.
mosaicplasty t.
Mubarak-Hargens decompression t.
Mueller t.
muscle energy t.
Nalebuff-Millender lateral band mobilization t.
neural arch resection t.
Neviaser acromioclavicular t.
Neviaser-Wilson-Gardner t.
Nicholas five-in-one reconstruction t.
Nicholas ligament t.
Niebauer-King t.
Nimmo receptor-tonus t.
Nirschl t.
noninvasive t.
no-touch t.
OATS t.
Ober-Barr transfer t.

Ober tendon t.
Obwegeser sagittal mandibular osteotomy t.
Ogata t.
Ollier t.
Omer-Capen t.
open palm t.
O'Phelan t.
Osborne-Cotterill elbow t.
Osgood modified t.
Osmond-Clarke t.
Ostrup harvesting t.
outside-in t.
outside-to-outside arthroscopy t.
Pack t.
Palmer t.
Palmer-Widen shoulder t.
pants-over-vest t.
Papineau t.
Parrish-Mann hammertoe t.
Parvin gravity t.
passive gliding t.
Paterson t.
Paulos ligament t.
Pauwels t.
Peacock transposing t.
Perry t.
Perry-Nickel t.
Perry-O'Brien-Hodgson t.
Perry-Robinson cervical t.
Pheasant elbow t.
Phemister-Bonfiglio t.
Phemister onlay bone graft t.
Pierrot-Murphy tendon t.
PNF t.
Porter-Richardson-Vainio t.
posterior flap t.
posterior iliofemoral t.
posterolateral costotransversectomy t.
postganglionic t.
postisometric relaxation traction t.
postisometric stretch t.
Pratt t.
preemptive blockade t.
preganglionic t.
press-fit acetabular implant insertion t.
Puddu tendon t.
Pulvertaft weave t.
Quénu nail plate removal t.
Ralston-Thompson pseudarthrosis t.
Ranawat-DeFiore-Straub t.
Ray-Clancy-Lemon t.
Rayhack t.
reduction t.
Reichenheim t.
reverse wedge t.
rhythmic initiation t.

Rideau t.
Riordan tendon transfer t.
Risser t.
Roberts t.
Robinson-Southwick fusion t.
Rockwood-Green t.
Rogers cervical fusion t.
Rood t.
Royle-Thompson transfer t.
Russe t.
Ryerson t.
sacral bar t.
sacrooccipital t. (SOT)
Sage-Clark t.
Saha transfer t.
Sakellarides-Deweese t.
Salter t.
Sammarco-DiRaimondo modification
  of Elmslie t.
Sarmiento trochanteric fracture t.
Scaglietti closed reduction t.
Schaberg-Harper-Allen t.
Schauwecker patellar wiring t.
Schepsis-Leach t.
Schnute wedge resection t.
Schober t.
Scott glenoplasty t.
screw insertion t.
Scuderi t.
second-generation cementing t.
Seddon t.
Sell-Frank-Johnson extensor shift t.
semitendinosus t.
Serafin t.
Sever modification of Fairbank t.
Sharrard transfer t.
Sherk-Probst t.
shish kebab t.
short lever accessory movement t.
Silfverskiöld t.
silver dollar t.
Simultaneous Interview T. (SIT)
single proximal portal t.
Skoog t.
sling and reef t.
slit catheter t.
Slocum fusion t.
Smith t.
Smith-Petersen t.
Smith-Robinson t.
Sofield femoral deficiency t.
Somerville t.

SOTO t.
Spälteholz t.
Speed-Boyd radial-ulnar t.
spinal fusion t.
spinal mobilization t.
spiral t.
Sprague arthroscopic t.
spray and stretch t.
Staheli t.
Stanisavljevic t.
Staples t.
STAR t.
Stark-Moore-Ashworth-Boyes t.
Steffee instrumentation t.
Stiles-Bunnell transfer t.
Stimson anterior shoulder
  reduction t.
strain/counterstrain t.
Straub t.
Strayer tendon t.
Strickland t.
strut fusion t.
suction-irrigation t.
surgical t.
sustained pressure t.
suture anchor t.
Swanson t.
Tajima suture t.
Taylor t.
Taylor-Daniel-Weiland t.
tension band wiring t.
Teuffer t.
third-generation cementing t.
Thomas-Thompson-Straub transfer t.
Thompson-Henry t.
Thompson-Loomer t.
thoracolumbar spondylosis
  surgical t.
threaded-hole-first t.
three-portal t.
Tohen tendon t.
Torg t.
Torgerson-Leach modified t.
transiliac bar t.
Trethowan-Stamm-Simmonds-
  Menelaus-Haddad t.
triangulation t.
triple-wire t.
Tullos t.
Turco clubfoot release t.
two-portal t.
two-sleeve t.

T

NOTES

technique *(continued)*
  two-stage tendon grafting t.
  two-strut tibial graft t.
  unitunnel t.
  unlocking spiral t.
  vasomotor t.
  Vastamäki t.
  Veleanu-Rosianu-Ionescu t.
  Verdan t.
  Vidal-Adrey fracture t.
  Viladot surgical t.
  Volz-Turner reattachment t.
  Vulpius-Compere tendon t.
  Wadsworth t.
  Wagner open reduction t.
  Wagoner cervical t.
  Warner-Farber ankle fixation t.
  Watkins fusion t.
  Watson t.
  Watson-Cheyne t.
  Weaver-Dunn acromioclavicular t.
  Weber-Brunner-Freuler-Boitzy t.
  Weber-Vasey traction-absorption
    wiring t.
  Weckesser t.
  Weinstein-Ponseti t.
  Wertheim-Bohlman t.
  West and Soto-Hall patella t.
  West-Soto-Hall patellar t.
  Whitesides t.
  Whitesides-Kelly cervical t.
  wick t.
  Wick catheter t.
  Williams-Haddad t.
  Wilson t.
  Wilson-Jacobs tibial fracture
    fixation t.
  Wilson-McKeever shoulder t.
  Windson-Insall-Vince grafting t.
  Winograd ingrown nail t.
  Winter spondylolisthesis t.
  wire removal t.
  Wirth-Jager tendon t.
  Woodward t.
  Zancolli rerouting t.
  Zariczny ligament t.
  Zarins-Rowe ligament t.
  Zazepen-Gamidov t.
  Zeier transfer t.
  Zielke t.
  Zoeller-Clancy t.
technology
  Cascading Tower T.
  GADS t.
  VSL t.
  work evaluation systems t. (WEST)
Tectonic magnet

tectora
  membrane t.
tectoral ligament
TED
  thromboembolic disease
    TED hose
    TED stockings
TEE
  transesophageal echocardiography
teeth
  Hutchinson t.
Teflon
  T. cannula
  T.-coated driver
  T. tri-leaflet prosthesis
Tegaderm dressing
Tegner
  T. activity scale
  T. activity score
Tegtmeier
  T. elevator
  T. hand board
Tei-Shin
Tekscan in-shoe monitoring device
telangiectasia
  t.-ataxia
  calcinosis, Raynaud, esophageal,
    sclerodactyly, t. (CREST)
telangiectatic osteosarcoma
TeleCaption decoder
Telectronics
  T. electrical stimulation apparatus
  T. electrical stimulation device
telemetry
telescopic
  t. rod
  t. view guide
telescoping
  t. brace
  t. medullary rod
  t. nail
telethermography
telethermometer
Telfa
  T. bolster
  T. gauze
  T. gauze dressing
Telos fracture table
TEM
  terminal extensor mechanism
temafloxacin
temazepam
Temper
  T. foam
  T. Foam cube
  T. Foam cushion

temperature
>body t.
>t. differential (TD)

Temperfoam

Temperlite saw blade

temper tantrum elbow

template
>acetabular cup t.
>Charnley t.
>femoral condylar t.
>malleable t.
>Moore t.
>Mueller t.
>Pedrialle t.
>prosthesis t.
>rod t.
>Stevens-Street elbow prosthesis t.
>templating t.
>thermoplastic t.
>tibial track t.
>transparent t.

templating
>t. roentgenogram
>t. template

Temple
>T. University nail
>T. University plate

temporal
>t. bone fracture
>t. dispersion
>t. fascia graft

temporalis fascia flap

temporary
>t. cavity phenomenon
>t. cerclage wire
>t. prosthetic fitting

temporomandibular
>t. joint (TMJ)
>t. joint arthralgia
>t. joint dislocation
>t. joint syndrome

Tempra

Tempur-Pedic
>T.-P. pressure relieving Swedish mattress
>T.-P. pressure relieving Swedish pillow

T.E.N.
>Vivomex T.E.N.

tenaculum

tenaculum-reducing forceps

TenderCloud pressure pad

Tenderlett device

tenderness
>bony t.
>costovertebral angle t.
>joint line t.
>myofascial t.
>percussion t.
>pillar t.
>point t.
>rebound t.

tender point (TeP)

tendinitis, tendonitis
>Achilles t.
>biceps t.
>bicipital t.
>birefringent lipid crystals in t.
>calcific t.
>de Quervain t.
>digital flexor t.
>infrapatellar t.
>infraspinatus t.
>patellar t.
>peripatellar t.
>peroneal t.
>posterior tibial t. (PTT)
>radial wrist extensor t.
>rotator cuff t.
>semimembranosus t.
>subscapular t.
>supraspinatus t.
>ulnar wrist extensor t.
>wrist extensor t.
>wrist flexor t.

tendinopathy
>insertion t.

tendinosis
>angiofibroblastic hyperplasia t.
>medial tennis elbow t.

tendinous
>t. attachment
>t. fiber

tendinum
>juncturae t.

tendo
>t. Achilles lengthening (TAL)
>t. Achillis
>t. Achillis mechanism
>t. calcaneus

tendon
>abductor digiti quinti t.
>abductor hallucis t.
>abductor pollicis brevis t.

NOTES

tendon *(continued)*
abductor pollicis longus t.
accessory communicating t.
Achilles t. (AT)
adductor hallucis t.
adductor pollicis brevis t.
adherent profundus t.
t. advancement
anchoring t.
anterior tibial t.
aponeurosis of t.
aponeurotic t.
attenuation of t.
attrition of t.
biceps brachialis t.
biceps brachii t.
biceps femoris t.
bicipital t.
brachialis t.
brachial plexus t.
brachioradialis t.
t.-braiding forceps
calcaneal t.
carpi radialis brevis t.
carpi radialis longus t.
t. centralization
common extensor t.
conjoined t.
digital extensor t.
digital flexor t.
digiti quinti proprius t.
t. disorder
t. displacement
ECRB t.
ECRL t.
EDB t.
EHL t.
elbow extensor t.
t. excursion
extensor carpi radialis brevis t.
extensor carpi radialis longus t.
extensor carpi ulnaris t.
extensor digiti minimi t.
extensor digiti quinti t.
extensor digitorum brevis t.
extensor digitorum communis t.
extensor digitorum longus t.
extensor hallucis longus t.
extensor indicis proprius t.
extensor pollicis brevis t.
extensor pollicis longus t.
extensor quinti t.
flexor carpi radialis t.
flexor carpi ulnaris t.
flexor digitorum communis t.
flexor digitorum longus t.
flexor digitorum profundus t.
flexor digitorum sublimis t.
flexor digitorum superficialis t.
flexor hallucis brevis t.
flexor hallucis longus t.
flexor pollicis brevis t.
flexor pollicis longus t.
flexor profundus t.
flexor sublimis t.
t. forceps
gastrocnemius t.
gastroc-soleus t.
G-lengthening of semitendinosus t.
Golgi t.
t. gouge
gracilis t.
t. graft (TG)
hamstring t.
hilus of t.
t.-holding forceps
iliopsoas t.
t. inflammation
infrapatellar t.
infraspinatus t.
interosseous t.
t. interposition arthroplasty
t. irregularity
t. jerk
t. lengthening
long head biceps t.
lumbrical t.
midpatellar t.
t. needle
t. nodularity
t. nodule
obturator internus t.
palmaris longus t.
t. passer
t.-passing forceps
patellar t.
patelloquadriceps t.
percutaneous lengthening of
  Achilles t.
peroneal t.
peroneus brevis t.
peroneus longus t.
peroneus tertius t.
plantaris t.
t. plate
popliteal t.
popliteus t.
posterior tibial t. (PTT)
postop flexor t. (PFT)
ProCol bovine bioprosthesis t.
profundus t.
pronator teres t.
proprius t.
t. prosthesis
t.-pulling forceps
quadriceps t.

rectus femoris t.
t. reflex
t. release
release of the flexor hallucis
 longus t.
t. repair
t.-retrieving forceps
t. rod
t. rupture
sartorius t.
t.-seizing forceps
semimembranosus t.
semitendinosus t.
t. sheath
slip of t.
snapping t.
t. snapping
split anterior tibial t. (SPLATT)
t. stripper
sublimis t.
subscapularis t.
t. substitution
superficialis t.
supraspinatus t.
t. thickening
thumb extensor t.
thumb flexor t.
tibial t.
tibialis anterior t.
tibialis posterior t.
t.-to-bone attachment
toe extensor t.
t. transfer
t. transposition
triceps brachii t.
t. tucker
t. tunneler
t.-tunneling forceps
wrist extensor t.
Z-lengthening of biceps t.
tendon-bearing
 patellar t.-b. (PTB)
tendon-bearing-supracondylar
 patella t.-b.-s.
tendon-bone
 t.-b. allograft
 bone-patellar t.-b. (BPB)
 t.-b. bridge
tendonitis (*var. of* tendinitis)
tendopathy
 plantar t.

tendosuspension
 Hibbs t.
 Jones t.
tendovaginitis
tenectomy
tennis
 t. elbow
 t. elbow splint
 t. elbow test
 t. heel
 t. leg
 t. toe
tenodesis
 Andrews iliotibial band t.
 Andrews lateral t.
 anterolateral femorotibial ligament t.
 calcaneal t.
 t. effect
 Eggers t.
 Ellison iliotibial band t.
 Evans t.
 extensor t.
 femorotibial ligament t.
 Fowler t.
 hallucis brevis t.
 t. of the heel cord
 iliotibial band t.
 interphalangeal t.
 key-grip t.
 keyhole t.
 MacIntosh extraarticular t.
 MacIntosh iliotibial band t.
 Moberg key-grip t.
 modified Watson-Jones ankle t.
 Mueller anterolateral femorotibial
  ligament t.
 Norwood iliotibial band t.
 Perry-O'Brien-Hodgson triple t.
 semitendinosus t.
 sublimis t.
 triple t.
 Watson-Jones ankle t.
 Westin t.
tenography
tenolysis
tenontagra
tenontophyma
tenoplastic reconstruction
tenosynovectomy
 dorsal t.
 flexor t.

T

NOTES

tenosynovial
t. giant cell tumor
t. injection
t. sheath
tenosynovitis
bicipital t.
de Quervain stenosing t.
flexor hallucis longus t.
stenosing t.
suppurative flexor t.
tuberculous peroneal t.
tenotomized
tenotomy
Achilles t.
adductor t.
Braun shoulder t.
extensor t.
flexor t.
Fowler central slip t.
t. knife
t. of metatarsophalangeal joint
percutaneous t.
semiopen sliding t.
sliding t.
subcutaneous tibialis posterior t.
transverse t.
Veleanu-Rosianu-Ionescu adductor t.
Z-plasty t.
tenovaginitis
inflammatory t.
tenoxicam
TENS
transcutaneous electrical nerve
stimulation
TENS unit
tensile
t. force
t. strain
t. strength
t. stress
Tensilon
T. test
T. test for myasthenia gravis
tensing test
tensiometer
Acufex t.
tensiometry
tension
t. band
t. band fixation
t. band plate
t. band plating
t. band wire
t. band wire tamp
t.-band wiring
t. band wiring technique
capsular-ligamentous t.
t. force

t. fracture
graft t.
heel t.
t. isometer
t. loading
t. myositis
neural t.
t. night splint (TNS)
oxygen t.
residual t.
tensioner
cable t.
Dwyer t.
Kirschner wire t.
tension-free
t.-f. Millesi nerve graft
t.-f. nerve graft
tensor
t. fasciae latae anchovy
t. fascia femoris flap
t. fascia lata (TFL)
t. fascia lata muscle flap
t. fascia lata syndrome
tent frame
tenuous vascularity
Tenzel elevator
TeP
tender point
Tepperwedge wedge
TEPP repair
Teq-Trode electrode
terbinafine
t. HCl
t. hydrochloride cream
t., oral
t., topical
teres
anterior pronator t.
ligamentum t.
t. major muscle
pronator t. (PT)
terminal
t. device (TD)
t. extensor mechanism (TEM)
t. head
t. knee extension
t. latency
t. overgrowth
t. Syme procedure
terminale
ossiculum t.
terminalis
linea t.
terrae
Mycobacterium t.
territory
motor unit t.

Terry
>   T. nail
>   T. Thomas sign

Terumo syringe

TES belt

Tesla magnet

test
>   abduction external rotation t.
>   abduction stress t.
>   accordion t.
>   Achilles squeeze t.
>   Achilles tendon t.
>   activated partial thromboplastin
>   time t. (APTT)
>   active bending t.
>   active knee extension t.
>   actual leg length t.
>   Adams forward-bending t.
>   Adams position t.
>   Adams scoliosis t.
>   Addis t.
>   adduction stress t.
>   Adson t.
>   AKE t.
>   Allen t.
>   Alli t.
>   ALRI t.
>   ankle dorsiflexion t.
>   ankle jerk reflex t.
>   anterior drawer t. (ADT)
>   anterior rotary drawer t.
>   anteroposterior stress t.
>   antinuclear antibody t.
>   anvil t.
>   AO pseudoisochromatic color
>   plate t.
>   Apley compression t.
>   Apley distraction t.
>   Apley grinding t.
>   Apley scratch t.
>   apprehension t.
>   ARA T.
>   arch-up t.
>   arm fossa t.
>   axial compression t.
>   axial load t.
>   axial manual traction t.
>   Babinski t.
>   ballottement t.
>   Barlow provocative t.
>   Beals t.
>   Bechterew t.

>   Beery T. for Visual-Motor
>   Integration
>   Bekhterev t.
>   belly-press t.
>   bench t.
>   Berg balance t.
>   biceps jerk reflex t.
>   Biodex t.
>   block t.
>   Booth t.
>   bounce home t.
>   bowstring t.
>   bracelet t.
>   brachial plexus tension t.
>   Bragard t.
>   break t.
>   British t.
>   *Brucella* agglutination t.
>   Brudzinski t.
>   brush t.
>   Bunnell t.
>   Bunnell-Littler t.
>   Burn bench t.
>   calf squeeze t.
>   Callaway t.
>   carpal compression t.
>   catch and clunk t.
>   cervical compaction t.
>   cervical sidegliding t.
>   Chaddock t.
>   Chiene t.
>   Childress duck waddle t.
>   chin-to-chest t.
>   chi-square t.
>   clunk t.
>   coccidioidin skin t.
>   cold pressor t.
>   Coleman lateral block t.
>   Combat Task t.
>   compression t.
>   concealed straight leg raising t.
>   conduction velocity t.
>   confrontational t.
>   confusion t.
>   contralateral straight leg raising t.
>   costoclavicular syndrome t.
>   Coton t.
>   cough t.
>   Cozen t.
>   Cram t.
>   crank t.
>   Crawford small parts dexterity t.

T

NOTES

test *(continued)*

crossover t.
Cybex t.
D'Ambrosia t.
Deerfield t.
de Kleyn t.
Deyerle sciatic tension t.
dial t.
digital response t.
disk diffusion t.
disk space saline acceptance t.
distraction t.
Doppler bidirectional t.
Downey object recognition t.
Downey texture discrimination t.
drawer t.
drop-arm t.
dual photon densitometry t.
duck waddle t.
Dugas t.
Duncan prone rectus t.
Dunn multiple comparison t.
Durkan carpal compression t.
Dvorak t.
Dynatron 2000 muscle t.
Eden t.
eighty-nine-newton t.
elbow flexion t.
elbow jerk reflex t.
Elihorn Maze T.
Ely t.
empty can t.
eversion stress t.
external rotation-abduction stress t.
  (EAST)
external rotation-recurvatum t.
external rotation stress t.
extrinsic entrapment t.
fabere t.
fadir t.
Fairbanks apprehension t.
Favort-Feder t.
Feagin shoulder dislocation t.
femoral nerve stretch t.
femoral nerve traction t.
figure-of-eight t.
figure-of-four t.
fingertips-to-floor t.
finger-to-nose t.
Finkelstein t.
first metatarsus rise t.
Fisher exact t.
Fisher Protected Least Significant
  Difference t.
Fist-Palm-Side T.
Fist-Ring T.
flexion-rotation-drawer knee
  instability t.

flexion spinal radiography t.
flip t.
fluctuation t.
fluorescein dye t.
fluoroallergosorbent t. (FAST)
foot placement t.
foraminal compression t.
forearm supination t.
Fournier t.
FRD t.
fulcrum t.
Gaenslen t.
Galant t.
Galeazzi t.
George t.
Gilchrist t.
Gillet marching t.
gluteus maximus tensing t.
golfer's elbow t.
Gordon squeeze t.
gracilis t.
graded exercise t. (GXT)
gravity drawer t.
gravity stress t.
grimace t.
grinding t.
Grooved Pegboard T.
Hamilton ruler t.
Harris Infant Neuromotor T.
  (HINT)
Hautant t.
Hawiva t.
Hawkins t.
heel-palm t.
heel-tip t.
heel-to-knee t.
heel-to-shin t.
Helfet t.
Hoffa t.
Hoffmann t.
Homans t.
Hoover t.
hop t.
Houle t.
Hughston external rotation
  recurvatum t.
Hughston knee jerk t.
Hughston-Losee jerk t.
Hughston plica t.
Hughston posterolateral drawer t.
Hughston posteromedial drawer t.
hyperabduction syndrome t.
hyperextension t.
iliac compression t.
iliopsoas t.
impingement t.
T. of Infant Motor Performance
  (TIMP)

Ingram-Withers-Speltz motor t.
inhibition t.
intrinsic t.
inversion stress t.
iodine starch t.
ischemic forearm exercise t.
Ishihara Color Blindness T.
jackknife t.
Jackson compression t.
Jacob shift t.
Jakob t.
Jamar t.
Jansen t.
Jebsen hand t.
Jebsen-Taylor hand function t.
jerk t.
jogging in place t.
Johnson-Zuck-Wingate motor t.
Jolly t.
Kaplan t.
Kemp t.
Kernig t.
Kleiger t.
Kleinmant t.
knee jerk reflex t.
knee laxity t.
Kolmogorov-Smirov t.
Kruskal-Wallis t.
Lachman t.
Lasègue rebound t.
lateral pivot shift t.
leaning hop t.
Lewin-Gaenslen t.
Lewin punch t.
Lewin reverse Lasègue t.
Lewin snuff t.
Lewin standing t.
Lewin supine t.
Lewis-Prusik t.
lift-off t.
ligamentous instability t.
light touch t.
Lippman t.
load and shift t.
locking-position t.
Losee knee instability t.
Ludington t.
Luekens wrinkle t.
lumbar extension t.
lumbar lateral flexion t.
lumbar protective mechanism t.
lumbar rotation t.

lunotriquetral shear t.
MacIntosh lateral pivot shift t.
Maddox rod t.
Maigne t.
Mann-Whitney U t.
manual muscle t.
matchstick t.
McMurray t.
Mennell t.
MicroFET2 muscle t.
middle-finger t.
military posture t.
Mills t.
Minnesota Manual Dexterity T.
Minnesota Rate of Manipulation t.
Minnesota Spatial Relations T.
Moberg Picking Up T.
monofilament pressure t.
Morton t.
Murphy punch t.
MyoForce t.
Naffziger t.
navicular drop t.
Neer impingement t.
nerve compression t. (NCT)
nerve conduction t. (NCT)
nerve conduction velocity t.
neuropsychologic t.
Ninhydrin print t.
Noyes flexion rotation drawer t.
Ober t.
oblique retinacular ligament
  tightness t.
O'Connor finger dexterity t.
O'Connor tweezer dexterity t.
O'Donoghue t.
one-leg hop for distance t.
one-leg stance t.
Oppenheim stroke t.
opposition t.
Ortolani t.
overhead exercise t.
pain provocation t.
palm-up t.
parachute t.
passive accessory motion t.
passive patellar glide t.
passive patellar tilt t.
passive physiological t.
patellar apprehension t.
patellar retraction t.
patellar tap t.

T

NOTES

test *(continued)*
   Patrick t.
   Patrick/fabere t.
   Perkins t.
   Perthes t.
   Phalen wrist flexion t.
   Physical Ability T. (PAT)
   pick-up t.
   pinprick t.
   pivot-shift t.
   plantarflexion-inversion t.
   plica t.
   polo t.
   polymerase chain reaction t.
   posterior drawer t.
   posterolateral drawer t.
   posteromedial pivot-shift t.
   prone extension t.
   prone knee-bend t.
   prone knee flexion t.
   prone rectus t.
   pulmonary function t.
   pulse status-pull t.
   push-up t.
   quadrant t.
   quadriceps contraction t.
   RA t.
   recurvatum t.
   relocation t.
   reverse Lasègue t.
   reverse pivot shift t.
   Romberg t.
   Roos overhead exercise t.
   rotary drawer t.
   rotary instability t.
   rotation drawer t.
   rotation recurvatum t.
   saline acceptance t.
   scaphoid lift t.
   scaphoid shift t.
   scapular approximation t.
   Scheffé t.
   Schirmer t.
   Schober t.
   seated root t.
   Seddon coin t.
   Semmes-Weinstein monofilament
    pressure t.
   shear t.
   Sherman block t.
   shift t.
   shoulder abduction t.
   shoulder depression t.
   shuck t.
   side-glide t.
   side-jump t.
   side-lying iliac compression t.
   Silfverskiöld t.

   Simmonds t.
   single-heel rise t.
   sit-and-reach t.
   sitting flexion t.
   sitting root t.
   sit-to-stand t.
   sit-up t.
   six-minute walk t.
   skin-gliding t.
   skin resistance t.
   Slocum ALRI t.
   Slocum anterior rotary drawer t.
   Slocum lateral pivot-shift t.
   Slocum rotary instability t.
   SLR with Bragard t.
   SLR with external rotation t.
   SLR with Kernig t.
   slump t.
   somatosensory t.
   Soto-Hall t.
   Spearman rank-order t.
   Speed t.
   sponge t.
   spring t.
   Spurling t.
   squat t.
   squatting t.
   squeeze t.
   Stagnara wake-up t.
   Staheli t.
   stair-running t.
   stairs hopple t.
   standing flexion t.
   standing Gillet t.
   starch t.
   station t.
   Steinmann t.
   t. stimulus
   Stinchfield t.
   straight leg raising t. (SLRT)
   stress t.
   stretch t.
   stroke t.
   Student-Newman-Keuls t.
   sudomotor activity t.
   supine iliac gapping t.
   supine long sitting t.
   supine straight leg raising t.
   suprascapular nerve entrapment t.
   supraspinatus t.
   sweat t.
   tandem gait t.
   tennis elbow t.
   Tensilon t.
   tensing t.
   Thomas t.
   Thomasen t.
   Thompson t.

thumbnail t.
tight retinacular ligament t.
tilt-up t.
timed Allen t.
tissue compression t.
Toglia Category Assessment T. (TCAT)
tourniquet t.
transverse humeral ligament t.
treadmill t.
Trendelenburg t.
triceps jerk reflex t.
triceps skinfold t.
triketohydrindene hydrate t.
triple-jump t.
Tromner t.
trunk incurvation t.
Tukey t.
tuning fork t.
two-point discrimination t.
Underburger t.
unilateral standing t.
valgus stress t.
Valpar Whole Body Range of Motion T.
Valsalva t.
varus stress t.
vertebral artery t.
vertical compression t.
vibration threshold t.
vibrometer t.
volitional muscle action t.
VonFrey hair t.
Voshell t.
wake-up t.
Waldron t.
walk t.
Wallenberg t.
water acceptance t.
Watson t.
Weber t.
Weinstein enhanced sensory t. (WEST)
well-leg raising t.
Western blot t.
Wilcoxon matched-pairs signed-rank t.
Wilson t.
wipe t.
Wright t.
Wright-Adson t.
wrinkle t.

wrist flexion t.
Yeager t.

tester

Cybex t.
grip t.
Jamar grip t.
Nicholas manual muscle t.
OSI laxity t.
WEST-foot nerve t.
West nerve t.

testing

active motion t. (AMT)
active movement t.
angle isometric t.
aquatic cardiac evaluation and t. (ACET)
arthrometer t.
biomechanical t.
compression t.
confirmatory t.
Cybex t.
Disk-Criminator sensory t.
Doppler ultrasound segmental blood pressure t.
dynametric t.
FootTrak t.
isokinetic t.
isometric strength t.
manual muscle t. (MMT)
mobility t.
Model 810 axial closed-loop hydraulic mechanical t.
motion t.
MRI t.
muscle t. (MT)
nerve involvement t.
neurological t.
NUTRI-SPEC t.
Omnitron exercise t.
palpation t.
passive mobility t.
pincer t.
PIVM t.
premanipulative t.
psychologic t.
quantitative sensory t. (QST)
radioallergosorbent t. (RAST)
range-of-motion t.
reciprocal isokinetic t.
rotation t.
segmental mobility t.
shear t.

NOTES

testing *(continued)*
    strength t.
    stress t.
    susceptibility t.
    TACTICON quantitative sensory t.
testosterone
tetanic contraction
tetanolysin
tetanospasmin
tetanus
    t. immune globulin
    t. prophylaxis
tetany
tethered
    t. cord syndrome
    t. spinal cord
tethering effect
tetracaine and dextrose
tetracalcium phosphate
tetracycline
tetraphasic action potential
tetraplegia
    traumatic t.
Tetrapolar
    Electro-Diagnostic Instruments
        Model 720 Bilateral T.
Teufel cervical brace
Teuffer
    T. technique
    T. tendo calcaneus repair
Teurlings wrist brace
TEV
    talipes equinovarus
Tevdek suture
Texas Scottish Rite Hospital (TSRH)
"Texas T" incision
Texon sole
TFA
    tibiofemoral angle
TFB-PS
    tibial fracture brace proximal support
TFC
    triangular fibrocartilage complex
        TFC tear
TFCC
    triangular fibrocartilage complex
T-finger splint
TFL
    tensor fascia lata
T-Foam
    T-F. bed pad
    T-F. cushion
    T-F. mattress
    T-F. pillow
TG
    tendon graft
T-Gel cushion
T-Gesic

TGF
    transforming growth factor
THA
    total hip arthroplasty
Thackray hip prosthesis
thalamic fracture
thalamotomy
thalidomide
thallium
    201 radioisotope t.
    t. scan
Than anaerobic threshold
T-handle
    T-h. curette
    T-h. Zimmer chuck
T-handled
    T-h. awl
    T-h. hook
    T-h. nut wrench
    T-h. reamer
    T-h. screw wrench
    T-h. trocar
Tharies
    T. femoral resurfacing component
    T. hip component
    T. hip replacement
    T. hip replacement prosthesis
Thatcher
    T. nail
    T. screw
The
    T. Backstroke
    T. Early Amnion Rupture Spectrum
    (TEARS)
    T. Healthy Back System
    T. Heeler inflatable heel protector
    T. Knee Society clinical-rating
    scale
    T. Original Backknobber muscle
    massager
    T. Original Backnobber massage
    tool
    T. Original Index Knobber II
    T. Original Index Knobber II
    massage tool
    T. Richie brace
    T. Rope stretching device
    T. Rope stretch and traction
    device
    T. Unloader
theater
    t. ache
    t. sign
theca
    digital t.
thecal
    t. injection
    t. sac

themoplastic ankle-foot orthosis
thenar
- t. atrophy
- t. creaking
- t. eminence
- t. flap
- t. muscle
- t. palmar crease (TPC)
- t. palsy
- t. space

theory
- Denis Browne three-column spine t.
- kinetic energy t.
- Maisel suppression t.
- Neviaser t.
- three-column spine t.

Thera
- T. Cane massager
- T. Cane shoulder exerciser
- T. Pulse bed

Thera-Back
Thera-Band
- T.-B. ASSIST
- T.-B. ASSIST exerciser
- T.-B. exercise ball
- T.-B. Exercise System for Golfers
- T.-B. handle
- T.-B. Max
- T.-B. Max resistive exercise
- T.-B. resistive exerciser
- T.-B. resistive therapy system
- T.-B. strip
- T.-B. System of Progressive Resistance
- T.-B. tubing

Therabath paraffin heat therapy system
TheraBeads microwaveable moist heat pack
Therabite
- T. jaw exerciser
- T. jaw motion rehabilitation system
- T. mobilizer

Thera-Boot bandage
TheraCane cane
Thera-Ciser
- T.-C. light exercise system
- T.-C. therapeutic exercise system

Theracloud pillow
Thera-Fit
Theraflex wrist exerciser
Theraform Selectives

Thera-Gesic cream
Theragloves
Theragym ball
Ther-A-Hoop exerciser
TheraKnit
Thera-Loop exerciser
Thera-Med cold pack
Thera-Medic shoe
Theramini 1, 2 electrotherapy stimulator
therapeutic
- t. light
- t. splint

Therapeutica Sleeping Pillow
Thera-P exercise bar
therapist
- industrial physical t. (IPT)

Thera-Plast putty
Therap-Loop
- T.-L. door anchor
- T.-L. door handle

Thera-Pos elbow orthosis
therapy
- active-assistive motion t.
- amplitude-summation interferential current t. (ASICT)
- anticoagulant t.
- anticonvulsant t.
- antithrombotic t.
- t. ball
- bee venom t.
- Bragg-peak photon-beam t.
- brisement t.
- T. Carrot Finger Orthosis (TCFO)
- cell t.
- chelation t.
- cold t.
- conservative t.
- Cool-Aid continuous controlled cold t.
- corticosteroid t. (CS)
- craniosacral t. (CST)
- deliberate t.
- diet t.
- Diversified chiropractic manipulative t.
- electrical stimulation t.
- electric differential t. (EDit)
- Electri-Cool continuous controlled cold t.
- electron beam t.
- fad t.

T

NOTES

therapy *(continued)*
    fomentation t.
    frequency-difference interferential current t. (FDICT)
    HBO t.
    heat t.
    herbal t.
    high-voltage t. (HVT)
    hot fomentation t.
    hyperbaric oxygen t.
    inferential t.
    InFerno moist heat t.
    infrared t.
    interferential t.
    intravenous t.
    Kelsey unloading exercise t.
    Livingstone t.
    magnet t.
    magnetic t.
    manipulative t.
    manual t.
    massage t.
    microcurrent t.
    mind-body t.
    motion t.
    Moxa heat t.
    moxibustion heat t.
    occupational t. (OT)
    orthomolecular medicine/megavitamin t.
    outpatient physical t.
    oxygen t.
    pancreatic enzyme t.
    parachute t.
    paraffin heat t.
    perioperative antibiotic t.
    physical t. (PT)
    piperacillin/tazobactam t.
    Polar wrap t.
    pool t.
    positional release t.
    postoperative t.
    ProFlo vascular compression t.
    prophylactic antibiotic t.
    pulsed short-wave t.
    T. Putty
    range of motion t., ROM t.
    reflex t.
    spinal manipulative t. (SMT)
    spinal manual t.
    steroid t.
    Synvisc injection t.
    Task Force on Standards of Physical T.
    transfusion t.
    transverse friction t.
    trial of conservative t.
    trigger point t. (TPT)
    tumor t.
    ultrasound t.

TheraSeed implant
Ther-A-Shapes positioner
Therasleep Cervical Pillow
Therasound transducer
Theratotic
    T. firm foot orthosis
    T. soft foot orthosis
Theratouch 4.7 stimulator
thermal
    t. agent
    t. anesthesia
    t. injury
    T. Pack
thermalator
    Whitehall t.
Thermalator heating unit
Thermapad pad
Thermasonic gel warmer
ThermaSplint heating bath
Thermo
    T. hand comforter
    T. HK/Rohadur orthotic
    T. HK/Tepefom orthotic
    T. knee comforter
ThermoCork
thermocouple
    t. instrument
    low impedance t.
    t. skin temperature device
ThermoFlex
    Maramed T.
thermogram
thermographic
    t. examination
    t. finding
    t. scanner
thermography
    infrared t.
    liquid crystal t. (LCT)
thermolabile plastic
thermomechanical implant metal prosthesis
thermomoldable
    t. insert
    t. material
Thermophore
    T. heat pack
    T. hot pack
thermoplastic
    DynaPrene splinting t.
    t. elastomer (TPE)
    t. template
thermoregulate
thermoregulatory sign

Thermoskin
- T. brace
- T. heat retainer

Thermosport hot/cold wrap
thermotherapy
Thero-Skin gel padding
thickened synovial membrane
thickening
- cortical t.
- ligamentous t.
- tendon t.

thickness
- lumbosacral junction cortical t.

thick patella sign
Thiemann disease
Thiersch
- T. medium split free graft
- T. thin split free graft
- T. wire

thigh
- t. corset
- t. cuff
- t.-foot angle
- t. holder
- t.-shank plane
- t. shell
- t. tourniquet

thimerosal
Thinline uncovered orthotic
thin osteotome
THINSite dressing
thin-wire Ilizarov fixator
thiomalate
- gold sodium t.

thiopental sodium
thioridazine
thiosulfate
- sodium t.

third
- t. digit
- distal t. (D/3, distal/3)
- t.-generation cementing technique
- middle t. (M/3, middle/3)
- proximal t. (P/3, proximal/3)
- t. toe

THKAFO
- trunk-hip-knee-ankle-foot orthosis

Thomas
- T. cervical collar brace
- T. classification
- T. collar
- T. collar cervical orthosis

- T. extrapolated bar graft
- T. fixator
- T. frame
- T. full-ring splint
- T. heel
- T. heel orthosis
- T. hinged splint
- T. knee splint
- T. Kodel sling
- T. leg splint
- T. needle
- T. posterior splint
- T. procedure
- T. sign
- T. splint with Pearson attachment
- T. suspension splint
- T. test
- T. walking brace
- T. walking caliper

Thomasen test
Thomas-Thompson procedure
Thomas-Thompson-Straub
- T.-T.-S. transfer
- T.-T.-S. transfer technique

Thompson
- T. anterolateral approach
- T. anteromedial approach
- T. excision
- T. femoral neck prosthesis
- T. frame
- F. R. T. endoprosthesis
- F. R. T. femoral prosthesis
- T. hemiarthroplasty hip prosthesis
- T. hip endoprosthesis system
- T. hip prosthesis forceps
- T. leg check system
- T. modification of Denis Browne splint
- T. posterior radial approach
- T. quadricepsplasty
- T. resection
- T. sign
- T. splint
- T. telescoping V osteotomy
- T. test

Thompson-Epstein
- T.-E. classification
- T.-E. classification of femoral fracture

Thompson-Henry technique
Thompson-Loomer technique
Thomsen disease

NOTES

thoraces (*pl. of* thorax)
thoracic
- t. approach
- t. curve
- t. curve scoliosis
- t. duct
- t. duct injury
- t. facet fusion
- t. hypokyphosis
- t. inlet syndrome
- t. kyphosis
- t. manual traction
- t. microtrauma
- t. nerve
- t. nerve injury
- t. outlet syndrome (TOS)
- t. pedicle
- t. pedicle marker
- t. plane
- t. spinal fusion
- t. spine (T-spine)
- t. spine biopsy
- t. spine decompression
- t. spine fracture
- t. spine kyphotic deformity
- t. spine lordosis
- t. spine orthosis
- t. spine pedicle diameter
- t. spine scoliotic deformity
- t. spine (T1 to T12)
- t. spine vertebral osteosynthesis
- t. and thoracolumbar spine surgery

thoracoabdominal
- t. approach
- t. artery injury
- t. incision

thoracoacromial artery
thoracodorsal
- t. artery transfer
- t. nerve injury

thoracoepigastric flap
thoracolumbar
- t. burst fracture
- t. curve
- t. degenerative disease
- t. erector spinae
- t. fracture-dislocation
- t. idiopathic scoliosis
- t. junction
- t. junction surgical exposure
- t. kyphoscoliosis
- t. kyphosis
- t. pedicle screw
- t. retroperitoneal approach
- t. spinal injury
- t. spine
- t. spine anterior exposure
- t. spine decompression

- t. spine flexion-distraction injury
- t. spine fracture-dislocation
- t. spine scoliosis
- t. spine stabilization
- t. spine vertebral osteosynthesis
- t. spondylosis
- t. spondylosis surgical technique
- t. standing orthosis brace
- t. trauma

thoracolumbosacral
- t. orthosis (TLSO)
- t. orthosis - flexion, extension, lateral bending, and transverse rotation (TLSO-FELR)
- t. plate
- t. spine

thoracoscapular arthrodesis
thoracotomy
- t. approach
- left-sided t.
- right-sided t.
- standard t.

thorax, pl. thoraces
Thorazine shuffle gait
thorn sign
Thornton
- T. bar
- T. nail
- T. nail plate
- T. screw

Thornwald antral drill
THR
- total hip replacement

threaded
- t. cancellous screw
- t. cortical dowel
- t. fusion cage
- t. guidepin
- t. rod
- t. Steinmann pin
- t. titanium acetabular prosthesis (TTAP)
- t. wire

threaded-hole-first technique
three
- t.-beat clonus
- t.-body wear
- t.-bone forearm
- T. Color Concept of wound classification
- t.-edge cutting forceps
- t.-finger spica cast
- t.-hole plate
- t.-jaw chuck
- t.-joint complex
- t.-part fracture
- t.-phase bone scan
- t.-plane deformity

t.-portal technique
t.-quarters prone position
t.-wheel walker

three-column
t.-c. cervical spine injury
t.-c. concept
t.-c. spine
t.-c. spine theory

three-dimensional (3D)
t.-d. analysis

three-point
t.-p. bending moment
t.-p. gait
t.-p. pressure cast
t.-p. pressure system
t.-p. skeletal traction

three-prong
t.-p. headrest
t.-p. rake blade retractor

threshold
anaerobic t. (AT)
experimental t.
lactate t. (LT)
lactic acidosis t. (LAT)
mechanical pain t. (MPTh)
pressure t.
reflex t.
t. stimulus
Than anaerobic t.
vibration perception t. (VPT)

thrombectomy
thrombin
t. powder
t.-soaked Gelfoam

thrombocytopenia
thrombocytopenia-absent
t.-a. radius (TAR)
t.-a. radius syndrome

thromboembolic disease (TED)
thromboembolism
thromboembolus
thrombogenesis
thrombophilia
thrombophlebitis
femoroiliac t.

thrombosed
thrombosis
deep vein t. (DVT)
deep venous t. (DVT)
iliofemoral t.
t. radial artery
venous t.

Thrombostat
through-and-through
t.-a.-t. fracture
t.-a.-t. tear
t.-a.-t. V-shaped horizontal
osteotomy

through-knee amputation
thrower's
t. elbow
t. fracture

throwing
t. function
t. injury

thrust
adjustive t.
double-thumb t.
lateral-to-medial t.
t. manipulation
pattern of t.
t. plate prosthesis (TPP)

THSP
titanium hollow screw plate
THSP system

thumb (1st digit)
abducted t.
absent t.
adducted t.
adductor sweep of t.
Bennett fracture of t.
bifid t.
bowler's t.
breakdancer's t.
clasped t.
congenital clasped t.
t. deformity
duplicate t.
t. duplication
t. extensor tendon
t. flexor tendon
floating t.
Flotan t.
t. forceps
gamekeeper's t.
hypoplastic t.
t.-in-palm deformity
jeweler's t.
t. loop
mallet t.
t. metacarpal
t. metacarpophalangeal joint
approach
t. opposition

NOTES

T

thumb *(continued)*
    t.-pinch grasp
    t. pinch power
    t. polydactyly
    t. post
    proximal annular pulley of the t.
    t. reconstruction
    t. screw
    short t.
    skier's t.
    spatulate t.
    t. spica
    t. spica cast
    spring swivel t.
    supernumerary t.
    surgeon's t.
    trigger t.
    triphalangeal t.
    t. web
    t. web splint
Thumbkeeper
    FREEDOM T.
thumbnail test
Thumper device
ThumZ'Up thumb splint
Thurston-Holland flag sign
thyroid
    t. cartilage
    t. gland
thyrotropin-releasing hormone
thyroxine
Ti-6A1-4V
    T. alloy
    T. implant metal
Ti-Bac
    T.-B. acetabular component
    T.-B. II hip prosthesis
tibia, pl. **tibiae**
    corticotomy of proximal t.
    distal t.
    groove distal t.
    t.-hindfoot osteomusculocutaneous
      rotationplasty with calcaneopelvic
      arthrodesis
    lip of t.
    osteochondrosis deformans tibiae
    Phemister medial approach to t.
    proximal t.
    transmetaphyseal amputation of t.
    t. valga
    t. vara
tibial
    t. acceleration
    t. aimer
    t. aligner
    t. artery
    t. base plate
    t. bending fracture

    t. bolt
    t. bone defect regeneration
    t. bone graft
    t. bowing
    t. channel
    t. collateral ligament (TCL)
    t. Collet
    t. component
    t. condyle
    t. condyle fracture
    t. cutter guide
    t. cutting block
    t. cutting guide
    t. defect
    t. diaphyseal fracture
    t. diaphyseal shortening
    t. driver
    t. eminence
    t. endoprosthesis
    t. epiphysis
    t. footprint
    t. fracture brace proximal support
      (TFB-PS)
    t. guidepin
    t. hemimelia
    t. hindfoot osteomusculocutaneous
      rotationplasty
    t. insert
    t. jig
    t. lengthening
    t. lift-off
    t. metaphysis
    t. muscle
    t. nerve
    t. nerve injury
    t. open fracture
    t. pin
    t. plafond
    t. plafond fracture
    t. plateau
    t. plateau fracture
    t. plateau fracture-dislocation
    t. plateau prosthesis
    t.-profibular synostosis
    t. pseudarthrosis
    t. punch
    t. retroflexion
    t. retrotorsion
    t. retroversion
    t. rim
    t. sesamoid
    t. sesamoid ligament
    t. sesamoid position (TSP)
    t. shaft fracture
    t. stylus
    t. talar tilt/tibiotalar tilt (TTT)
    t. tendon
    t. torsion

t. torsion system
t. track holder
t. track template
t. tray
t. triplane fracture
t. tubercle
t. tubercle avulsion
t. tubercle prominence
t. tuberosity
t. tuberosity fracture
t. tuberosity osteotomy
t. tunnel
t. vein

tibiale
ligamentum collateral t.

tibialis
t. anterior
t. anterior muscle
t. anterior tendon
t. posterior dislocation
t. posterior function
t. posterior muscle
t. posterior tendon
t. sign

tibiocalcaneal
t. arthrodesis
t. fusion
t. ligament
t. medullary nailing

tibiofemoral
t. alignment
t. angle (TFA)
t. articulation
t. joint

tibiofibular
t. articulation
t. clear space
t. diastasis
t. fracture
t. fusion
t. joint
t. joint dislocation
t. ligament
t. line
t. overlap
t. subluxation
t. synchondrosis
t. syndesmosis
t. synostosis

tibionavicular ligament
tibiotalar
t. angle

t. arthritis
t. arthrodesis
t. fusion
t. impingement
t. joint
t. stability

tibiotalocalcaneal
t. arthrodesis
t. fusion

Tibone posterior capsulorrhaphy
tibular pseudarthrosis
tic
ticarcillin/clavulanate
ticarcillin and clavulanate potassium
ticlike pain
Ti/CoCr hip prosthesis
Ticonium splint
Ti-Con prosthesis
tie
free t.
t.-over bolster
table t.

Tiemann nail
tier
Harris wire t.

Tietze syndrome
Ti-Fit total hip system
Tiger blade
tightener
Kirschner t.
Sklar wire t.
wire t.

tightness
adductor hamstring t.
hamstring t.

tight retinacular ligament test
Tikhoff-Linberg
T.-L. radical arm procedure
T.-L. shoulder girdle resection

Tilastin hip prosthesis
tile
T. classification
t. plate facet replacement
T. polytrauma algorithm
T. view

Tillaux-Chaput
T.-C. fracture
T.-C. tubercle

Tillaux fracture
Tillaux-Kleiger fracture
Tillman prosthesis

T

NOTES

tilt
>angular t.
>anterior pelvic t.
>anteroposterior t.
>cock-robin head t.
>mediolateral t.
>palmar t.
>pelvic lateral t.
>posterior pelvic t.
>sacral t.
>subtalar t.
>superoinferior t.
>t. table (TT)
>talar t.
>tibial talar tilt/tibiotalar t. (TTT)
>T. and Turn Paragon bed
>t.-up test
>varus t.
>t. wrist

tilting
>coronal t.

Tilt-In-Space wheelchair conversion
tiludronate
TIME
>toddler and infant motor evaluation

time
>capillary filling t.
>capillary refill t.
>conduction t.
>cycle t.
>double support t.
>echo t. (TE)
>intercritical t.
>loading t.
>operating t.
>partial thromboplastin t. (PTT)
>procedure t.
>prothrombin t. (PT)
>reaction t.
>repetition t. (TR)
>rise t.
>step t.
>stride t.
>swing t.
>tincture of t. (TOT)
>total tourniquet t.
>tourniquet t.
>warm ischemic t.

timed Allen test
Timentin
TiMesh implantable hardware fixation
timing
>t. of decompression
>right-left t.

timolol
TIMP
>Test of Infant Motor Performance

tin
>baking t.

Tinactin for Jock Itch
tincture
>t. of belladonna
>t. of benzoin
>opium t.
>t. of time (TOT)

tinea pedis
Tinel-Hoffmann sign
Tinel sign
Tinetti gait assessment
Ting
tingle
tingling
Ti-Nidium alloy
Tiobi transfer
tip
>Cloward cervical drill t.
>Fragmatome t.
>Frazier suction t.
>t. of medial malleolus
>t.-pinch dynamometry
>screw t.
>Woodruff t.

tiptoe gait
Ti-spacer
>Cohort T.-s.

Tisseel fibrin glue
Tissucol
tissue
>adipose t.
>adjustment of the articulations and adjacent t.
>bursal t.
>capsular support t.
>capsuloligamentous t.
>cartilaginous t.
>t. compression test
>connective t.
>devitalized t.
>t. expander
>exuberant granulation t.
>fatty t.
>fibrous scar t.
>t. forceps
>granulation t.
>hypertrophic granulation t.
>intervening connective t.
>ligamentous support t.
>t. mandrel implant material
>muscular t.
>necrotic t.
>neural t.
>t. nutrition
>osseous t.
>periarticular t.
>perineural t.

periosteal t.
pharyngeal t.
t. pressure
t. pressure measurement
pressure-sensitive t.
pressure-tolerant t.
t. protector
t. repair
revascularized t.
scar t.
skeletal t.
t. slack
soft t.
subcutaneous t.
t. texture abnormality (TTA)
t. transfer
t. transplant
t.-type plasminogen activator
vascular t.
viable t.
viscoelastic t.

Titan
T. Apollo electric flexion table
T. cemented hip prosthesis
T. Meridian Intersegmental Traction table
T. Nova manual flexion-extension multi flex table

titanium
t. alloy
t.-alloy implant
t. cable
t. circumferential grommet
t. half pin
t. hollow screw plate (THSP)
t. hollow screw plate system
t. implant
t. implant material
t. implant prosthesis
t. microsurgical bipolar forceps
t. plate
t. screw

titer
antistreptolysin-O t. (ASOT)

Ti-Thread prosthesis
Titian hip prosthesis
Titus
T. forearm splint
T. wrist splint

Tivanium
T. cancellous bone screw
T. hip prosthesis

T. implant metal
T. implant metal prosthesis

tizanidine
TJ
triceps jerk
TJR
total joint replacement
TKA
total knee arthroplasty
trochanter-knee-ankle
TK Optimizer knee prosthesis
TKR
total knee replacement
TLSO
thoracolumbosacral orthosis
TLSO brace
TLSO-FELR
thoracolumbosacral orthosis - flexion, extension, lateral bending, and transverse rotation
TMA
transmalleolar axis
transmetatarsal amputation
true metatarsus adductus
TMA prosthesis
TMA-thigh angle
TMJ
temporomandibular joint
TMJ halter
TMT
tarsometatarsal
T-nail
TNS
tension night splint
Toad finger splint
tobramycin
tobramycin-impregnated PMMA implant
Tobruk splint
toddler and infant motor evaluation (TIME)
toddler's fracture
Todd-Wells guide
toe
t. amputation
t.-block anesthesia
t. box
Butler procedure to correct overlapping t.'s
clubbed t.
clubbing of t.
cock-up t.
t. comb

NOTES

T

toe *(continued)*
crossover second t.
curly t.
downgoing t.
t.-drop brace
DuVries technique for
  overlapping t.
t. extensor
t. extensor muscle
t. extensor tendon
extra t.
fifth t.
flail t.
t. flexor muscle
floating t.
floppy t.
great t.
t. gripping exercise
t.-ground purchase
t. implant
lesser t.
t. loop
mallet t.
marathoner's t.
Morton t.
t.-off phase of gait
t.-out angle
overlapping fifth t.
overriding fifth t.
t.-phalanx transplantation
t. plate
t. plate extension
t. pressure
t. prosthesis
push-off by great t.
t. raises exercise
t. reflex
runner's t.
sausage t.
searching big t.
second t.
set angle of t.
t. spica cast
splaying of t.
t. spread sign
supernumerary t.
tennis t.
third t.
t.-to-hand transfer
t.-to-midthigh cast
t.-touch weightbearing
turf t.
underlapping t.
upgoing t.
V-Y plasty correction of varus t.
t. walk
t. walking

t.-walking gait
webbed t.
toeing
t.-in gait
t. in
t. out
t.-out gait
toenail
dystrophic t.
ingrown t.
onychomycotic t.
Toennis tumor forceps
Toes Protector
toe-to-groin
t.-t.-g. cast
t.-t.-g. modified Jones dressing
Tofranil
toggle-recoil adjustment
toggle sign
Toglia Category Assessment Test
(TCAT)
Tohen-Carmona-Barrera transfer
Tohen tendon technique
tolazoline
Tolectin DS
tolerance
fatigue t.
host t.
pressure t.
tolmetin
tolnaftate
Tomasini brace
Tomberlin-Alemdaroglu splint
Tommy trapeze bar
tomo
tomogram
tomogram (tomo)
tomograph
tomography
computed t. (CT)
computerized axial t. (CAT)
conventional t.
helical computed t.
hypocycloidal ankle t.
positron emission t. (PET)
preoperative t.
quantitative computed t. (QCT)
single photon emission computed t.
  (SPECT)
transpiral t.
trispiral t.
Tom Smith arthritis
tone
t.-inhibiting leg cast
muscle t.
t.-reducing ankle-foot orthosis
  (TRAFO)

tongs
 Barton t.
 Barton-Cone t.
 Böhler t.
 cervical fracture t.
 Cherry t.
 cranial t.
 Crutchfield-Raney t.
 Gardner-Wells t.
 Raney-Crutchfield t.
 skull t.
 traction t.
 Trippi-Wells traction t.
 Vinke skull traction t.
tongue
 t. fracture
 t.-in-groove recession
 t.-type fracture
tonicity
tonic neck reflex
tonus
 myogenic t.
tool
 Backnobber II massage t.
 Gore smoother crucial t.
 Index Knobber II massage t.
 Magnassager massage t.
 OsteoStat disposable power t.
 The Original Backnobber
  massage t.
 The Original Index Knobber II
  massage t.
too-many-toes sign
toothed
 t. cutter
 t. tissue forceps
 t. washer
top
 circular laminar hook with offset t.
 t.-entry (open body) hook
Topaz flexion table
TOP ejector punch
tophaceous
 t. deposit
 t. gout
tophectomy
tophus, pl. **tophi**
 gouty t.
topical
 Achromycin T.
 Akne-Mycin T.
 A/T/S T.

 Baciguent T.
 BactoShield T.
 Caldesene T.
 Del-Mycin T.
 Dyna-Hex T.
 Elase T.
 Elase-Chloromycetin T.
 Emgel T.
 Eryderm T.
 Erygel T.
 Erymax T.
 erythromycin, t.
 E-Solve-2 T.
 ETS-2% T.
 Exelderm T.
 Garamycin T.
 G-myticin T.
 Hibiclens T.
 Hibistat T.
 MetroGel T.
 Micatin T.
 Monistat-Derm T.
 Mycifradin Sulfate T.
 Mycitracin T.
 NeoDecadron T.
 Neomixin T.
 Oxistat T.
 Pedi-Pro T.
 Polysporin T.
 Staticin T.
 terbinafine, t.
 Topicycline T.
 Triple Antibiotic T.
 T-Stat T.
Topicycline Topical
topography
 internal t.
Toposar Injection
Toradol
 T. Injection
 T. Oral
Torg
 T. classification
 T. knee reconstruction
 T. technique
Torgerson-Leach modified technique
torn
 t. meniscotibial ligament
 t. meniscus
tornado injury
Tornwaldt bursitis
Torode-Zieg classification

NOTES

Toronto
    T. brace
    T. Medical CPM exerciser
    T. parapodium orthosis
    T. pelvic fracture classification
    T. splint
TORP
    total ossicular replacement
    Plastiport TORP
    TORP prosthesis
torque
    t. curve
    t. force
    frictional t.
    t. heel shoe
    t. load
    t. production
    rotatory t.
    t. screwdriver
    unwanted screw t.
    t. wrench
torque-meter
    Compudriver digital t.-m.
Torres syndrome
torsion
    t. bar splint
    femorotibial t.
    t. fracture
    internal tibial t. (ITT)
    internal tibiofibular t.
    tibial t.
    t. wedge fracture nonunion
torsional
    t. abnormality
    t. alignment
    t. fracture
    t. gripping strength
    t. load
    t. overload
    t. stiffness
    t. stress
torticollis
    acquired t.
    congenital t.
    muscular t.
    nonspasmodic t.
    spasmodic t.
torus
    t. fracture
    regeneration t.
TOS
    thoracic outlet syndrome
TOT
    tincture of time
total
    t. active motion (TAM)
    t. ankle arthroplasty
    t. arthrodesis of the wrist

    t. articular replacement arthroplasty (TARA)
    t. articular replacement arthroplasty prosthesis
    t. articular resurfacing arthroplasty (TARA)
    t. condylar knee
    t. condylar knee prosthesis
    t. condylar semiconstrained tricompartmental prosthesis
    t. contact bivalve ankle-foot orthosis
    t. contact cast (TCC)
    t. contact casting (TCC)
    t. contact orthosis (TCO)
    t. contact socket
    t. elbow arthroplasty
    t. eversion range of motion
    t. gym
    T. Gym Exercise Program
    t. hip arthroplasty (THA)
    t. hip replacement (THR)
    t. hip replacement prosthesis
    t. joint replacement (TJR)
    t. joint replacement prosthesis
    t. knee arthroplasty (TKA)
    T. Knee for children
    t. knee instrumentation
    T. Knee 2100 prosthetic knee
    t. knee replacement (TKR)
    t. knee replacement prosthesis
    t. meniscectomy
    t. mesenteric apron method
    t. ossicular replacement (TORP)
    t. parenteral nutrition (TPN)
    t. passive motion (TPM)
    t. patellectomy
    t. patellofemoral joint arthroplasty
    t. replacement joint
    t. shoulder arthroplasty
    t. tourniquet time
    t. transfer (TT)
    t. wrist arthroplasty
TotalGym
Totallift-II
Toti trephine drill
toto
tottering gait
touchdown weightbearing
touch sensation
Touch-Test sensory evaluator
tourniquet
    Accuflate t.
    Bodenstab t.
    t. control
    Digikit finger t.
    digital t.
    double t.

Esmarch t.
finger t.
forearm t.
t. gauge
t. ischemia
t. palsy
t. paralysis
pneumatic ankle t.
t. pressure
Profex arthroscopic t.
TCPM pneumatic t.
t. test
thigh t.
t. time
upper arm t.

towel
Charnley t.
t. clamp
t. clip
huck t.
t. roll
sterile t.

Townley
T. anatomic knee system
T. bone graft screw
T. femur caliper
T. TARA prosthesis
T. tibial plateau plate
T. total knee prosthesis

Townsend brace
Townsend-Gilfillan
T.-G. plate
T.-G. screw

toxemia
toxicity
aluminum t.
methotrexate t.

toxin
botulinum t. A (BtA)

Toygar angle
TPC
thenar palmar crease

TPE
thermoplastic elastomer
TPE ankle-foot orthosis
TPE biomechanical foot orthosis

T-pin
Delitala T.-p.
T.-p. handle

TPL-6
T. hip system
T. total hip replacement

T-plasty modification of Bankart shoulder operation
TPM
total passive motion
TPN
total parenteral nutrition
TPP
thrust plate prosthesis
TPP hip endoprosthesis
TPR ankle prosthesis prosthesis
TPT
trigger point therapy
TR
repetition time
TR-28
T. hip prosthesis
T. total hip replacement
trabecula, pl. trabeculae
partially necrotic osseous t.
trabecular
t. bone
t. index of Singh
t. traction
tracer catheter
tracheal injury
tracheostomy
tracing
nerve t.
t. paper
track
t.-bound joint
pin t.
tracker
T. knee brace
Palumbo patella t.
patella t.
tracking
patellar t.
Trackmaster treadmill
Tracrium
tract
gastrointestinal t.
iliotibial t.
pyramidal t.
sinus t.
spinocerebellar t.
spinothalamic t.
urinary t.
traction (tx)
90-90 t.
ambulatory t.
Anderson t.

T

NOTES

traction *(continued)*
AOA halo cervical t.
Apley t.
t. application
autologous t.
axial t.
axis t.
Baker trabecular t.
balanced skeletal t.
banjo t.
Barton-Cone tong t.
Bendixen-Kirschner t.
bipolar vertebral t.
Blackburn t.
Böhler tong t.
Borchgrevin t.
t. bow
Bremer halo cervical t.
Bryant t.
Buck t.
t. cast
cervical AOA halo t.
cervical halter t.
cervical manual t.
C-Flex supine cervical t.
Cherry tong t.
Cotrel t.
Crego-McCarroll t.
Crile head t.
Crutchfield skeletal tong t.
device for transverse t. (DTT)
Dunlop t.
elastic t.
t. epiphysis
t. epiphysitis
Exo-Static t.
t. exostosis
fingertrap t.
floating t.
t. footpiece
t. fracture
Freiberg t.
Frejka t.
Gallo t.
Gardner-Wells tong t.
gentle t.
Georgiade visor cervical t.
Graham t.
Granberry t.
halo-dependent t.
halo-extension t.
halo-femoral t.
halo-hyperextension t.
halo-pelvic t.
halo-wheelchair t.
halter t.
Hamilton t.
t. handle

Handy-Buck t.
Hare t.
head-halter t.
Hoke-Martin t.
Holter t.
Houston halo cervical t.
Hoyer t.
Ingebrightsen t.
inhibitive t.
intermittent t.
intermittent cervical t. (ICT)
Jones suspension t.
Kessler t.
Keys-Kirschner t.
King cervical t.
Kirschner skeletal t.
Kuhlman t.
Logan t.
longitudinal t.
low-profile halo t.
Lyman-Smith t.
manual t.
McBride tripod pin t.
Miami acute collar cervical t.
Miami J collar cervical t.
Necktrac t.
Neufeld t.
ninety-ninety t.
Orr-Buck t.
Ortho-Vent t.
overhead olecranon t.
Pease-Thomson t.
pelvic hyperextension t.
Perkins t.
Peterson t.
Philadelphia collar cervical t.
t. pin
Pugh t.
pulp t.
Quigley t.
Raney-Crutchfield tong t.
Roger Anderson t.
rubber band t.
Russell skeletal t.
Saunders t.
Sayre t.
skeletal t.
snug t.
t. splint
split Russell skeletal t.
t. spur
static t.
Steinmann t.
t. stirrup
sugar-tong t.
supine C-Trax t.
suspension t.
Syms t.

tape t.
thoracic manual t.
three-point skeletal t.
t. tongs
t. tongs screw
trabecular t.
transverse t.
vertical t.
Vinke tong t.
Watson-Jones t.
well-leg t.
Wells t.
Whitman t.
Zimfoam splint t.
traction-absorption
Weber-Vasey t.-a.
tractograph
MOM t.
Tracto-Halter
T.-H. gait
T.-H. training
tractor
Hamilton pelvic traction screw t.
Zim-Trac traction splint t.
tractotomy
TRAFO
tone-reducing ankle-foot orthosis
TRAFO orthosis
Trager method
Tragerwork
trailers
leaders and t.
train
near-constant frequency t.'s
trainer
athletic t.
impulse inertial exercise t.
Kinesthetic Ability T. (KAT)
Monark Rehab T.
Posture Pump Spine T.
Sprint cross t.
training
activity t. (AT)
bowel t.
DAPRE strength t.
Fartlek t.
flexibility t.
gait t.
neurodevelopmental t.
physical t. (PT)
proprioceptive t.
propriosensory t.

prosthetic gait t.
sensory-motor t.
stabilization t.
strength t.
Tracto-Halter t.
weight t.
tramadol
t. HCl
t. hydrochloride
trampoline injury
tranexamic acid
transacromial approach
transaminase
glutamic-oxaloacetic t.
glutamic-pyruvic t.
transarticular
t. pin
t. screw
t. screw fixation
t. wire fixation
transaxial
t. gradient recalled image
t. spoiled gradient recalled image
transaxillary approach
transbrachioradialis approach
transcalcaneal approach
transcapitate
t. fracture
t. fracture-dislocation
transcapitellar
t. pin
t. wire fixation
transcarpal amputation
transcervical femoral fracture
transchondral fracture
transclavicular approach
transcondylar
t. amputation
t. axis (TCA)
t. fracture
transcutaneous
t. crush injury
t. electrical nerve stimulation (TENS)
t. fixation of fracture
t. oxygen tension determination
Transdermal
Alora T.
Climara T.
Duragesic T.
Esclim T.

T

NOTES

Transdermal *(continued)*
    Estraderm T.
    Vivelle T.
transducer
    force t.
    FT03C t.
    Hall-effect strain t.
    linear-variable-differential t.
    magnetic motion t.
    mechanical two-dimensional echo t.
    rotatory-variable-differential t.
    Therasound t.
transection
    step-cut t.
transepicondylar axis
transepiphyseal
    t. fracture
    t. separation
transesophageal
    t. echocardiography (TEE)
    t. echocardiography scan
transfemoral
    t. alignment
    t. amputation
transfer
    anterior t.
    anteromedial tubercle t.
    Baker lateral semitendinosus t.
    Barr anterior t.
    bed-to-chair t.
    biceps brachialis muscle t.
    bone t.
    Boyes t.
    Boyle-Thompson tendon t.
    brachioradialis t.
    Brooker-Jones tendon t.
    Brooks-Jones tendon t.
    Brooks-Seddon pectoralis major tendon t.
    Brooks-Seddon tendon t.
    Brown fibular t.
    Buncke t.
    Bunnell posterior tibial tendon t.
    Caldwell-Durham tendon t.
    Camitz tendon t.
    Campbell t.
    Chandler tendon t.
    Chaves muscle t.
    Chaves-Rapp muscle t.
    Clark pectoralis major t.
    Columbus McKinnon assist for lifting or t.
    composite free tissue t.
    coracoacromial ligament t.
    Couch-Derosa-Throop t.
    crossed intrinsic t.
    distal t.
    Drennan posterior t.

    dynamic muscle t.
    Eggers t.
    extensor digitorum t.
    extensor hallucis longus t.
    fibular t.
    Flatt tendon t.
    flexor digitorum longus tendon t.
    Fowler tendon t.
    free flap t.
    free gracilis muscle t.
    free tissue t.
    Gage distal t.
    gastrocnemius tendon t.
    Girdlestone tendon t.
    Green t.
    Green-Banks t.
    Harmon t.
    Hiroshim t.
    His-Haas muscle t.
    Hoffer split t.
    Hovanian latissimus dorsi muscle t.
    Huber abductor digiti quinti t.
    Ikuta pectoralis major t.
    iliopsoas t.
    iliotibial band t.
    independent t.
    ion t.
    Johnson-Spiegl tendon t.
    Jones t.
    Kessler posterior tibial tendon t.
    Lamb muscle t.
    lateral t.
    Littler-Cooley abductor digiti quinti t.
    Littler-Cooley muscle t.
    Manktelow pectoralis major t.
    McLaughlin subscapularis t.
    Menelaus triceps t.
    t. metatarsalgia
    microvascular osseous t.
    Moberg deltoid muscle t.
    Moberg deltoid-to-triceps t.
    muscle t.
    Mustard iliopsoas t.
    neuromuscular t.
    Neviaser-Wilson-Gardner t.
    Ober anterior t.
    Ober-Barr procedure for brachioradialis t.
    opponens t.
    patellar tendon t. (PTT)
    pedicled fibular t.
    peroneus brevis t.
    posterior deltoid-to-triceps t.
    posterior tibial tendon t.
    semitendinosus tendon t.
    Sharrard posterior t.
    single-stage tissue t.

split anterior tibialis tendon t.
split anterior tibial tendon t.
  (SPLATT)
static tendon t.
stress t.
subscapularis tendon t.
Sutherland lateral t.
tendon t.
Thomas-Thompson-Straub t.
thoracodorsal artery t.
Tiobi t.
tissue t.
toe-to-hand t.
Tohen-Carmona-Barrera t.
total t. (TT)
vascularized osseous t.
wraparound neurovascular composite
  free tissue t.
transfibular
t. approach
t. arthrodesis
t. fusion
transfixing pin
transfixion
t. bolt
t. pin
t. screw
transformation
transforming
t. growth factor (TGF)
t. growth factor beta
transfusion
autologous blood t.
blood t.
t. therapy
transhamate
t. fracture
t. fracture-dislocation
transient
t. lesion
t. osteoporosis
transiliac
t. amputation
t. bar technique
t. fracture
t. lengthening
t. rod fixation
transition
cervicothoracic t.
transitional vertebra
translation
anterior t.

anteroposterior t.
caudal t.
cephalad t.
coronal plane deformity sagittal t.
dorsal t.
t. injury
t. mobility
t. motion
posterior t.
ulnar t.
vertical t.
translational
t. osteotomy
t. position
translatory
t. force
t. motion
translocation
ulnar t.
translumbar amputation
transmalleolar
t. ankle
t. ankle arthrodesis
t. axis (TMA)
t. portal
transmetaphyseal amputation of tibia
transmetatarsal
t. amputation (TMA)
t. capsulotomy
transmission
impulse-based nerve t.
nerve t.
nociceptive t.
nonimpulsed base nerve t.
transmitter
chest-band t.
transmitter-receiver
Itrel programmed t.-r.
transolecranon approach
transoral
t. approach
t. odontoid resection
transosseus suture
transparent template
transpatellar tendon portal
transpedicular
t. approach
t. convex anterior hemipiphysiodesis
t. fixation
t. fixation effective pedicle
  diameter

T

NOTES

transpedicular *(continued)*
    t. fixation system design
    t. screw
transpedicularly implanted anterior spinal support device
transpelvic amputation
transperitoneal
    t. approach
    t. exposure
transphenoidal dissector
transpiral tomography
Transpire wrist orthosis
transplant
    Bosworth femoroischial t.
    d'Aubigne patellar t.
    Elmslie-Trillat t.
    fibular t.
    free vascularized bone t.
    one-half patellar tendon t.
    patellar t.
    pedicled t.
    pes anserinus t.
    Slocum pes anserinus t.
    tissue t.
    vascularized bone t.
    whole bone t.
    whole fibular t.
transplantation
    allograft t.
    t. antigen
    Bosworth femoroischial t.
    Cowen-Loftus toe-phalanx t.
    femoroischial t.
    muscle-tendon t.
    osteoarticular allograft t.
    toe-phalanx t.
transport
    axoplasmic t.
transposing index ray
transposition
    dorsal subcutaneous nerve t.
    t. flap
    intramuscular nerve t.
    intraosseous nerve t.
    subcutaneous anterior t.
    subfascial t.
    tendon t.
transpositional
transsacral fracture
transscaphoid
    t. dislocation fracture
    t. perilunate dislocation
transsternal approach
transsyndesmotic
    t. bolt in tibiofibular diastasis
    t. screw fixation
transtendo calcaneus portal

transthoracic
    t. approach
    t. echocardiography (TTE)
transtibial
    t. amputation
transtriquetral
    t. fracture
    t. fracture-dislocation
transtrochanteric
    t. approach
    t. rotational osteotomy
transversalis
    arcus pedis t.
    t. fascia
transversarium
    foramen t.
transverse (TV)
    t. acetabular ligament
    t. approach
    t. atlantal ligament
    t. axis
    t. axis knee flexion
    t. capsulotomy
    t. carpal ligament
    t. chevron osteotomy
    t. connector
    t. deficiency
    t. diaphyseal osteotomy
    t. fixation
    t. fixator application
    t. friction massage
    t. friction therapy
    t. humeral ligament test
    t. incision
    t. intertarsal ligament
    t. ligament of acetabulum
    t. ligament of atlas
    t. ligament of knee
    t. ligament rupture
    t. lines of Park
    t. loading device
    t. metatarsal ligament
    t. metatarsal osteotomy
    t. myelopathy
    t. pedicle angle
    t. pedicle diameter
    t. plane
    t. plane alignment
    t. plane motion insufficiency
    t. process
    t. process fracture
    t. retinacular ligament
    t. scapular ligament
    t. screw
    t. spinal ligament
    t. supracondylar osteotomy
    t. tarsal joint
    t. tear

t. tenotomy
t. traction
transversely
transversospinalis syndrome
transversum
ligamentum carpi t.
transversus abdominis muscle
Tranxene
TRAP
tartrate resistant acid phosphatase
trap
trapdoor
trapezial
t. area
t. arthrosis
t. prosthesis
trapeziectomy
trapeziodeltoid interval
trapeziometacarpal
t. capsule
t. fusion
t. joint
t. joint replacement prosthesis
trapeziotrapezoidal joint
trapezium
Burton-Pelligrini excising t.
t. fracture
t. implant prosthesis
t. ossification
trapezius
t. fiber analysis
t. muscle
trapezoid
t. ligament
t. line
t. ossification
Trapezoidal-28 (T28)
T.-28 hip prosthesis
T.-28 internal prosthesis
trapezoidal osteotomy
trapezoideum
ligamentum t.
trapped meniscus
trapping
Conrad-Bugg t.
optical t.
trauma
arterial t.
birth t.
cervical spine t.
craniospinal t.
high-energy t.

hyperextension t.
hyperflexion t.
lumbar spine t.
multiple t.
musculoskeletal t.
T. Score
thoracolumbar t.
Traumafix apparatus
traumatic
t. amputation
t. anterior instability
t. arthritis
t. cervical disk herniation
t. compartment syndrome
t. dislocation
t. disorder disease
t. displacement
t. neuroma
t. paraplegia
t. prepatellar neuralgia
t. spondylolisthesis
t. tetraplegia
t., unidirectional instability and Bankart lesion (TUBS)
traumatized ligament
Trautman Locktite prosthetic hook
Trautmann chisel
Travase
tray
Alcon Instrument Delivery System t.
Bucky x-ray t.
CAPIS screw assortment t.
Denis Browne t.
glenoid metal t.
one-time sharp debridement t.
tibial t.
x-ray t.
Treace stapes drill
treadmill
Aquaciser underwater t.
AquaGaiter t.
Hydrotrack underwater t.
Lifestride t.
Orbiter t.
t. running
t. test
Trackmaster t.
Woodway t.
treatment (tx)
active t.
adjustive t.

NOTES

645

treatment *(continued)*
    bone cyst t.
    Boyd-Ingram-Bourkhard t.
    closed t.
    compression rod t.
    distraction/compression scoliosis t.
    dual compression scoliosis t.
    Head & Shoulders Intensive T.
    Keesay t.
    low-friction ion t. (LFIT)
    manual t.
    neurodevelopmental t.
    neuromuscular reflex t.
    neuromuscular scoliosis orthotic t.
    nonoperative t.
    Parabath paraffin heat t.
    poliomyelitis t.
    ReJuveness scar t.
    SB+ testing and t.
    SB– testing and t.
    t. for scoliosis
    shock t.
Tredex
    Universal T.
tree
    BTE Assembly T.
    pinch t.
    pipe t.
trellis formation
tremor
    action t.
    contraction t.
    intention t.
    postural t.
    resting t.
tremulousness
Trendelenburg
    T. gait
    T. limp
    T. lurch
    T. position
    T. test
Trental
trephine
    bone t.
    Castroviejo t.
    t. drill
    t. needle biopsy
    Phemister biopsy t.
Trethowan metatarsal osteotomy
Trethowan-Stamm-Simmonds-Menelaus-
    Haddad technique
Triacet
triacetin
triad
    t. knee repair
    t. of O'Donoghue
    O'Donoghue unhappy t.

    T. prosthesis
    Waddell t.
trial
    t. acetabular cup
    t. base plate
    clinical t.
    component t.
    t. of conservative therapy
    t. driver
    t. femoral component
    t. fit
    t. implant
    lower hook t.
    t. prosthesis
    radial t.
    t. range of motion
    t. reduction
    t. seating
    t. spacer
    t. stem
    ulnar t.
    upper hook t.
trialkylphosphine gold complex
Triam-A
triamcinolone
    t. acetate
    t. acetonide
Triam Forte
triamterene/hydrochlorothiazide
triangle
    anal t.
    anterior t.
    aponeurotic t.
    Burow t.
    cervical t.
    clavipectoral t.
    Codman t.
    Hardy-Joyce t.
    IMP knee positioning t.
    infraclavicular t.
    Kager t.
    knee positioning t.
    Langenbeck t.
    metal measuring t.
    Middeldorpf t.
    neutral t.
    Petit t.
    posterior t.
    sacral t.
    von Weber t.
    Ward t.
Tri-angle shoulder abduction brace
triangular
    t. advancement flap
    t. ankle fusion frame
    t. arm sling
    t. base transverse bar configuration
    t. compression device

t. defect
t. external ankle fixation
t. fibrocartilage
t. fibrocartilage complex (TFC, TFCC)
t. fibrocartilage complex tear
t. ligament
t. medullary nail
t. pillow splint
t. rasp
t. wrist bone
triangulated pedicle screw
triangulate triple frame
triangulating
triangulation
indirect t.
t. technique
t. technique for arthroscope
triaxial
t. motion
t. semiconstrained elbow prosthesis
t. total elbow arthroplasty
Tri-Axial prosthesis
triazolam
tricalcium phosphate
triceps
t. brachii tendon
t. jerk (TJ)
t. jerk reflex test
t. skinfold test
t. surae jerk
t. surae muscle
t. surae reflex
t. surae release
tricepsplasty
trichilemmal cyst
trichloromonofluoromethane
dichlorodifluoromethane and t.
Trichophyton
T. mentagrophytes
T. rubrum
trick
t. knee
t. movement
Tricodur
T. compression support bandage
T. Epi compression bandage
T. Epi compression dressing
T. Omos compression bandage
T. Omos compression dressing
T. Talus compression bandage
T. Talus compression dressing

tricompartmental
t. implant
t. knee prosthesis
Tri-Con component
Tricon-M
T.-M. component
T.-M. cruciate-sparing prosthesis
T.-M. patellar prosthesis
Tri-Core cervical support pillow
tricorrectional bunionectomy
tricortical
t. iliac crest bone graft
t. ilial strip graft
tricyclic antidepressant
triethanolamine salicylate
triethiodide
gallamine t.
triflanged
t. Lottes nail
t. medullary nail
Tri-Flex auxiliary suspension belt
Tri-Float pressure reduction mattress
trifluoperazine
trifurcation
trigeminal neuralgia
trigger
t. digit
t. finger
t. finger release
t. point
t. point injection
t. point therapy (TPT)
t. thumb
t. thumb release
TriggerWheel
T. device
T. Wand
trigonum
os t.
triketohydrindene hydrate test
Trilafon
trilaminate cushion
trilateral knee-ankle-foot orthosis
trileaflet prosthesis
Trilisate
Trillat
T. osteotomy
T. procedure
Tri-Lock total hip prosthesis with Porocoat
Trilogy acetabular cup system
trimalleolar ankle fracture

NOTES

T

Trimedyne Omnipulse homium laser
trimethoprim sulfamethoxazole
trimipramine
Trimline knee immobilizer
trimmer
    motorized t.
Tri-Motion Knee System
Trinkle
    T. bone drill
    T. brace
    T. brace and adapter
    T. chuck adapter
    T. power drill
    T. screwdriver
    T. Super-Cut twist drill
triode
tripartite muscle origin
triphalangeal
    t. thumb
    t. thumb deformity
triphase technetium scintigraphy
triphasic action potential
triplanar
    t. protractor
    t. protractor apparatus
triplane
    t. construct
    t. motion
    t. osteotomy
    t. tibial fracture
triple
    T. Antibiotic Topical
    t. arthrodesis
    t. diapering
    t. discharge
    t. envelope system
    t. frame
    t. hemisection
    t.-injection cinearthrography
    t. innominate osteotomy
    t.-jump test
    t. ligamentous repair
    t. reamer
    t. tarsal fusion
    t. tenodesis
triplegia
triplet
triple-wire
    t.-w. fusion
    t.-w. procedure
    t.-w. technique
triploscope
tripod
    t. cane
    t. foot
    McBride t.
tripoding
Trippi-Wells traction tongs

triquetral fracture
triquetrolunate
    t. dislocation
    t. instability
triquetrum
    t. bone
    t.-lunate arthrodesis
    t. ossification
triradial cartilage
tri-radial resector blade
triradiate
    t. acetabular extensile approach
    t. cartilage
    t. transtrochanteric approach
trisalicylate
    choline magnesium t.
triscaphe
    t. arthrodesis
    t. fusion
    t. joint
trismus
trisomy
    t. 21
trispiked
trispiral tomography
TriStander
Tristoject
Tritin
    Dr Scholl's Maximum Strength T.
triton tumor
Tri-Wedge total hip system
Tri W-G table
trocar
    blunt t.
    sharp t.
    T-handled t.
trochanter
    greater t.
    t. holder
    t.-holding clamp
    lesser t.
trochanteric
    t. advancement
    t. bolt
    t. bursa
    t. bursitis
    t. migration
    t. osteotomy
    t. pin
    t. reamer
    t. shift
    t. slide
    t. spine
    t. wire
trochanter-knee-ankle (TKA)
trochlea
trochlear
    t. defect

t. groove
t. notch

troika
aponeurotic t.

trolley
Bolero lift bath t.
Tupper t.

tromethamine
ketorolac t.

Tromner test

Tronzo
T. classification of intertrochanteric fracture
T. elevator
T. fracture classification
T. prosthesis

trophic
t. change
t. fracture
t. joint disorder
t. ulcer
t. ulceration

tropism
facet t.

trough
bone t.
t. line

trousers
military antishock t. (MAST)

Trowbridge
T. TerraRound foot
T. TerraRound sports limb
T. triple-speed drill

Trowbridge-Campau bone drill

true
t. acetabular region
t. acetabulum
T. Blue exercise band
t. lateral view
t. metatarsus adductus (TMA)
t. rib
t. spacer

TRUE/FLEX Intramedullary nail

Tru-Fit custom molded shoe

Trumble
T. arthrodesis
T. talectomy

Trümmerfeld zone

Tru-Mold shoe

truncated tarsometatarsal wedge arthrodesis

truncated-wedge
t.-w. arthrodesis
t.-w. tarsometatarsal arthrodesis vertical talus

trunk
t. control
t. curl
t. incurvation test
t. righting
t. shift
sympathetic t.

Trunkey fracture classification system

trunk-hip-knee-ankle-foot orthosis (THKAFO)

trunnion-bearing hip prosthesis

Tru-Support
T.-S. EW bandage
T.-S. SA bandage

try
DiChiara hand t.

Trypanosoma gambiense

trypsin, balsam peru, and castor oil

Tsai-Stillwell procedure

Tscherne classification

Tscherne-Gotzen tibial fracture classification

T-shaped
T-s. AO plate
T-s. capsulotomy
T-s. incision
T-s. inserter

TSP
tibial sesamoid position

T-spine
thoracic spine

TSPP
technetium stannous pyrophosphate

TSRH
Texas Scottish Rite Hospital
TSRH buttressed laminar hook
TSRH circular laminar hook
TSRH corkscrew device
TSRH crosslink
TSRH crosslink stabilization
TSRH crosslink system
TSRH double-rod construct
TSRH eyebolt spreader
TSRH hook holder
TSRH hook inserter
TSRH hook-rod
TSRH implant
TSRH instrumentation

T

NOTES

TSRH *(continued)*
 TSRH L-bolt
 TSRH mini-corkscrew device
 TSRH pedicle hook
 TSRH pedicle screw
 TSRH plate
 TSRH rod fixation
 TSRH spinal implant system
 TSRH trial hook
 TSRH Universal spinal
  instrumentation system
 TSRH wrench
T-Stat Topical
T-Stick adhesive
T-strap
 medial T-s.
Tsuge
 T. debulking
 T. tendon repair
Tsuji laminaplasty
TT
 tilt table
 total transfer
101T/201T
 EMG 101T/201T
TTA
 tissue texture abnormality
TTAP
 threaded titanium acetabular prosthesis
 TTAP prosthesis
TTAP-ST acetabular prosthesis
TTE
 transthoracic echocardiography
t-test
 paired t-t.
 Student's t-t.
TTR
 tarsal tunnel release
TTS
 tarsal tunnel syndrome
TTT
 tibial talar tilt/tibiotalar tilt
tube
 Adson suction t.
 Baron suction t.
 chest t.
 Dawson-Yuhl suction t.
 digit t.
 Dynamic digit extensor t.
 endoneural t.
 Esmarch t.
 Ferguson-Frazier suction t.
 t. flap graft
 Gillquist suction t.
 t. guide
 Hemovac suction t.
 irrigation t.
 Jergesen t.

 stockinette t.
 suction t.
 t.-to-film distance
 vent t.
TubeGauz bandage
tuber angle
tubercle
 t. avulsion
 Chaput t.
 conoid t.
 Gerdy t.
 Ghon t.
 lateral tibial t.
 Lisfranc t.
 Lister t.
 medial t.
 t. osteotomy
 tibial t.
 Tillaux-Chaput t.
 Wagstaff t.
tubercular granuloma
tuberculosis
 diaphyseal t.
 extraarticular t.
 t. of hip
 metaphyseal t.
 Mycobacterium t.
 osteoarticular t.
 skeletal t.
 spinal t.
 t. spondylitis
tuberculous
 t. arthritis
 t. dactylitis
 t. lesion
 t. peroneal tenosynovitis
 t. trochanteric bursitis
 t. vertebral osteomyelitis
tuber-joint angle
tuberosity
 bicipital t.
 t. fragment
 greater t.
 ischial t.
 lesser t.
 posterior t.
 radial t.
 tibial t.
 ungual t.
 ununited tibial t.
tuberous xanthoma
Tubersitz amputee gait
Tubex gauze dressing
Tubigrip
 T. bandage
 T. dressing
tubing
 Dakin t.

foam t.
gel t.
medullary vent t.
PVC t.
Silipos mesh t.
Thera-Band t.

TUBS
    traumatic, unidirectional instability and
      Bankart lesion
      TUBS procedure

Tubsider Kneeling Seat

tubular
    t. plate
    t. punch
    t. stockinette

tubularization of the graft

tubulization

tucker
    Bishop-Black tendon t.
    Bishop-DeWitt tendon t.
    Bishop-Peter tendon t.
    Burch-Greenwood tendon t.
    tendon t.

Tudor-Edwards bone-cutting forceps

Tuf Nex neck exerciser

Tuf-Skin tape adherent

TufStuf II cast tape

tuft
    distal t.
    finger t.
    t. fracture

tuftal resorption

Tui Na

Tuinal

Tuke saw

Tukey test

Tuli
    T. gel-heel cup
    T. heel cup

tulip pedicle screw

Tullos technique

Tumble
    T. Forms feeder
    T. Forms roll

tumbler graft

tumefaction

tumor
    Abrikossoff t.
    aggressive t.
    ball-valve t.
    t.-bearing bone
    Bednar t.

benign t.
blood vessel t.
bone t.
bone-forming t.
brown fat t.
cartilaginous t.
cerebellopontine angle t.
Codman t.
cortical desmoid t.
cystic t.
desmoid t.
dumbbell t.
Enneking staging of malignant soft
    tissue t.
Ewing t.
extraabdominal desmoid t.
fatty tissue t.
fibroblastic t.
fibroid t.
fibrous t.
giant cell t. (GCT)
glomus t.
t.-grasping forceps
histiocytic t.
Hodgkin t.
hyperparathyroidism t.
intraosseous t.
lipid t.
lumbar t.
lymph vessel t.
mesenchymal t.
metastatic spinal t.
t. metastatic to spine
nerve sheath t.
neural t.
neuroectodermal t.
occult primary malignant t.
pluripotential mesenchymal t.
primary t.
t.-replacement endoprosthesis
t. resection
retinal anlage t.
Schwann t.
soft tissue t.
spinal t.
superior sulcus t.
synovial t.
tenosynovial giant cell t.
t. therapy
triton t.
vascular t.
vertebral body t.

T

NOTES

tumor *(continued)*
    t. vessel
    xanthomatous giant cell t.
tumoral calcinosis
tumorous
    t. condition
    t. involvement
Tums
    T. E-X Extra Strength Tablet
    T. Extra Strength Liquid
tuning fork test
tunnel
    t.-and-sling fixation
    carpal t.
    cubital t.
    t. drill guide
    femoral t.
    fibroosseous t.
    Gaynor-Hart x-ray position of
      carpal t.
    t. locator guide
    osseous t.
    radial t.
    subsartorial t.
    tarsal t.
    tibial t.
    ulnar t.
    t. view
tunneler
    tendon t.
Tunturi hand exerciser
Tuohy needle
Tupman plate
Tupper
    T. arthroplasty
    T. trolley
turbo-spin-echo imaging sequence
turbulence
Turco
    T. clubfoot release
    T. clubfoot release technique
    T. posteromedial release
    T. repair of talipes equinovarus
Turco-Spinella tendo calcaneus repair
turf
    t. toe
    t. toe injury
turgor
TurnAide therapeutic system
turnbuckle
    t. ankle brace
    t. cast
    t. distractor
    t. elbow splint
    t. jack
    t. knee brace
    t. wrist orthosis
turn-down tendon flap

Turn-Easy transfer aid
turned-up pulp deformity
turner
    T. pin
    T. prosthesis
    rotating t.
    T. syndrome
Turning Board Exercise System
turnstile casting stand
turret exostosis
Turyn sign
TUWAVE galvanic stimulator/TENS unit
TV
    transverse
Twilite Oral
twin-blade oscillating saw
Twin Cities Lo-Profile halo
twist
    t. drill
    t. drill point
twister
    Axel wire t.
    Batzdorf cervical wire t.
    t. cable
    cerclage wire t.
    Cooley-Baumgarten wire t.
    Miltex wire t.
    orthotic coiled spring t.
    Shifrin wire t.
two
    t.-column cervical spine injury
    t.-hole plate
    t.-inclinometer method
    t.-part fracture
    t.-portal technique
    t.-sleeve technique
    t.-strut tibial graft technique
two-plane
    t.-p. bilateral external fixator
    t.-p. bilateral frame
    t.-p. deformity
    t.-p. fluoroscopy
    t.-p. roentgenogram
    t.-p. unilateral external fixator
    t.-p. unilateral frame
two-point
    t.-p. discrimination
    t.-p. discrimination test
    t.-p. gait
    t.-p. nerve block
    t.-p. step-to gait pattern
two-poster
    t.-p. brace
    t.-p. cervical orthosis
two-prong
    t.-p. rake retractor
    t.-p. stem finger prosthesis

Tworek screw guide
two-stage
    t.-s. hip fusion
    t.-s. Syme amputation
    t.-s. tendon grafting technique
    t.-s. tendon graft reconstruction
tx
    traction
    treatment
TX-1, TX-7 traction table
Tycron suture
tying forceps
Tylenol
    T. Extended Relief
    T. With Codeine

Tylok high-tension cable system
tyloma
Tylox
type
    T. C-50, C-90 AFO
    contraction t.
    t. 501, 502, 504, 602 finger splint
    foot t.
    t. II curve pattern
    t. I, II, III, IIIA, IIIB, IIIC open
      fracture
    sleeve t.
Tyrell hook

NOTES

T

653

UBC
University of British Columbia
UBC brace
UBE
upper body ergometer
UBP
universal bone plate
UBP system
UCB
unilateral calcaneal brace
University of California, Berkeley
UCB. foot orthosis
UCB shoe insert
UCBI
University of California, Berkeley insert
UCBL
University of California, Berkeley
Laboratory
UCBL foot plate
UCI ankle prosthesis
UCL
ulnar collateral ligament
UCLA
U. anatomic shoulder arthroplasty
U. CAPP TD hook
U. functional long leg brace
U. Shoulder Rating scale
UCOheal orthotic
UCO Quick-Sil silicone system
UCP compression plate
Ueba release
Uematsu shoulder arthrodesis
UE Tech Weight Well Exercise System
UFO
Universal Plantar Fasciitis Orthosis
universal plantar fasciitis orthosis
Orthomerica UFO
UFOS
universal frame outer socket
UHMWPE
ultrahigh molecular weight polyethylene
UHMWPE prosthesis
UHR locking ring mechanism
UID/S
unilateral interfacetal dislocation or
subluxation
UKA
unicompartmental knee arthroplasty
ulcer
decubitus u.
diabetic neurotrophic u.
ischemia foot u.
ischemic u.
neuropathic u.
neurotrophic food u.

peptic u.
pressure u.
stasis u.
supramalleolar venous u.
trophic u.
Wagoner u.
ulceration
neuropathic forefoot u.
neurotrophic u.
sublesional u.
trophic u.
Ullman line
Ullrich
U. drill guard
U. drill-guard drill
ulna
absent u.
distal u.
Monteggia fracture-dislocation of u.
proximal u.
ulnar
u. anlage
u. artery
u. artery injury
u. bearing
u. bursa
u. carpal collateral ligament
u. clubhand
u. collateral ligament (UCL)
u. collateral ligament injury
u. collateral ligament rupture
u. column
u. convexity
u. creaking
u. cubital tunnel syndrome
u. deviation
u. deviation deformity
u. dimelia
u. drift
u. drift deformity
u. fracture
u. gutter splint
u. head
u. head excision
u. head implant prosthesis
u. hemiresection interposition
arthroplasty
u.-humeral angle
u. impaction syndrome
u. lengthening
midcarpal u. (MCU)
u. minus variance
u. motor neurectomy
u. nerve (UN)
u. nerve block

U

ulnar *(continued)*
  u. nerve entrapment syndrome
  u. nerve injury
  u. nerve palsy
  u. nerve release
  u. neuropathy
  u. rasp
  u. recession
  u. reflex
  u. ruler
  u. side grip
  u. translation
  u. translocation
  u. trial
  u. tunnel
  u. wrist extensor tendinitis
ulnare
  ligamentum collaterale u.
  ligamentum collaterale carpi u.
ulnaris
  extensor carpi u. (ECU)
  flexor carpi u. (FCU)
ulnarward
ulnocarpal
  u. abutment
  u. abutment syndrome
  u. arthrodesis
  u. impingement
  u. joint
  u. ligament
ulnohumeral joint
ulnolunate
  u. articulation
  u. ligament
ulnotriquetral ligament
ulnotriquetrum articulation
ULO
  upper limb orthosis
ULP
  upper limb prosthesis
Ulrich
  U. bone-holding clamp
  U. bone-holding forceps
Ulrich-St. Gallen forceps
Ulson fixator system
Ultec thin dressing
Ultima
  U. calcar stems
  U. Fx stems
  U. hip replacement system
  U. total hip system
Ultiva
Ultra
  Grisactin U.
  U. Mide 25 lotion
  U. Stim silver electrode
Ultrabrace brace

Ultra-Drive
  U.-D. bone cement removal system
  U.-D. ultrasonic revision system
Ultrafix
  U. apparatus
UltraFix RC suture anchor system
Ultraflex Dynamic Joint
Ultra-Flex orthopaedic bed
Ultra-Guard
  U.-G. FS hip bracing system
  U.-G. hip orthosis system
ultrahigh molecular weight polyethylene (UHMWPE)
Ultra-Light athletic tape
Ultram
UltraPower drill system
Ultraprin
ultrasonic probe
ultrasonography
  compression u.
  duplex Doppler u.
ultrasound (US)
  AMREX therapeutic u.
  compression u.
  duplex u.
  Dynatron 150 u.
  u. electrotherapy
  u. phonophoresis
  pulsed u.
  Sonicator 720 u.
  Sonicator Plus u.
  u. therapy
ultrasound-guided
  u.-g. echo biopsy
  u.-g. stereotactic biopsy
ultraviolet light (UV)
Ultra-X external fixation system
umbilical tape
UMS
  upper fossa active, medial knee pain, and short leg on the side ipsilateral to the week fossa
UN
  ulnar nerve
Unasyn
unbalanced
  u. depolymerization
  u. hemivertebra
uncemented femoral component
uncinate
  u. hypertrophy
  u. process fracture
uncoarthrosis
uncommitted metaphyseal lesion
uncompensated rotary scoliosis
unconditional stimulus (US)

unconstrained
- u. shoulder arthroplasty
- u. tricompartmental knee prosthesis

uncoordinated gait

uncovertebral
- u. arthrosis
- u. joint
- u. spur

undecylenic acid and derivatives

undeRAP

underarm
- u. body jacket
- u. brace
- u. cast
- u. orthosis

Underburger test

under direct vision

undergrowth

underlapping toe

undermined skin

underscoring

undersurface of patella

underwater Bovie

undisplaced fracture

undyed suture

ungual tuberosity

unguarded osteotome

unguis incarnatus

Uni-Ace

uniaxial structure

unicameral bone cyst

unicompartmental
- u. knee arthroplasty (UKA)
- u. knee implant
- u. knee prosthesis

unicondylar
- u. fracture
- U. Geomedic hemi-knee system
- u. prosthesis

Uniflex
- U. calibrated step drill
- U. dressing
- U. drill bushing
- U. humeral nail
- U. nailing system

Unilab
- U. Surgibone
- U. Surgibone surgical implant

unilateral
- u. acute radicular syndrome
- u. calcaneal brace (UCB)
- u. chronic radicular syndrome

- u. interfacetal dislocation
- u. interfacetal dislocation or subluxation (UID/S)
- u. pedicle cannulation
- u. posterior-anterior movement
- u. sacroiliac approach
- u. standing test
- u. variable screw placement system

Unilink system for hand surgery

uninhibited ankle motion

union
- bone u.
- bony u.
- u. broach retention drill
- u. broach retention pin
- callous bone u.
- delayed fracture u.
- European Chiropractic U. (ECU)
- osteonal bone u.
- Osteotron stimulator for bone u.
- primary bone u.
- secondary bone u.
- slow u.

Uni-Patch electrode gel

Unipen
- U. Injection
- U. Oral

Uniplane
- U. rocker

unipolar
- u. cauterization
- u. cautery
- u. needle electrode
- u. release

uniportal arthroscopic microdiskectomy

Unique Vitamin E

unisegmental mobility

unit
- AME microcurrent TENS u.
- Autoflex II, III CPM u.
- Back Bubble gravity traction u.
- basic multicellular remodeling u.
- BioMed TENS u.
- bone metabolic u.
- bone remodeling u.
- Bovie coagulating u.
- C-arm fluoroscopy u.
- Cybex Torso Rotation Testing and Rehabilitation U.
- Cybex Trunk Extension Flexion u.
- DynaLator ultrasound u.
- Dystrophile exercise u.

U

NOTES

unit *(continued)*
    Eclipse TENS u.
    Econo 90 traction u.
    ElastaTrac home lumbar traction u.
    Exo-Bed traction u.
    Exo-Overhead traction u.
    functional spinal u. (FSU)
    G5 Fleximatic
      massage/percussion u.
    G5 Vibramatic
      massage/percussion u.
    home cervical traction u. (HCTU)
    Hydra-Cadence gait-control u.
    hydraulic knee u.
    Hydrocollator heating u.
    intervertebral motor u.
    JACE hand continuous passive
      motion u.
    Magnatherm and Magnatherm SSP
      electromagnetic therapy u.
    MENS u.
    motor u.
    musculotendinous u.
    myofascial u.
    myotatic u.
    Orthodyne Enhancer u.
    over-the-door traction u.
    Pebax counter u.
    postanesthesia care u. (PACU)
    rotator u.
    single-axis knee u.
    Solitens TENS u.
    u. spinal rod
    Systems 2000 TENS u.
    TENS u.
    Thermalator heating u.
    TUWAVE galvanic
      stimulator/TENS u.
    vertebral motion u. (VMU)
unitary plastic
United States Vocational Rehabilitation
  Act
Unitek steel crown
unitunnel technique
univalve cast
univalved
universal
    U. acromioclavicular splint
    U. AerobiCycle
    u. bone plate (UBP)
    U. bone plate system
    u. canvas body restraint
    U. ComputeRow
    u. coronal movement
    U. distal radius fracture
      classification
    U. drill point
    U. femoral head prosthesis

    U. Fitstep
    u. frame outer socket (UFOS)
    u. full-circle manual goniometer
    U. gutter splint
    U. hex screwdriver
    U. hip prosthesis
    u. incision
    U. instrumentation
    u. intelligence
    U. knee positioner
    U. lateral positioner
    U. modular femoral hip component
      extractor
    U. nail
    U. Plantar Fasciitis Orthosis (UFO)
    u. plantar fasciitis orthosis (UFO)
    u. precautions
    U. proximal femur (UPF)
    U. radial component
    u. sling
    U. Spine System (USS)
    U. support splint
    U. Tredex
    U. two-speed hand drill
    U. wire clamp
Uni-Versatil sling
University
    U. of British Columbia (UBC)
    U. of British Columbia brace
    U. of California, Berkeley (UCB)
    U. of California, Berkeley insert
      (UCBI)
    U. of California, Berkeley SACH
      foot
    U. of California cuff suspension
      PTB socket
    U. of Florida LINAC
    Louisiana State U. (LSU)
    University of California, Berkeley
      Laboratory (UCBL)
Unloader
    U. Adj. knee brace
    The U.
unlocking spiral technique
unmineralized osteoid
unmyelinated
Unna
    U. boot cast
    U. boot wrap
    U. paste
    U. paste boot
    U. paste shell
Unna-Flex Plus venous ulcer kit
unopposed
unplanned valgus osteotomy
unreduced dislocation
unremodeled defect

unrestricted closed and open chain knee extension exercise
unscher wire
unsegmented vertebral bar
unstable
    u. cervical spine injury
    u. fracture
    u. fracture-dislocation
    u. joint
unsteadiness of gait
unsteady gait
unsustained clonus
unthreaded wire
ununited
    u. fracture
    u. tibial tuberosity
unusual infection
unwanted screw torque
unwinding
U osteotomy
up
    U. and About system
    u.-angle hook
    press u.
upbiting
    u. basket forceps
    u. rongeur
upcurved punch forceps
upcut rongeur
Update
    Orthopaedic Knowledge U. (OKU)
UPF
    Universal proximal femur
    UPF prosthesis
upgoing toe
6U portal
upper
    u. arm tourniquet
    u. body ergometer (UBE)
    u. cervical spine anterior construct
    u. cervical spine anterior exposure
    u. cervical spine fusion
    u. cervical spine posterior construct
    u. cervical spine procedure
    u. extremity
    u. extremity myoelectric prosthesis
    u. fossa active, medial knee pain, and short leg on the side ipsilateral to the week fossa (UMS)
    u. hand retractor
    U. 7 head halter

    u. hook trial
    u. limb orthosis (ULO)
    u. limb prosthesis (ULP)
    u. limits of normal
    u. motor neuron disease
    u. motor neuron lesion
    u. thoracic spine
uppercycle
uprights
    orthosis overlapped u.
upright-Y incision
uptake
    maximal oxygen u.
    myo-inositol u.
upward-cutting triangular knife
Uracel
Urban
    U. Walker
    U. Walkers shoe
Urbaniak
    U. neurovascular free flap
    U. scapular flap
Urbanwalkers shoe insert
Ureacin-20
    U. cream
    U. creme
Ureacin-10 lotion
ureter injury
urethane
    Poron cellular u.
urethra
urethrogram
urethrography
Urias
    U. air splint
    U. pressure splint
uric acid crystal
uricosuric agent
urinalysis
urinary
    u. incontinence
    u. obstruction
    u. output
    u. retention
    u. tract
urine
    u. culture
    u. protein myeloma
urist view
urodynamic
urogenital diaphragm
urokinase

U

NOTES

urologic
 u. complication
 u. injury
US
 ultrasound
 unconditional stimulus
 US manufacturing air castaway
U.S.
 U.S. Army bone chisel
 U.S. Army gouge
 U.S. Army osteotome
U-shaped
 U.-s. incision
 U.-s. retractor
Uslenghi
 U. drill guide
 U. plate

USMC
 USMC multi axis ankle
 USMC stance locking safety knee
USP#2 suture
U-splint splint
USS
 Universal Spine System
Utah
 U. artificial arm
 U. artificial limb
utensil
 swivel u.
uterus
Utrata forceps
UV
 ultraviolet light
UVEX eye protector

V

V blade plate
V nail plate
V osteotomy

V40

V40 femoral head implant component
V40 forged femoral head

V1 halo ring
V-A alignment rod
Vac

Sani V.

vacant glenoid sign
Vac-Pac positioner
vacuolar myelopathy
vacuum

v. disk
M-PACT cast v.

vagal reaction
vaginal

v. hand ligament
v. ligament of hand
v. pack

vagoglossopharyngeal neuralgia
vagus nerve
Vainio arthroplasty
Valenti arthroplasty
Valentine splint
Valeo back support
valerian
valeriana officinalis
valga

coxa v.
tibia v.

valgum

genu v.
idiopathic genu v. (IGV)

valgus

v. angle
v. angulation
v. bar
calcaneal v.
congenital convex pes plano v.
v. contracture
convex pes v.
v. deformity
v. extension osteotomy
v. extension overload syndrome
flexible pes v.
v. foot
forefoot v.
genu v.
hallux v.
heel v.
v. high tibial osteotomy

hindfoot v.
idiopathic hallux v.
v. instability
v. intertrochanteric-wedge osteotomy
juvenile hallux v.
v. knee
v. knee motion
McBride bunion hallux v.
metatarsus v.
pes plano v.
physiologic v.
rearfoot v.
senile hallux v.
v. stress
v. stress test
v. subtrochanteric osteotomy
talipes convex pes v.
v. wedge-prop osteotomy
v. Y-shaped prop osteotomy

Valium Oral
Valls hip prosthesis
Valls-Ottolenghim-Schajowicz needle biopsy
Valorin

V. Extra
V. Super

Valpar

V. component work sample series
V. Whole Body Range of Motion Test

Valpius-Compere procedure
valproate
valproic acid
Valrelease
Valsalva

V. maneuver
V. test

value

mean v.

valve

bulb and thumb screw v.
Quadtro cushion with Isoflap v.

Van

V. Arsdale triangular splint
V. Beek nerve approximator
V. Buren sequestrum forceps
V. Geesen stain
V. Neck disease
V. Ness procedure
V. Ness rotationplasty
V. Rosen splint

vanadium
Vancocin
Vancoled
vancomycin

V

Vanghetti limb prosthesis
Vantage Performance monitor (VPM)
Vanzetti sign
VAPC dorsiflexion assist orthosis
Vapo coolant spray and stretch
vapor
    Mitek v.
vara
    coxa v.
    developmental coxa v.
    infantile tibia v. (ITV)
    tibia v.
variabilis
    Dermacentor v.
variable
    v. axis knee system
    v. circumference suprapatellar
      socket (VCSPS)
    v. flexion overhinge (VFO)
    metabolic v.
    v. screw placement (VSP)
    v. screw placement system
    v. screw placement system
      instrumentation
    v. screw placement system-
      instrumented lumbar spine
    v. screw placement system-plated
      patient
    v. screw plate (VSP)
    v. spinal plating (VSP)
variance
    analysis of v. (ANOVA)
    multivariate analysis of v.
      (MANOVA)
    negative ulnar v. (NUV)
    positive ulnar v. (PUV)
    ulnar minus v.
vari-angle clip applier
Varian LINAC
variant
    four-part v.
variation
    coefficient of v. (CV)
    hindfoot anatomic v.
    postural v.
vari-balance board set
varices (*pl. of* varix)
varicosity
    superficial v.
Vari-Duct hip and knee orthosis
Varikopf hip prosthesis
varix, pl. varices
Varney
    V. acromioclavicular brace
    V. pin
Varni-Thompson Pediatric Pain
  Questionnaire

varum
    genu v.
varus
    calcaneal v.
    v. contracture
    cubitus v.
    v. derotational osteotomy
    dynamic hallux v.
    forefoot v.
    genu v.
    hallux v.
    heel v.
    v. hindfoot
    v. hindfoot deformity
    v. knee
    v. malalignment
    v. malunion
    metatarsus v. (MTV)
    metatarsus primus v., metatarsus
      primus adductus (MPV)
    v. MTP angle
    rearfoot v.
    v. rotational osteotomy (VRO)
    v. rotation shortening osteotomy
    v. stress test
    v. supramalleolar osteotomy
    v. tilt
varus-valgus
    v.-v. adjustment screw
    v.-v. angulation
    v.-v. instability
    knee v.-v.
    v.-v. lift-off
    v.-v. plane
varus/valgus stress of the elbow
VAS
    visual analog scale
vasa nervorum
vascular
    v. accident
    v. assessment
    v. bundle implantation into bone
    v. endothelium
    v. forceps
    v. gangrene
    v. inflow
    v. injury
    v. invasion
    v. nonunion
    v. surgery
    v. tissue
    v. tumor
vascularity
    tenuous v.
vascularized
    v. bone graft
    v. bone transplant
    v. fibular graft

v. free flap
v. osseous transfer
v. osteoseptocutaneous fibular
autogenous graft
v. rib strut graft
vasculature
vasculitis
mesenteric v.
rheumatoid v.
vasculopathy
vasculosis
circulus articuli v.
vasocillator frame
vasoconstriction
vasodilation
vasodilator
vasogenic shock
vasomotor
v. startle reflex
v. technique
vasopneumatic intermittent compression
vasopressor
vasospasm
vasospastic ischemia
Vastamäki
V. paralysis
V. technique
vastus
v. intermedius
v. lateralis (VL)
v. lateralis muscle
v. lateralis ridge
v. medialis
v. medialis advancement (VMA)
v. medialis muscle
v. medialis obliquus (VMO)
v. medialis obliquus muscle
v. medialis obliquus:vastus lateralis
electromyographic ratio (VMO:VL
EMG ratio)
VATER
vertebral (defcts), (imperforate) anus,
tracheoesophageal (fistula), radial and
renal dysplasia
vertebral (defects), (imperforate) anus,
tracheoesophageal (fistula), radial and
renal (dysplasia)
VATER syndrome
Vater-Pacini corpuscle
VAX-D
vertebral axial decompression
VAX-D therapy table

VC
voluntary closing
voluntary control
VCSPS
variable circumference suprapatellar
socket
VDA
video-dimensional analysis
VDDR
vitamin D-dependent rickets
VDRR
vitamin D-resistant rickets
VDS
ventral derotating spinal
ventral derotation spondylodesis
vector
V. low back analysis system
major injury v. (MIV)
v. quantity
vehicle
all-terrain v. (ATV)
vehicular accident
Veillonella
vein
anterior jugular v.
axillary v.
v.'s of Batson
brachiocephalic v.
carotid v.
cephalic v.
common iliac v.
v. graft
grafting v.
iliac v.
iliolumbar v.
innominate v.
intercostal v.
internal iliac v.
internal jugular v.
lingual v.
lumbar v.
middle sacral v.
middle thyroid v.
peroneal v.
popliteal v.
saphenous v.
subclavian v.
superficial temporal v.
superior thyroid v.
tibial v.
vertebral v.
vela (*pl. of* velum)

V

NOTES

velar
fronting of v.
Velcro
V. extenders splint
V. fitting
V. Hand Exerboard
V. immobilization
V. immobilizer
V. strap
Veleanu-Rosianu-Ionescu
V.-R.-I. adductor tenotomy
V.-R.-I. technique
velocity
angular v.
conduction v. (CV)
maximum conduction v.
maximum eversion v.
maximum inversion v.
motion v.
motor nerve conduction v.
  (MNCV)
muscle fiber conduction v.
nerve conduction v. (NCV)
propagation v.
sensory nerve conduction v.
Velpeau
V. axillary lateral view
V. axillary radiograph
V. bandage
V. cast
V. deformity
V. dressing
V. shoulder immobilizer
V. sling
V. sling-dressing
V. stockinette
V. wrap
velum, pl. **vela**
vena
v. cava
v. comitans
Venable
V. plate
V. screw
Venable-Stuck
V.-S. fracture pin
V.-S. nail
V.-S. screw
vena cava
inferior v. c.
superior v. c.
venae comitantes
Venn-Watson classification
Venodyne boot
venography
epidural v.
intraosseous v.
magnetic resonance v.

Venosan
V. support hose
V. support sock
venous
v. cleft
v. compression
v. foot pump
v. impulse
v. thromboembolic disease (VTED)
v. thrombosis
ventilation
high-frequency oscillatory v.
  (HFOV)
maximal voluntary v. (MVV)
mechanical v.
ventral
v. derotating spinal (VDS)
v. derotating spinal wrench
v. derotation spondylodesis (VDS)
ventriculography
ventriculoperitoneal shunt
vent tube
VEP
visual evoked potential
VePesid
V. Injection
V. Oral
VER
visual evoked response
vera
aloe v.
rubra v.
verapamil
Verb ColorCards
Verbrugge
V. bone clamp
V. bone-holding forceps
V. needle
Verdan
V. osteoplastic thumb reconstruction
V. technique
Veress needle
Verlow brace
Vermont
V. pedicle fixation system
V. spinal fixator (VSF)
V. spinal fixator articulation
Vernier
V. caliber gauge
V. caliper
Verocay body
verruca, pl. **verrucae**
v. cryotherapy
v. plantaris
v. vulgaris
Verruca-Freeze
V.-F. freezing system
verrucous lesion

VersaClimber exercise machine
VersaFlex tubing kit
Versa-Fx femoral fixation
Versa-Helper floor stand
Versalok low back fixation system
VersaPulse holmium laser
Versa-Stim self-adhering electrode
versatility
    attachment v.
Versa-Trac lumbar spine retractor system
Versa-Trainer exerciser
version
    external v.
    femoral neck v.
    Gait Abnormality Rating Scale Modified v. (GARS-M)
    internal v.
Versi-Splint carry bag
VerSys hip system
vertebra, pl. **vertebrae**
    apex v.
    apical v.
    arcus vertebrae
    bioconcave v.
    butterfly v.
    cleft v.
    codfish v.
    end v.
    first cervical v.
    inferior v.
    last normal v. (LNV)
    lumbar v.
    lumbosacral v.
    malposed v.
    olisthetic v.
    v. plana fracture
    v. prominens reflex
    scalloping of v.
    second cervical v.
    stable v.
    transitional v.
    wedge-shaped v.
    wedging of olisthetic v.
vertebral
    v. adjustment
    v. ankylosis
    v. artery
    v. artery involvement
    v. artery test
    v. axial decompression (VAX-D)
    v. body

    v. body anterior cortex
    v. body corpectomy
    v. body decompression
    v. body fracture
    v. body impactor
    v. body tumor
    v. border
    v. collapse
    v. column
    v. compression
    v. derangement
    v. end plate
    v. exposure
    v. fascia
    v. instability
    v. lesion
    v. level
    v. medicine
    v. motion segment
    v. motion unit (VMU)
    v. osteomyelitis
    v. osteosynthesis
    v. osteosynthesis fusion rate
    v. resection
    v. rib
    v. ring apophysis
    v. rotation
    v. stable burst fracture
    v. subluxation
    v. subluxation complex (VSC)
    v. subluxation syndrome
    v. vein
    v. wedge compression fracture
vertebral (defcts), (imperforate) anus, tracheoesophageal (fistula), radial and renal dysplasia (VATER)
vertebralis
    arcus v.
vertebrectomy
    Bohlman anterior cervical v.
    cervical spondylotic myelopathy v.
    microsurgical thoracoscopic v.
vertebrobasilar
    v. injury
    v. insufficiency
vertebrogenic interference
vertebroligamentous sprain strain
Verteflex
    V. arthrotonic stabilizer
    V. Intersegmental Traction Table
Vertetrac ambulatory traction system

NOTES

vertical

anatomical v.
v. axis
v. compression
v. compression test
v. loading
v. longitudinal tear
v. mattress suture
v. midline incision
v. pedicle diameter
v. plane
v. sacral compaction
v. shear (VS)
v. shear fracture
v. shock pylon
v. subsidence
v. suspension reflex
v. symphyseal mobility
v. talus
v. traction
v. translation

verticality control
Vertstreken closed medullary nailing
very

v. low birth weight infant
V. Special Arts (VSA)

vesalianum

os v.

Vesely-Street

V.-S. splint
V.-S. split nail

vesicocutaneous fistula
vesicostomy
Vess chair
vessel

v. clamp
v. dilator
endosteal v.
great v.
haversian v.
humeral circumflex v.
lymph v.
milking of v.
periosteal v.
popliteal v.
v. shifting
tumor v.

vest

halo v.
Little cargo v.
Standard E-Z-On V.
Vitrathene v.

vestibular ball
Vestibulator positioning tumble form
VFO

variable flexion overhinge

V-groove hollow-ground connection design

viability
viable tissue
Vibram

V. rockerbottom shoe
V. sole

Vibramat
vibration

v. glove
v. perception threshold (VPT)
v. sensation
v. threshold test
whole-body v.

vibrator

v. hand syndrome
Magic Wand v.

vibratory
vibrogram

digital v.

vibrometer test
Vicodin

V. ES
V. HP

Vicoprofen
Vicryl suture
victim

multiple trauma v.

Victorian brace
Vidal-Adrey

V.-A. fracture technique
V.-A. modified Hoffman external fixation device apparatus
V.-A. modified Hoffmann external fixation device
V.-A. modified Hoffmann fixation

video-dimensional analysis (VDA)
videofluoroscopy
video-gate analysis
videoradiography
Videx
vidian neuralgia
Vidicon vacuum chamber pickup tube for video camera
Vi-Drape dressing
view

Adams v.
Alexander v.
anteroposterior v.
apical lordotic v.
axial calcaneus v.
axial sesamoid v.
axillary v.
baseline v.
Beath v.
bicipital tuberosity v.
Böhler calcaneal v.
Böhler lumbosacral v.
Broden v.
Canale-Kelly v.

carpal tunnel v.
Carter-Rowe v.
cine v.
coalition v.
coned-down v.
cross-table v.
dens x-ray v.
Didiee v.
dorsoplantar v.
Dunlop-Shands v.
Ferguson v.
Ficat v.
frog-leg lateral v.
Harris v.
Harris-Beath axial calcaneus v.
Hermodsson tangential v.
Hill-Sachs v.
Hobb v.
Hughston v.
iliac oblique v.
infrapatellar v.
inlet v.
intraoperative v.
inversion ankle stress v.
Jones v.
Judet pelvic x-ray v.
lateral oblique v.
Lauren v.
Lowell v.
magnification v.
Merchant v.
mortise v.
nonstanding lateral oblique v.
notch v.
oblique v.
obturator oblique v.
odontoid x-ray v.
outlet v.
plantar axial v.
push-pull ankle stress v.
push-pull hip v.
Robert v.
scapulolateral v.
skijump v.
skyline v.
spot v.
standing dorsoplantar v.
standing lateral v.
standing weightbearing v.
stress v.
Stryker-Notch v.
sunrise v.

sunset v.
swimmer's v.
tangential x-ray v.
Tile v.
true lateral v.
tunnel v.
urist v.
Velpeau axillary lateral v.
von Rosen v.
Waters x-ray v.
weightbearing dorsoplantar v.
West Point axillary lateral v.
x-ray v.
Zanca v.
Vigilon dressing
Vigorimeter
Martin V.
vigorimeter
Viladot
V. prosthesis
V. surgical technique
Vilex
V. cannulated screw system
V. Ouchless Hook
villonodular synovitis
villous
v. lipomatous proliferation
v. synovitis
vinblastine
Vincasar PFS Injection
vincristine
vinculum
v. breve
v. longum
Vinertia
V. implant metal
V. implant metal prosthesis
Vinke
V. skull traction tongs
V. tong traction
Vioform
viral
v.-associated arthritis
v. monarthritis
v. myositis
Virgin hip screw
Virilitrac
Virtual hip joint
Virtullene brace material
virus
human immunodeficiency v. (HIV)
visceral tendon sheath

NOTES

V

visceroptosis
viscerosomatic reflex
Visclas orthosis
viscoelastic
    v. creep
    v. heel insert
    v. material
    v. polymer
    v. tissue
viscoelasticity
Viscoheel
    V. K heel cushion
    V. K, N orthosis
    V. N cushion
    V. SofSpot orthosis
    V. SofSpot viscoelastic heel
      cushion
Viscol
Viscolas heel cushion
Viscoped S insole
viscosity
viscous
vise
    allograft bone v.
    AlloGrip bone v.
    v.-like pain
    pin v.
    Starrett pin v.
VISI
    volar flexed intercalated segment
    instability
vision
    V. Epic wheelchair
    under direct v.
visor halo fixation device
Vistacon
Vistaquel
Vistaril
Vistazine
Vistec x-ray detectable sponge
visual
    v. analog scale (VAS)
    v. assessment
    v. closure
    v. evoked potential (VEP)
    v. evoked response (VER)
    v. neglect
    V. Neglect Board
    v. orientation
    v. perception
visualized
Vita ADE cream
Vitallium
    V. alloy
    V. cup arthroplasty
    V. drill
    V. equipment
    V. humeral replacement prosthesis

    V. implant
    V. implant material
    V. implant metal
    V. Küntscher nail
    V. plate
    V. screw
    V. staple
Vitallium-W implant metal prosthesis
Vitalock
    V. cluster acetabular component
    V. solid-back acetabular component
vitamin
    v. C, D, K deficiency
    v. D-dependent rickets (VDDR)
    v. D-resistant rickets (VDRR)
    Unique V. E
Vitox
    V. alumina ceramic material
    V. femoral head
Vitrathene
    V. jacket
    V. vest
Viva shoe
Vivelle Transdermal
Vivomex T.E.N.
VL
    vastus lateralis
VLC compression screw
VMA
    vastus medialis advancement
V-medullary nail
VMO
    vastus medialis obliquus
VMO:VL EMG ratio
    vastus medialis obliquus:vastus lateralis
    electromyographic ratio
VMO:VL ratio
VMU
    vertebral motion unit
V. Mueller screwdriver
VO
    voluntary opening
VO$_{2max}$
vocal cord
vocational
    v. assessment
    v. feasibility
Vogue arm sling
void
    signal v.
volar
    v. angulation deformity
    v. aspect
    v. beak ligament
    v. carpal ligament
    v. compartment syndrome
    v. condyle
    v. digital artery

v. epineurolysis
v. finger approach
v. flexed intercalated segment
instability (VISI)
v. glide
v. midline approach
v. midline oblique incision
v. plaster splint
v. plate
v. plate arthroplasty
v. plate arthroplasty technique
fracture-dislocation
v. plate repair
v. radial approach
v. semilunar wrist dislocation
v. shear fracture
v. surface
v. synovectomy
v. ulnar approach
v. wrist
v. zigzag finger incision

volare
ligamentum carpi v.

volarly

volarward approach

volitional
v. activity
v. contraction
v. exercise
v. fatigue
v. muscle action test

volitionally

Volkmann
V. bone curette
V. bone hook
V. canal
V. claw hand
V. clawhand deformity
V. fracture
V. ischemia
V. ischemic contracture
V. ischemic paralysis
V. rake retractor
V. splint

Volkov-Oganesian
V.-O. elbow distraction device
V.-O. external fixation
V.-O. external fixation apparatus
V.-O. external fixation device

**Volkov-Oganesian-Povarov hinged
distraction apparatus**

volleys of pain

Volpicelli functional ambulation scale

voltage

Voltaren
V. Ophthalmic
V. Oral
V.-XR Oral

volume conduction

volumeter
Ableware V.
foot v.
hand v.
v. set

voluntary
v. activity
v. closing (VC)
v. closing terminal device
v. control (VC)
v. control 4-bar knee
v. opening (VO)
v. opening terminal device

Volz
V. total wrist arthroplasty
V. wrist
V. wrist prosthesis

Volz-Turner
V.-T. reattachment
V.-T. reattachment technique

vomer

von
v. Bekhterev reflex
v. Hippel-Lindau syndrome
v. Lackum transection shift jacket
v. Lackum transection shift jacket
brace
v. Langenbeck periosteal elevator
v. Recklinghausen disease
v. Rosen abduction splint
v. Rosen cruciform splint
v. Rosen splint hip orthosis
v. Rosen view
v. Saal medullary pin
v. Schwann law
v. Weber triangle
v. Willebrand disease

VonFrey hair test

VonMises stress

Voorhoeve disease

Voshell
V. bursa
V. sign
V. test

V

NOTES

Vostal
>   V. classification of radial fracture
>   V. radial fracture classification

V-osteotomy
>   Japas V-o.
>   offset V-o.

VOS wrench

VPM
>   Vantage Performance monitor

VPT
>   vibration perception threshold

VRO
>   varus rotational osteotomy

VS
>   vertical shear

VSA
>   Very Special Arts

VSC
>   vertebral subluxation complex

VSF
>   Vermont spinal fixator
>   VSF clamp

V-shaped
>   V-s. incision
>   V-s. osteotomy

"V" sign

VSL technology

VSP
>   variable screw placement

variable screw plate
variable spinal plating
>   VSP fixation
>   VSP plate
>   VSP plate instrumentation
>   VSP system

VTED
>   venous thromboembolic disease

vulgaris
>   verruca v.

Vulpius
>   V. Achilles tendon reconstruction
>   V. equinus deformity operation
>   V. lengthening
>   V. procedure

Vulpius-Compere
>   V.-C. gastrocnemius lengthening
>   V.-C. tendon technique

Vulpius-Stoffel procedure

VuRyser monitor lift

V-Y
>   V-Y advancement flap
>   V-Y Kutler flap
>   V-Y plasty
>   V-Y plasty correction of varus toe
>   V-Y quadricepsplasty

WACH orthopaedic shoe
wad
    flexor w.
    mobile w.
Waddell
    W. Chronic Back Pain Disability
      index
    W. triad
wadding
    cotton sheet w.
    shot w.
waddling gait
Wadsworth
    W. elbow approach
    W. posterolateral approach
    W. technique
    W. unconstrained elbow prosthesis
wafer procedure
Wagdy double-V osteotomy
Wagner
    W. acetabular reamer
    W. approach
    W. classification
    W. closed pinning
    W. device external fixator
    W. distractor
    W. external fixation apparatus
    W. external fixation device
    W. femoral lengthening
    W. femoral metaphyseal shortening
    W. frame
    W. leg-lengthening apparatus
    W. limb lengthening method
    W. modification of Syme
      amputation
    W. open reduction technique
    W. profundus advancement
    W. prosthesis
    W. retractor
    W. revision hip system
    W. skin incision
    W. tibial lengthening
    W. trochanteric advancement
    W. two-stage Syme amputation
Wagner-Schanz
    W.-S. screw
    W.-S. screw apparatus
    W.-S. screw device
wagon
    dumbbell w.
    w. wheel fracture
Wagoner
    W. cervical technique
    W. posterior approach
    W. ulcer

Wagstaffe fracture
Wagstaff tubercle
Wainwright plate
waist
    w. of the phalanx
    w. suspension belt
wake-up test
Waldenstrom macroglobulinemia
Waldron test
WALK
    weight-activated locking knee
walk
    w. test
    toe w.
Walkabout walker
WalkAide system
Walk-A-Matic walker
walker
    air w.
    ATO w.
    w. basket
    Cam w.
    cast w.
    Castaway ankle w.
    Castaway leg w.
    Charcot restraint orthotic w.
      (CROW)
    Comfy w.
    controlled ankle w.
    Delta w.
    DH pressure relief w.
    EasyStep pressure relief w.
    Equalizer air w.
    four-point w.
    Guardian w.
    hemiambulator w.
    Hi-Top foot/ankle w.
    W. hollow quill pin
    Lumex w.
    Merry W.
    Moon W.
    obese w.
    ORLAU swivel w.
    ProROM w.
    Rolator w.
    Rollator Nova w.
    rubber sole cast w.
    rubber wedge w.
    W. ruptured disk curette
    Sabel cast w.
    short leg w.
    w. skis
    w. sleds
    swivel w.
    three-wheel w.

W

walker *(continued)*
 Urban W.
 Walkabout w.
 Walk-A-Matic w.
walking
 aerobic w.
 w. biomechanics
 bipedal w.
 w. boot cast
 w. brace
 crutch w.
 w. heel
 heel and toe w.
 nonweightbearing crutch w.
 w. program
 toe w.
Walk-'n-Tone exerciser
wall
 medial w.
 w.-slide exercise
Walldius Vitallium mechanical knee prosthesis
Wallenberg
 W. procedure
 W. syndrome
 W. test
wallerian degeneration
Wal-Pil-O neck pillow
Walter-Liston forceps
Walther fracture
Walton
 W. maneuver
 W. meniscal clamp
 W. wire-pulling forceps
Walton-Ruskin forceps
Wanchik
 W. neutral position splint
 W. writer
wand
 Arthrocare w.
 TCFO placement w.
 TriggerWheel W.
wandering alarm
Wangensteen
 W. needle
 W. needle holder
waning discharge
Ward
 W. periosteal elevator
 W. triangle
Ward-Tomasin-Vander-Griend fixation
warfarin sodium
warm
 w. ischemia
 w. ischemic time
 W.-Up active wound therapy system

warm-and-form
 w.-a.-f. cast
 w.-a.-f. insert
warmer
 gel w.
 Thermasonic gel w.
Warm Springs brace
warmth
 joint w.
Warner-Farber
 W.-F. ankle fixation
 W.-F. ankle fixation technique
Warren-Mack rotating drill
Warren-Marshall classification
Warren White Achilles tendon lengthening
Warsaw hip prosthesis
wart
 mosaic w.
 plantar w. (PW)
Wartenberg
 W. disease
 W. pinwheel
 W. sign
washboard syndrome
washer
 C w.
 contoured w.
 w. crimper
 w. holder
 male/female w.
 oval w.
 plate spacer w.
 Synthes ligament w.
 toothed w.
wash mitt
Wassel
 W. classification of thumb polydactyly
 W. thumb duplication classification
 W. type IV thumb duplication
Wasserstein fixation device
wasting
 quadriceps w.
Watanabe
 W. classification of discoid meniscus
 W. discoid meniscus classification
 W. pin
 W. pin holder
 W. retractor
Watco
 W. brace
 W. knee immobilizer
water acceptance test
Waterman osteotomy
waterpick
Water Pik irrigation

Waterpillow
Mediflow W.
water-soluble contrast agent
Waters x-ray view
Watkins
W. fusion
W. fusion technique
WATSMART stereography system
Watson
W. scaphotrapeziotrapezoidal fusion
W. technique
W. test
Watson-Cheyne-Burghard procedure
Watson-Cheyne technique
Watson-Jones
W.-J. ankle tenodesis
W.-J. anterior approach
W.-J. arthrodesis
W.-J. bone gouge
W.-J. classification of tibial
tubercle avulsion fracture
W.-J. fracture repair
W.-J. frame
W.-J. guidepin
W.-J. incision
W.-J. lateral approach
W.-J. nail
W.-J. procedure
W.-J. reconstruction
W.-J. spinal fracture classification
W.-J. tibial fracture classification
W.-J. traction
Waugh
W. knee prosthesis
W. total ankle replacement
prosthesis
wave
A w.
axon w.
double flexion w.
F w.
H w.
w. keyboard
M w.
positive w.
positive sharp w.
T w.
W. Web
waveform
biphasic (low-volt) w.
bipolar IF w.
electrical stimulator w.

micro w.
monophasic (high-volt) w.
quadpolar IF w.
Russian w.
wax
bone w.
Horsley bone w.
Wayfarer prosthesis
Wayne County reduction
WC
wheelchair
WCS
Wisconsin Compression System
WCS-90
Clorpactin W.
WD
wrist disarticulation
WD, WN
well developed, well nourished
weakness
breakaway w.
motor w.
overstretch w.
wear
abnormal shoe w.
asymmetric w.
w. debris
shoe w.
Softflex Wrist W.
three-body w.
wear-and-tear degeneration
weaver
W. rockerbottom shoe
Weaver-Dunn
W.-D. acromioclavicular operation
W.-D. acromioclavicular technique
W.-D. procedure
W.-D. resection
weaver's bottom
web
w. area of hand
w. border of hand
w. contracture
w. corn
finger w.
w. space
w. space creep
w. space flap
w. space infection
thumb w.
Wave W.

NOTES

W

Webb
- W. bolt nail
- W. fixation
- W. pin
- W. stove bolt

Webb-Andreesen condylar bolt

webbed
- w. finger
- w. toe

Weber
- W. C fracture
- W. classification
- W. classification of physeal injury
- W. fracture classification system
- W. frame
- W. hip implant
- W. humeral osteotomy
- W. Permalock
- W. procedure
- W. static two-point discrimination
- W. subcapital osteotomy
- W. syndrome
- W. test

Weber-Brunner-Freuler-Boitzy technique
Weber-Brunner-Freuler open reduction
Weber-Danis ankle injury classification
Weber-Vasey
- W.-V. traction-absorption
- W.-V. traction-absorption wiring technique

Webril
- W. bandage
- W. cotton padding
- W. dressing
- W. immobilization

webspace incision
Webster
- W. needle
- W. needle holder

Weck
- W. knife
- W. osteotome

Weckesser technique
Wedeen wire passer
wedge
- abduction w.
- w. adjustable cushioned heel
- w. adjustable cushioned heel shoe
- Ballert Buildup foot w.
- bone w.
- bumper w.
- cast w.
- closing base w.
- compensatory w.
- w. compression fracture
- Duo-Cline Dual Support contoured bed w.
- Good 'N Bed w.

- w. graft
- inner heel w. (IHW)
- medial heel w. (MHW)
- medial heel-and-sole w.
- medial sole w.
- w. nonunion
- open w. (OW)
- w. osteotomy
- Positex knee w.
- w. posting
- w. resection
- roof w.
- Saunders mobilization w.
- seating w.
- self-adhering varus/valgus w.
- super w.
- W. TAG suture anchor system
- Tepperwedge w.
- Yancy cast w.

wedge-shaped
- w.-s. osteotomy
- w.-s. uncomminuted fragment
- w.-s. uncomminuted tibial plateau fracture
- w.-s. vertebra

wedging
- w. cast
- w. of olisthetic vertebra

Wegener granulomatosis
weight
- w. acceptance
- w.-activated locking knee (WALK)
- w.-bearing rotation injury
- w. boot
- distal segment w.
- lean body w. (LBW)
- w. training

weightbearing
- w. acetabular dome
- w. axis
- w. brace
- w. crutch
- w. dome of acetabulum
- w. dorsoplantar view
- full w. (FWB)
- w. ground reaction force
- w. joint
- pain with w.
- partial w.
- progression to full w.
- w. surface
- w. symmetry
- w. tangential radiograph
- toe-touch w.
- touchdown w.

weighted
- w. pen
- w. walking stick

weightlifter's clavicle
weight-relieving
    w.-r. caliper
    w.-r. Forte harness
    w.-r. orthosis
weights and pulleys
Weil
    W. implant
    W. pelvic sling
    W. splint
Weiland
    W. classification
    W. harvesting
    W. iliac crest bone graft
Weil-modified Swanson implant
Weinstein enhanced sensory test (WEST)
Weinstein-Ponseti technique
Weinstock desyndactylization
Weise jack screw
Weissman classification
Weiss spring
Weit-Arner retractor
Weitbrecht
    W. ligament
    W. retinaculum
Weitlaner retractor
weld
    callus w.
    cold w.
    hot w.
    spot w.
well developed, well nourished (WD, WN)
well-differentiated myxoid liposarcoma
Weller
    W. cartilage forceps
    W. total hip joint prosthesis
well-leg
    w.-l. cast
    w.-l. holder
    w.-l. raising
    w.-l. raising test
    w.-l. splint
    w.-l. support
    w.-l. traction
Wells
    W. pedicle clamp
    W. traction
well-seated prosthesis
Wenger plate
Werdnig-Hoffmann disease

Werenskiold sign
Wertheim-Bohlman technique
Wertheim splint
WEST
    Weinstein enhanced sensory test
    work evaluation systems technology
West
    W. bone chisel
    W. bone gouge
    W. hand dissector
    W. nerve tester
    W. osteotome
    W. Point Ankle Grading System
    W. Point axillary lateral radiograph
    W. Point axillary lateral view
    W. Shur cartilage clamp
    W. and Soto-Hall patella technique
Westcott Pyramid Program
Westergren sedimentation rate
Wester meniscal clamp
Western
    W. blot test
    W. Ontario and McMaster University osteoarthritis index
"western boot" in open fracture
Westfield acromioclavicular immobilizer
Westfield-style envelope sling
WEST-foot nerve tester
Westhaven Yale Multidimensional Pain Inventory (WHYMPI)
Westin-Hall incision
Westin tenodesis
Westin-Turco category
West-Soto-Hall
    W.-S.-H. patellar technique
    W.-S.-H. patellectomy
wet gangrene
wet-to-dry dressing
WFE
    Williams flexion exercise
What's Wrong ColorCards
Wheaton brace
WHECS
    wrist hand extension compression support
wheel
    Carborundum grinding w.
    pin w.
    shoulder w.
wheelchair (WC)
    Action Jr. w.
    Amigo mechanical w.
    antitipper w.

W

NOTES

wheelchair *(continued)*
Applause Super-Hemi w.
Epic w.
HiRider motorized/lift w.
Invacare w.
Jay J2 w.
Lumex lightweight w.
manual w.
Nitro w.
power w.
Quickie Carbon w.
Quickie EX w.
Quickie GPS w.
Quickie GP Swing-Away w.
Quickie GPV w.
Quickie Kidz w.
Quickie Recliner w.
Quickie Ti w.
self-propelling w.
Skil-Care reclining w.
Slam'r w.
Vision Epic w.
4XP Tilt System w.
Zippie 2 w.
Zippie P500 w.
whiplash
acute w.
whiplash-shaken infant syndrome
Whipple disease
whirlpool bath (WPB)
whiskering
white
w. blood cell count
W. chisel
W. epiphysiodesis
w. fixation
w. matter
W. posterior ankle fusion
W. posterior arthrodesis
W. screwdriver
W. slide procedure
w. tendo calcaneus lengthening
Whitecloud-LaRocca
W.-L. cervical arthrodesis
W.-L. fibular strut graft
Whitehall
W. Glacier Pack
W. thermalator
White-Kraynick tendo calcaneus
Whitesides
W. knee prosthesis
W. line
W. Ortholoc II condylar femoral
prosthesis
W. technique
W. tissue pressure determination
Whitesides-Kelly cervical technique
Whitfield's Ointment

whitlow
herpetic w.
Whitman
W. arch support
W. femoral neck reconstruction
W. frame
W. osteotomy
W. paralysis
W. plate
W. talectomy procedure
W. traction
Whitman-Thompson procedure
Whitney single-use plastic curette
WHO
wrist-hand orthosis
whole
w.-body vibration
w. bone transplant
w. fibular transplant
whorled pattern
WHYMPI
Westhaven Yale Multidimensional Pain
Inventory
Wiberg
center-edge angle of W.
W. center edge angle
W. fracture staple
W. fracture stapler
W. patellar classification
W. periosteal elevator
W. type II patellar contour
Wichman retractor
wick
W. catheter technique
w. technique
wicking catheter
wide
w.-based gait
w. excision
w.-mesh petroleum gauze dressing
w. periosteal elevator
w. toebox shoe
width
step w.
Wiet
W. cup forceps
W. graft-measuring instrument
Wikco ankle machine
Wilco ankle exerciser
Wilcoxon matched-pairs signed-rank test
Wilde
W. ethmoid forceps
W. rongeur forceps
Wiley-Galey classification
Wilke
W. boot
W. boot brace
Wilkie syndrome

Wilkinson synovectomy
Wilkins radial fracture classification
Willauer-Gibbon periosteal elevator
William
    W. Harris hip prosthesis
    W. microlumbar disk excision
Williams
    W. Advantage table
    W. brace
    W. diskectomy
    W. diskography
    W. exercise program
    W. flexion exercise (WFE)
    W. interlocking Y nail
    W. Model 170 table
    W. orthosis
    W. procedure
    W. rod
    W. screwdriver
    W. self-retaining retractor
Williams-Haddad
    W.-H. release
    W.-H. technique
Williger
    W. bone curette
    W. bone mallet
    W. periosteal elevator
willow fracture
Wilmington
    W. plastic jacket
    W. scoliosis brace
Wilson
    W. ankle fusion
    W. bolt
    W. bone graft
    W. bunionectomy
    W. cone arthrodesis
    W. convex frame
    W. disease
    W. double oblique osteotomy
    W. fracture
    W. gonad retractor
    W. oblique displacement osteotomy
    W. plate
    W. procedure for extraarticular
      fusion of elbow
    W. sign
    W. splint
    W. technique
    W. test
Wilson-Burstein hip internal prosthesis

Wilson-Cook prosthesis repositioner
Wilson-Jacobs
    W.-J. patellar graft
    W.-J. tibial fixation
    W.-J. tibial fracture fixation
      technique
Wilson-Johansson-Barrington
    W.-J.-B. cone arthrodesis
Wilson-McKeever
    W.-M. arthroplasty
    W.-M. shoulder technique
Wiltberger anterior cervical approach
Wiltse
    W. ankle osteotomy
    W. approach
    W. bilateral lateral fusion
    W. diskectomy
    W. fixator
    W. osteotomy of ankle
    W. pedicle screw fixation system
    W. system aluminum master rod
    W. system cross-bracing
    W. system double-rod construct
    W. system H construct
    W. system single-rod construct
    W. system spinal rod
    W. varus supramalleolar osteotomy
Wiltse-Spencer paraspinal approach
Wiltze angle
Winberger
    W. line
    W. sign
wince
wincing
Winco
    W. Adjusting Bench
    W. Folding Treatment Table
windblown
    w. deformity
    w. hand, whistling face syndrome
    w. hip
    w. knee
Windlass mechanism
window
    cast w.
    cortical w.
    femoral cortical w.
windowed cast
windowing
    cortical w.
windshield wiper sign

NOTES

W

Windson-Insall-Vince
    W.-I.-V. bone graft
    W.-I.-V. grafting technique
windswept
    w. deformity
    w. hip
wind-up
    w.-u. injury
    w.-u. phenomenon
wing
    Badgley resection of iliac w.
    dorsal w.
    w. excision of Littler
    iliac w.
    w. of ilium
    w. plate
Wingfield frame
winging
    w. motion
    w. of scapula
    scapular w.
wink
    40 W.'s
    anal w.
    W. retractor
    w. sign
Winkelmann rotationplasty
winking
    Gunn jaw w.
    w. owl sign
Winograd
    W. ingrown nail technique
    W. nail plate removal
    W. partial matrixectomy
    W. technique for ingrown nail
Winquist femoral shaft fracture
  classification
Winquist-Hansen
    W.-H. classification of femoral
      fracture
    W.-H. femoral fracture classification
    W.-H. fracture comminution
      classification system
Winquist-Hansen-Pearson closed femoral
  diaphyseal shortening
Winter
    W. convex fusion
    W. splint
    W. spondylolisthesis
    W. spondylolisthesis technique
wipe test
wire
    bayonet-point w.
    w. bending pliers
    Brooker w.
    Bunnell pullout w.
    calibrated guide w.
    cerclage w.

circular w.
circumferential w.
Compere w.
compression w.
w. contour preparation
w. crimper
w. cutter
Dall-Miles cerclage w.
definitive cerclage w.
w. drill
w. and drill guide
w. driver
Drummond w.
w.-extracting forceps
w. fixation bolt
w.-fixation buckle
W.-Foam Orthotic
guide w.
w.-holding forceps
Ilizarov w.
interfragmentary w.
intraosseous w.
Isola w.
K-w.
Kirschner w. (K-wire)
w. knot
w. loop
loop circumferential w.
w. loop fixation
Luque cerclage w.
Magnuson w.
Martin loop circumferential w.
monofilament w.
nonthreaded w.
olive w.
Oppenheimer spring w.
Outrigger w.
over-tying w.
w. passage
w. passer
w. penetration depth
w. prosthesis-crimping forceps
w.-pulling forceps
w. removal technique
Schauwecker patellar tension
  band w.
sharp-pointed w.
smooth transfixion w.
spinous process w.
w. splint
w. stabilization
stainless steel w.
sublaminar w.
w. suture
temporary cerclage w.
tension band w.
Thiersch w.
threaded w.

w. tightener
trochanteric w.
w.-twisting forceps
unscher w.
unthreaded w.
Wisconsin button w.

wire-cutting
    w.-c. forceps
    w.-c. scissors

wire-tightening
    w.-t. clamp
    w.-t. forceps

wiring
    cervical oblique facet w.
    circumferential w.
    compression w.
    facet fracture stabilization w.
    facet subluxation stabilization w.
    figure-of-eight w.
    interfacet w.
    interspinous w.
    intraosseous w.
    Luque w.
    oblique facet w.
    posterior interspinous w.
    Schauwecker patellar w.
    spinous process w.
    sublaminar w.
    tension-band w.
    Wisconsin w.

Wirth-Jager tendon technique

Wisconsin
    W. button
    W. button wire
    W. Compression System (WCS)
    W. interspinous segmental spinal
      instrumentation
    W. wire fixation
    W. wiring

Wissinger rod
Wister wire/pin cutter
Wit portable TENS system
Wixson hip positioner
wobble
    w. board
    Wooden W.

Wolf
    W. arthroscope
    W. full-thickness free graft
    W. light source

Wolfe-Böhler
    W.-B. cast breaker
    W.-B. mallet

Wolfe-Kawamoto bone graft
Wolferman drill
wolffii
    Acinetobacter w.

Wolff law
Wolfson frame
Wolin meniscoid lesion
Wolvek sternal approximation fixation
Women
    Selsun Gold for W.

Wonder-Cup heel cup
Wonderflex silicone
Wonder-Spur heel cup
Wonderzorb
    W. heel cup
    Soft Silicones W.

wood
    W. alloy
    W. lamp

wooden
    w. postoperative clogs
    w. shoe
    w.-soled shoe
    W. Wobble

Woodruff
    W. screw
    W. screwdriver
    W. tip

woodscrew (*var. of* wood screw)
wood screw
Woodson
    W. elevator
    W. probe

Woodward
    W. operation wound
    W. procedure
    W. technique

Woodway treadmill
Woofry-Chandler classification of
   Osgood-Schlatter lesion
Woringer-Kolopp disease
work
    concentric w.
    w. conditioning
    eccentric w.
    w. evaluation systems technology
      (WEST)
    w. hardening
    w. hardening exercise

NOTES

W

work *(continued)*
    w. hardening program
    negative w.
    physical w.
    sedentary w.
Workers' Compensation
worm drive
wormian bone
Wort
    Saint John's W.
wound
    closed w.
    w. closure
    w. culture
    w. dehiscence
    foot puncture w.
    gunshot w.
    Gustilo classification of
      puncture w.
    incised w.
    w. irrigation
    joint w.
    w. measuring guide
    open w.
    w. packing
    puncture w.
    self-inflicted gunshot w.
    shotgun w.
    stab w.
    Woodward operation w.
Wound-Evac drain
woven bone
WPB
    whirlpool bath
W-plasty
wrap
    Ace w.
    AquaWrap coding compression w.
    BodyIce w.
    boot w.
    Coban elastic w.
    Coflex w.
    Coopercare Lastrap support w.
    digit w.
    Dura-Kold reusable compression
      ice w.
    Dura-Soft soft-compression reusable
      ice or heat w.
    Elasto-Gel hot/cold w.
    Elasto-Gel shoulder therapy w.
    Elasto-Link joint w.
    Electro-Link joint w.
    gauze w.
    gel w.
    Ice Wedge hot/cold therapy w.
    joint w.
    kastRAP w.
    Kerlix w.

    kneeRAP w.
    Kold W.
    loop-over w.
    neck w.
    Nylatex w.
    shoulderRAP w.
    Stimprene w.
    super w.
    Thermosport hot/cold w.
    Unna boot w.
    Velpeau w.
wraparound
    w. flap bone graft
    w. neurovascular composite free
      tissue transfer
    w. neurovascular free flap
    w. splint
wrapping
    compressive centripetal w.
    nerve w.
    stump w.
wrench
    Allen w.
    beaded-pin w.
    box-end w.
    cannulated w.
    Fox w.
    Harrington flat w.
    hex w.
    Key-loc w.
    Kurlander orthopaedic w.
    locknut w.
    Mueller w.
    open-end w.
    w. pin
    socket w.
    T-handled nut w.
    T-handled screw w.
    torque w.
    TSRH w.
    ventral derotating spinal w.,
      VOS w.
wrenched knee
wrestler's elbow
Wright
    W. knee prosthesis
    W. maneuver
    W. plate
    W. test
    W. Universal brace
Wright-Adson test
Wrightlock
    W. posterior fixation system
    W. spinal fixation system
wringer
    w. arm
    w. injury
wrinkle test

Wrisberg
> W. lesion
> ligament of W.
> W. ligament type of discoid
> meniscus

wrist
> w. creaking
> w. curl
> w. deformity
> w. disarticulation (WD)
> w. drop
> w. extensor
> w. extensor tendinitis
> w. extensor tendon
> w. flexion test
> w. flexor tendinitis
> w. gauntlet
> gymnast's w.
> w. hand extension compression
> support (WHECS)
> w.-hand orthosis (WHO)
> w. joint implant prosthesis
> w. pain syndrome
> W. Pro wrist support device

> slack w.
> w. speed profile
> tilt w.
> total arthrodesis of the w.
> volar w.
> Volz w.

wrist-driven
> w.-d. flexor hinge orthosis
> w.-d. prehension orthosis
> w.-d. wrist-hand orthosis

Wristiciser
> W. exerciser

WristJack wrist splint

Wristlet
> FREEDOM USA W.

writer
> Wanchik w.

wryneck
> congenital w.

Wu bunionectomy

Wullstein drill

Wurzburg plate

Wygesic

Wylie lumbar bulldog clamp

NOTES

W

X

X axis
X clamp
X plate

X-Act podiatric marker
Xanax
xanthogranuloma

juvenile x.

xanthoma

fibrous x.
malignant fibrous x.
tuberous x.

xanthomatous giant cell tumor
xenograft
Xenophor femoral prosthesis
Xerac
Xercise

X. band
X. tube resistive device

Xeroform

X. gauze dressing

xerography
xeroradiography
xerotic
Xertube
XIP

x-ray in plaster

xiphoid process
Xi-scan

X.-s. fluoroscope
X.-s. fluoroscopy
X.-s. image

XiScan mini-C-arm
XL

Lodine XL
Procardia XL

X-long cement forceps
XMB tibial reaming guide
Xomed drill
XOP

x-ray out of plaster

XO-soft-sole orthotic
XPE foot orthosis
4XP Tilt System wheelchair
x-ray

artifact on x-r.
Cedell-Magnusson classification of
  arthritis on x-r.
intraoperative x-r.
x-r. out of plaster (XOP)
x-r. overlay
penciling of ribs on x-r.
x-r. photogrammetry
x-r. in plaster (XIP)
postreduction x-r.
x-r. tray
x-r. view

X-shaped plate
XTB knee extension device
X-TEND-O knee flexor
X-Y

X-Y plotter
X-Y sensor system

(XY)

frontal plane (XY)

Xylocaine

X. with epinephrine

(X,Y,Z)

cardinal axes (X,Y,Z)
coordinate system (X,Y,Z)

X

Y

Y axis
Y bone plate
Y B Sore cushion
Y fracture
Y incision
Yale brace
Yamanda myelotomy knife
Yancey osteotomy
Yancy cast wedge
Yankauer periosteal elevator
Yasargil
Y. elevator
Y. Leyla retractor arm
Y. ligature carrier
Y. ligature guide
Y. needle holder
Y. spring hook
Y-axis translatory displacement
Yeager test
Years
Disability Adjusted Life Y.
(DALYs)
Yee posterior shoulder approach
yellow
y. ligament
y. marrow
y. nail syndrome
Yergason
Y. sign
Y. test of shoulder subluxation

YIS knee prosthesis
Y-knot tying system
Y nail
Williams interlocking Y n.
Yochum chiropractic software
yoga
yoke
Billington y.
Yoke transposition procedure
Young
Y. hinged knee prosthesis
Y. modulus
Y. pelvic fracture classification
Y. procedure
Young-Vitallium hinged prosthesis
Youngwhich modification
Yount
Y. fasciotomy
Y. procedure
Y-shaped
Y.-s. incision
Y.-s. plate
Y-strap knee immobilizer
Y-T fracture
Yuan screw
yucca
Y. board
y. wood splint
Yu osteotomy
Y-V plasty
Y-V-plasty incision

Y

Z

Z axis
Z band
Z fixation nail
Z line
Z pin
Z retractor
Z stent prosthesis

z

z foot

Zadik

Z. foot operation
Z. total matrixectomy
Z. total nail bed ablation

Zahn

lines of Z.

Zaias nail biopsy
zalcitabine
Zanca view
Zancolli

Z. biceps tendon rerouting
Z. capsuloplasty
Z. flexion capsulodesis
Z. procedure for clawhand
    deformity
Z. reconstruction
Z. rerouting technique
Z. static lock procedure

Zancolli-Lasso procedure
Zang

Z. metatarsal cap
Z. metatarsal cap implant

Zariczny ligament technique
Zarins-Rowe

Z.-R. ligament technique
Z.-R. procedure

Zarontin
Zazepen-Gamidov technique
Zeasorb-AF Powder
zebra body myopathy
Zefazone
Zeichner implant
Zeier transfer technique
Zelicof orthopaedic awl
Zel-X
Zenith

Z. ACS table
Z. Hylos table
Z. stationary table
Z. Thompson table
Z. Verti-Lift table

Zenith-Cox flexion/distraction table
Zenker diverticulum
Zenotech biomaterial-synthetic ligament

Zickel

Z. classification
Z. fracture
Z. fracture classification system
Z. medullary apparatus
Z. nail fixation
Z. nailing
Z. rod
Z. subcondylar nail
Z. subtrochanteric fracture fixation
Z. subtrochanteric fracture operation
Z. subtrochanteric nail
Z. supracondylar device
Z. supracondylar fixation apparatus
Z. supracondylar medullary nail

zidovudine-induced myopathy
Zielke

Z. bifid hook
Z. derotator bar
Z. distraction device
Z. gouge
Z. instrumentation for scoliosis
    spinal fusion
Z. pedicular instrumentation
Z. rod
Z. technique

zigzag

z. approach
z. compensatory deformity
z. finger incision

Zimalate twist drill
Zimalite

Z. implant metal
Z. implant metal prosthesis

Zimaloy

Z. femoral head prosthesis
Z. implant metal
Z. implant metal prosthesis
Z. staple

Zimeldine
Zimfoam

Z. head halter
Z. pad
Z. pin
Z. splint
Z. splint traction

Zimmer

Z. airplane splint
Z. Anatomic hip prosthesis system
Z. antiembolism stockings
Z. bone cement
Z. bone stem
Z. cartilage clamp
Z. Centralign Precoat hip prosthesis
Z. Cibatome Cement Eater

Z

Zimmer *(continued)*
    Z. Cibatome cement eater
    Z. clavicular cross splint
    Z. compression hip screw
    Z. continuous anatomical passive exerciser
    Z. crossover instrumentation system
    Z. driver-extractor
    Z. electrical stimulation apparatus
    Z. electrical stimulation device
    Z. extractor
    Z. femoral canal broach
    Z. femoral condyle blade plate
    Z. fracture frame
    Z.-Gigli saw blade
    Z. goniometer
    Z. gouge
    Z. hand drill
    Z. head halter
    Z. hip implant system
    Z. impaction screw-plate
    Z. knee immobilizer
    Z. laminectomy frame
    Z. low viscosity adhesive
    Z. low-viscosity cement
    Z. NexGen LPS knee femoral component
    Z. Orthair ream driver
    Z. oscillating saw
    Z. pin
    Z. PMMA precoat process
    Z. protractor
    Z. Pulsavac wound debridement system
    Z. reamer brace
    Z. rotary bur
    Z. screwdriver
    Z. shoulder prosthesis
    Z. side plate
    Z. skin graft mesher
    Z. snare
    Z. telescoping nail
    Z. tibial bolt
    Z. tibial nail cap
    Z. tibial prosthesis
    Z. Universal drill
    Z. Y plate
Zimmer-Hall drive system
Zimmer-Hoen forceps
Zimmer-Hudson shank
Zimmer-Kirschner hand drill
Zimmerman pericyte
Zimmer-Schlesinger forceps
Zim-Trac
    Z.-T. traction splint
    Z.-T. traction splint tractor

Zim-Zip
    Z.-Z. rib belt
    Z.-Z. rib belt splint
Zinacef Injection
zinc
    Dermagran wound cleanser with z.
Zinco
    Z. ankle orthosis
    Z. CAM walker brace
    Z. thumb-wrist immobilizer
zipper
    Z. anti-disconnect device
    z. cast
Zippie
    Z. P500 wheelchair
    Z. 2 wheelchair
Ziramic femoral head
Zirconia
    Z. femoral head prosthesis
    Z. orthopaedic prosthetic head
    Z. orthopedic prosthesis
zirconium
    z. oxide arthroplasty material
    z. oxide ceramic prosthesis
Z-lengthening of biceps tendon
Zlotsky-Ballard
    Z.-B. acromioclavicular injury classification
    Z.-B. classification of acromioclavicular injury
ZMC
    zygomatic-malar complex
    ZMC fracture
ZMS intramedullary fixation system
Zodiac TM Manual Flexion-Distraction table
Zoeller-Clancy
    Z.-C. procedure
    Z.-C. technique
Zohar shoe
Zolicef
Zollinger
    Z. legholder
    Z. splint
Zoloft
zolpidem
Zonas porous tape
zone
    autonomous z.
    dorsal root entry z. (DREZ)
    elastic z.
    endplate z.
    growth z.
    Gruen z.
    isolated z.
    neutral z. (NZ)
    paraphysiologic z.
    z. of Ranvier

z.-specific cannula
Trümmerfeld z.
zonography
zooplastic graft
Zoradol
Zorbacel shock-absorbing material
Zoroc plaster
ZORprin
Zostrix
Zostrix-HP
Z-plasty
Z-p. approach
Broadbent-Woolf four-limb Z-p.
Cozen-Brockway Z-p.
four-limb Z-p.
Gudas scarf Z-p.
Z-p. incision
Z-p. local flap graft
Peet Z-p.
Z-p. release
scarf Z-p.
Z-p. tenotomy
Z-shaped plate
Z-slide
Z-s. lengthening
Z-s. lengthening in hallux limitus

Z-Stim stimulator
ZTT
Z. acetabular cup
Z. I, II cup
Zucker splint
Zuelzer
Z. awl
Z. hook
Z. hook plate
Z. screw
Zung Depression Index
Zuni
Z. exercise system
Z. gym
Z. harness
Zweymuller
Z. hip prosthesis
Z. hip system
Zydone
zygapophyseal
z. joint
z. joint injection
zygomatic-malar complex (ZMC)
Zyloprim
Zymderm collagen implant
Zyranox femoral head

NOTES

Z

Appendix 1
Anatomical Illustrations

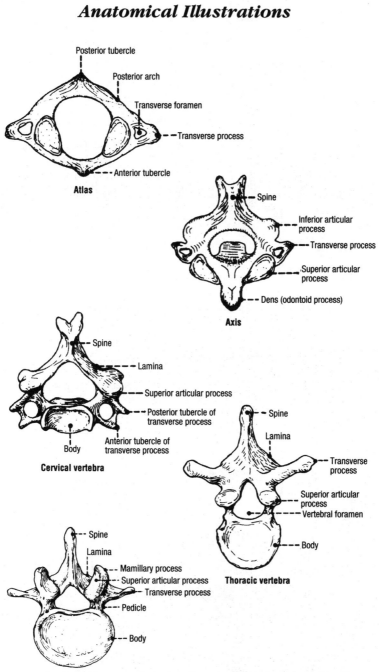

Figure 1. Typical cervical, thoracic, and lumbar vertebrae.

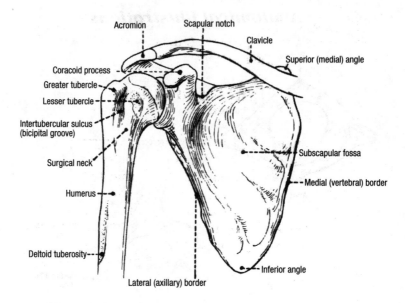

Figure 2. Pectoral girdle and humerus, anterior view.

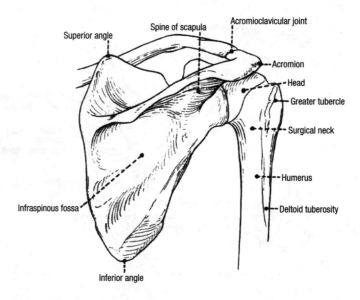

Figure 3. Pectoral girdle and humerus, posterior view.

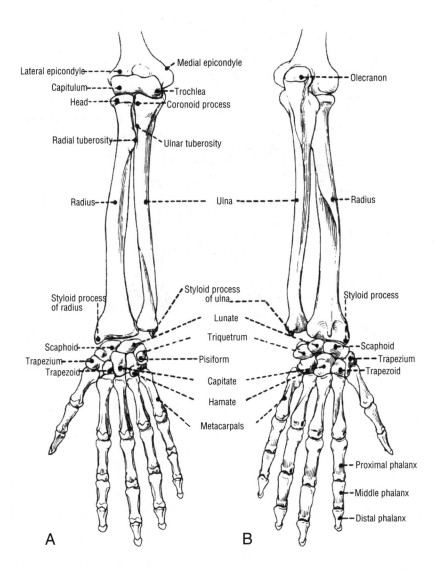

Figure 4. Bones of the forearm and hand. Anterior view (left) and posterior view (right).

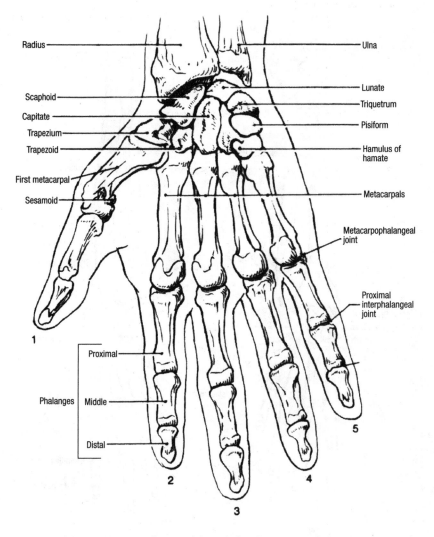

Figure 5. Bones and joints of the right hand, anterior (palmar) view.

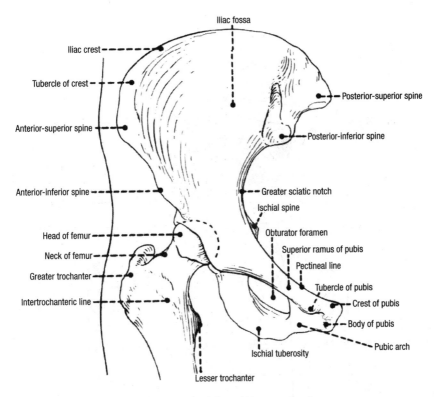

Figure 6. Bones of pelvis and hip, anterior view.

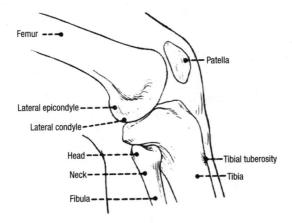

Figure 7. Bones of the knee region, lateral view.

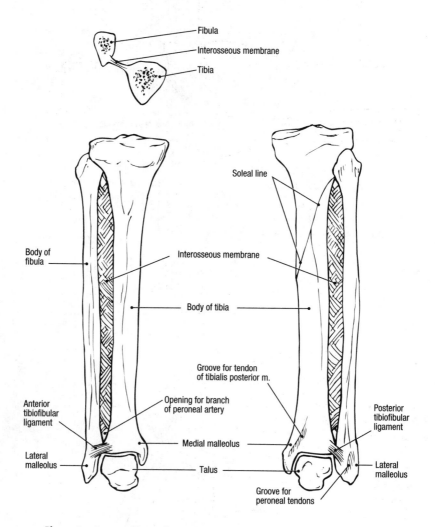

Figure 8. Bones of lower leg. Anterior view (left) and posterior view (right).

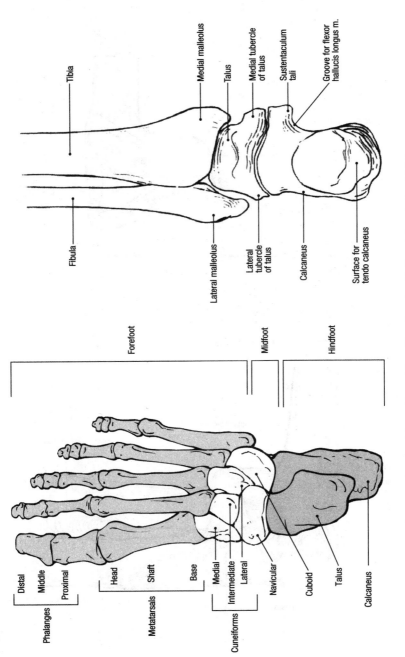

Figure 9. Bones of the ankle and foot. Superior view (left) and dorsal view (right).

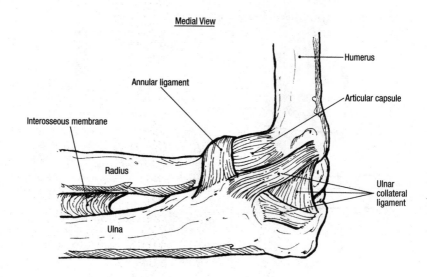

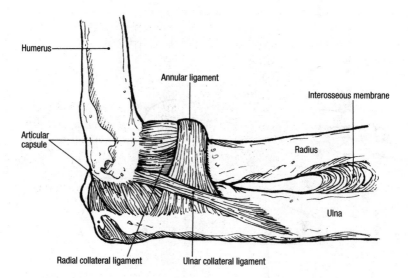

Figure 10. Ligaments of the elbow. Lateral view (above) and medial view (below).

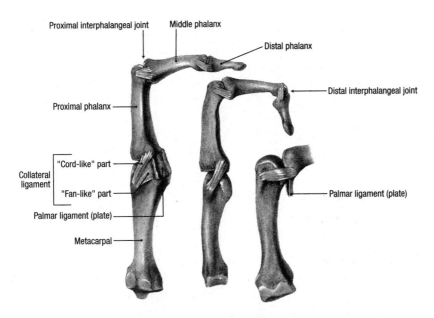

Figure 11. Ligaments of metacarpophalangeal and interphalangeal joints.

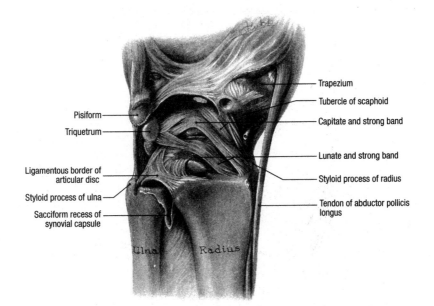

Figure 12. Ligaments of the distal radioulnar, radiocarpal, and intercarpal joints.

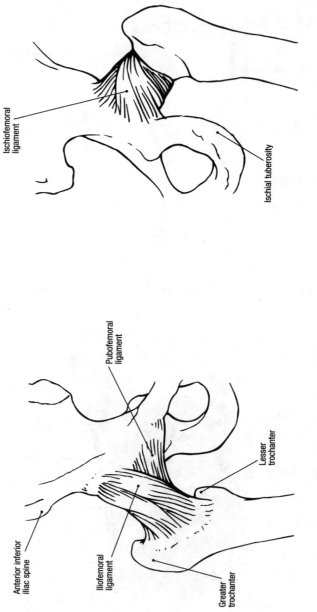

Figure 13. Ligaments of the hip. Anterior (left) and posterior (right) views.

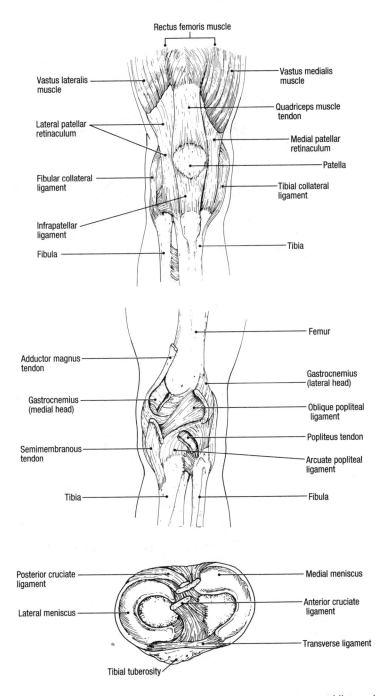

Figure 14. Ligaments of the knee. Anterior view (above), posterior view (middle), and superior view (bottom).

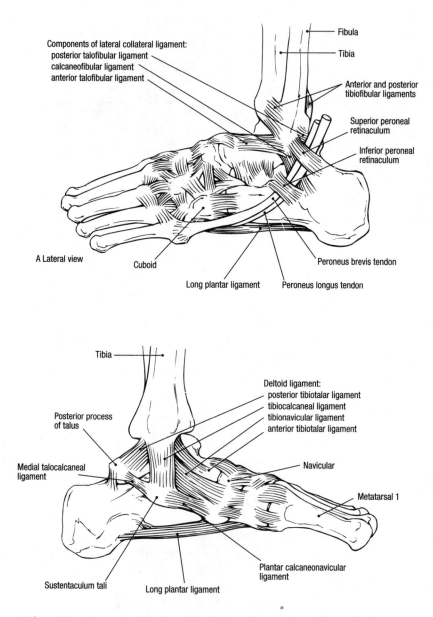

Figure 15. Ligaments of the foot. Lateral view (above) and medial view (below).

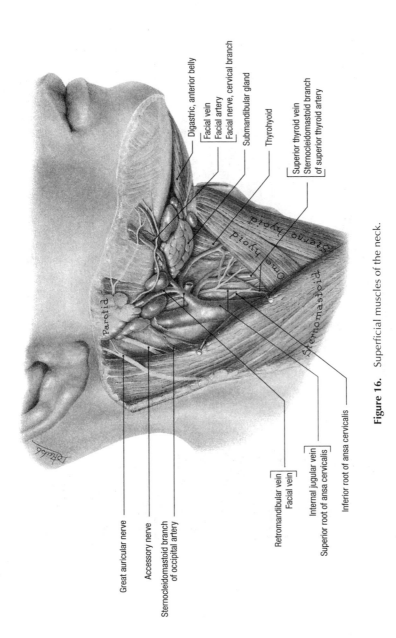

Figure 16. Superficial muscles of the neck.

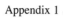

Common trunk of facial and lingual arteries
Stylohyoid
Fascia enveloping submandibular gland

Facial artery
Submental artery
Nerve to Mylohyoid
Hyoid bone
Mylohyoid
Internal laryngeal nerve
Inferior constrictor
Thyrohyoid
External laryngeal nerve
Superior thyroid artery
Sternothyroid
Sternohyoid
Anterior jugular vein

External cartoid artery
Occipital artery
Hypoglossal nerve
Accessory nerve
Superior root of ansa cervicalis
Sternocleidomastoid artery
Internal cartoid artery
External cartoid artery
Ansa cervicalis
Common cartoid artery
Internal jugular vein
Sternocleidomastoid branch
Sternocleidomastoid
"Fascial carpet" of posterior triangle
Transverse cervical vein
Omohyoid fascia
Sternocleidomastoid

Omohyoid
Sternal head
Clavicular head
Clavicle

Figure 17. Deep muscles of the neck.

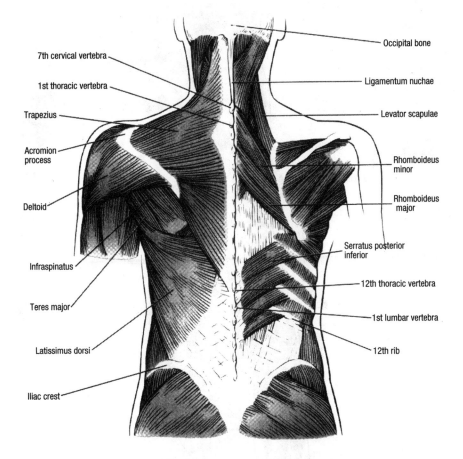

Figure 18. Superficial muscles of the back, posterior view.

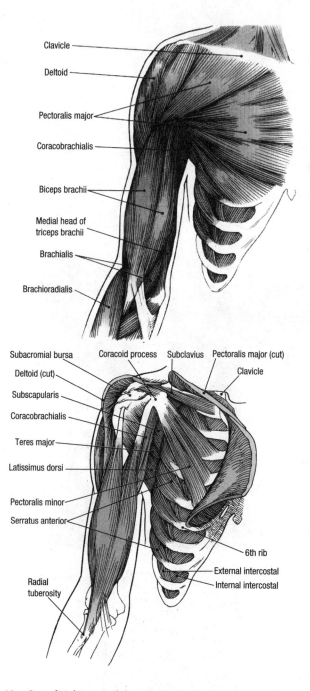

Figure 19. Superficial (top) and deep (bottom) muscles of the shoulder and chest.

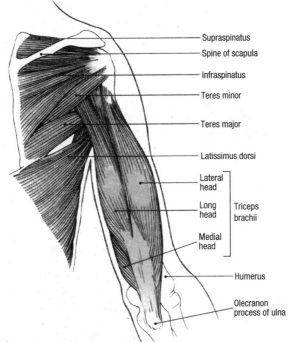

Figure 20. Muscles of the arm, posterior view.

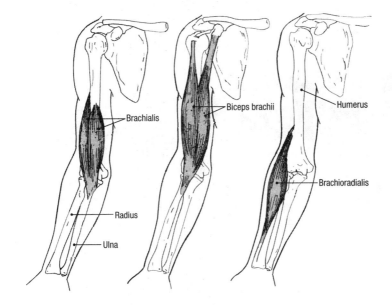

Figure 21. Muscles of the arm, anterior view.

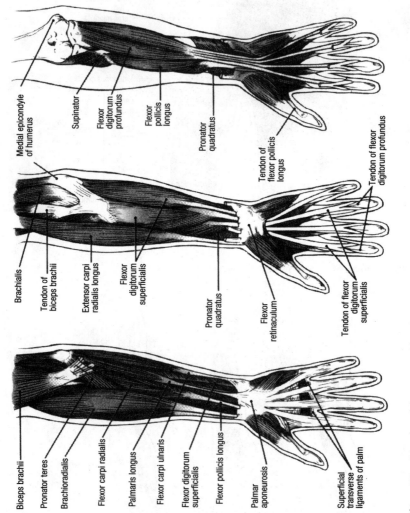

Figure 22. Muscles of the wrist and hand, anterior view. Superficial (left), mid-level (middle), and deep (right).

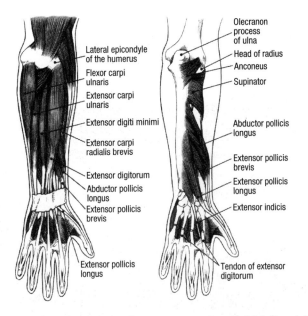

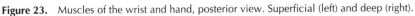

Figure 23. Muscles of the wrist and hand, posterior view. Superficial (left) and deep (right).

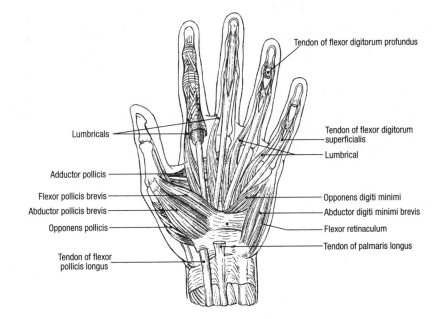

Figure 24. Muscles of the hand, anterior (palmar) view.

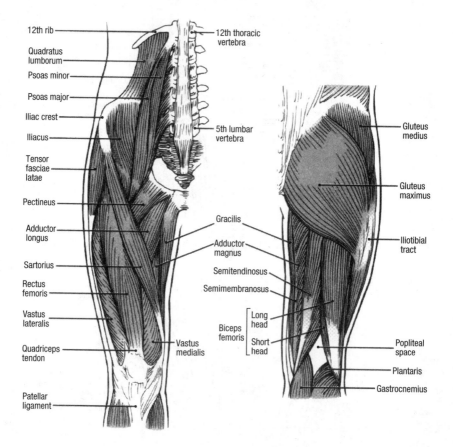

Figure 25. Superficial muscles of the hip and thigh. Anterior view (left) and posterior view (right).

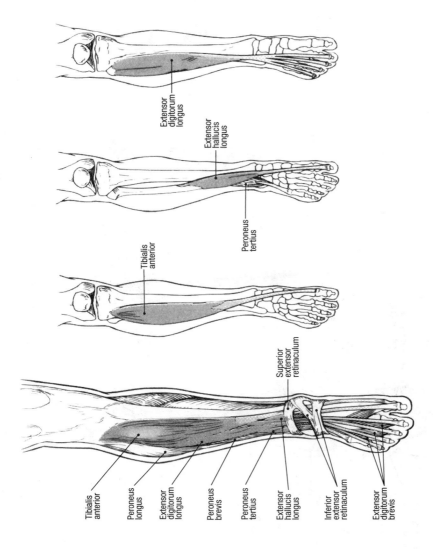

Figure 26. Muscles of the lower leg, anterior compartment.

Extensor digitorum longus

Extensor hallucis longus

Peroneus tertius

Tibialis anterior

Superior extensor retinaculum

Tibialis anterior

Peroneus longus

Extensor digitorum longus

Peroneus brevis

Peroneus tertius

Extensor hallucis longus

Inferior extensor retinaculum

Extensor digitorum brevis

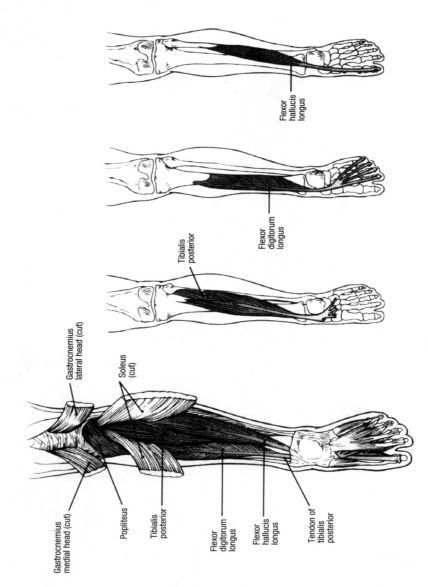

Figure 27. Muscles of the lower leg, deep compartment, posterior view.

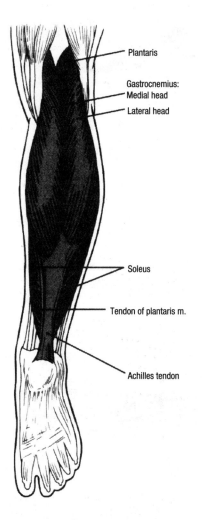

Plantaris

Gastrocnemius:
Medial head
Lateral head

Soleus

Tendon of plantaris m.

Achilles tendon

Figure 28. Muscles of lower leg, superficial compartment, posterior view.

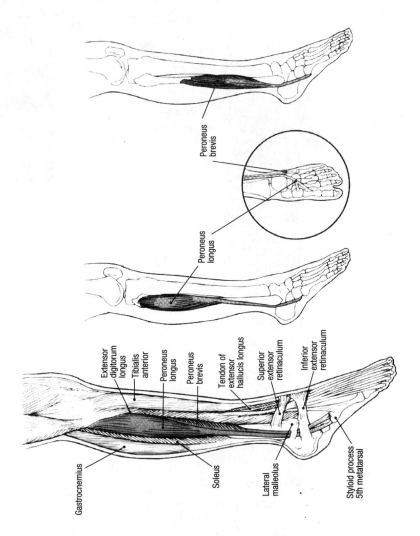

Figure 29. Muscles of the lower leg, lateral compartment.

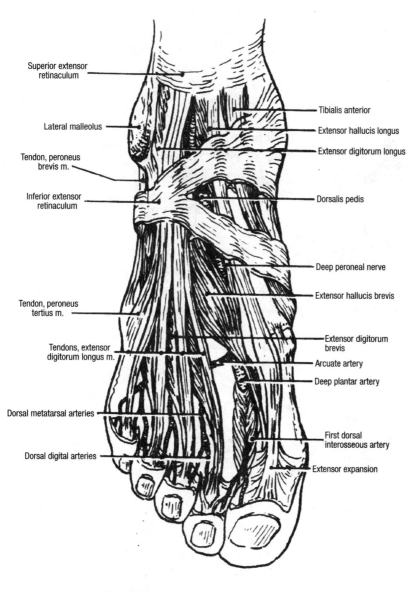

Superior extensor
retinaculum

Lateral malleolus

Tendon, peroneus
brevis m.

Inferior extensor
retinaculum

Tendon, peroneus
tertius m.

Tendons, extensor
digitorum longus m.

Dorsal metatarsal arteries

Dorsal digital arteries

Tibialis anterior

Extensor hallucis longus

Extensor digitorum longus

Dorsalis pedis

Deep peroneal nerve

Extensor hallucis brevis

Extensor digitorum
brevis

Arcuate artery

Deep plantar artery

First dorsal
interosseous artery

Extensor expansion

Figure 30.   Muscles of the dorsum of the foot.

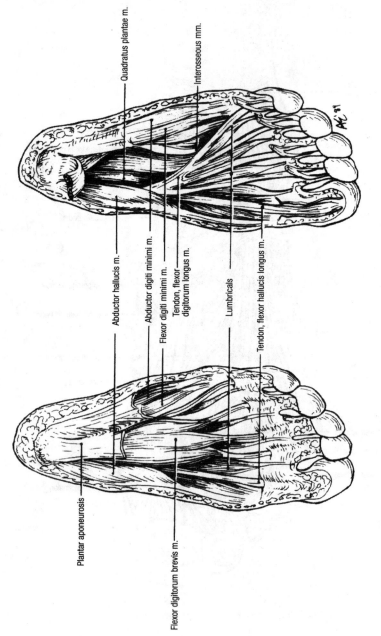

Figure 31. Superficial muscles of the plantar foot. First layer (left) and second layer (right).

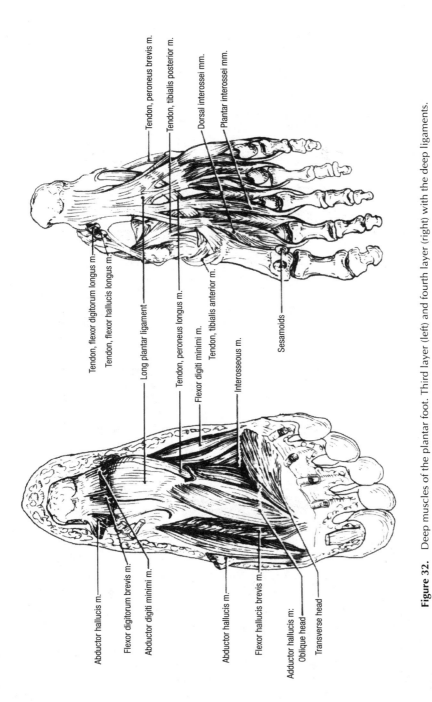

Figure 32. Deep muscles of the plantar foot. Third layer (left) and fourth layer (right) with the deep ligaments.

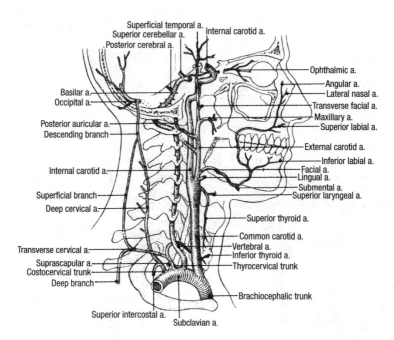

Figure 33. Subclavian and carotid arteries and their branches.

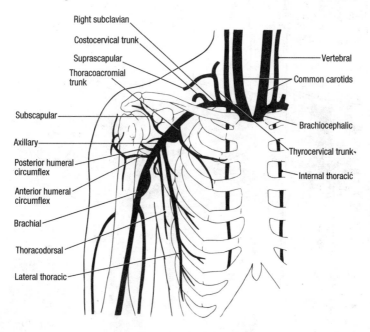

Figure 34. Blood supply to the shoulder.

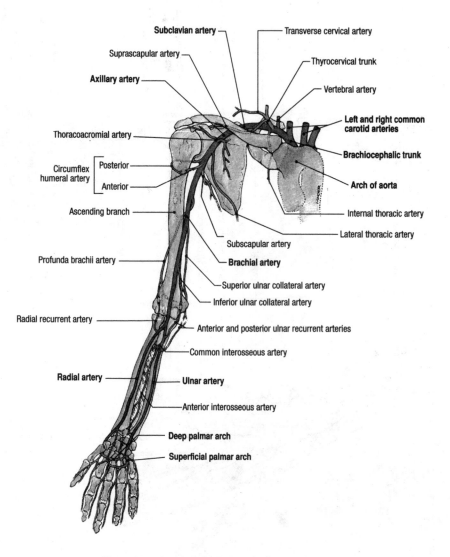

Figure 35. Arteries of the upper limb, anterior view.

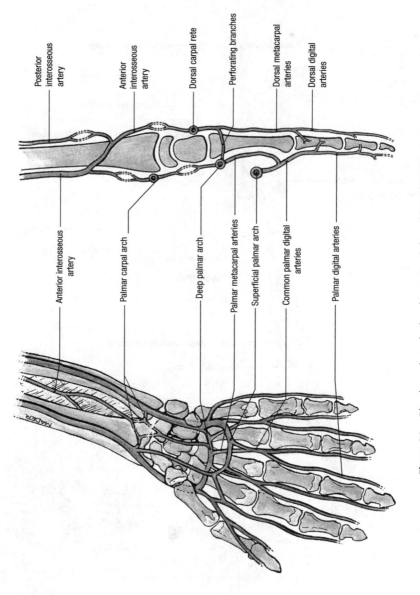

Figure 36. Blood supply to the hand, anterior (left) and lateral (right) views.

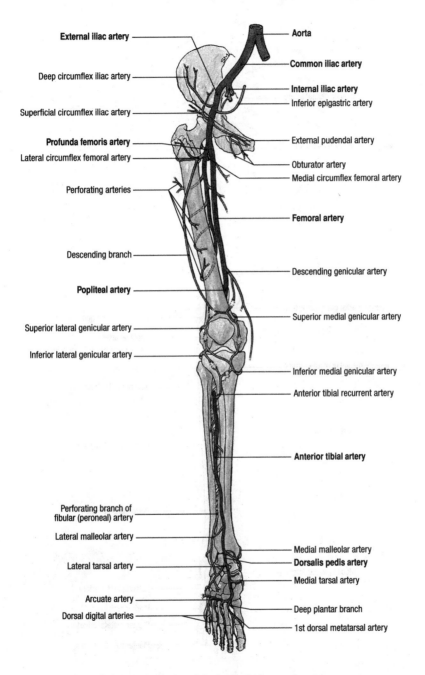

Figure 37. Arteries of the lower limb, anterior view.

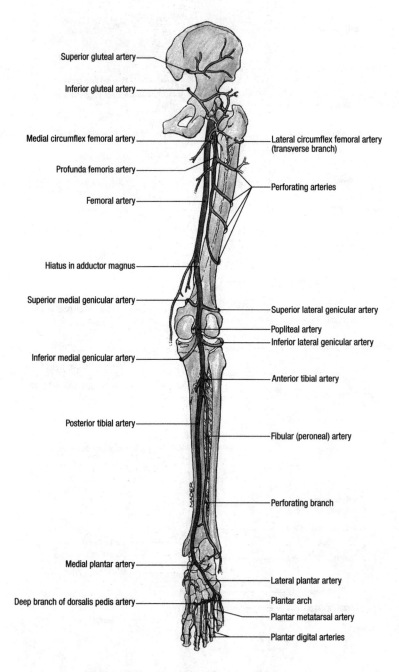

Figure 38. Arteries of the lower limb, posterior view.

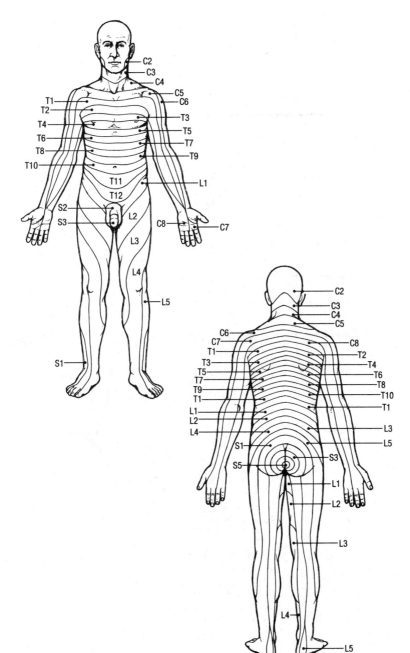

Figure 39. Dermatomes.

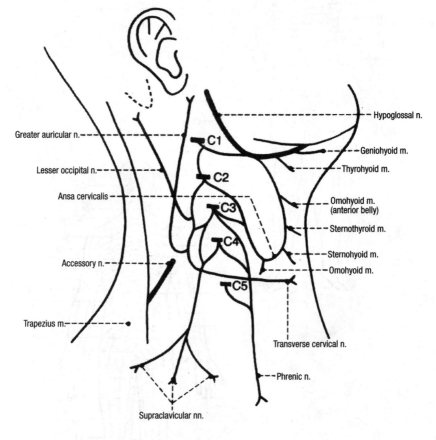

Figure 40. Cervical plexus.

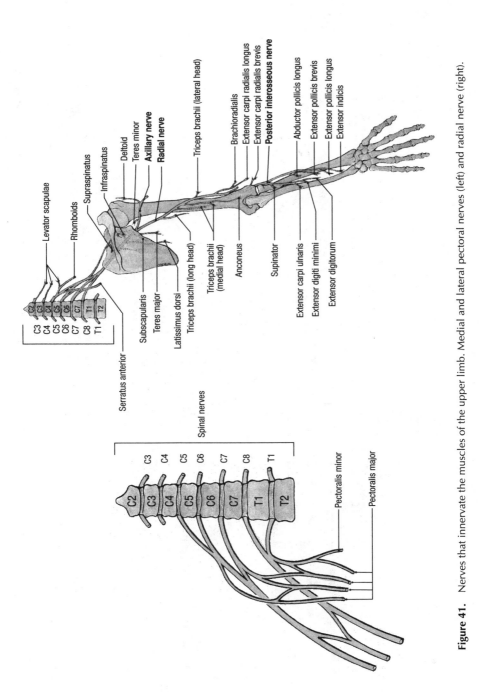

Figure 41. Nerves that innervate the muscles of the upper limb. Medial and lateral pectoral nerves (left) and radial nerve (right).

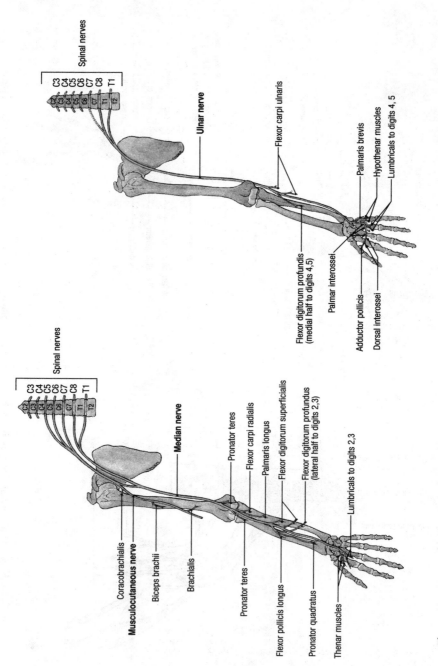

Figure 42. Nerves that innervate the muscles of the upper limb. Median and musculocutaneous nerves (left) and ulnar nerve (right).

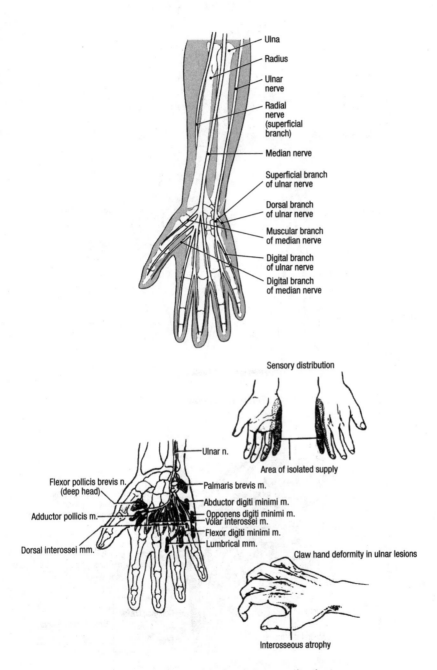

Figure 43. Nerves of the hand—sensory distribution.

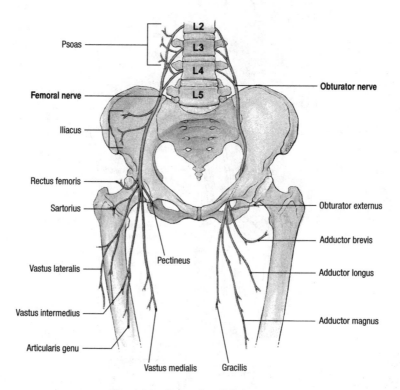

Figure 44. Femoral and obturator nerves.

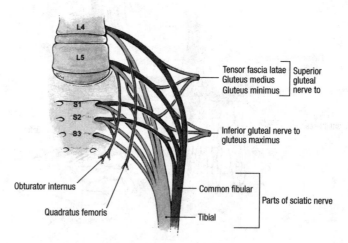

Figure 45. Formation of the sciatic nerve in the pelvis.

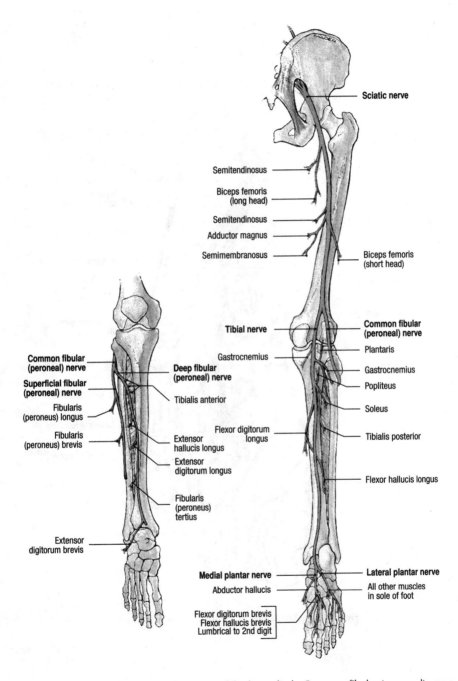

Figure 46. Motor distribution of the nerves of the lower limb. Common fibular (peroneal) nerve (left) and sciatic nerve (right).

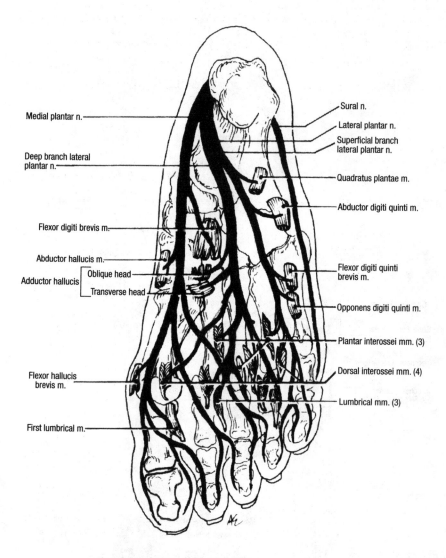

Medial plantar n.

Sural n.

Lateral plantar n.

Superficial branch lateral plantar n.

Deep branch lateral plantar n.

Quadratus plantae m.

Abductor digiti quinti m.

Flexor digiti brevis m.

Abductor hallucis m.

Adductor hallucis — Oblique head

Transverse head

Flexor digiti quinti brevis m.

Opponens digiti quinti m.

Plantar interossei mm. (3)

Dorsal interossei mm. (4)

Flexor hallucis brevis m.

Lumbrical mm. (3)

First lumbrical m.

Figure 47. Distribution of the tibial nerve in the foot.

Appendix 2

Fracture Illustrations

Salter-Harris Classification Table

Type I.	A Type I epiphyseal separation occurs when the fracture extends through the epiphyseal plate, resulting in displacement of the epiphysis.
Type II.	In this injury, the direction of the fracture is similar to the Type I injury; however, a triangular segment of metaphysis is fractured and accompanies the separated epiphyseal fragment.
Type III.	In a Type III epiphyseal fracture, the fracture line extends from the joint through the epiphysis to the epiphyseal plate, and then along the plate, dislodging a segment of epiphysis.
Type IV.	In the Type IV injury, the fracture line passes from the joint surface, through the epiphysis, the epiphyseal plate, and the adjacent metaphysis.
Type V.	This variety of epiphyseal injury results from a crushing type of force applied to the epiphysis, and the epiphyseal plate is injured.

Direction of Fracture Lines

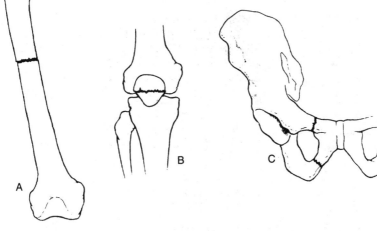

Figure 48. Transverse fractures. **A,** Transerve fracture of the middle third of the femur. **B,** Transverse fracture of the midpatella. **C,** Transverse fracture of the superior and inferior pubic rami.

Figure 49. Oblique fractures. **A,** Oblique fracture of the proximal third of metacarpal. **B,** Oblique fracture of the medial malleolus.

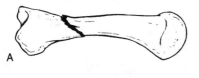

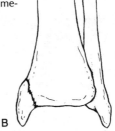

Spinal Fractures

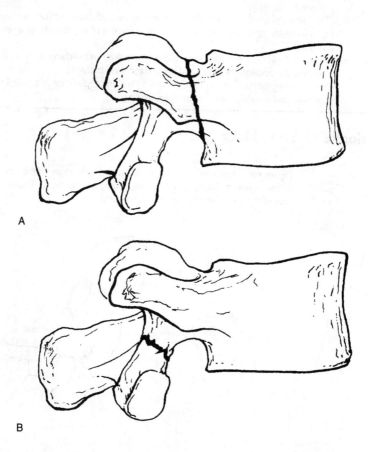

A

B

Figure 50. **A,** Fracture through the pedicle. **B,** Fracture through the pars interarticularis.

Shoulder Fractures

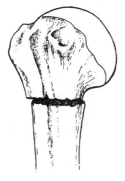

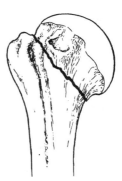

Figure 51. Transverse fracture of the surgical neck of the humerus.

Figure 52. Fracture of the anatomic neck of the humerus.

Elbow Fractures

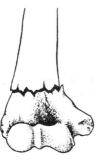

Figure 53. Supracondylar fractures are fractures that occur above the level of the condyles.

Figure 54. Transcondylar fracture. Note that the fracture extends through both condyles.

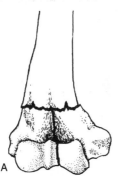

A

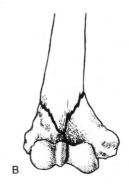

B

Figure 55. Comminuted intraarticular fractures of the distal humerus. **A,** T-shaped fracture. **B,** Y-shaped fracture.

Elbow Fractures (continued)

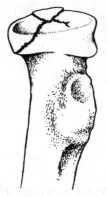

Figure 56. Comminuted fracture of the head of the radius.

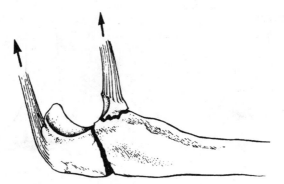

Figure 57. Fracture of the olecranon and coronoid process. Muscle contraction can cause distraction of fracture fragments.

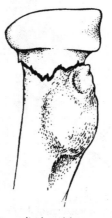

Figure 58. Transverse nondisplaced fracture of the neck of the radius.

Pelvic Fractures

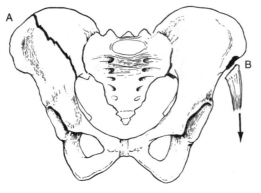

Figure 59. Fractures of the ilium. **A,** Oblique fracture through the wing of the ilium. **B,** Avulsion fracture of the anteroinferior iliac spine.

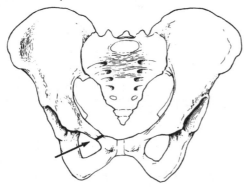

Figure 60. Oblique fracture of the superior pubic ramus.

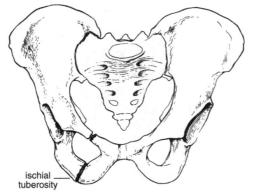

Figure 61. Transverse fractures of the inferior ischial ramus and superior pubic ramus.

Hip Fractures

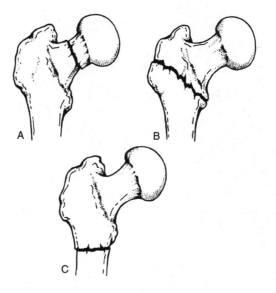

Figure 62. Fractures of the hip are described by the location in which they occur. **A,** Transverse intracapsular fracture. **B,** Oblique intertrochanteric fracture. **C,** Transverse subtrochanteric fracture.

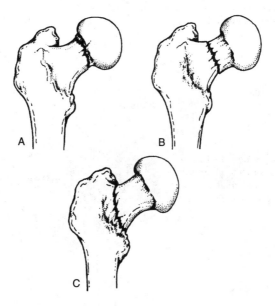

Figure 63. Subclassification of intracapsular fractures. **A,** Subcapital fracture. **B,** Transcervical fracture. **C,** Base of neck fracture.

Knee Fractures

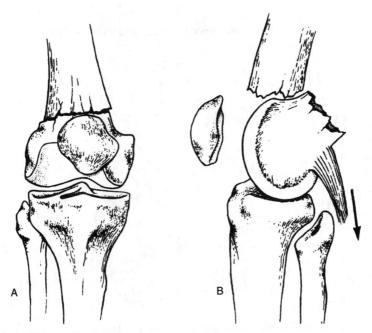

Figure 64.   Supracondylar fracture. **A** and **B,** Transverse supracondylar fracture of the femur. Note the pull of the gastrocnemius muscle, causing the distal fragment to be rotated posteriorly.

Figure 65.   A valgus force applied to the knee causes the hard femoral condyle to be driven into the softer tibial plateau, resulting in depression of the tibial plateau.

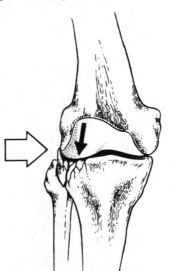

Leg Fractures

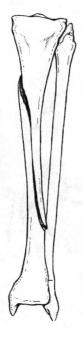

Figure 66. Spiral fractures. Spiral fractures of the middle third of the tibia.

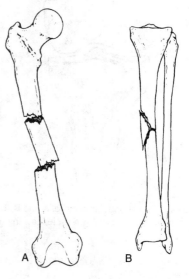

Figure 67. **A,** Segmental fracture of the femur. **B,** Butterfly fragment.

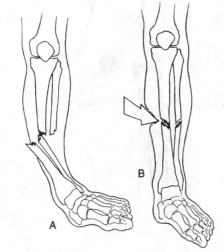

Figure 68. **A,** Compound fracture caused by an inside-out injury. The skin defect is caused, following the fracture, by the bone perforating the skin from within. **B,** Outside-in compound fracture. In this injury, the skin defect is produced by the fracturing agent entering from without.

Ankle Fractures

Figure 69. Fracture of the posterior malleolus.

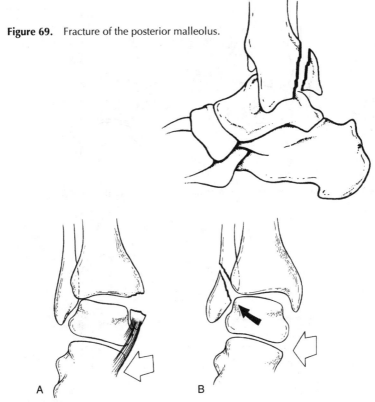

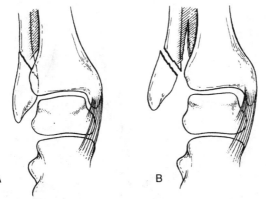

Figure 70. **A,** Avulsion fracture of the medial malleolus. **B,** Oblique fracture of the lateral malleolus.

Figure 71. **A,** Fracture of the lateral malleolus occurring above its articular surface, thus the ankle mortise is not involved. **B,** Similar fracture as in **A,** above the articular surface with disturbance of the mortise due to separation of the syndesmosis.

Ankle Fractures (continued)

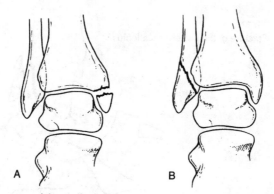

Figure 72. Fractures of the malleoli. **A,** Transverse fracture of the medial malleolus. **B,** Oblique fracture of the lateral malleolus.

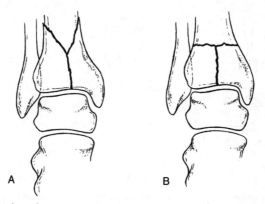

Figure 73. **A,** Y-shaped comminuted intraarticular fracture of the distal tibia. **B,** T-shaped comminuted intraarticular fracture of the distal tibia.

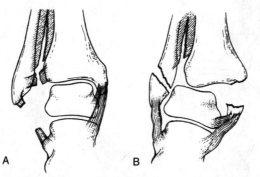

Figure 74. Separation of the distal tibiofibular syndesmosis. **A,** Separation of the tibiofibular syndesmosis without an accompanying fracture. **B,** Separation of the syndesmosis associated with fracture of the medial and lateral malleoli.

Foot Fractures

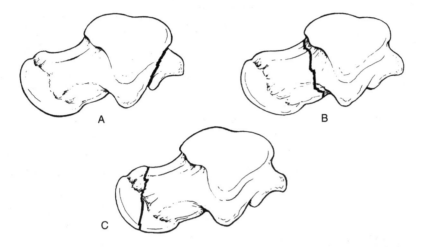

Figure 75. Fractures of the talus can be described by the anatomic area involved. **A,** Fracture of the posterior process. **B,** Fracture of the body. **C,** Fracture of the head.

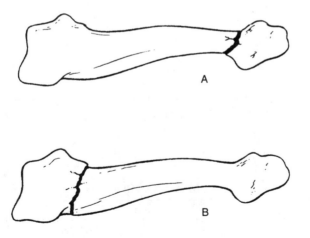

Figure 76. **A,** Fracture of the head of a metatarsal. **B,** Fracture of the base of a metatarsal.

Appendix 3
Table of Muscles

1. Muscles of the Shoulder

Muscle	Origin	Insertion	Nerve	Action
Deltoid	Lateral third of clavicle, acromion, and spine of scapula	Deltoid tuberosity of humerus	Axillary n.	Abducts, adducts, flexes, extends, and rotates arm medially
Supraspinatus	Supraspinous fossa of scapula	Superior facet of greater tubercle of humerus	Suprascapular n.	Abducts arm
Infraspinatus	Infraspinous fossa	Middle facet of greater tubercle of humerus	Suprascapular n.	Rotates arm laterally
Subscapularis	Subscapular fossa	Lesser tubercle of humerus	Upper and lower subscapular n.	Rotates arm medially
Teres major	Dorsal surface of inferior angle of scapula	Medial lip of intertubercular groove of humerus	Lower subscapular n.	Adducts and rotates arm medially
Teres minor	Upper portion of lateral border of scapula	Lower facet of greater tubercle of humerus	Axillary n.	Rotates arm laterally
Latissimus dorsi	Spines of T7–T12 thoracolumbar fascia, iliac crest, ribs 9–12	Floor of bicipital groove of humerus	Thoracodorsal n.	Adducts, extends, and rotates arm medially

2. Muscles of the Arm

Muscle	Origin	Insertion	Nerve	Action
Coracobra-chialis	Coracoid process	Middle third of medial surface of humerus	Musculocuta-neous n.	Flexes and adducts arm
Biceps brachii	Long head, supraglenoid tubercle; short head, coracoid process	Radial tuberosity of radius	Musculocuta-neous n.	Flexes arm and forearm, supinates forearm

(continued)

Muscle	Origin	Insertion	Nerve	Action
Brachialis	Lower anterior surface of humerus	Coronoid process of ulna and ulnar tuberosity	Musculocutaneous n.	Flexes forearm
Triceps	Long head, infraglenoid tubercle; lateral head, superior to radial groove of humerus; medial head, inferior to radial groove	Posterior surface of olecranon process of ulna	Radial n.	Extends forearm
Anconeus	Lateral epicondyle of humerus	Olecranon and upper posterior surface of ulna	Radial n.	Extends forearm

3. Muscles of the Anterior Forearm

Muscle	Origin	Insertion	Nerve	Action
Pronator teres	Medial epicondyle and coronoid process of ulna	Middle of lateral side of radius	Median n.	Pronates forearm
Flexor carpi radialis	Medial epicondyle of humerus	Bases of second and third metacarpals	Median n.	Flexes forearm, flexes and abducts hand
Palmaris longus	Medial epicondyle of humerus	Flexor retinaculum, palmar aponeurosis	Median n.	Flexes hand and forearm
Flexor carpi ulnaris	Medial epicondyle, medial olecranon, and posterior border of ulna	Pisiform, hook of hamate, and base of fifth metacarpal	Ulnar n.	Flexes and adducts hand, flexes forearm
Flexor digitorum superficialis	Medial epicondyle, coronoid process, oblique line of radius	Middle phalanges of finger	Median n.	Flexes proximal interphalangeal joints, flexes hand and forearm

(continued)

Muscle	Origin	Insertion	Nerve	Action
Flexor digitorum profundus	Anteromedial surface of ulna, interosseous membrane	Bases of distal phalanges of fingers	Ulnar and median nn.	Flexes distal interphalangeal joints and hand
Flexor pollicis longus	Anterior surface of radius, interosseous membrane, and coronoid process	Base of distal phalanx of thumb	Median n.	Flexes thumb
Pronator quadratus	Anterior surface of distal ulna	Anterior surface of distal radius	Median n.	Pronates forearm

4. Muscles of the Posterior Forearm

Muscle	Origin	Insertion	Nerve	Action
Brachioradialis	Lateral supracondylar ridge of humerus	Base of radial styloid process	Radial n.	Flexes forearm
Extensor carpi radialis longus	Lateral supracondylar ridge of humerus	Dorsum of base of second metacarpal	Radial n.	Extends and abducts hand
Extensor carpi radialis brevis	Lateral epicondyle of humerus	Posterior base of third metacarpal	Radial n.	Extends fingers and abducts hands
Extensor digitorum	Lateral epicondyle of humerus	Extensor expansion, base of middle and digital phalanges	Radial n.	Extends fingers and hand
Extensor digiti minimi	Common extensor tendon and interosseous membrane	Extensor expansion, base of middle and distal phalanges	Radial n.	Extends little finger
Extensor carpi ulnaris	Lateral epicondyle and posterior surface of ulna	Base of fifth metacarpal	Radial n.	Extends and adducts hand

(continued)

Muscle	Origin	Insertion	Nerve	Action
Supinator	Lateral epicondyle, radial collateral and annular ligaments	Lateral side of upper part of radius	Radial n.	Supinates forearm
Abductor pollicis longus	Interosseous membrane, middle third of posterior surfaces of radius and ulna	Lateral surface of base of first metacarpal	Radial n.	Abducts thumb and hand
Extensor pollicis longus	Interosseous membrane and middle third of posterior surface of ulna	Base of distal phalanx of thumb	Radial n.	Extends distal phalanx of thumb and abducts hand
Extensor pollicis brevis	Interosseous membrane and posterior surface of middle third radius	Base of proximal phalanx of thumb	Radial n.	Extends proximal phalanx of thumb and abducts hand
Extensor indicis	Posterior surface of ulna and interosseous membrane	Extensor expansion of index finger	Radial n.	Extends index finger

5. Muscles of the Hand

Muscle	Origin	Insertion	Nerve	Action
Abductor pollicis brevis	Flexor retinaculum, scaphoid, and trapezium	Lateral side of base of proximal phalanx of thumb	Median n.	Abducts thumb
Flexor pollicis brevis	Flexor retinaculum and trapezium	Base of proximal phalanx of thumb	Median n.	Flexes thumb
Opponens pollicis	Flexor retinaculum and trapezium	Lateral side of first metacarpal	Median n.	Opposes thumb to other digits

(continued)

Muscle	Origin	Insertion	Nerve	Action
Adductor pollicis	Capitate and bases of second and third metacarpals (oblique head); palmar surface of third metacarpal (transverse head)	Medial side of base of proximal phalanx of the thumb	Ulnar n.	Adducts thumb
Palmaris brevis	Medial side of flexor retinaculum, palmar aponeurosis	Skin of medial side of palm	Ulnar n.	Wrinkles skin on medial side of palm
Abductor digiti minimi	Pisiform and tendon of flexor carpi ulnaris	Medial side of base of proximal phalanx of little finger	Ulnar n.	Abducts little finger
Flexor digiti minimi brevis	Flexor retinaculum and hook of hamate	Medial side of base of proximal phalanx of little finger	Ulnar n.	Flexes proximal phalanx of little finger
Opponens digiti minimi	Flexor retinaculum and hook of hamate	Medial side of fifth metacarpal	Ulnar n.	Opposes little finger
Lumbricals (4)	Lateral side of tendons of flexor digitorum profundus	Lateral side of extensor expansion	Median (two lateral) and ulnar (two medial) nn.	Flex metacar-pophalangeal joints and extend interphalangeal joints
Dorsal interossei (4)	Adjacent sides of metacarpal bones	Lateral sides of bases of proximal phalanges; extensor expansion	Ulnar n.	Abduct fingers; flex metacar-pophalangeal joints; extend interphalangeal joints

(continued)

Muscle	Origin	Insertion	Nerve	Action
Palmar interossei (3)	Medial side of second metacarpal; lateral sides of fourth and fifth metacarpals	Bases of proximal phalanges in same sides as their origins; extensor expansion	Ulnar n.	Adduct fingers; flex metacarpo-phalangeal joints; extend interphalangeal joints

6. Anterior Muscles of the Thigh

Muscle	Origin	Insertion	Nerve	Action
Iliacus	Iliac fossa; ala of sacrum	Lesser trochanter	Femoral n.	Flexes and rotates thigh medially (with psoas major)
Sartorius	Anterior–superior iliac spine	Upper medial side of tibia	Femoral n.	Flexes and rotates thigh laterally; flexes and rotates leg medially
Rectus femoris	Anterior–inferior iliac spine; posterior–superior rim of acetabulum	Base of patella; tibial tuberosity	Femoral n.	Flexes thigh; extends leg
Vastus medialis	Intertro-chanteric line; linea aspera; medial intermuscular septum	Medial side of patella; tibial tuberosity	Femoral n.	Extends leg
Vastus lateralis	Intertro-chanteric line; greater trochanter; linea aspera; gluteal tuberosity; lateral intermuscular septum	Lateral side of patella; tibial tuberosity	Femoral n.	Extends leg
Vastus intermedius	Upper shaft of femur; lower lateral intermuscular septum	Upper border of patella; tibial tuberosity	Femoral n.	Extends leg

7. Medial Muscles of the Thigh

Muscle	Origin	Insertion	Nerve	Action
Adductor longus	Body of pubis below its crest	Middle third of linea aspera	Obturator n.	Adducts, flexes, and rotates thigh laterally
Adductor brevis	Body and inferior pubic ramus	Pectineal line; upper part of linea aspera	Obturator n.	Adducts, flexes, and rotates thigh laterally
Adductor magnus	Ischiopubic ramus; ischial tuberosity	Linea aspera; medial supracondylar line; adductor tubercle	Obturator and sciatic nn.	Adducts, flexes, and extends thigh
Pectineus	Pectineal line of pubis	Pectineal line of femur	Obturator and femoral nn.	Adducts and flexes thigh
Gracilis	Body and inferior pubic of ramus	Medial surface of upper quarter of tibia	Obturator n.	Adducts and flexes thigh; flexes and rotates leg medially
Obturator externus	Margin of obturator foramen and obturator membrane	Intertrochanteric fossa of femur	Obturator n.	Rotates thigh laterally

8. Muscles of the Gluteal Region

Muscle	Origin	Insertion	Nerve	Action
Gluteus maximus	Ilium; sacrum; coccyx; sacrotuberous ligament	Gluteal tuberosity; iliotibial tract	Inferior gluteal n.	Extends and rotates thigh laterally
Gluteus medius	Ilium between iliac crest, and anterior and posterior gluteal lines	Greater trochanter	Superior gluteal n.	Abducts and rotates thigh medially
Gluteus minimus	Ilium between anterior and inferior gluteal lines	Greater trochanter	Superior gluteal n.	Abducts and rotates thigh medially
Tensor fasciae latae	Iliac crest; anterior–superior iliac spine	Iliotibial tract	Superior gluteal n.	Flexes, abducts, and rotates thigh medially

(continued)

Muscle	Origin	Insertion	Nerve	Action
Piriformis	Pelvic surface of sacrum; sacrotuberous ligament	Upper end of greater trochanter	Sacral n. (S1–S2)	Rotates thigh medially
Obturator internus	Ischiopubic rami; obturator membrane	Greater trochanter	N. to obturator internus	Abducts and rotates thigh laterally
Superior gemellus	Ischial spine	Obturator internus tendon	N. to obturator internus	Rotates thigh laterally
Inferior gemellus	Ischial tuberosity	Obturator internus tendon	N. to quadratus femorus	Rotates thigh laterally
Quadratus femoris	Ischial tuberosity	Intertro-chanteric crest	N. to quadratus femoris	Rotates thigh laterally

9. Posterior Muscles of the Thigh*

Muscle	Origin	Insertion	Nerve	Action
Semitendinosus	Ischial tuberosity	Medial surface of upper part of tibia	Tibial portion of sciatic n.	Extends thigh; flexes and rotates leg medially
Semimembra-nosus	Ischial tuberosity	Medial condyle of tibia	Tibial portion of sciatic n.	Extends thigh; flexes and rotates leg medially
Biceps femoris	Long head from ischial tuberosity; short head from linea aspera and upper supracondylar line	Head of fibula	Tibial (long head) and common peroneal (short head) divisions of sciatic n.	Extends thigh; flexes and rotates leg medially

*These three muscles collectively are called hamstrings.

10. Anterior and Lateral Muscles of the Leg

Muscle	Origin	Insertion	Nerve	Action
Anterior:				
Tibialis anterior	Lateral tibial condyle; interosseous membrane	First cuneiform; first metatarsal	Deep peroneal n.	Dorsiflexes and inverts foot

(continued)

Muscle	Origin	Insertion	Nerve	Action
Extensor hallucis longus	Middle half of anterior surface of fibula; interosseous membrane	Base of distal phalanx of big toe	Deep peroneal n.	Extends big toe; dorsiflexes and inverts foot
Extensor digitorum longus	Lateral tibial condyle; upper two-thirds of fibula; interosseous membrane	Bases of middle and distal phalanges	Deep peroneal n.	Extends toes; dorsiflexes foot
Peroneus tertius	Distal one-third of fibula; interosseous membrane	Base of fifth metatarsal	Deep peroneal n.	Dorsiflexes and everts foot
Lateral:				
Peroneus longus	Lateral tibial condyle; head and upper lateral side of fibula	Base of first metatarsal; medial cuneiform	Superficial peroneal n.	Everts and plantar flexes foot
Peroneus brevis	Lower lateral side of fibula; intermuscular septa	Base of fifth metatarsal	Superficial peroneal n.	Everts and plantar flexes foot

11. Posterior Muscles of the Leg

Muscle	Origin	Insertion	Nerve	Action
Superficial group:				
Gastrocnemius	Lateral (lateral head) and medial (medial head) femoral condyles	Posterior aspect of calcaneus via tendo calcaneus	Tibial n.	Flexes knee; plantar flexes foot
Soleus	Upper fibula head; soleal line on tibia	Posterior aspect of calcaneus via tendo calcaneus	Tibial n.	Plantar flexes foot
Plantaris	Lower lateral supracondylar line	Posterior surface of calcaneus	Tibial n.	Flexes and rotates leg medially

(continued)

Muscle	Origin	Insertion	Nerve	Action
Deep group:				
Popliteus	Lateral condyle of femur; popliteal ligament	Upper posterior side of tibia	Tibial n.	Flexes and rotates leg medially
Flexor hallucis longus	Lower two-thirds of fibula; interosseous membrane; intermuscular septa	Base of distal phalanx of big toe	Tibial n.	Flexes distal phalanx of big toe
Flexor digitorum longus	Middle posterior aspect of tibia	Distal phalanges of lateral four toes	Tibial n.	Flexes lateral four toes; plantar flexes foot
Tibialis posterior	Interosseous membrane; upper parts of tibia and fibula	Tuberosity of navicular; sustentacula tali; three cuneiforms; cuboid; bases of metatarsals 2–4	Tibial n.	Plantar flexes and inverts foot

12. Muscles of the Foot

Muscle	Origin	Insertion	Nerve	Action
Dorsum of foot:				
Extensor digitorum brevis	Dorsal surface of calcaneus	Tendons of extensor digitorum longus	Deep peroneal n.	Extends toes
Extensor hallucis brevis	Dorsal surface of calcaneus	Base of proximal phalanx of big toe	Deep peroneal n.	Extends big toe
Sole of foot:				
Abductor hallucis	Medial tubercle of calcaneus	Base of proximal phalanx of big toe	Medial plantar n.	Abducts big toe

(continued)

Muscle	Origin	Insertion	Nerve	Action
Flexor digitorum brevis	Medial tubercle of calcaneus	Middle phalanges of lateral four toes	Medial plantar n.	Flexes middle phalanges of lateral four toes
Abductor digiti minimi	Medial and lateral tubercles of calcaneus	Proximal phalanx of little toe	Lateral plantar n.	Abducts little toe
Quadratus plantae	Medial and lateral side of calcaneus	Tendons of flexor digitorum longus	Lateral plantar n.	Aids in flexing toes
Lumbricals (4)	Tendons of flexor digitorum longus	Proximal phalanges; extensor expansion	First by medial plantar n.; lateral three by lateral plantar n.	Flex metatarso-phalangeal joints and extend interphalangeal joints
Flexor hallucis brevis	Cuboid; third cuneiform	Proximal phalanx of big toe	Medial plantar n.	Flexes big toe
Adductor hallucis:				
Oblique head	Bases of metatarsals 2–4	Proximal phalanx of big toe	Lateral plantar n.	Adducts big toe
Transverse head	Capsule of lateral four metatarso-phalangeal joints			
Flexor digiti minimi brevis	Base of metatarsal 5	Proximal phalanx of little toe	Lateral plantar n.	Flexes little toe
Plantar interossei (3)	Medial sides of metatarsals 3–5	Medial sides of base of proximal phalanges 3–5	Lateral plantar n.	Adduct toes; flex proximal, and extend distal phalanges
Dorsal interossei (4)	Adjacent shafts of metatarsals	Proximal phalanges of second toes (medial and lateral sides), and third and fourth toes (lateral sides)	Lateral plantar n.	Abduct toes; flex proximal, and extend distal phalanges

(continued)

13. Muscles of the Thoracic Wall

Muscle	Origin	Insertion	Nerve	Action
External intercostals	Lower border of ribs	Upper border of rib below	Intercostal n.	Elevate ribs in inspiration
Internal intercostals	Lower border of ribs	Upper border of rib below	Intercostal n.	Depress ribs; interchondral part elevates ribs
Innermost intercostals	Lower border of ribs	Upper border of rib below	Intercostal n.	Elevate ribs
Transverse thoracic	Posterior surface of lower sternum and xiphoid	Inner surface of costal cartilages 2–6	Intercostal n.	Depresses ribs
Subcostalis	Inner surface of lower ribs near their angles	Upper borders of ribs 2 or 3 below	Intercostal n.	Elevates ribs
Levator costarum	Transverse processes of T7–T11	Subjacent ribs between tubercle and angle	Dorsal primary rami of C8–T11	Elevates ribs

14. Muscles of the Anterior Abdominal Wall

Muscle	Origin	Insertion	Nerve	Action
External oblique	External surface of lower eight ribs (5–12)	Anterior half of iliac crest; anterior–superior iliac spine; pubic tubercle; linea alba	Intercostal n. (T7–T11); subcostal n. (T12)	Compresses abdomen; flexes trunk; active in forced expiration
Internal oblique	Lateral two-thirds of inguinal ligament; iliac crest; thoracolumbar fascia	Lower four costal cartilages; linea alba; pubic crest; pectineal line	Intercostal n. (T7–T11); subcostal n. (T12); iliohypogastric and ilioinguinal nn. (L1)	Compresses abdomen; flexes trunk; active in forced expiration
Transversus abdominis	Lateral one-third of inguinal ligament; iliac crest; thoracolumbar fascia; lower six costal cartilages	Linea alba; pubic crest; pectineal line	Intercostal n. (T7–T12); subcostal n. (T12); iliohypogastric and ilioinguinal nn. (L1)	Compresses abdomen; depresses ribs

(continued)

Muscle	Origin	Insertion	Nerve	Action
Rectus abdominis	Pubic crest and pubic symphysis	Xiphoid process and costal cartilages 5–7	Intercostal n. (T7–T11); subcostal n. (T12)	Depresses ribs; flexes trunk
Pyramidalis	Pubic body	Linea alba	Subcostal n. (T12)	Tenses linea alba
Cremaster	Middle of inguinal ligament; lower margin of internal oblique muscle	Tubercle and pubic crest	Genitofemoral n.	Retracts testis

15. Muscles of the Posterior Abdominal Wall

Muscle	Origin	Insertion	Nerve	Action
Quadratus lumborum	Transverse processes of LV3–LV5; iliolumbar ligament; iliac crest	Lower border of last rib; transverse processes of LV1–LV3	Subcostal n.; L1–L3	Depresses twelfth rib; flexes trunk laterally
Psoas major	Transverse processes, intervertebral disks and bodies of TV12–LV5	Lesser trochanter	L2–L3	Flexes thigh and trunk
Psoas minor	Bodies and intervertebral disks of TV12–LV1	Pectineal line; iliopectineal eminence	L1	Aids in flexing of trunk

LV = lumbar vertebra; TV = thoracic vertebra

16. Superficial Back

Muscle	Origin	Insertion	Nerve	Action
Trapezius	External occipital protuberance, superior nuchal line, ligamentum nuchae, spines of C7–T12	Spine of scapula, acromion, and lateral third of clavicle	Spinal accessory n., C3–C4	Adducts, rotates, elevates, and depresses scapula

(continued)

Muscle	Origin	Insertion	Nerve	Action
Levator scapulae	Transverse processes of C1–C4	Medial border of scapula	Nerves to levator scapulae, C3–C4, dorsal scapular n.	Elevates scapula
Rhomboid minor	Spines of C7–T1	Root of spine of scapula	Dorsal scapular n., C5	Adducts scapula
Rhomboid major	Spines of T2–T5	Medial border of scapula	Dorsal scapular n.	Adducts scapula
Latissimus dorsi	Spines of T5–T12, thoracodorsal fascia, iliac crest, ribs 9–12	Floor of bicipital groove of humerus	Thoracodorsal n.	Adducts, extends, and rotates arm medially
Serratus posterior–superior	Ligamentum nuchae, supraspinal ligament, and spines of C7–T3	Upper border of ribs 2–5	Intercostal n., T1–T4	Elevates ribs
Serratus posterior–inferior	Supraspinous ligament and spines of T11–L3	Lower border of ribs 9–12	Intercostal n., T9–T12	Depresses ribs

17. Suboccipital Muscles

Muscle	Origin	Insertion	Nerve	Action
Rectus capitis posterior major	Spine of axis	Lateral portion of inferior nuchal line	Suboccipital n.	Extends, rotates, and flexes head laterally
Rectus capitis posterior minor	Posterior tubercle of atlas	Occipital bone below inferior nuchal line	Suboccipital n.	Extends and flexes head laterally
Obliquus capitis superior	Transverse process of atlas	Occipital bone above inferior nuchal line	Suboccipital n.	Extends, rotates, and flexes head laterally
Obliquus capitis inferior	Spine of axis	Transverse process of atlas	Suboccipital n.	Extends head and rotates it laterally

18. Muscles of the Neck

Muscle	Origin	Insertion	Nerve	Action
Cervical muscles:				
Platysma	Superficial fascia over upper part of deltoid and pectoralis major	Mandible; skin and muscles over mandible and angle of mouth	Facial n.	Depresses lower jaw and lip and angle of mouth; wrinkles skin of neck
Sterno-cleidomastoid	Manubrium sterni and medial one-third of clavicle	Mastoid process and lateral one-half of superior nuchal line	Spinal accessory n.; C2-C3 (sensory)	Singly turns face toward opposite side; together flex head, raise thorax
Suprahyoid muscles:				
Digastric	Anterior belly from digastric fossa of mandible; posterior belly from mastoid notch	Intermediate tendon attached to body of hyoid	Posterior belly by facial n.; anterior belly by mylohyoid n. of trigeminal n.	Elevates hyoid and tongue; depresses mandible
Mylohyoid	Mylohyoid line of mandible	Median raphe and body of hyoid bone	Mylohyoid n. of trigeminal n.	Elevates hyoid and tongue; depresses mandible
Stylohyoid	Styloid process	Body of hyoid	Facial n.	Elevates hyoid
Geniohyoid	Genial tubercle of mandible	Body of hyoid	C1 via hypoglossal n.	Elevates hyoid and tongue
Infrahyoid muscles:				
Sternohyoid	Manubrium sterni and medial end of clavicle	Body of hyoid	Ansa cervicalis	Depresses hyoid and larynx
Sternothyroid	Manubrium sterni; first costal cartilage	Oblique line of thyroid cartilage	Ansa cervicalis	Depresses thyroid cartilage and larynx
Thyrohyoid	Oblique line of thyroid cartilage	Body and greater horn of hyoid	C1 via hypoglossal n.	Depresses and retracts hyoid and larynx

(continued)

Muscle	Origin	Insertion	Nerve	Action
Omohyoid	Inferior belly from medial lip of suprascapular notch and suprascapular ligament; superior belly from intermediate tendon	Inferior belly to intermediate tendon; superior belly to body of hyoid	Ansa cervicalis	Depresses and retracts hyoid and larynx

19. Prevertebral Muscles

Muscle	Origin	Insertion	Nerve	Action
Lateral vertebral:				
Anterior scalene	Transverse processes of CV3–CV6	Scalene tubercle on first rib	Lower cervical (C5–C8)	Elevates first rib; bends neck
Middle scalene	Transverse processes of CV2–CV7	Upper surface of first rib	Lower cervical (C5–C8)	Elevates first rib; bends neck
Posterior scalene	Transverse processes of CV4–CV6	Outer surface of second rib	Lower cervical (C6–C8)	Elevates second rib; bends neck
Anterior vertebral:				
Longus capitus	Transverse processes of CV3–CV6	Basilar part of occipital bone	C1–C4	Flexes and rotates head
Longus colli (L. cervicis)	Transverse processes and bodies of CV3–TV3	Anterior tubercle of atlas; bodies of CV2–CV4; transverse process of CV5–CV6	C2–C6	Flexes and rotates head
Rectus capitis anterior	Lateral mass of atlas	Basilar part of occipital bone	C1–C2	Flexes and rotates head
Rectus capitis lateralis	Transverse process of atlas	Jugular process of occipital bone	C1–C2	Flexes head laterally

(continued)

20. Muscles of Facial Expression

Muscle	Origin	Insertion	Nerve	Action
Occipito-frontalis	Superior nuchal line; upper orbital margin	Epicranial aponeurosis	Facial n.	Elevates eyebrows; wrinkles forehead (surprise)
Corrugator supercilii	Medial supraorbital margin	Skin of medial eyebrow	Facial n.	Draws eyebrows downward medially (anger)
Orbicularis oculi	Medial orbital margin; medial palpebral ligament; lacrimal bone	Skin and rim of orbit; tarsal plate; lateral palpebral raphe	Facial n.	Closes eyelids (squinting)
Procerus	Nasal bone and cartilage	Skin between eyebrows	Facial n.	Wrinkles skin over bones (sadness)
Nasalis	Maxilla lateral to incisive fossa	Ala of nose	Facial n.	Draws ala of nose toward septum
Depressor septi*	Incisive fossa of maxilla	Ala and nasal septum	Facial n.	Constricts nares
Orbicularis oris	Maxilla above incisor teeth	Skin of lip	Facial n.	Closes lips
Levator anguli oris	Canine fossa of maxilla	Angle of mouth	Facial n.	Elevates angle of mouth medially (disgust)
Levator labii superioris	Maxilla above infraorbital foramen	Skin of upper lip	Facial n.	Elevates upper lip; dilates nares (disgust)
Levator labii superioris alaeque nasi*	Frontal process of maxilla	Skin of upper lip	Facial n.	Elevates ala of nose and upper lip
Zygomaticus major	Zygomatic arch	Angle of mouth	Facial n.	Draws angle of mouth backward and upward (smile)
Zygomaticus minor	Zygomatic arch	Angle of mouth	Facial n.	Elevates upper lip

(continued)

Muscle	Origin	Insertion	Nerve	Action
Depressor labii inferioris	Mandible below mental foramen	Orbicularis oris and skin of lower lip	Facial n.	Depresses lower lip
Depressor anguli oris	Oblique line of mandible	Angle of mouth	Facial n.	Depresses angle of mouth
Risorius	Fascia over masseter	Angle of mouth	Facial n.	Retracts angle of mouth (false smile)
Buccinator	Mandible; pterygomandibular raphe; alveolar processes	Angle of mouth	Facial n.	Presses cheek to keep it taut
Mentalis	Incisive fossa of mandible	Skin of chin	Facial n.	Elevates and protrudes lower lip
Auricularis anterior, superior, and posterior*	Temporal fascia; epicranial aponeurosis; mastoid process	Anterior, superior, and posterior sides of auricle	Facial n.	Retract and elevate ear

*Indicates less important muscles.

21. Muscles of Mastication

Muscle	Origin	Insertion	Nerve	Action
Temporalis	Temporal fossa	Coronoid process and ramus of mandible	Trigeminal n.	Elevates and retracts mandible
Masseter	Lower border and medial surface of zygomatic arch	Lateral surface of coronoid process, ramus and angle of mandible	Trigeminal n.	Elevates mandible
Lateral pterygoid	Superior head from infratemporal surface of sphenoid; inferior head from lateral surface of lateral pterygoid plate	Neck of mandible; articular disk and capsule of temporo-mandibular joint	Trigeminal n.	Protracts (protrudes) and depresses mandible

(continued)

Nerve	Cranial Exit	Cell Bodies	Components	Chief Functions
Medial pterygoid	Tuber of maxilla; medial surface of lateral pterygoid plate; pyramidal process of palatine bone	Medial surface of angle and ramus of mandible	Trigeminal n.	Protracts (protrudes) and elevates mandible

22. Cranial Nerves

Nerve	Cranial Exit	Cell Bodies	Components	Chief Functions
I: Olfactory	Cribriform plate	Nasal mucosa	SVA	Smell
II: Optic	Optic canal	Ganglion cells of retina	SSA	Vision
III: Oculomotor	Superior orbital fissure	Nucleus CN III (midbrain)	GSE	Eye movements (superior, inferior, and medial recti, inferior oblique, and levator palpebrae superioris mm.)
		Edinger-Westphal nucleus (midbrain)	GVE	Constriction of pupil (sphincter pupillae m.) and accommodation (ciliary m.)
IV: Trochlear	Superior orbital fissure	Nucleus CN IV (midbrain)	GSE	Eye movements (superior oblique m.)
V: Trigeminal	Superior orbital fissure; foramen rotundum and foramen ovale	Motor nucleus CN V (pons)	SVE	Muscles of mastication, (mylohyoid, anterior belly of digastric, tensor veli palatini, and tensor tympani mm.)

(continued)

Nerve	Cranial Exit	Cell Bodies	Components	Chief Functions
		Trigeminal ganglion	GSA	Sensation in head (skin and mucous membranes of face and head)
VI: Abducens	Superior orbital fissure	Nucleus CN VI (pons)	GSE	Eye movement (lateral rectus m.)
VII: Facial	Stylomastoid foramen	Motor nucleus CN VII (pons)	SVE	Muscle of facial expression (posterior belly of digastric stylohyoid, and stapedius mm.)
		Salivatory nucleus (pons)	GVE	Lacrimal and salivary secretion
		Geniculate ganglion	SVA	Taste from anterior two-thirds of tongue and palate
		Geniculate ganglion	GVA	Sensation from palate
		Geniculate ganglion	GSA	Sensation from external acoustic meatus
VIII: Vestibulococh-lear	Does not leave skull	Vestibular ganglion Spiral ganglion	SSA SSA	Equilibrium Hearing
IX: Glossopharyn-geal	Jugular foramen	Nucleus ambiguus (medulla)	SVE	Elevation of pharynx (stylo-pharyngeus m.)
		Dorsal nucleus (medulla)	GVE	Secretion of saliva (parotid gland)
		Inferior ganglion	GVA	Sensation in carotid sinus and body, tongue, and pharynx
		Inferior ganglion	SVA	Taste from posterior one-third of tongue

(continued)

A71

Nerve	Cranial Exit	Cell Bodies	Components	Chief Functions
		Inferior ganglion	GSA	Sensation in external and middle ear
X: Vagus	Jugular foramen	Nucleus ambiguus (medulla)	SVE	Muscles of movements of pharynx, larynx, and palate
		Dorsal nucleus (medulla)	GVE	Involuntary muscle and gland control in thoracic and abdominal viscerae
		Inferior ganglion	GVA	Sensation in pharynx, larynx, and other viscerae
		Inferior ganglion	SVA	Taste from root of tongue and epiglottis
		Superior ganglion	GSA	Sensation in external ear and external acoustic meatus
XI: Accessory	Jugular foramen	Spinal cord (cervical)	SVE	Movement of head and shoulder (sternocleido-mastoid and trapezius mm.)
XII: Hypoglossal	Hypoglossal canal	Nucleus CN XII (medulla)	GSE	Muscles of movements of tongue

23. Muscles of Eye Movement

Muscle	Origin	Insertion	Nerve	Action
Superior rectus	Common tendinous ring	Sclera just behind cornea	Oculomotor n.	Elevates eyeball
Inferior rectus	Common tendinous ring	Sclera just behind cornea	Oculomotor n.	Depresses eyeball
Medial rectus	Common tendinous ring	Sclera just behind cornea	Oculomotor n.	Adducts eyeball

(continued)

Muscle	Origin	Insertion	Nerve	Action
Lateral rectus	Common tendinous ring	Sclera just behind cornea	Abducens n.	Abducts eyeball
Levator palpebrae superioris	Lesser wing of sphenoid above and anterior to optic canal	Tarsal plate and skin of upper eyelid	Oculomotor n.	Elevates upper eyelid
Superior oblique	Body of sphenoid bone above optic canal	Sclera beneath superior rectus	Trochlear n.	Rotates downward and medially; depresses adducted eye
Inferior oblique	Floor of orbit lateral to lacrimal groove	Sclera beneath lateral rectus	Oculomotor n.	Rotates upward and laterally; elevates adducted eye

24. Muscles of the Palate

Muscle	Origin	Insertion	Nerve	Action
Tensor veli palatini	Scaphoid fossa; spine of sphenoid; cartilage of auditory tube	Tendon hooks around hamulus of medial pterygoid plate to insert into aponeurosis of soft palate	Mandibular branch of trigeminal n.	Tenses soft palate
Levator veli palatini	Petrous part of temporal bone; cartilage of auditory tube	Aponeurosis of soft palate	Vagus n. via pharyngeal plexus	Elevates soft palate
Palatoglossus	Aponeurosis of soft palate	Dorsolateral side of tongue	Vagus n. via pharyngeal plexus	Elevates tongue
Palato-pharyngeus	Aponeurosis of soft palate	Thyroid cartilage and side of pharynx	Vagus n. via pharyngeal plexus	Elevates pharynx; closes nasopharynx
Musculus uvulae	Posterior nasal spine of palatine bone; palatine aponeurosis	Mucous membrane of uvula	Vagus n. via pharyngeal plexus	Elevates uvula

(continued)

25. Muscles of the Tongue

Muscle	Origin	Insertion	Nerve	Action
Styloglossus	Styloid process	Side and inferior aspect of tongue	Hypoglossal n.	Retracts and elevates tongue
Hyoglossus	Body and greater horn of hyoid bone	Side and inferior aspect of tongue	Hypoglossal n.	Depresses and retracts tongue
Genioglossus	Genial tubercle of mandible	Inferior aspect of tongue; body of hyoid bone	Hypoglossal n.	Protrudes and depresses tongue
Palatoglossus	Aponeurosis of soft palate	Dorsolateral side of tongue	Vagus n. via pharyngeal plexus	Elevates tongue

26. Muscles of the Pharynx

Muscle	Origin	Insertion	Nerve	Action
Circular muscles:				
Superior constrictor	Medial pterygoid plate; pterygoid hamulus; pterygo-mandibular raphe; mylohyoid line of mandible; side of tongue	Median raphe and pharyngeal tubercle of skull	Vagus n. via pharyngeal plexus	Constricts upper pharynx
Middle constrictor	Greater and lesser horns of hyoid; stylohyoid ligament	Median raphe	Vagus n. via pharyngeal plexus	Constricts lower pharynx
Inferior constrictor	Arch of cricoid and oblique line of thyroid cartilages	Median raphe of pharynx	Vagus n. via pharyngeal plexus, recurrent and external laryngeal n.	Constricts lower pharynx

(continued)

Muscle	Origin	Insertion	Nerve	Action
Longitudinal muscles:				
Stylo-pharyngeus	Styloid process	Thyroid cartilage and muscles of pharynx	Glossopharyngeal n.	Elevates pharynx and larynx
Palato-pharyngeus	Hard palate; aponeurosis of soft palate	Thyroid cartilage and muscles of pharynx	Vagus n. via pharyngeal plexus	Elevates pharynx and closes nasopharynx
Salpingo-pharyngeus	Cartilage of auditory tube	Muscles of pharynx	Vagus n. via pharyngeal plexus	Elevates nasopharynx; opens auditory tube

27. Muscles of the Larynx

Muscle	Origin	Insertion	Nerve	Action on Vocal Cords
Cricothyroid	Arch of cricoid cartilage	Inferior horn and lower lamina of thyroid cartilage	External laryngeal n.	Tenses
Posterior cricoarytenoid	Posterior surface of lamina of cricoid cartilage	Muscular process of arytenoid cartilage	Recurrent laryngeal n.	Abducts
Lateral cricoarytenoid	Arch of cricoid cartilage	Muscular process of arytenoid cartilage	Recurrent laryngeal n.	Adducts
Transverse arytenoid	Posterior surface of arytenoid cartilage	Opposite arytenoid cartilage	Recurrent laryngeal n.	Adducts
Oblique arytenoid	Muscular process of arytenoid cartilage	Apex of opposite arytenoid	Recurrent laryngeal n.	Adducts
Aryepiglottic	Apex of arytenoid cartilage	Side of epiglottic cartilage	Recurrent laryngeal n.	Adducts

(continued)

Ganglion	Location	Parasympathetic Fibers	Sympathetic Fibers	Chief Distribution
Thyroarytenoid	Inner surface of thyroid lamina	Anterolateral surface of arytenoid cartilage	Recurrent laryngeal n.	Adducts
Thyroepiglottic	Anteromedial surface of lamina of thyroid cartilage	Lateral margin of epiglottic cartilage	Recurrent laryngeal n.	Adducts
Vocalis	Anteromedial surface of lamina of thyroid cartilage	Vocal process	Recurrent laryngeal n.	Adducts and tenses

28. Summary of Autonomic Ganglia of the Head and Neck

Ganglion	Location	Parasympathetic Fibers	Sympathetic Fibers	Chief Distribution
Ciliary	Lateral to optic n.	Oculomotor n. and its inferior division	Internal carotid plexus	Ciliary muscle, and sphincter pupillae (parasympathetic); dilator pupillae and tarsal mm. (sympathetic)
Pterygopalatine	In pterygopalatine fossa	Facial n., greater petrosal n., and n. of pterygoid canal	Internal carotid plexus	Lacrimal gland and glands in palate and nose
Submandibular	On hyoglossus	Facial n., chorda tympani, and lingual n.	Plexus on facial a.	Submandibular and sublingual glands
Otic	Below foramen ovale	Glosso-pharyngeal n., its tympanic branch, and lesser petrosal n.	Plexus on middle meningeal a.	Parotid gland

From Chung KW. Gross anatomy, 2nd ed. Malvern: Harwal Publishing Company, 1991.

Appendix 4

Table of Ligaments and Tendons

Shoulder/Upper Arm

Latin name	English name	Articulation
La. acromioclaviculare	acromioclavicular l.	Connects acromion to clavicle; strengthens articular capsule.
La. collaterale ulnare	Collateral ulnar l.	Connects medial epicondyle to humerus and coronoid process of ulna and olecranon.
La. conoideum	Conoid l.	Connects coracoid process of scapula to clavicle.
La. coracoacromiale	Coracoacromial l.	Connects coracoid process to acromion.
La. coracoclaviculare	Coracoclavicular l.	Connects coracoid process of scapula to clavicle.
La. coracohumerale	Coracohumeral l.	Connects coracoid process of scapula to humerus.
La. costoclaviculare	Costoclavicular l.	Connects 1st costal cartilage to clavicle.
La. glenohumeralia	Glenohumeral ligs.	Connect articular capsule of humerus to glenoid cavity and anatomical neck of humerus.
La. interclaviculare	Interclavicular l.	Connects clavicle to opposite clavicle.
La. transversum scapulae inferius	Inferior transverse l.	Connects scapula to glenoid cavity; creates foramen of scapula for vessels/nerves.
La. transversum scapulae superius	Superior transverse l.	Connects coracoid process to scapular notch.
La. trapezoideum	Trapezoid l.	Connects coracoid process to clavicle.

Hand/Forearm

Latin name	English name	Articulation
La. anulare radii	Annular l. of radius	Connects radius to ulna.
La. carpi radiatum	Radiate l. of wrist	Multiple fibrous bands on palmar surface of metacarpal joint.
La. carpi transversum	Transverse carpal l.	Continuous with antebrachial fascia.

(continued)

Abbreviations used: l., ligament; La. ligamenta; ligs., ligament.

Hand/Forearm

Latin name	English name	Articulation
La. carpi volare	Transverse carpal l.	Reinforcing fibers in antebrachial fascia, palmar surface of wrist.
La. carpometacarpalia dorsalia	Dorsal carpometacarpal ligs.	Join carpal bones to bases of metacarpals.
La. carpometacarpalia palmaria	Palmar carpometacarpal metacarpals.	Join carpal bones to ligs.
La. collateralia articulationum interphalangealium manus	Collateral ligs. of interphalangeal articulations	Fibrous bands on each side of interphalangeal joints of fingers.
La. collateralia articulationum metacarpophalangealium	Collateral ligs. of metacarpophalangeal articulations	Fibrous bands on sides of each metacarpophalangeal joint.
La. collaterale carpi radiale	Radial carpal collateral l.	Connects styloid process of radius to scaphoid.
La. collaterale carpi ulnare	Ulnar carpal collateral l.	Connects styloid process of ulna to triquetral and pisiform bones.
La. collaterale radiale	Collateral radial l.	Connects lateral epicondyle of humerus to annular l. of radius.
La. intercarpalia dorsalia interossea	Dorsal intercarpal ligs.	Connect carpal bones together.
La. intercarpalia interossea	Interosseous intercarpal ligs.	Connect various carpal bones.
La. intercarpalia palmaria	Palmar intercarpal ligs.	Connect various carpal bones.
La. metacarpalia dorsalia	Dorsal metacarpal ligs.	Interconnect bases of metacarpal bones.
La. metacarpalia interossea	Interosseous metacarpal ligs.	Interconnect bases of metacarpal bones.
La. metacarpalia palmaria	Palmar metacarpal ligs.	Interconnect bases of metacarpals.
La. metacarpeum transversum profundum	Deep transverse metacarpal l.	Interconnect heads of metacarpals.
La. metacarpale transversum superficiale	Superficial transverse metacarpal l.	Between longitudinal bands of palmar aponeurosis.
La. palmaria articulationum interphalangealium	Palmar ligs. of interphalangeal articulations	Interphalangeal articulations of hand between collateral
La. pisohamatum	Pisohamate l.	Connects pisiform bone to hook of hamate bone.

(continued)

Hand/Forearm

Latin name	English name	Articulation
La. pisometacarpeum	Pisometacarpal l.	Connects pisiform bone to bases of metacarpals.
La. quadratum	Quadrate l.	Connects radial notch of ulna to neck of radius.
La. radiocarpale dorsale	Dorsal radiocarpal l.	Connects radius to carpal bones.
La. radiocarpale palmare	Palmar radiocarpal l.	Connect radius to lunate, triquetral, capitate, and hamate bones.
La. ulnocarpale palmare	Palmar ulnocarpal l.	Connects styloid process of ulna to carpal bones.

Spine

Latin name	English name	Articulation
La. alaria	Alar l.	Connects axis to occiput; limits rotation of head.
La. apicis dentis axis	Apical dental l.	Connects axis to occiput.
La. atlantooccipitale laterale	Lateral atlantooccipital l.	Connects occiput to atlas.
La. capitis costae intraarticulare	Interarticular l. of head of rib	Connects crest of rib to intervertebral disk.
La. capitis costae radiatum	Radiate l. of head of rib	Connects head of rib to adjacent vertebrae/disks.
La. caudale integumenti communis	Caudal retinaculum	Forms coccygeal foveola.
La. costotransversarium	Costotransverse l.	Connects neck of rib to transverse process of corresponding vertebra.
La. costotransversarium laterale	Lateral costotransverse l.	Connects transverse process of vertebra to corresponding rib.
La. costotransversarium superius	Superior costotransverse l.	Connects neck of rib to transverse process of vertebra above.
La. cruciforme atlantis	Cruciform l. of atlas	Connects transverse l. of atlas to longitudinal fascicles.
La. flava	Yellow ligs.	Join laminae of 2 adjacent vertebrae.
La. iliofemorale	Iliofemoral l.	Connects ant./inf. iliac spine and intertrochanteric femur.
La. iliolumbale	Iliolumbar l.	Connects L4-L5 to iliac crest.

(continued)

Spine

Latin name	English name	Articulation
La. interspinalia	Interspinal ligs.	Interconnect spinous processes.
La. intertransversaria	Intertransverse ligs.	Interconnect vertebral transverse processes.
La. longitudinale anterius	Ant. longitudinal l.	Extends from occiput/atlas to sacrum.
La. longitudinale posterius	Post. longitudinal l.	Extends from occiput to coccyx.
La. lumbocostale	Lumbocostal l.	Connects 12th rib to transverse processes of L1-L2.
La. nuchae	Nuchal l.	Extends from cervical spinous processes to occipital crest.
La. sacrococcygeum anterius	Anterior sacrococcygeal l.	Connects sacrum to coccyx.
La. sacrococcygeum laterale	Lateral sacrococcygeal l.	Connects 1st coccygeal vertebra to sacrum; completes foramen of S-5.
La. sacrococcygeum posterius profundum	Deep posterior sacrococcygeal l.	Terminal portion of post. longitudinal l.; unites S-5 and coccyx.
La. sacrococcygeum posterius superficiale	Superficial posterior sacrococcygeal l.	Connects sacral hiatus to coccyx.
La. sacroiliaca anteriora	Anterior sacroiliac ligs.	Connect sacrum to ilium
La. sacroiliaca interossea	Interosseous sacroiliac ligs.	Numerous bundles connecting tuberosities of sacrum to those of ilium.
La. sacroiliaca posteriora	Posterior sacroiliac ligs.	Connect ilium and iliac spines to sacrum.
La. sacrospinalum	Sacrospinal l.	Connects ischium to lateral margins of sacrum.
La. sacrotuberale	Sacrotuberal l.	Connects ischial tuberosity to sacrum and coccyx and iliac spine.
La. supraspinale	Supraspinal l.	Interconnects tips of spinous processes of vertebrae.
La. transversum atlantis	Transverse l. of atlas	Horizontal portion of cruciform l. of atlas.

Hip/Thigh

Latin name	English name	Articulation
La. capitis femoris	l. of head of femur round l. of femur	Connects femur, acetabular notch, and transverse l. of acetabulum.
La. inguinale	Inguinal l.	Connects ilium to pubis.
La. ischiofemorale	Ischiofemoral l.	Connects ischium to femur.
La. transversum acetabuli	Transverse l. of acetabulum	Connects acetabular lip of hip joint to acetabular notch.

Knee/Calf

Latin name	English name	Articulation
La. capitis fibulae anterius	Anterior l. of head of fibula	Connects head of fibula to lateral condyle of tibia.
La. capitis fibulae posterius	Posterior l. of head of fibula	Connects head of fibula to lateral condyle of tibia.
La. collaterale fibulare	Collateral fibular l.	Connects lateral epicondyle of femur to head of fibula.
La. collateral tibiale	Collateral tibial l.	Connects medial epicondyle of femur to medial meniscus and tibia.
La. cruciatum anterius genus	Anterior cruciate l. of knee.	Connects lateral condyle of femur to condylar eminence of tibia.
La. cruciata genus	Cruciate ligaments of knee	Bundles in knee joint between condyles of femur.
La. cruciatum posterius genus	Posterior cruciate l. of knee	Connects medial condyle of femur to intercondylar area of tibia.
La. meniscofemorale anterius	Anterior meniscofemoral l.	Connects lateral meniscus to posterior cruciate l.
La. meniscofemorale posterius	Posterior meniscofemoral l.	Connects lateral meniscus to medial condyle of femur.
La. patellae	Patellar l.	Connects patella to tibial tuberosity.
La. popliteum arcuatum	Arcuate popliteal l.	Connects fibula to articular capsule.
La. popliteum obliquum	Oblique popliteal l.	Connects medial condyle of tibia to lateral epicondyle of femur.
La. tibiofibulare anterius	Anterior tibiofibular l.	Connects tibia to fibula.
La. tibiofibulare posterius	Posterior tibiofibular l.	Connects tibia to distal fibula.
La. transversum genus	Transverse. of knee	Connects lateral meniscus to medial meniscus.

Appendix 4

Foot and Ankle

Latin name	English name	Articulation
La. bifurcatum	Bifurcate ligament	Dorsum of foot; comprises calcaneonavicular and calcaneocuboid ligaments.
La. calcaneocuboideum	Calcaneocuboid l.	Connects calcaneus to cuboid.
La. calcaneocuboideum plantare	Plantar calcaneocuboid l. Short plantar l.	Connects calcaneus to cuboid.
La. calcaneofibulare	Calcaneofibular l.	Connects fibula to calcaneus.
La. calcaneonaviculare	Calcaneonavicular l.	Connects calcaneus to navicular bone.
La. calcaneonaviculare dorsale	Dorsal calcaneonavicular l.	Connects calcaneus to navicular bone.
La. calcaneonaviculare plantare	Plantar calcaneonavicular l.	Connects sustentaculum tali to navicular. Supports talus.
La. calcaneotibiale	Calcaneotibial l.	Connect medial malleolus to sustentaculum tali of calcaneus.
La. collateralia articulationum interphalangealium pedis	Collateral ligs. of interphalangeal articulations	Fibrous bands on each side of interphalangeal joints of toes.
La. collateralia articulationum metatarsophalangealium	Collateral ligs. of metatarsophalangeal articulations	Fibrous bands on sides of each etatarsophalangeal joint.
La. cruciatum cruris	Inferior extensor of foot	Joins malleolus to dorsum of foot.
La. cuboideonaviculare dorsale	Dorsal cuboideonavicular l.	Connects cuboid and navicular bones.
La. cuboideonaviculare plantare	Plantar cuboideonavicular l.	Connects cuboid and navicular bones.
La. cuneocuboideum dorsale	Dorsal cuneocuboid l.	Connects cuboid and lateral cuneiform bones.
La. cuneocuboideum interosseum	Interosseus cuneocuboid l.	Connects cuboid and lateral cuneiform bones.
La. cuneocuboideum plantare	Plantar cuneocuboid l.	Connects cuboid and lateral cuneiform bones.
La. cuneometatarsalia interossea	Interosseous cuneometatarsal ligs.	Connect cuneiform and metatarsal bones.
La. cuneonavicularia dorsalia	Dorsal cuneonavicular ligs.	Connect navicular and cuneiform bones.
La. cuneonavicularia plantaria	Plantar cuneonavicular ligs.	Connect navicular to cuneiform bones.

(continued)

Foot and Ankle

Latin name	English name	Articulation
La. intercuneiformia dorsalia	Dorsal intercuneiform ligs.	Connect dorsal surfaces of cuneiform bones.
La. intercuneiformia interossea	Interosseous intercuneiform ligs.	Connect adjacent cuneiform bones.
La. intercuneiformia plantaria	Plantar intercuneiform ligs.	Join plantar surfaces of cuneiform bones.
La. laterale articulationis talocruralis	Lateral l. of ankle joint	Lateral side of ankle joint.
La. mediale articulationis talocruralis	Medial l. of ankle	Connects medial malleolus of tibia to tarsal bones.
La. metatarsale transversum profundum	Deep transverse metatarsal l.	Joins heads of metatarsals.
La. metatarsale transversum superficiale	Superficial transverse metatarsal l.	Lies on sole of foot beneath heads of metatarsals.
La. metatarsalia dorsalia	Dorsal metatarsal ligs.	Interconnect bases of metatarsal bones.
La. metatarsalia interossea	Interosseous metatarsal ligs.	Interconnect bases of metatarsal bones.
La. metatarsalia plantaria	Plantar metatarsal ligs.	Plantar surface of metatarsal bones.
La. plantaria articulationum interphalangealium pedis	Plantar ligs. of interphalangeal articulations	Interphalangeal articulations of foot between collateral ligs.
La. plantaria articulationum metatarsophalangeal	Plantar ligs. of metatarsophalangeal articulations	Plantar surface of metatarsophalangeal articulations between collateral ligs.
La. plantare longum	Long plantar l.	Connects calcaneus to bases of metatarsal bones.
La. talocalcaneare laterale	Lateral talocalcaneal l.	Connects talus to calcaneus.
La. talocalcaneare mediale	Medial talocalcaneal l.	Connects tubercle of talus to sustentaculum tali of calcaneus.
La. talocalcaneu interosseum	Interosseous talocalcaneal l.	Connects calcaneus to talus.
La. talofibulare anterius	Anterior talofibular l.	Connects lateral malleolus of fibula to posterior process of talus.
La. talonaviculare	Talonavicular l.	Connects neck of talus to navicular bone.
La. tarsi	Ligs. of tarsus	Connect bones of tarsus.

(continued)

Foot and Ankle

Latin name	English name	Articulation
La. tarsi dorsalia	Dorsal ligs. of tarsus	Collectively, bifurcate, dorsal cuboideonavicular, cuneocuboid, cuneonavicular, intercuneiform, and talonavicular ligaments.
La. tarsi interossea	Interosseous ligaments of tarsus	Collectively, interosseous, cuneocuboid, intercuneiform, and talocalcaneal ligs.
La. tarsi plantaria	Plantar ligs. of tarsus	Inferior ligs. of foot (long plantar, plantar calcaneocuboid, calcaneonavicular, cuneonavicular, cuboideonavicular, intercuneiform, cuneocuboid).
La. tarsometatarsalia dorsalia	Dorsal tarsometatarsal ligs.	Connect bases of metatarsals to dorsal cuboid and cuneiform bones.
La. tarsometatarsalia plantaria	Plantar tarsometatarsal ligs.	Connect metatarsal bones to cuboid and cuneiform bones.
La. transversum cruris	Superior extensor retinaculum of foot	Connects tibia to fibula. Holds extensor tendons in place.
Tendo calcaneus	Achilles tendon calcaneal tendon	Connects triceps surae muscle to tuberosity of calcaneus.

Anatomy Words (English-Latin)

Arteries

anterior radial collateral artery . . . . arteria collateralis radialis

anterior spinal artery . . . . arteria spinalis anterior

anterior tibial artery . . . . arteria tibialis anterior

ascending cervical artery . . . . arteria cervicalis ascendens

axillary artery . . . . arteria axillaris

brachial artery . . . . arteria brachialis

carotid artery . . . . arteria carotis (communis, externa, interna)

circumflex scapular artery . . . . arteria circumflexa scapulae

common carotid artery . . . . arteria carotis communis

common iliac artery . . . . arteria iliaca communis

deep circumflex iliac artery . . . . arteria circumflexa iliaca profunda

dorsalis pedis artery . . . . arteria dorsalis pedis

dorsal metatarsal artery . . . . arteria metatarsea dorsalis

facial artery . . . . arteria facialis

femoral artery . . . . arteria femoralis

femoral circumflex artery . . . . arteria circumflexa femoris (lateralis, medialis)

hypogastric artery . . . . ganglia pelvina

iliac artery . . . . arteria iliaca (communis, externa, interna)

iliolumbar artery . . . . arteria iliolumbalis

inferior thyroid artery . . . . arteria thyroidea inferior

internal carotid artery . . . . arteria carotis interna

internal iliac artery . . . . arteria iliaca interna

lingual artery . . . . arteria lingualis

metatarsal artery . . . . arteria metatarsae (dorsalis, plantaris)

middle sacral artery . . . . arteria sacralis mediana

nutrient artery . . . . arteria nutricia

obturator artery . . . . arteria obturatoria

peroneal artery . . . . arteria peronea

plantar artery . . . . arteria plantaris (lateralis, medialis)

popliteal artery . . . . arteria poplitea

posterior tibial artery . . . . arteria tibialis posterior

pudendal artery . . . . arteria pudenda (interna, externa)

radial artery . . . . arteria radialis

radicular artery . . . . ramus spinalis

rectal artery . . . . arteria rectalis (inferior, media, superior)

sacral artery . . . . arteria sacralis (lateralis, medialis)
segmental artery . . . . arteria segmenti
spinal artery . . . . ramus spinalis
subclavian artery . . . . arteria subclavia
superficial circumflex iliac artery. . . . . . . arteria circumflexa ilium superficialis
superficial temporal artery . . . . arteria temporalis superficialis
superior laryngeal artery . . . . arteria laryngea superior
superior thyroid artery . . . . arteria thyroidea superior
tibial artery. . . . . arterai tibialis (anterior, posterior)
ulnar artery. . . . . arteria ulnaris
vertebral artery . . . . arteria vertebralis

Bones

cancellous bone . . . . substantia spongiosa
carpal bone. . . . . os carpalis
collar bone . . . . clavicula
compact bone . . . . substantia compacta
cortical bone. . . . . substantia corticalis
cuboid bone . . . . os cuboideum
cuneiform bone . . . . os cuneiforme (intermedium, laterale,
                                        mediale)
flat bone . . . . os planum
hamate bone . . . . os hamatum
hook of hamate bone . . . . hamulus ossis hamati
hyoid bone . . . . os hyoideum
innominate bone. . . . . os coxae
long bone . . . . os longum
lunate bone. . . . . os lunatum
bone marrow . . . . medulla ossium
metacarpal bone . . . . os metacarpale
metatarsal bone . . . . os metatarsale
navicular bone . . . . os naviculare
pisiform bone . . . . os pisiforme
scaphoid bone. . . . . os scaphoideum
semilunar bone . . . . os lunatum
sesamoid bone . . . . os sesamoideum
short bone. . . . . os breve
spongy bone . . . . substantia spongiosa
tarsal bone . . . . os tarsalis
trabecular bone. substantia spongiosa

Ligaments

acromioclavicular ligament . . . . ligamentum acromioclaviculare
annular ligament. . . . . ligamentum annulare

anterior cruciate ligament. . . . . ligamentum cruciatum anterius
anterior talofibular ligament. . . . . ligamentum talofibulare anterius
arcuate ligament. . . . . ligamentum arcuatum (lateralis, medi-
                               ale, medianum, pubis)
atlantal transverse ligament . . . . ligamentum transversum atlantis
calcaneofibular ligament . . . . ligamentum calcaneofibulare
calcaneonavicular ligament . . . . ligamentum calcaneonaviculare
capsular ligament. . . . . ligamentum caplulare
collateral ligament . . . . ligamentum collaterale
conoid ligament . . . . ligamentum conoideum
coracoacromial ligament . . . . ligamentum coracoacromiale
coracoclavicular ligament . . . . ligamentum coracoclaviculare
coracohumeral ligament. . . . . ligamentum coracohumerale
costoclavicular ligament . . . . ligamentum costoclaviculare
cruciate ligament . . . . ligamentum cruciatum (anterius,
                               atlantis, cruris, posterius)
deep transverse metacarpal ligament . . . . ligamentum metacarpale transversum
                               profundum
deltoid ligament . . . . ligamentum deltoideum
fibular collateral ligament . . . . ligamentum collaterale fibulare
glenohumeral ligament. . . . . ligamentum glenohumalium
intercarpal ligament . . . . ligamentum intercarpalium
interclavicular ligament . . . . ligamentum interclaviculare
interspinous ligament. . . . . ligamentum interspinale
intertranverse ligament. . . . . ligamentum intertransversarium
lacinate ligament . . . . retinaculum musculorum flexorum
longitudinal ligament . . . . ligamentum longitudinale
meniscofemoral ligament. . . . . ligamentum meniscofemorale
                               (anterius, posterius)
nuchal ligament . . . . ligamentum nuchae
oblique popliteal ligament . . . . ligamentum popliteum obliquum
patellar ligament. . . . . ligamentum patellae
plantar ligament . . . . ligamentum plantaris
posterior cruciate ligament. . . . . ligamentum cruciatum posterius
posterior longitudinal ligament . . . . ligamentum longitudinale posterius
posterior talofibular ligament. . . . . ligamentum talofibulare posterius
quadrate ligament. . . . . ligamentum quadratum
radial collateral ligament . . . . ligamentum collaterale carpi radiale
radiate ligament . . . . ligamentum radiatum
radiate sternocostal ligament . . . . ligamentum sternocostalium radiatum
radiocarpal ligament. . . . . ligamentum radiocarpale (dorsalis,
                               palamare)
sacrospinous ligament . . . . ligamentum sacrospinale

sacrotuberous ligament . . . . ligamentum sacrotuberale
sternoclavicular ligament . . . . ligamentum sternoclaviculare
talofibular ligament . . . . ligamentum talofibulare (anterius, posterius)
tibial collateral ligament . . . . ligamentum collaterale tibiale
tibiofibular ligament . . . . ligamentum tibiofibulare (anterius, posterius)
transverse acetabular ligament . . . . ligamentum transversum acetabuli
transverse atlantal ligament . . . . ligamentum transversum atlantis
transverse scapular ligament . . . . ligamentum transversum scapulae (inferius, superius)
trapezoid ligament . . . . ligamentum trapezoideum
triangular ligament . . . . ligamentum triangulare
ulnar collateral ligament . . . . ligamentum collaterale ulnare

Muscles

abductor digiti minimi muscle . . . . musculus abductor digiti minimi (manus, pedis)
abductor digiti quinti muscle . . . . musculus abductor digiti quinti
abductor hallucis muscle . . . . musculus abductor hallucis
abductor pollicis brevis muscle . . . . musculus abductor pollicis brevis
abductor pollicis longus muscle . . . . musculus abductor pollicis longus
anterior scalene muscle . . . . musculus scalenus anterior
anterior serratus muscle . . . . musculus serratus anterior
anterior tibial muscle . . . . musculus tibialis anterior
biceps brachii muscle . . . . musculus biceps brachii
biceps femoris muscle . . . . musculus biceps femoris
brachialis muscle . . . . musculus brachialis
brachioradialis muscle . . . . musculus brachioradialis
deltoid muscle . . . . musculus deltoideus
digastric muscle . . . . musculus digastricus
dorsal interosseous muscle . . . . musculus interosseus dorsalis (manus, pedis)
extensor carpi radialis brevis muscle . . . . musculus extensor carpi radialis longus
extensor carpi radialis longus muscle . . . musculus extensor carpi radialis brevis
extensor carpi ulnaris muscle . . . . musculus extensor carpi ulnaris
extensor digiti minimi muscle . . . . musculus extensor digiti minimi
extensor digitorum brevis muscle . . . . . . musculus extensor digitorum brevis
extensor digitorum communis muscle . . . musculus extensor digitorum communis
extensor digitorum longus muscle . . . . . . musculus extensor digitorum longus
extensor hallucis brevis muscle . . . . musculus extensor hallucis brevis

extensor hallucis longus muscle........ musculus extensor hallucis longus
extensor pollicis brevis muscle .... musculus extensor pollicis brevis
extensor pollicis longus muscle........ musculus extensor pollicis longus
external intercostal muscle............ musculus intercostalis externus
flexor carpi radialis muscle .... musculus flexor carpi radialis
flexor carpi ulnaris muscle............ musculus flexor carpi ulnaris
flexor digitorum longus muscle .... musculus flexor digitorum longus
flexor digitorum profundus muscle ..... musculus flexor digitorum profundus
flexor digitorum sublimis muscle........ musculus flexor digitorum sublimis
flexor digitorum superficialis muscle.... musculus flexor digitorum super-
           ficialis
flexor hallucis brevis muscle .... musculus flexor hallucis brevis
flexor hallucis longus muscle.......... musculus flexor hallucis longus
flexor pollicis brevis muscle .... musculus flexor pollicis brevis
flexor pollicis longus muscle .... musculus flexor pollicis longus
gastrocnemius muscle .... musculus gastrocnemius
gluteus maximus muscle .... musculus gluteus maximus
gluteus medius muscle............... musculus gluteus medius
gluteus minimus muscle.............. musculus gluteus minimus
greater rhomboid muscle .... musculus rhomboideus major
iliacus muscle...................... musculus iliacus
iliocostal muscle.................... musculus iliocostalis
iliopsoas muscle.................... musculus iliopsoas
infraspinatus muscle................. musculus infraspinatus
latissimus dorsi muscle .... musculus latissimus dorsi
levator scapulae muscle .... musculus levator scaplulae
longus capitus muscle .... musculus longissimus capitas
longus colli muscle.................. musculus longus colli
lumbrical muscle .... musculus lumbricalis (manus, pedis)
obturator internus muscle............. musculus obturator internus
omohyoid muscle................... musculus omohyoideus
opponens digiti quinti muscle .... musculus opponens digiti minimi
opponens pollicis muscle............. musculus opponens pollicis
palmar interosseous muscle .... musculus interosseus palmaris
palmaris longus muscle .... musculus palmaris longus
pectoralis major muscle .... musculus pectoralis major
peroneus brevis muscle .... musculus peroneus brevis
peroneus longus muscle.............. musculus peroneus longus
peroneus tertius muscle .... musculus peroneus tertius
plantaris muscle .... musculus plantaris
platysma muscle.................... musculus platysma
popliteus muscle.................... musculus popliteus
pronator quadratus muscle .... musculus pronator quadratus

pronator teres muscle . . . . musculus pronator teres
psoas muscle . . . . musculus psoas (major, minor)
quadratus femoris muscle. . . . . musculus quadratus femoris
quadratus lumborum muscle . . . . musculus quadratus lumborum
quadriceps femoris muscle. . . . . musculus quadriceps femoris
rectus abdominis muscle . . . . musculus rectus abdominis
rectus femoris muscle. . . . . musculus rectus femoris
sartorius muscle . . . . musculus sartorius
scalenus anticus muscle . . . . musculus scalenus anticus
semimembranosus muscle . . . . musculus semimembranosus
semitendinosus muscle. . . . . musculus semitendinosus
serratus anterior muscle . . . . musculus serratus anterior
sternocleidomastoid muscle. . . . . musculus sternocleidomastoideus
sternohyoid muscle . . . . musculus sternohyoideus
sternomastoid muscle. . . . . see: sternocleidomastoid muscle
sternothyroid muscle . . . . musculus sternothyroideus
strap muscle . . . . see infrahyoid muscle
subscapularis muscle . . . . musculus subscapularis
supinator muscle . . . . musculus supinator
supraspinatus muscle . . . . musculus supraspinatus
teres major muscle . . . . musculus teres major
tibialis anterior muscle. . . . . musculus tibialis anterior
tibialis posterior muscle . . . . musculus tibialis posterior
transversus abdominis muscle . . . . musculus transversus abdominis
trapezius muscle. . . . . musculus trapezius
triceps surae muscle . . . . musculus triceps surae
vastus lateralis muscle . . . . musculus vastus lateralis
vastus medialis muscle. . . . . musculus vastus medialis

Nerves

accessory nerve . . . . nervus accessorius
articular nerve . . . . nervus articularis
axillary nerve . . . . nervus axillaris
common peroneal nerve. . . . . nervus peroneus communis
cutaneous nerves . . . . nervus cutaneus
deep peroneal nerve . . . . nervus peroneus profundus
dorsal scapular nerve . . . . nervus dorsalis scapulae
femoral nerve . . . . nervus femoralis
femoral cutaneous nerve . . . . nervus cutaneus femoris (lateralis,
                                                           medialis)
genitofemoral nerve . . . . nervus genitofemoralis
hypoglossal nerve. . . . . nervus hypoglossus
iliohypogastric nerve . . . . nervus iliohypogastricus
ilioinguinal nerve . . . . nervus ilioinguinalis

inferior laryngeal nerve . . . . nervus laryngeus inferior
intercostal nerve . . . . nervus intercostalis
intercostobrachial nerve . . . . nervus intercostobrachialis
intermediate dorsal cutaneous nerve . . . . nervus cutaneus dorsalis intermedius
lateral antebrachial cutaneous nerve . . . . nervus cutaneus antebrachii lateralis
lateral anterior thoracic nerve . . . . nervus pectoralis lateralis
lateral femoral cutaneous nerve . . . . nervus cutaneus femoris lateralis
lateral plantar nerve . . . . nervus plantaris lateralis
mandibular nerve . . . . nervus mandibularis
medial antebrachial cutaneous nerve . . . . nervus cutaneus anttebrachii medialis
medial dorsal cutaneous nerve . . . . nervus cutaneus dorsalis medialis
median nerve . . . . nervus medianus
musculocutaneous nerve . . . . nervus musculocutaneus
obturator nerve . . . . nervus obturatorius
phrenic nerve . . . . nervus phrenicus
posterior interosseous nerve . . . . nervus interosseus posterior
radial nerve . . . . nervus radialis
recurrent laryngeal nerve . . . . nervus laryngeus recurrens
sacral nerve . . . . nervus sacralis
saphenous nerve . . . . nervus saphenus
sciatic nerve . . . . nervus ischiadicus
spinal nerve . . . . nervus spinalis
spinal accessory nerve . . . . nervus accessorius
superficial peroneal nerve . . . . nervus peroneus superficialis
superior gluteal nerve . . . . nervus gluteus superior
superior laryngeal nerve . . . . nervus laryngeus superior
suprascapular nerve . . . . nervus suprascapularis
sural nerve . . . . nervus suralis
thoracic nerve . . . . nervus thoracis
tibial nerve . . . . nervus tibialis
ulnar nerve . . . . nervus ulnaris
vagus nerve . . . . nervus vagus

Veins

anterior jugular vein . . . . vena jugularis anterior
axillary vein . . . . vena axillaris
brachiocephalic vein . . . . vena bradhiocephalica
cephalic vein . . . . vena cephalica
common iliac vein . . . . vena iliaca communis
iliolumbar vein . . . . vena iliolumbalis
innominate vein . . . . vena brachioceplhalica
internal iliac vein . . . . vena iliaca interna
internal jugular vein . . . . vena jugularis interna
lingual vein . . . . vena lingualis

Appendix 5

lumbar vein . . . . vena lumbalis
middle thyroid vein . . . . vena thyroidea media
peroneal vein . . . . vena peronea
popliteal vein . . . . vena poplitea
subclavian vein. . . . . vena subclavia
superficial vein. . . . . vena cutanea
superficial temporal vein . . . . vena temsporalis superficialis
superior thyroid vein . . . . vena thyroidea superior
vertebral vein . . . . vena vertebralis

Appendix 6
Common Terms by Procedure

Amputation Terms

4 × 4
ABD pad
Achilles tenotomy
adductor magnus flap
air-driven oscillating saw
Ambulator® Chukka Boot
anterior myocutaneous flap
Bailey Saw guide
bone hook
Chopart amputation
demarcation
disarticulation
extensor digitorum transfer
femoral nerve
fishmouth incision
flexor digitorum communis (FDC)
free tie
Gigli saw
Gigli-Strully saw
guillotine amputation
heel pad
Hibbs osteotome
Langenbeck periosteal elevator
Lisfranc amputation
Liston amputation knife
Liston bone cutting forceps
Luer bone ronguer
Marquardt osteotomy
metatarsal phalangeal (MP) crease
metatarsal shaft
parajugular line
periosteal elevator
plantar flap
profunda femoris
Putti bone rasp
rasp
ray amputation
Satterlee saw
short-leg plaster cast
skew flap
slow cautery
staged
stockinette
superficial femoral artery (SFA)
supracondylar
Syme amputation
talar neck
tibialis anterior
transmetatarsal amputation (TMA)
vastus medialis muscle
volar condyle
Xeroform dressing

Arthroscopic Instrumentation Terms

AcuDriver osteotome
Axel wire twister
Axis fixation system
bone graft shoe horn
bone punch rongeur
bone hole punch
cerclage wire twister
CurvTek TSR bone drill
Delrin-handle bone saw
extraction pliers
Harmon chisel
James wound forceps
King wound forceps
Lagenbeck bone saw
Miltex bone saw
Miltex wire twister
needle-nose pliers
needle-nose vise-grip pliers
Orthocomp cement
OrthoPak bone growth stimulator
patella bone saw
pin crimper
Puka chisel
single-sided bone saw

Sklar ligature needle
Sklar bone drill/saw
slip-joint pliers
Sontec pliers
spanner gauge
Sparta wire cutter
Spartan jaw wire cutter
T-C ring-handle wire extractor
Universal bone plate (UBP) system

Cervical Diskectomy and Fusion with Bone Graft (Spine Surgery) Terms

allograft
annulus fibrosus
anterior cervical fascia
anterior and posterior (AP) fusion
anterior longitudinal ligament
anterosuperior iliac spine
autograft
autologous blood
bacitracin solution
benzoin
Betadine scrub, paint, solution
bipolar cautery
bleeding bone
bone plug
bone wax
bone dollop
bur hole, burr hole
cadaver bone graft
carotid artery
carotid sheath
cervical traction
corticocancellous bone
countersunk
cricothyroid membrane
cutting current
decompression
decortication
disk extrusion
disk space
disk protrusion

dry sterile dressing (DSD)
dura mater graft
dura
end plate
epidural space
epinephrine
facet, facetectomy
fascia lata graft
femoral shaft
fingerbreadth
flexion distraction
foraminotomy
harvest site
herniated nucleus pulposus (HNP)
herniated disk
hypertrophic ligament
iliac crest
interbody fusion
intercalary graft
interspace
lamina, pl. laminae
laminotomy
longus colli muscle
lumbodorsal fascia
methyl methacrylate
methylene blue dye
microneurosurgical technique
morcellate
nerve root decompression
neural foraminotomy
neural foramen
osteoarticular graft
osteopenia
osteophyte
pericardium graft
periosteum
platysma
posterior sacroiliac spine (PSIS)
posterior longitudinal ligament (PLL)
prevertebral space
purchase
radiculopathy
Sensorcaine

somatosensory evoked potentials
(SSEP)
spinal cord compression
spinous process
Steri-Strips
sternocleidomastoid muscle
strap muscle
subfascial incision
subperiosteal
thrombin-soaked Gelfoam
tricortical
vocal cord

Oblique Osteotomy and Arthroplasty (Podiatry) Terms

4×4
Ace wrap
Adaptic
Allis forceps
Ancef
Babcock forceps
Betadine solution
bone stock
bone-cutting forceps
Chevron osteotomy
Coban
contracture
Darco Wedge shoe
Deschamp needle
diamond pin cutter
digital block
double-action cutter
drill bit
Esmarch bandage
exsanguinate
extensor tendon
Felt shears
Hall sagittal saw
hyperkeratotic lesion
Inge spreader
K-wire driver
Kerlix
King forceps

Kirschner wire (K-wire)
Kling dressing
Lowman clamp
Mayo block
metatarsophalangeal (MTP) joint
obturator
Osteomed screw
Owens silk
Piffard curette
plug cutters
pneumatic ankle tourniquet
power rasp
rasp
rongeur
sagittal saw
side-cut pin cutter
Sklar wire tightener
Sklar pin cutter
Snap Lock wire/pin extractor
square-end pliers
Steinmann pin
T-C ring handle pin and wire extractor
T-C pin cutter
transverse capsulotomy
transverse tenotomy

Open Reduction and Internal Fixation of Hip Terms

abduction pillow
acetabular cup
acetabulum
Acufex grasper
Ancef
Arthro-sew
articular surface
axilla
Bennett retractor
bipolar cup
bipolar prosthesis
C-arm fluoroscopy unit
canal finder
capsular layer
Caspari shuttle

Caspari punch
cerclage wire
compression hip screw
cookie cutter
derotational pin
DHS hip screw
drive-through sign
DuraPrep
fascia lata
femoral shaft
femoral guide pin
femoral head
four tap screws
four-hole side plate
fracture table
greater trochanter
image intensifier
inferior glenohumeral ligament (IGHL)
    insertion
Innomed arthroplasty measuring system
intertrochanteric fracture
Jackson bone clamp
lag screw
leg length
longitudinal incision
outside-in technique
Press-Fit
pulsatile lavage
purchase
reamer
Revo knot
Revo suture anchor
Revo loop handle knot pusher
Ringer lactate
sideplate barrel
sliding knot
subcapital fracture
subchondral bone
Suretac bioabsorbable fixation device
Telos table
tensor fascia lata
vastus lateralis muscle
VerSys hip system

Open Reduction and Internal Fixation of the Radius (Wrist Surgery) Terms

1-2 portal
14-gauge Angiocath
3-4 portal
4-5 portal
6U portal
AO technique
axillary block anesthesia
bulky hand dressing
buttress-type plate
carpometacarpal (CMC) joint
Coban
dorsal splint
dorsal radial slope
dorsal ulnar cutaneous branch
eburnate
Esmarch bandage
extensor carpi radialis longus (ECRL)
extensor carpi radialis brevis (ECRB)
extensor pollicis longus (EPL)
extensor carpi ulnaris (ECU)
extensor digitorum communis (EDC)
extensor digiti quinti (EDQ)
external fixator
extraarticular
extravasation
finger trap
Henry approach
hockey-stick incision
image intensifier
intraarticular fragment
Lister tubercle
Mersilene suture
midcarpal portal
morcellate
no-touch technique
oscillating saw
pronator quadratus
radial sensory nerve
radial artery
scaphocapitate interval

scaphotrapezoid interosseous ligament
Silastic standard elastometer prosthesis
snuffbox
superficial radial nerve
Synthes plate, screw
T-shaped incision
trial fit
triangular fibrocartilage complex (TFC)
    tear
triangular rasp
venae comitantes
volar splint

Physical Therapy Terms

arc pain
Codman cane
cortisone
dexamethasone
end-range pain
extension
iontophoresis
isotonic exercise
joint mobilization
joint protection
moist heat
Neer impingement sign
opposite arm-assisted range of motion
    exercise
posture protection
pulley exercise
radiation
range of motion (ROM) exercise
rotation
surgical tubing
therapeutic exercise
tubing program
ultrasound
upper body ergometer (UBE)

Shoulder Acriomioplasty and Arthroscopy Terms

5.5-mm shaver
abduction

acromioclavicular ligament
adduction
adhesive capsulitis
anterior triangle
anterolateral raphe
Apex Universal Drive and Irrigation
    System
arthroscopic syovector
arthroscopic shaver
Balfour self-retaining retractor
Bankart repair
beach chair position
bevel
bicipital groove
bite
blunt arthroscopic cannula
bursal debridement
calcific tendinitis
Charnley retractor
clavipectoral fascia
compression dressing
coracoacromial ligament
coracobrachialis
coracohumeral ligament
coracoid
Depo-Medrol
Fukuda humeral head retractor
Gelpi retractors
glenohumeral joint
glenoid cavity
glenoid labrum
Hagl lesion
Hill-Sachs lesion
Homan retractor
impingement syndrome
joker
lateral acromial border
McConnel shoulder positioner
musculocutaneous nerve
purse-string suture
Rockwood anterior acromioplasty
rotator cuff
self-sealing cannula

Sharpey fiber
subacromial space
subacromial decompression
subscapularis
suction irrigation system
supraspinatus
synovectomy
synovitis
thoracoacromial artery
through-and-through tear
triangulation
vertical axis
Wissinger rod

Spinal Instrumentation Terms

Adcon adhesive control gel
Adcon-L antiadhesion barrier gel
Andrews table
angled curette
Apofix cervical instrumentation
Atlantis cervical plate system
Atlas cable system
BacFix System
BAK cage
blunt hook dissector
C-arm fluoroscopy
Capner gouge
Caspar retractor
cervical/lumbar hammer
Clarus SpineScope
Cloward rongeur
Cloward surgical saddle
Cloward retractor, spreader
Codman anterior cervical plate (ACP) system
Codman Ti-frame posterior fixation system
Cohort bone screw
Cohort Ti-spacer
Cohort bone brush
Cohort anterior plate system (APS)
Cohort spinal impactors

crank frame retractor
Crosslink plate
deep retractor
demineralized bone matrix (DBM)
diskogram needle
distraction screw
distraction pin
distractor
doughnut headrest
dual nerve root suction retractor
DynaFix external fixation system
EBIce
Elan drill
flat-bottomed Kerrison rongeur
fusion cage
Gardner-Wells tongs
GDLH posterior spinal system
graft driver
halo vest
halo brace
Holter traction
interlaminar clamp
interspinous cable
Jackson table
Kerrison rongeur
lag screw
Leksell rongeur
Liberty spinal system
LIFEC (lumbar intersomatic fusion expandable cage)
Magnum chisel, curette
mallet
Mayfield head rest
MDS microdebrider
Miami collar
Miami J collar
Microsect curette, shaver
Midas Rex drill, burr
Mini-ALIF
multiaxial screw
neck roll
oscillating saw
OsteoGen implantable stimulator

OsteoSet-T medicated bone graft
   substitute
osteotome
PEAK Fixation System
pedicle sounder
Penrose drain
PercScope
Philadelphia collar
pituitary rongeur
plastic end caps
polyaxial cervical screws
Preclude spinal membrane
segmental spinal correction system
   (SSCS)
self-retaining retractor
Shadow-Line ACF spine retractor system
Silhouette spinal system
SITElite
SITEprobe
SITEtrac
Sofwire cable system
SpF spinal stimulator
spinal needle
Steinmann pin
stereolithography (SL) cage
straight curette
Super Cut laminectomy ronguer
Tacoma sacral plate
tamp
Tang retractor
threaded cortical dowels
TOP ejector punch
Tuohy needle
Universal Spine System (USS)
Versa-Trac lumbar spine retractor system
Versalok low back fixation system
Wrightlock spinal fixation system
Wrightlock posterior fixation system

Total Knee Replacement Terms

Ace bandage
Adaptic gauze

alignment guide rod
anterior cruciate ligament (ACL)
aspirated fat
biceps femoris
bolster
bone plug
bone-on-bone
broach
C-clamp
cancellous surface
cement gun
centralizing rod
chamfer cut
ConstaVac drainage
continuous passive motion (CPM)
cooling machine
Coumadin
cruciate punch
cruciate-sacrificing
cruciform tibial base plate
crystalloid
curved osteotome
cutting jig, cutting block
deep venous thrombosis (DVT)
   prophylaxis
Dexon sutures
digital impaction
distal femur
distal tuft
drill point
eburnation of cartilage
elastic stockings
electrocoagulation
Esmarch bandage
eversion
extensor mechanism
extramedullary guide
fat pad
femoral component
femoral condyle
femoral head
femoral jig
flexion valgus deformity

flexion/extension gap
Foley catheter
footrest
four-in-one block
free-hand cut
gastrocnemius soleus
Hemovac drain
Howmedica Duracon implant
hyperplasia
iliotibial band
intercondylar notch
intramedullary canal
intramedullary (IM) rod
Johnson & Johnson P.F.C. Cruciate-
  Substituting insert
Kerlix
keyhole punch
knee immobilizer
Kocher clamp
KT1000/s surgical arthrometer
laminar air flow
LH1000 arthroscopic leg holder
medial compartment
medial parapatellar arthrotomy
medial collateral ligament
medial/lateral femoral condyle
medial/lateral meniscus
medial tubercle
medullary canal
meniscectomy
methyl methacrylate
notch cutting guide, notch cut
Osteonics Scorpio insert
Osteonics jig
parapatellar incision
patellar groove
patellar tracking
patient-controlled anesthesia (PCA)
plain gauze
plastic patella
polo test
polyethylene component

Polysorb suture
posterior cruciate ligament (PCL)
Press-Fit femoral component
Pulsavac irrigation
PVC drain
quadriceps tendon
range of motion
respiratory exhaust system
Rowe blanket
S-cutting block
sandbag
Sapphire View arthroscope
sequential compression device (SCD)
spacer
step drill
subluxation
subperiosteal
superior pole of patella
Systec irrigation
tibial insert
tibial plateau
tibial base plate
tibial cutting guide
tibial liftoff
tibial tubercle
tibial tray
Toradol
tourniquet
towel clip
trial spacer
trial reduction
true spacer
uncemented femoral component
valgus
varus
vastus medialis obliquus
Venodyne boot
warfarin sodium
wedge
weightbearing surface
Zimmer NexGen LPS knee femoral
  component

Appendix 7
Sample Reports,
Including Sample Physical Therapy Note

Sample Above-Knee Amputation

TITLE OF OPERATION: Above-knee amputation of the left leg.

PROCEDURE IN DETAIL: The patient was brought to the operating room and placed in the supine position. A left parajugular line was inserted and secured by the anesthesiologist, and after this was done, anesthesia was induced through the IV. She initially had the esophageal airway for general anesthesia ventilation. After this was done, the left leg was prepped using Betadine solution and draped. The area of the ulceration was protected using stockinette. Sterile drapes were placed and a fishmouth incision was fashioned at the distal aspect of the left thigh. Using the scalpel, the line of demarcation was incised through the skin and subcutaneous, and the Bovie was also used intermittently with the scalpel to incise the area. The subcutaneous and the muscle groups were noted to be edematous. The vessels were noted to be very atherosclerotic. The vessels were secured and doubly ligated using free ties of 0 Vicryl. The femoral nerve was secured, and a clamp was placed proximally while it was pulled on tension, and then it was transected and the stump was tied. After leaving the clamp, I cut proximally.

The femur was transected using the Gigli saw, and after transection, the edges were rasped smooth using the rasp. After that, hemostasis was achieved with free ties of 0 Vicryl. The wound was washed out and, after washing, the muscle groups, the hamstrings, and the quadriceps were approximated using interrupted sutures of 0 Vicryl. This approximation was at the edge of the femur. After reapproximating the muscle groups to the fascia, the subcutaneous was then reapproximated using interrupted sutures of 0 Vicryl. This brought the subcutaneous together. Then the skin was closed with staples. Xeroform dressings were applied over the wound, and 4 × 4s and an ABD were applied. A specially made stump cap was placed over the dressing to hold it in place. The patient tolerated this procedure very well. Estimated blood loss was about 25 cc.

Sample Cervical Diskectomy and Fusion with Bone Graft

TITLE OF OPERATION: Anterior cervical diskectomy and fusion at left C6-C7 with allograft from the patient's right iliac crest.

PROCEDURE IN DETAIL: The patient was brought to the operating room, and after induction of satisfactory general endotracheal anesthesia, he was placed on the operating table in supine position with the head resting on a doughnut headrest and neck slightly extended by placing a roll underneath the neck. Shaving, prepping, and draping of the anterior cervical region and right anterosuperior iliac spine was performed in the usual sterile fashion. The incision line was then marked over the right anterosuperior iliac spine and also on the right side of the neck starting from the midline and extending obliquely toward the right side for about 3 cm in length. The incision line was infiltrated at both sides with dilute solution of epinephrine. Incision was taken down initially in the neck to the platysmal layer. Platysmal fiber was then separated along the lines of the fibers, and a self-retaining retractor was inserted. We then dissected medial to the sternocleidomastoid muscle border in the plane between the SVM and carotid sheath laterally and the trachea and esophagus medially. Steering through this plane, we reached the prevertebral space. Intraoperative fluoroscopy equipment had already been placed, as had cervical traction using traction with 10 pounds. Fluoroscopy was used to confirm the level of C6-C7 disk space.

After confirmation of the exact level by placing a needle into this space, we put the distraction screw in the body of C6-C7 under direct fluoroscopy. After placing distraction screws, a distractor was placed and disk space was entered using a #15 blade, cutting through the anterior longitudinal ligament and annulus fibrosus. A large amount of degenerated disk material was then removed with multiple sizes of pituitary rongeurs. After removal of degenerated disk material for the most of the disk space, the posterior longitudinal ligament was identified and a hole in the posterior longitudinal ligament on the left side was noted through which the disk herniation has occurred; pieces were lying in the epidural space. The free segment of disk material was then removed and the posterior longitudinal ligament was resected. The posterior longitudinal ligament portion on the left half was then removed with Cloward rongeurs. This confirmed the satisfactory decompression of the nerve root, and a blunt hook dissector was then passed to remove any further fragments which might be lying in the neural foramen. Neural foraminotomy was then performed using multiple sizes of small Cloward rongeurs. After neural foraminotomy was performed, wound and disk space were thoroughly irrigated with normal saline and bacitracin solution. Hemostasis was secured by placing Gelfoam soaked in thrombin in the epidural space.

Disk space measurements were then taken. It was noted to 7 mm high, 15 mm deep, and 14 mm wide. Based on these measurements, bone plug was then planned.

Allograft harvesting was then performed from the right anterosuperior iliac spine where the incision line had already been covered with diluted solution of epinephrine. The incision was taken down to the deeper fascial layer, and the self-retaining retractor was then placed. Cutting current was then used to cut through the deep fascia and periosteum. The muscle was then dissected off the bone, and after dissecting off the muscle satisfactorily, we placed deeper retractors. Using a 7-mm wide beveled oscillating saw blade, we cut a few pieces of bone from the anterosuperior iliac spine using an Elan drill. The inferior portion of the bone was then cut by using a small sharp osteotome and mallet. After removing the piece of bone, we used the bone wax to apply on the rough surfaces of bone for hemostasis. The wound was thoroughly irrigated with normal saline and bacitracin solution. After satisfactory hemostasis was accomplished using unipolar and bipolar cautery, we placed pieces of Gelfoam, and closure was then performed in layers using 0 Vicryl suture for deeper muscular and fascial layers, subcutaneous fat was closed with 4-0 Vicryl suture, and subcuticular layer was closed with 3-0 Vicryl stitch. Steri-Strips were applied to approximate the skin.

The bone plug was then cleaned from periosteum and was fashioned with a high-speed drill. After fashioning the bone plug appropriately, we placed the bone plug under direct fluoroscopy in the disk space. After the bone plug had been found to fit appropriately, we irrigated the wound with normal saline and bacitracin solution. Hemostasis was secured with bipolar cautery, the distraction pin was then removed, and bone wax was applied at the site of the distraction pin for satisfactory hemostasis. Closure was then performed after removing the retractor and the Cottonoid. A 3-0 Vicryl suture was used to approximate the platysma and 4-0 Vicryl sutures were used for subcuticular closure. Steri-Strips were applied to approximate the skin. Sterile dressing was then placed. The patient was then placed in a Philadelphia collar and taken to the recovery room in stable neurologic condition.

Sample Excision of Trapezium and Excisional Arthroplasty of Scaphotrapezoidal Joint

TITLE OF OPERATION:
1. Excision of the trapezium with #1-Swanson Silastic implant, trapeziometacarpal joint.
2. Excisional arthroplasty, scaphotrapezoidal joint.

PROCEDURE IN DETAIL: The patient was successfully induced under axillary block anesthesia on the left. A well-padded pretested pneumatic tourniquet was applied to the left upper extremity. The arm was exsanguinated and the tourniquet inflated to 250 mmHg. After routine sterile preparation, a reverse hockey-stick incision was made at the base of the first metacarpal. Under optical magnification, dissection was carried through subcutaneous tissues. A branch of the radial sensory nerve was retracted out of harm's way throughout the procedure. T-shaped incision was made in the capsule which was reflected to expose the base of the first metacarpal. The CMC joint was noted to be completely eburnated. Using the oscillating saw, the base of the metacarpal was transected and removed. The trapezium was then removed in a morcellated fashion. Upon removal of the trapezium, the scaphotrapezoidal joint was noted also to be eburnated and arthritic. It was decided to proceed with a scaphotrapezoidal excisional arthroplasty in addition to the trapeziometacarpal arthroplasty of the CMC joint. Using the oscillating saw, the base of the trapezoid was sharply transected and excised leaving a gap of approximately 1 cm. The wound was then copiously irrigated and the base of the first metacarpal rasped with the appropriate triangular rasps. Trial fit was performed with a #1 prosthesis and found to be satisfactory. Thereafter, three 4-0 Mersilene sutures were placed, two in the remnants of the scaphotrapezoid interosseous ligament and the last in the base of the first metacarpal through two previously drilled holes. These were to be used for ligamentous reconstruction. Now the wound was irrigated and a #1-Silastic standard elastomer prosthesis was inserted in a no-touch fashion. The joint was reduced and found to fit appropriately. A capsular reconstruction was then effected using the aforementioned Mersilene sutures. This offered a stable capsular reconstruction. The joint was reduced without difficulty after this reconstruction. The skin was closed with 5-0 nylon placed in a running fashion. The wound was instilled with a mixture of 0.5% plain Marcaine and 2% plain Xylocaine. Xeroform was applied to the wound followed by a bulky hand dressing and dorsal and volar splints. The patient tolerated the procedure well and left the room in satisfactory condition.

Sample Oblique Osteotomy and Arthroplasty

TITLE OF OPERATION:
1. Oblique osteotomy of the second metatarsal head, dorsiflexory and shortening with 2.4 8-10 mm Osteomed screw fixation.
2. Arthroplasty fourth proximal interphalangeal joint, left.

PROCEDURE IN DETAIL: After satisfactory preoperative evaluation, the patient was brought into the operating room and placed on the operating room table in the supine position. Ancef 1 g was administered preoperatively prophylactically per the anesthesia department. After adequate IV sedation, a local infiltrative block using 0.5% Marcaine plain was infiltrated in a Mayo block fashion about the second metatarsal, in a digital block fashion about the fourth metatarsal. A pneumatic ankle tourniquet was then placed around the patient's well-padded left foot 1 cm proximal to the malleolus. It was then prepped and draped in the usual aseptic manner. An Esmarch bandage was used to exsanguinate the left lower extremity prior to elevation of the left pneumatic ankle tourniquet to 250 mmHg.

Attention was first directed to the dorsal aspect of the second metatarsal where a linear incision measuring approximately 3 cm was performed centered over the metatarsophalangeal joint of the second metatarsal. It was incised with a #10 blade, deepened with a #15 blade to the level of the extensor tendon, which was reflected laterally. Capsulotomy was performed dorsally longitudinally and carefully resected. The metatarsal head was easily visualized. Next, using the sagittal saw and two blades, an oblique osteotomy from dorsal to plantar, proximal to distal was performed just proximal to the level of the dorsal articular surface of the second metatarsal. The osteotomy was through and through. The area was then flushed with copious amounts of sterile saline. Next, the 2.4 drill bit was inserted into the metatarsal perpendicular to the osteotomy cut. Then a radiograph of the left foot was taken to ascertain the position of the osteotomy and the fixation. It was shown that it was in good position and of proper length, and the drill bit was removed and a 2.4 8-10 mm Osteomed screw was placed in the area. This allowed rigid fixation, which was ascertained. The area was then flushed with copious amounts of sterile saline. The capsule was closed with 4-0 Vicryl in a simple interrupted manner, the subcu with 4-0 Vicryl in a simple interrupted manner. The skin was closed with 5-0 nylon in a horizontal mattress stitch.

Attention was then directed to the fourth toe, where a linear incision was inscribed over the proximal interphalangeal joint, deepened with a #15 blade. A transverse capsulotomy was performed. The capsule and tendon were resected to visualize the proximal phalangeal head. Then, using the sagittal saw, it was resected perpendicularly along the axis of the proximal phalanx. The area was then rasped smooth and flushed with copious amounts of sterile saline. The wound was reapproximated with 4-0

Vicryl in a simple interrupted manner. The skin was closed with 5-0 nylon in a horizontal mattress stitch.

Pneumatic ankle tourniquet was deflated for a total tourniquet time of approximately 40 minutes. The patient tolerated the procedure well. No complications occurred during the procedure. The foot was dressed with Adaptic saline-soaked 4 × 4's, dry 4 × 4's, Kerlix, and Coban. Vascularity was maintained after tourniquet release for a capillary fill time of all digits of approximately 3 seconds to the left foot. The patient will be maintained nonweightbearing with a Darco Wedge shoe.

Sample Open Reduction and Internal Fixation of Hip

TITLE OF OPERATION: Open reduction and internal fixation of intertrochanteric fracture, left hip, with DHS hip screw
and four-hole sideplate.

PROCEDURE IN DETAIL: Under satisfactory spinal anesthesia, the patient was
placed on the Telos table, and I was able to do some traction with some manipulation
and reduction. This was checked in the AP and lateral position. She was then prepped
and draped in this position. A 6-inch incision was made beginning at the tip of the
greater trochanter and going distally along the lateral thigh. Sharp dissection was used
to go down through the subcutaneous fat. Hemostasis was achieved with electrocoagulation. The fascia was incised in line with the incision, and the vastus lateralis
muscle was split by sharp resection down to the underlying femur and a Bennett retractor placed. Under C-arm control, I placed a guidewire up into the neck. It hap-
pened to be that the greater trochanter had fractured right at the place where the
guidewire went, so this made placement rather easy. This was checked on the AP and
lateral, and I used the 135° angle guide. I then measured and determined I needed a
90-mm compression hip screw. The wire was then driven in a little further, and the
drill for the hip screw and sideplate barrel was then run over the screw under x-ray
control. This was then removed, and the 90-mm compression hip screw was then
placed over the guidewire and again checked in the AP and lateral projections. It was
found to be in good position, and I had very good purchase in the head.

Next, the 135° angle, four-hole sideplate, the barrel of which was slipped over the
shaft of the screw and fixed to the femoral shaft. It was held in place with a Jackson
bone clamp. Four screws were then placed by drilling, measuring, and putting in four
tap screws; one 40-mm, two 38-mm, and a 6-mm screw. Finally, all of them were
tightened down. The Jackson clamp was removed, and the wound was irrigated. The
vastus lateralis muscle was allowed to fall back together. The fascia was closed with
#1-Vicryl interrupted sutures. The subcutaneous fat was closed with 0-Vicryl inter-
rupted inverted sutures, and the skin was closed with skin staples. A Betadine dressing was applied. The patient left the operating room in satisfactory condition with no
drains and no complications. The patient received 1 g of Ancef IV prior to the start
of the procedure.

Sample Open Reduction and Internal Fixation of the Radius

TITLE OF OPERATION: Left distal radius open reduction and internal fixation and application of internal fixator.

PROCEDURE IN DETAIL: After the patient was identified and after adequate anesthesia, he was positioned supine on the operating table. The left arm was placed on the arm table. It was prepped and draped in a sterile fashion. The arm was exsanguinated with an Esmarch bandage and then tourniquet was inflated to 250 mmHg. A volar approach was done, distal modified Henry approach. Care was taken to protect the superficial radial nerve and also the radial artery and its venae comitantes. The pronator quadratus was incised longitudinally and elevated off the bone. The fracture was identified, reduced, and the joint was also visualized. Intraarticular fragment was also reduced. Once the fracture had been reduced, it was plated with a Synthes plate. Using AO technique, the plate was applied. The fracture was controlled in both AP and lateral planes using image intensifier. It was found to be well reduced, and the screws and the tips of the screws were not impinging any vital structures and were extraarticular. After that was done, the wound was irrigated copiously with antibiotic normal saline solution. It was closed in layers using 2-0 Vicryl and 3-0 nylon. Next, an external fixator was placed dorsolaterally in order to provide additional stability. Since this is a very large gentleman, the plate that was used was a buttress type. Dressings were applied without difficulty again using standard AO technique. The incision was closed with 3-0 nylon after it had been irrigated copiously. A dressing was applied and the patient was aroused from anesthesia without any complications.

Sample Physical Therapy Note

TREATMENT:	Treatment today consisted of iontophoresis, moist heat, and ultrasound of the cervical spine; joint mobilization of the neck and shoulder; therapeutic exercise to the neck and shoulder $\times$ 45 minutes.
CHIEF COMPLAINT:	Cervical neck pain and right shoulder pain.
PROGRESS:	The patient states that he is the same as he was the last time he was in for therapy.
COMPLIANCE:	He states 75%.
AGGRAVATING FACTORS:	Working.
PAIN/DISCOMFORT LEVEL:	The patient states that the pain is 5/10.

PATIENT'S PROGRESS: The patient is doing well with his cervical spine exercises. His neck retraction and neck extension and rotation are relatively improved. His radiating pain is reduced. His right shoulder is very painful. He has a positive Neer impingement sign. He has pain and pressure on flexion and abduction. He has pain on resisted abduction. He has a rotator cuff tendinitis, probable impingement.

The patient was put on a four-step treatment approach. He was advised to use ice for pain and antiinflammatories for pain. He was started on a shoulder mobilization program. He did fairly with this today. He had less shoulder pain. He had better motion following his therapy. He is advised to use the exercise program on a regular basis.

HOME PROGRAM: The patient is able to do home program with no difficulties. The patient was advised to call the clinic to report if there are any difficulties with the home program.

FOLLOWUP: The patient will be seen back in the clinic on Thursday. The patient did well with his therapy today. I will talk to orthopedics about his shoulder pathology. He may need to be referred to orthopedics as he appears to have a stage II right shoulder impingement.

Sample Shoulder Arthroscopy with Synovectomy and Debridement

TITLE OF OPERATION:
1. Manipulation of the shoulder under general anesthesia for range of motion in the shoulder.
2. Arthroscopic examination of the right shoulder.
3. Arthroscopic synovectomy of the right shoulder.
4. Debridement of the undersurface of the rotator cuff muscle.
5. Debridement of the glenoid labrum.

PROCEDURE IN DETAIL: The patient was placed on the operating table in supine position. After satisfactory general endotracheal anesthesia was administered, the patient was placed in the left lateral position. Perioperative intravenous antibiotics were given. The arm and the right shoulder were prepped and draped in a sterile fashion. The arm was kept in a position of 40 degrees of abduction from the vertical axis of the body with 15 degrees of forward flexion, with the patient tilted posteriorly. The landmarks were made on the shoulder area, and a standard arthroscopic examination was performed using a posterior portal, anterior portal, and lateral portals. The posterior portal was created about 1.5 cm distal and medial to the posterior lateral corner of the acromion. A small skin incision was made at that level, and the cannula was inserted in to the shoulder joint against the bony surface of the glenoid cavity. The arthroscope was inserted, and the joint was visualized. There was a quite thick labrum present in the superior, and superoanterior aspect of the labrum, but the anterior half of the labrum was torn in several jagged pieces. The biceps tendon also revealed some synovitis present on the superior aspect of the biceps, as well as the inferior aspect of the tendon. The arthroscope was then moved over along the passage of the biceps tendon until the bicipital groove in the humerus. The undersurface of the rotator cuff was visualized. There was erosion of the articular surface of the rotator cuff with a partial tear, and the tear was covered with fatty tissue.

The synovectomy was first performed. The arthroscope was then brought into the interval between the biceps tendon and the subscapularis. At this level, the arthroscope was removed from the sheath and a Wissinger rod was inserted to pierce the anterior capsule and then up to the skin edge. A small skin incision was made and the rod was brought out of the skin wound. The arthroscopic synovector was hooked up to the arthroscopic cannula, and the arthroscopic synovector was used to complete the synovectomy of the shoulder joint, debridement of the rotator cuff, and removal of the fatty tissue; then beveling of the ruptured edges of rotator cuff was done. Debridement of the glenoid labrum and its anterior and inferior aspect was also performed. No degenerative changes were present in the glenohumeral joint. After this was performed all the joint cavity was cleaned out of loose bodies and tissue with the suction irrigation system.

The subacromial decompression was performed with a lateral portal created about 2 cm lateral to the lateral border of the acromion, and a blunt arthroscopic cannula was inserted through this portal into the subacromial space. The arthroscope was removed from the posterior portal and was redirected into the subacromial space, where it could visualize the arthroscopic cannula. The arthroscopic shavers were used to clean out the bursal tissue, as well as the superior surface of the rotator cuff. The acromio-clavicular ligament was identified as a shiny structure from the anterior aspect of the acromion, and the ligament was taken off the acromion along with a bite of the acromion in anterior and lateral aspect. The subacromial space was then injected with 20 cc of 0.5% Marcaine solution mixed with 80 mg of Depo-Medrol. There was a small tear in the superior surface of the rotator cuff also, which was not a through-and-through tear; that tear was debrided.

All the portals were closed with 3-0 nylon sutures, and a sterile compression dressing was applied.

The patient tolerated the procedure well and was transferred from the operating room to the recovery room in stable condition.

Sample Total Knee Replacement

TITLE OF OPERATION: Total knee replacement, left.

PROCEDURE IN DETAIL: The patient was brought to the operating room as an a.m. admit, following the usual preoperative preparation. He was given 1 g of Ancef intravenously and in the presence of appropriate anesthetic monitoring, intravenous fluids and epidural anesthesia were given by the anesthesiologist without complication. Supplementary sedation was also applied. A Foley catheter was placed. A Venodyne boot was placed on the right lower extremity, on the right calf, and a Rowe blanket was placed underneath the left presacrum, internally rotating the left knee. A sandbag was placed on the exam table to allow a footrest with flexion on the knee. A tourniquet was placed high on the thigh, and the entire left leg, from ankle to tourniquet, was sterilely prepped and draped in the usual manner. The leg was exsanguinated using an Esmarch bandage, and the tourniquet was inflated to 300 mmHg.

With the knee flexed, a straight anterior incision was made from the tibial tubercle to 4 cm proximal to the superior pole of the patella and brought down to the extensor mechanism. A medial parapatellar arthrotomy was made from medial to the tibial tubercle, into the medial aspect of the quadriceps tendon. The patella was everted. Advanced arthritic changes with completed eburnation of cartilage were seen in the medial compartment, both weightbearing surface and femoral condyle and tibial plateau. Limited meniscectomies were performed. The medullary canal was entered with a large drill point just superior to the intercondylar notch and an intramedullary guide rod with attached distal cutting jig, set to 7°, was inserted into the femoral canal. When a 12-mm distal tuft was fixed, the cutting block was held with drill points. Using oscillating saw, distal femur was resected 12 mm. Thereupon, an AP cutting jig was applied, after measurements verified an extra large femur. Anterior-posterior chamfer cuts were then made.

Attention was then turned to the tibia. Remnants of medial and lateral meniscus were removed. The anterior cruciate ligament was removed. The external tibial cutting guide was applied, and, when appropriate alignment was verified, a 3° posterior cutting block was fixed to the tibial plateau with drill points and set to remove 11 mm of tibial articular surface as measured from the lateral tibial plateau. This was performed with an oscillating saw.

Attention was then turned to the patella, which measured a total of 26 mm in thickness. An 11-mm cut was made and drill holes were placed to accept a large patellar component. A trial reduction was performed at this time. It was found that an extra large 2 tibial base plate gave appropriate fit, and an 11-mm tibial trial insert allowed for appropriate medial lateral stability. The polo test was positive; that is, the component could easily be pulled out with the knee in extension and with the knee in flexion; there was no tibial liftoff. External alignment guide rods were used to verify appropriate rotation of the tibial base plate and that it was fixed with two pins, and the cut surface of the tibial plateau was prepared with a cruciate punch.

While the assistant copiously lavaged and dried the cancellous surfaces, the surgeon went to the back table and mixed methyl methacrylate under vacuum conditions and it was placed in the cement gun. It was brought to the table and the tibial component was cemented into place and impacted. All extraneous metal was removed. A porous coat Press-Fit femoral component was impacted into place, and the knee was pressurized in extension with a trial 11-mm plastic insert. The patella was also cemented into place and held with a clamp. Thereupon, after cement had hardened, all extraneous metal was removed. The knee was brought through a range of motion with the 11-mm trial tibial insert, and again, its stability was found to be appropriate with a positive polo test. Thereupon, after again copiously lavaging the knee and removing all debris from the tibial baseplate, the permanent tibial insert, 11 mm in depth, was snapped into place. The knee was again copiously lavaged and brought through a range of motion. The patella tracked quite appropriately. Full extension was possible as well as flexion to beyond 120°. Bolsters were placed under the knee to place it in approximately 30° of flexion, and the extensor mechanism was closed using interrupted 0-Dexon sutures. Subcuticular tissue was closed using inverted 2-0 Dexon and a running 4-0 subcuticular Dexon was used to close skin. This was to reinforce the Steri-Strips. Marcaine 0.5% with epinephrine was infiltrated about the incision edges and Steri-Strips were applied followed by sterile dressing and then by high elastic stockings.

Postoperatively, prophylactic measures will be taken to prevent complications with intravenous antibiotics, which were started preoperatively and will be continued for 24 hours. Low-dose Coumadin will be begun for DVT prophylaxis and Venodyne boots will be used bilaterally. CPM will be started in the recovery room to gain early passive range of motion of the knee. Pain control will be continued with PCA and narcotics by mouth as needed.

Drugs by Indication

ARTHRITIS
Aminoquinoline (Antimalarial)
  Aralen® Phosphate
  chloroquine phosphate
  hydroxychloroquine
  Plaquenil®
Analgesic, Topical
  capsaicin
  Capsin® [OTC]
  Capzasin-P® [OTC]
  Dolorac™ [OTC]
  No Pain-HP® [OTC]
  R-Gel® [OTC]
  Zostrix® [OTC]
  Zostrix®-HP [OTC]
Antiinflammatory Agent
  Arava™
  leflunomide
Antineoplastic Agent
  cyclophosphamide
  Cytoxan® Injection
  Cytoxan® Oral
  Folex® PFS
  methotrexate
  Neosar® Injection
  Rheumatrex®
Antirheumatic, Disease Modifying
  Enbrel®
  etanercept
Chelating Agent
  Cuprimine®
  Depen®
  penicillamine
Gold Compound
  auranofin
  Aurolate®
  aurothioglucose
  gold sodium thiomalate
  Ridaura®
  Solganal®

Immunosuppressant Agent
  azathioprine
  cyclosporine
  Imuran®
  Neoral® Oral
  Sandimmune® Injection
  Sandimmune® Oral
Nonsteroidal Antiinflammatory Drug
  (NSAID)
  Actron® [OTC]
  Advil® [OTC]
  Aleve® [OTC]
  Anacin® [OTC]
  Anaprox®
  Ansaid® Oral
  Argesic®-SA
  Artha-G®
  Arthritis Foundation® Pain
    Reliever [OTC]
  Arthropan® [OTC]
  A.S.A. [OTC]
  Ascriptin® [OTC]
  aspirin
  Asprimox® [OTC]
  Bayer® Aspirin [OTC]
  Bayer® Buffered Aspirin [OTC]
  Bayer® Low Adult Strength [OTC]
  Bayer® Select® Pain Relief
    Formula [OTC]
  Bufferin® [OTC]
  Buffex® [OTC]
  Cama® Arthritis Pain Reliever
    [OTC]
  Cataflam® Oral
  Children's Advil® Oral
    Suspension [OTC]
  Children's Motrin® Oral
    Suspension [OTC]
  choline magnesium trisalicylate
  choline salicylate

Clinoril®
Daypro™
diclofenac
diflunisal
Disalcid®
Dolobid®
Dynafed® IB [OTC]
Easprin®
Ecotrin® [OTC]
Ecotrin® Low Adult Strength
    [OTC]
Empirin® [OTC]
Extra Strength Adprin-B® [OTC]
Extra Strength Bayer® Enteric
    500 Aspirin [OTC]
Extra Strength Bayer® Plus
    [OTC]
Extra Strength Doan's® [OTC]
Feldene®
fenoprofen
flurbiprofen
Genpril® [OTC]
Halfprin® 81® [OTC]
Haltran® [OTC]
Heartline® [OTC]
IBU®
Ibuprin® [OTC]
ibuprofen
Ibuprohm® [OTC]
Indochron E-R®
Indocin®
Indocin® SR
indomethacin
Junior Strength Motrin® [OTC]
ketoprofen
Magan®
magnesium salicylate
Marthritic®
meclofenamate
Menadol® [OTC]
Midol® IB [OTC]
Mobidin®
Mono-Gesic®

Motrin®
Motrin® IB [OTC]
nabumetone
Nalfon®
Naprelan®
Naprosyn®
naproxen
Nuprin® [OTC]
Orudis®
Orudis® KT [OTC]
Oruvail®
oxaprozin
piroxicam
Regular Strength Bayer® Enteric
    500 Aspirin [OTC]
Relafen®
Saleto-200® [OTC]
Saleto-400®
Saleto-600®
Saleto-800®
Salflex®
Salgesic®
salsalate
Salsitab®
St Joseph® Adult Chewable
    Aspirin [OTC]
sulindac
Tolectin®
Tolectin® DS
tolmetin
Trilisate®
Voltaren® Oral
Voltaren-XR® Oral
ZORprin®
BLASTOMYCOSIS
    Antifungal Agent
    itraconazole
    ketoconazole
    Nizoral®
    Sporanox™
BURSITIS
    Nonsteroidal Antiinflammatory Drug
        (NSAID)

Advil® [OTC]
Aleve® [OTC]
Anacin® [OTC]
Anaprox®
Arthritis Foundation® Pain
    Reliever [OTC]
Arthropan® [OTC]
A.S.A. [OTC]
Ascriptin® [OTC]
aspirin
Asprimox® [OTC]
Bayer® Aspirin [OTC]
Bayer® Buffered Aspirin [OTC]
Bayer® Low Adult Strength
    [OTC]
Bayer® Select® Pain Relief
    Formula [OTC]
Bufferin® [OTC]
Buffex® [OTC]
Cama® Arthritis Pain Reliever
    [OTC]
Children's Advil® Oral
    Suspension [OTC]
Children's Motrin® Oral
    Suspension [OTC]
choline magnesium trisalicylate
choline salicylate
Dynafed® IB [OTC]
Easprin®
Ecotrin® [OTC]
Ecotrin® Low Adult Strength
    [OTC]
Empirin® [OTC]
Extra Strength Adprin-B® [OTC]
Extra Strength Bayer® Enteric
    500 Aspirin [OTC]
Extra Strength Bayer® Plus
    [OTC]
Genpril® [OTC]
Halfprin® 81® [OTC]
Haltran® [OTC]
Heartline® [OTC]
IBU®

Ibuprin® [OTC]
ibuprofen
Ibuprohm® [OTC]
Indochron E-R®
Indocin®
Indocin® SR
indomethacin
Junior Strength Motrin® [OTC]
Menadol® [OTC]
Midol® IB [OTC]
Motrin®
Motrin® IB [OTC]
Naprelan®
Naprosyn®
naproxen
Nuprin® [OTC]
Regular Strength Bayer® Enteric
    500 Aspirin [OTC]
Saleto-200® [OTC]
Saleto-400®
Saleto-600®
Saleto-800®
St Joseph® Adult Chewable
    Aspirin [OTC]
Trilisate®
ZORprin®

DECUBITUS ULCERS
  Enzyme
    Biozyme-C®
    collagenase
    Elase-Chloromycetin® Topical
    Elase® Topical
    fibrinolysin and
        desoxyribonuclease
    Santyl®
  Protectant, Topical
    Granulex
    trypsin, balsam peru, and castor oil
  Topical Skin Product
    Debrisan® [OTC]
    dextranomer

DEEP VENOUS THROMBOSIS
  PROPHYLAXIS

ardeparin
Coumadin
dalteparin
danaparoid
enoxaparin
Fragmin
heparin
Lovenox Injection
Normiflo
Orgaran
warfarin
GOUT
  Antigout Agent
    colchicine
    colchicine and probenecid
  Nonsteroidal Antiinflammatory Drug
    (NSAID)
    Advil® [OTC]
    Aleve® [OTC]
    Anaprox®
    Bayer® Select® Pain Relief
      Formula [OTC]
    Cataflam® Oral
    Clinoril®
    diclofenac
    Dynafed® IB [OTC]
    Genpril® [OTC]
    Haltran® [OTC]
    IBU®
    Ibuprin® [OTC]
    ibuprofen
    Ibuprohm® [OTC]
    Indochron E-R®
    Indocin®
    Indocin® SR
    indomethacin
    Junior Strength Motrin® [OTC]
    Menadol® [OTC]
    Midol® IB [OTC]
    Motrin®
    Motrin® IB [OTC]
    Naprelan®
    Naprosyn®

naproxen
Nuprin® [OTC]
oxyphenbutazone
Saleto-200® [OTC]
Saleto-400®
Saleto-600®
Saleto-800®
sulindac
Voltaren® Oral
Voltaren-XR® Oral
  Uricosuric Agent
    Anturane®
    probenecid
    sulfinpyrazone
  Xanthine Oxidase Inhibitor
    allopurinol
    Zyloprim®
HERNIATED DISC
  Enzyme
    Chymodiactin®
    chymopapain
INFLAMMATION
  (NONRHEUMATIC)
  Adrenal Corticosteroid
    Acthar®
    Adlone® Injection
    A-methaPred® Injection
    Aristocort®
    Aristocort® Forte
    Articulose-50® Injection
    betamethasone
    Celestone®
    Celestone® Soluspan®
    Cortef®
    corticotropin
    cortisone acetate
    Cortone® Acetate
    Dalalone D.P.®
    Dalalone L.A.®
    Decadron®
    Decadron®-LA
    Decadron® Phosphate
    Decaject®

Decaject-LA®
Delta-Cortef® Oral
Deltasone®
depMedalone® Injection
Depoject® Injection
Depo-Medrol® Injection
dexamethasone
Dexasone®
Dexasone® L.A.
Dexone®
Dexone® LA
Flutex®
Hexadrol® Phosphate
H.P. Acthar® Gel
Hycort®
Hydrocort®
hydrocortisone
Hydrocortone® Acetate
Hydrocortone® Phosphate
Kenacort®
Kenaject-40®
Kenalog®
Kenalog-10®
Kenalog-40®
Kenalog® H
Liquid Pred®
Medrol® Oral
methylprednisolone
M-Prednisol® Injection
Orasone®
Pandel®
paramethasone acetate
Pediapred® Oral
Predcor-TBA® Injection
Prednicen-M®
prednisolone
Prednisol® TBA Injection
prednisone
Prelone® Oral
Solu-Cortef®
Solu-Medrol® Injection
Solurex®
Solurex L.A.®

S-T Cort®
Stemex®
Tac™-3
Tac™-40
Triacet™
Triam-A®
triamcinolone
Triam Forte®
Tristoject®
INSOMNIA
Antihistamine
AllerMax® Oral [OTC]
Anxanil®
Atarax®
Banophen® Oral [OTC]
Belix® Oral [OTC]
Benadryl® Oral [OTC]
Ben-Allergin-50® Injection
Compoz® Gel Caps [OTC]
Compoz® Nighttime Sleep Aid
    [OTC]
Diphenhist® [OTC]
diphenhydramine
Dormarex® 2 Oral [OTC]
Dormin® Oral [OTC]
Genahist® Oral
hydroxyzine
Hyzine-50®
Maximum Strength Nytol® [OTC]
Miles Nervine® Caplets [OTC]
Nytol® Oral [OTC]
Phendry® Oral [OTC]
QYS®
Siladryl® Oral [OTC]
Sleep-eze 3® Oral [OTC]
Sleepinal® [OTC]
Sleepwell 2-nite® [OTC]
Snooze Fast® [OTC]
Sominex® Oral [OTC]
Twilite® Oral [OTC]
Vistacon®
Vistaquel®
Vistaril®

Vistazine®
40 Winks® [OTC]
Barbiturate
  amobarbital
  amobarbital and secobarbital
  Amytal®
  butabarbital sodium
  Butalan®
  Buticaps®
  Butisol Sodium®
  Nembutal®
  pentobarbital
  phenobarbital
  secobarbital
  Seconal™ Injection
  Tuinal®
Benzodiazepine
  Ativan®
  Dalmane®
  diazepam
  Doral®
  estazolam
  flurazepam
  Halcion®
  lorazepam
  ProSom™
  quazepam
  Restoril®
  temazepam
  triazolam
  Valium® Oral
Hypnotic, Nonbarbiturate
  Ambien™
  Aquachloral® Supprettes®
  chloral hydrate
  ethchlorvynol
  glutethimide
  Placidyl®
  zolpidem
METABOLIC BONE DISEASE
  Vitamin D Analog
    calcifediol
    Calderol®

MUSCLE SPASM
  Skeletal Muscle Relaxant
    carisoprodol
    carisoprodol and aspirin
    carisoprodol, aspirin, and codeine
    chlorzoxazone
    cyclobenzaprine
    Flaxedil®
    Flexaphen®
    Flexeril®
    gallamine triethiodide
    metaxalone
    methocarbamol
    methocarbamol and aspirin
    Mivacron®
    mivacurium
    Norflex™
    Norgesic™
    Norgesic™ Forte
    orphenadrine
    orphenadrine, aspirin, and caffeine
    Paraflex®
    Parafon Forte™ DSC
    Robaxin®
    Robaxisal®
    Skelaxin®
    Soma®
    Soma® Compound
    Soma® Compound w/Codeine
NERVE BLOCK
  Local Anesthetic
    Anestacon®
    betamethasone
    bupivacaine
    Carbocaine®
    Celestone®
    chloroprocaine
    Citanest® Forte
    Citanest® Plain
    Depo-Medrol® Injection
    Dermaflex® Gel
    Dilocaine®
    etidocaine

Isocaine® HCl
lidocaine
lidocaine and epinephrine
Marcaine®
mepivacaine
methylprednisolone
Naropin®
Nervocaine®
Nesacaine®
Nesacaine®-MPF
Novocain® Injection
Octocaine®
Octocaine® Injection
Polocaine®
Pontocaine®
Pontocaine® With Dextrose
    Injection
prilocaine
procaine
ropivacaine
Sensorcaine®
Sensorcaine®-MPF
Solarcaine® Aloe Extra Burn
    Relief [OTC]
tetracaine
tetracaine and dextrose
Xylocaine®
Xylocaine® With Epinephrine
NEURALGIA
  Analgesic, Nonnarcotic
    Arthropan® [OTC]
    choline salicylate
  Analgesic, Topical
    capsaicin
    Capsin® [OTC]
    Capzasin-P® [OTC]
    Dolorac™ [OTC]
    Myoflex® [OTC]
    No Pain-HP® [OTC]
    R-Gel® [OTC]
    Sportscreme® [OTC]
    triethanolamine salicylate
    Zostrix® [OTC]

Zostrix®-HP [OTC]
Nonsteroidal Antiinflammatory Drug
    (NSAID)
  Anacin® [OTC]
  Arthritis Foundation® Pain
    Reliever [OTC]
  A.S.A. [OTC]
  aspirin
  Asprimox® [OTC]
  Bayer® Aspirin [OTC]
  Bayer® Buffered Aspirin [OTC]
  Bufferin® [OTC]
  Buffex® [OTC]
  Cama® Arthritis Pain Reliever
    [OTC]
  Easprin®
  Ecotrin® [OTC]
  Ecotrin® Low Adult Strength
    [OTC]
  Extra Strength Adprin-B® [OTC]
  Extra Strength Bayer® Enteric
    500 Aspirin [OTC]
  Extra Strength Bayer® Plus
    [OTC]
  Halfprin® 81® [OTC]
  St Joseph® Adult Chewable
    Aspirin [OTC]
  ZORprin®
NEUROLOGIC DISEASE
  Adrenal Corticosteroid
    Acthar®
    Adlone® Injection
    A-methaPred® Injection
    Aristocort®
    betamethasone
    Celestone®
    Cortef®
    corticotropin
    cortisone acetate
    Cortone® Acetate
    Dalalone®
    Decadron®
    Delta-Cortef® Oral

Deltasone®
depMedalone® Injection
Depoject® Injection
Depo-Medrol® Injection
Depopred® Injection
dexamethasone
Dexasone®
Dexasone® L.A.
Dexone®
Dexone® LA
D-Med® Injection
Duralone® Injection
Haldrone®
Hexadrol®
Hexadrol® Phosphate
H.P. Acthar® Gel
hydrocortisone
Hydrocortone® Acetate
Hydrocortone® Phosphate
Kenacort®
Kenaject-40®
Kenalog®
Kenalog-10®
Kenalog-40®
Key-Pred® Injection
Key-Pred-SP® Injection
Liquid Pred®
Medralone® Injection
Medrol® Oral
methylprednisolone
Meticorten®
M-Prednisol® Injection
paramethasone acetate
Pediapred® Oral
Predcor-TBA® Injection
prednisolone
Prednisol® TBA Injection
prednisone
Prelone® Oral
Solu-Cortef®
Solu-Medrol® Injection
Solurex®
Solurex L.A.®

Tac™-40
triamcinolone
ONYCHOMYCOSIS
Antifungal Agent
Fulvicin® P/G
Fulvicin-U/F®
Grifulvin® V
Grisactin® Ultra
griseofulvin
Gris-PEG®
Lamisil® Oral
terbinafine, oral
OSTEOARTHRITIS
Analgesic, Nonnarcotic
Arthrotec®
diclofenac and misoprostol
Analgesic, Topical
capsaicin
Capsin® [OTC]
Capzasin-P® [OTC]
Dolorac™ [OTC]
No Pain-HP® [OTC]
R-Gel® [OTC]
Zostrix® [OTC]
Zostrix®-HP [OTC]
Nonsteroidal Antiinflammatory Drug
(NSAID)
Actron® [OTC]
Advil® [OTC]
Aleve® [OTC]
Anacin® [OTC]
Anaprox®
Argesic®-SA
Artha-G®
Arthritis Foundation® Pain
Reliever [OTC]
Arthropan® [OTC]
A.S.A. [OTC]
Ascriptin® [OTC]
aspirin
Asprimox® [OTC]
Bayer® Aspirin [OTC]
Bayer® Buffered Aspirin [OTC]

Bayer® Select® Pain Relief
Formula [OTC]
Bufferin® [OTC]
Buffex® [OTC]
Cama® Arthritis Pain Reliever
[OTC]
Cataflam® Oral
Children's Advil® Oral
Suspension [OTC]
Children's Motrin® Oral
Suspension [OTC]
choline magnesium trisalicylate
choline salicylate
Clinoril®
Daypro™
diclofenac
diflunisal
Disalcid®
Doan's®, Original [OTC]
Dolobid®
Dynafed® IB [OTC]
Easprin®
Ecotrin® [OTC]
Empirin® [OTC]
etodolac
Extra Strength Adprin-B® [OTC]
Extra Strength Bayer® Enteric
500 Aspirin [OTC]
Extra Strength Bayer® Plus
[OTC]
Extra Strength Doan's® [OTC]
Feldene®
fenoprofen
Genpril® [OTC]
IBU®
Ibuprin® [OTC]
ibuprofen
Ibuprohm® [OTC]
Indochron E-R®
Indocin®
Indocin® I.V.
Indocin® SR
indomethacin

Junior Strength Motrin® [OTC]
ketoprofen
Lodine®
Lodine® XL
Magan®
magnesium salicylate
Marthritic®
meclofenamate
Menadol® [OTC]
Midol® IB [OTC]
Mobidin®
Mono-Gesic®
Motrin®
Motrin® IB [OTC]
nabumetone
Nalfon®
Naprelan®
Naprosyn®
naproxen
Nuprin® [OTC]
Orudis®
Orudis® KT [OTC]
Oruvail®
oxaprozin
piroxicam
Regular Strength Bayer® Enteric
500 Aspirin [OTC]
Relafen®
Saleto-200® [OTC]
Saleto-400®
Saleto-600®
Saleto-800®
Salflex®
Salgesic®
salsalate
Salsitab®
St Joseph® Adult Chewable
Aspirin [OTC]
sulindac
Tolectin®
Tolectin® DS
tolmetin
Trilisate®

Voltaren® Ophthalmic
Voltaren® Oral
Voltaren-XR® Oral
ZORprin®
Prostaglandin
Arthrotec®
diclofenac and misoprostol
OSTEODYSTROPHY
Vitamin D Analog
calcifediol
Calciferol™ Injection
Calciferol™ Oral
Calcijex™
calcitriol
Calderol®
DHT™
dihydrotachysterol
Drisdol® Oral
ergocalciferol
Hytakerol®
Rocaltrol®
OSTEOMALACIA
Vitamin D Analog
Calciferol™ Injection
Calciferol™ Oral
Drisdol® Oral
ergocalciferol
OSTEOMYELITIS
Antibiotic, Miscellaneous
Cleocin HCl®
Cleocin Pediatric®
Cleocin Phosphate®
clindamycin
Lyphocin®
Vancocin®
Vancoled®
vancomycin
Carbapenem (Antibiotic)
imipenem and cilastatin
meropenem
Merrem® I.V.
Primaxin®
Cephalosporin (First Generation)

Ancef®
Cefadyl®
cefazolin
cephalothin
cephapirin
Kefzol®
Zolicef®
Cephalosporin (Second Generation)
cefmetazole
cefonicid
Cefotan®
cefotetan
cefoxitin
Ceftin® Oral
cefuroxime
Kefurox® Injection
Mefoxin®
Monocid®
Zefazone®
Zinacef® Injection
Cephalosporin (Third Generation)
Cefizox®
Cefobid®
cefoperazone
cefotaxime
ceftazidime
ceftizoxime
ceftriaxone
Ceptaz™
Claforan®
Fortaz®
Rocephin®
Tazicef®
Tazidime®
Penicillin
ampicillin and sulbactam
bacampicillin
Bactocill®
dicloxacillin
Dycill®
Dynapen®
Nafcil™ Injection
nafcillin

A123

Nallpen® Injection
oxacillin
Pathocil®
Prostaphlin®
Spectrobid®
ticarcillin and clavulanate
    potassium
Timentin®
Unasyn®
Unipen® Injection
Unipen® Oral
Quinolone
ciprofloxacin
Cipro™ Injection
Cipro™ Oral
OSTEOPOROSIS
Bisphosphonate Derivative
alendronate
Aredia™
Didronel®
etidronate disodium
Fosamax®
pamidronate
Electrolyte Supplement
Alka-Mints®
Amitone®
Cal Carb-HD®
Calcichew™
Calciday-667®
Calci-Mix™
calcium carbonate
calcium glubionate
calcium lactate
calcium phosphate, dibasic
Cal-Plus®
Caltrate® 600
Caltrate, Jr.®
Chooz®
Dicarbosil®
Equilet®
Florical®
Gencalc® 600
Mallamint®

Nephro-Calci®
Os-Cal® 500
Oyst-Cal 500®
Oystercal® 500
Rolaids ® Calcium Rich
Tums®
Tums® E-X Extra Strength
    Tablet
Tums ® Extra Strength Liquid
Estrogen and Androgen Combination
Estratest®
Estratest® H.S.
estrogens and methyltestosterone
Premarin® With
Methyltestosterone
Estrogen and Progestin Combination
estrogens and
medroxyprogesterone
Premphase™
Prempro™
Estrogen Derivative
Alora® Transdermal
chlorotrianisene
Climara® Transdermal
depGynogen® Injection
Depo®-Estradiol Injection
Depogen® Injection
diethylstilbestrol
Dioval® Injection
Esclim® Transdermal
Estinyl®
Estrace® Oral
Estraderm® Transdermal
estradiol
Estra-L® Injection
Estratab®
Estring®
Estro-Cyp® Injection
estrogens, conjugated
estrogens, esterified
ethinyl estradiol
Gynogen L.A.® Injection
Menest®

Premarin®
Stilphostrol®
TACE®
Vivelle™ Transdermal
Mineral, Oral
  fluoride
Polypeptide Hormone
  Calcimar® Injection
  calcitonin
  Cibacalcin® Injection
  Miacalcin® Injection
  Miacalcin® Nasal Spray
  Osteocalcin® Injection
  Salmonine® Injection
Selective Estrogen Receptor
Modulator (SERM)
  Evista®
  raloxifene
OSTEOSARCOMA
Antineoplastic Agent
  Adriamycin PFS™
  Adriamycin RDF®
  cisplatin
  doxorubicin
  Folex® PFS
  methotrexate
  Platinol®
  Platinol®-AQ
  Rheumatrex®
  Rubex®
PAGET DISEASE OF BONE
Antidote
  Mithracin®
  plicamycin
Bisphosphonate Derivative
  alendronate
  Aredia™
  Didronel®
  etidronate disodium
  Fosamax®
  pamidronate
  Skelid®
  tiludronate

Polypeptide Hormone
  Calcimar® Injection
  calcitonin
  Cibacalcin® Injection
  Miacalcin® Injection
  Miacalcin® Nasal Spray
  Osteocalcin® Injection
  Salmonine® Injection
PAIN
Analgesic, Narcotic
  acetaminophen and codeine
  Alfenta® Injection
  alfentanil
  Alor® 5/500
  Anexsia®
  Anodynos-DHC®
  aspirin and codeine
  Astramorph™ PF Injection
  Azdone®
  Bancap HC®
  belladonna and opium
  Bexophene®
  B&O Supprettes®
  Buprenex®
  buprenorphine
  butalbital compound and codeine
  butorphanol
  Capital® and Codeine
  codeine
  Codoxy®
  Co-Gesic®
  Dalgan®
  Damason-P®
  Darvocet-N®
  Darvocet-N® 100
  Darvon®
  Darvon® Compound-65
    Pulvules®
  Darvon-N®
  Demerol®
  dezocine
  DHC Plus®
  dihydrocodeine compound

Dilaudid®
Dilaudid-5®
Dilaudid-HP®
Dolacet®
Dolene®
Dolophine®
droperidol and fentanyl
DuoCet™
Duragesic® Transdermal
Duramorph® Injection
Empirin® With Codeine
fentanyl
Fentanyl Oralet®
Fiorinal® With Codeine
Hydrocet®
hydrocodone and acetaminophen
hydrocodone and aspirin
hydrocodone and ibuprofen
Hydrogesic®
hydromorphone
HydroStat IR®
Hy-Phen®
Infumorph™ Injection
Innovar®
Kadian™ Capsule
Levo-Dromoran®
levorphanol
Lorcet®
Lorcet®-HD
Lorcet® Plus
Lortab®
Lortab® ASA
Margesic® H
Medipain 5®
Mepergan®
meperidine
meperidine and promethazine
methadone
morphine sulfate
MS Contin® Oral
MSIR® Oral
MS/L®
MS/S®

nalbuphine
Norcet®
Norco®
Nubain®
Numorphan®
OMS® Oral
opium alkaloids
opium tincture
Oramorph SR™ Oral
oxycodone
oxycodone and acetaminophen
oxycodone and aspirin
OxyContin®
OxyIR™
oxymorphone
Panasal® 5/500
Pantopon®
paregoric
pentazocine
pentazocine compound
Percocet®
Percodan®
Percodan®-Demi
Percolone™
Phenaphen® With Codeine
Propacet®
propoxyphene
propoxyphene and acetaminophen
propoxyphene and aspirin
remifentanil
RMS® Rectal
Roxanol™ Oral
Roxanol Rescudose®
Roxanol SR™ Oral
Roxicet® 5/500
Roxicodone™
Roxilox®
Roxiprin®
Stadol®
Stadol® NS
Stagesic®
Sublimaze® Injection
Sufenta® Injection

sufentanil
Synalgos®-DC
Talacen®
Talwin®
Talwin® Compound
Talwin® NX
T-Gesic®
Tylenol® With Codeine
Tylox®
Ultiva™
Vicodin®
Vicodin® ES
Vicodin® HP
Vicoprofen®
Wygesic®
Zydone®
Analgesic, Nonnarcotic
Acephen® [OTC]
Aceta® [OTC]
acetaminophen
acetaminophen and diphenhydramine
acetaminophen and
  phenyltoloxamine
acetaminophen, aspirin, and
  caffeine
Actron® [OTC]
Advil® [OTC]
Aleve® [OTC]
Anacin® [OTC]
Anaprox®
Ansaid® Oral
Apacet® [OTC]
Argesic®-SA
Artha-G®
Arthritis Foundation® Pain
  Reliever [OTC]
Arthropan® [OTC]
A.S.A. [OTC]
Ascriptin® [OTC]
Aspergum® [OTC]
aspirin
Aspirin Free Anacin® Maximum
  Strength [OTC]

Asprimox® [OTC]
Bayer® Aspirin [OTC]
Bayer® Buffered Aspirin [OTC]
Bayer® Low Adult Strength
  [OTC]
Bayer® Select® Pain Relief
  Formula [OTC]
Bufferin® [OTC]
Buffex® [OTC]
Cama® Arthritis Pain Reliever
  [OTC]
Cataflam® Oral
Children's Advil® Oral
  Suspension [OTC]
Children's Dynafed® Jr [OTC]
Children's Motrin® Oral
  Suspension [OTC]
Children's Silapap® [OTC]
choline magnesium trisalicylate
choline salicylate
Clinoril®
Daypro™
diclofenac
diflunisal
Disalcid®
Dolobid®
Dynafed® IB [OTC]
Easprin®
Ecotrin® [OTC]
Ecotrin® Low Adult Strength
  [OTC]
Empirin® [OTC]
etodolac
Excedrin®, Extra Strength [OTC]
Excedrin® P.M. [OTC]
Extra Strength Adprin-B® [OTC]
Extra Strength Bayer® Enteric
  500 Aspirin [OTC]
Extra Strength Bayer® Plus
  [OTC]
Extra Strength Dynafed® E.X.
  [OTC]
Feldene®

fenoprofen
Feverall™ [OTC]
Feverall™ Sprinkle Caps
   [OTC]
flurbiprofen
Gelpirin® [OTC]
Genapap® [OTC]
Genpril® [OTC]
Goody's® Headache Powders
Halenol® Childrens [OTC]
Halfprin® 81® [OTC]
Haltran® [OTC]
Heartline® [OTC]
IBU®
Ibuprin® [OTC]
ibuprofen
Ibuprohm® [OTC]
Indochron E-R®
Indocin®
Indocin® I.V.
Indocin® SR
indomethacin
Infants Feverall™ [OTC]
Infants' Silapap® [OTC]
Junior Strength Motrin® [OTC]
Junior Strength Panadol® [OTC]
ketoprofen
ketorolac tromethamine
Levoprome®
Liquiprin® [OTC]
Lodine®
Lodine® XL
Mapap® [OTC]
Maranox® [OTC]
Marthritic®
meclofenamate
mefenamic acid
Menadol® [OTC]
methotrimeprazine
Midol® IB [OTC]
Midol® PM [OTC]
Mono-Gesic®
Motrin®

Motrin® IB [OTC]
nabumetone
Nalfon®
Naprelan®
Naprosyn®
naproxen
Neopap® [OTC]
Norgesic™
Norgesic™ Forte
Nuprin® [OTC]
Ocufen® Ophthalmic
orphenadrine, aspirin, and caffeine
Orudis®
Orudis® KT [OTC]
Oruvail®
oxaprozin
oxyphenbutazone
Panadol® [OTC]
Percogesic® [OTC]
piroxicam
Ponstel®
Redutemp® [OTC]
Regular Strength Bayer® Enteric
   500 Aspirin [OTC]
Relafen®
Ridenol® [OTC]
Saleto-200® [OTC]
Saleto-400®
Saleto-600®
Saleto-800®
Salflex®
Salgesic®
salsalate
Salsitab®
sodium salicylate
St Joseph® Adult Chewable
   Aspirin [OTC]
sulindac
Tempra® [OTC]
Tolectin®
Tolectin® DS
tolmetin
Toradol® Injection

Toradol® Oral
tramadol
Trilisate®
Tylenol® [OTC]
Tylenol® Extended Relief [OTC]
Ultram®
Uni-Ace® [OTC]
Uracel®
Voltaren® Ophthalmic
Voltaren® Oral
Voltaren-XR® Oral
ZORprin®
Antitussive/Analgesic
acetaminophen and
dextromethorphan
Bayer® Select® Chest Cold
Caplets [OTC]
Drixoral® Cough & Sore Throat
Liquid Caps [OTC]
Decongestant/Analgesic
Advil® Cold & Sinus Caplets
[OTC]
Dimetapp® Sinus Caplets [OTC]
Dristan® Sinus Caplets [OTC]
Motrin® IB Sinus [OTC]
pseudoephedrine and ibuprofen
Sine-Aid® IB [OTC]
Local Anesthetic
AK-Taine®
Alcaine®
ethyl chloride
ethyl chloride and
dichlorotetrafluoroethane
Fluro-Ethyl® Aerosol
I-Paracaine®
Ophthetic®
proparacaine
Nonsteroidal Antiinflammatory Drug
(NSAID)
Doan's®, Original [OTC]
Extra Strength Doan's® [OTC]
Magan®
magnesium salicylate

Mobidin®
PAIN (LUMBAR PUNCTURE)
Analgesic, Topical
EMLA®
lidocaine and prilocaine
PAIN (MUSCLE)
Analgesic, Topical
dichlorodifluoromethane and
trichloromonofluoromethane
Fluori-Methane® Topical Spray
PHEOCHROMOCYTOMA
Alpha-Adrenergic Blocking Agent
Dibenzyline®
phenoxybenzamine
Beta-Adrenergic Blocker
Inderal®
propranolol
Diagnostic Agent
phentolamine
Regitine®
Tyrosine Hydroxylase Inhibitor
Demser®
metyrosine
PLANTAR WARTS
Keratolytic Agent
Duofilm® Solution
salicylic acid and lactic acid
Topical Skin Product
silver nitrate
PLANTARIS
Keratolytic Agent
Duofilm® Solution
Keralyt® Gel
salicylic acid and lactic acid
salicylic acid and propylene glycol
POLYMYOSITIS
Antineoplastic Agent
chlorambucil
cyclophosphamide
Cytoxan® Injection
Cytoxan® Oral
Folex® PFS
Leukeran®

methotrexate
Neosar® Injection
Rheumatrex®
Immunosuppressant Agent
  azathioprine
  Imuran®Agent
  chlorambucil
  cyclophosphamide
  Cytoxan® Injection
  Cytoxan® Oral
  Folex® PFS
  Leukeran®
  methotrexate
  Neosar® Injection
  Rheumatrex®
RHABDOMYOSARCOMA
  Antineoplastic Agent
    Alkeran®
    Cosmegen®
    cyclophosphamide
    Cytoxan® Injection
    Cytoxan® Oral
    dactinomycin
    etoposide
    melphalan
    Neosar® Injection
    Oncovin® Injection
    Toposar® Injection
    VePesid® Injection
    VePesid® Oral
    Vincasar® PFS™ Injection
    vincristine
RHEUMATIC DISORDERS
  Adrenal Corticosteroid
    Acthar®
    Adlone® Injection
    A-methaPred® Injection
    Aristocort®
    betamethasone
    Celestone®
    Celestone® Soluspan®
    Cortef®
    corticotropin

cortisone acetate
Cortone® Acetate
Decadron®
Decadron®-LA
Decadron® Phosphate
Delta-Cortef® Oral
Deltasone®
Depo-Medrol® Injection
dexamethasone
Dexasone®
Dexasone® L.A.
Dexone®
Dexone® LA
Hexadrol®
Hexadrol® Phosphate
H.P. Acthar® Gel
hydrocortisone
Hydrocortone® Acetate
Hydrocortone® Phosphate
Kenalog®
Kenalog-10®
Kenalog-40®
Medrol® Oral
methylprednisolone
Meticorten®
M-Prednisol® Injection
paramethasone acetate
Pediapred® Oral
prednisolone
prednisone
Prelone® Oral
Solu-Cortef®
Solu-Medrol® Injection
Solurex®
Solurex L.A.®
Tac™-3
Tac™-40
triamcinolone
RHEUMATIC FEVER
  Nonsteroidal Antiinflammatory Drug
    (NSAID)
    Argesic®-SA
    Artha-G®

Arthropan® [OTC]
choline magnesium trisalicylate
choline salicylate
Disalcid®
Doan's®, Original [OTC]
Extra Strength Doan's® [OTC]
Magan®
magnesium salicylate
Marthritic®
Mobidin®
Mono-Gesic®
Salflex®
Salgesic®
salsalate
Salsitab®
Trilisate®
Penicillin
   Bicillin® C-R 900/300 Injection
   Bicillin® C-R Injection
   penicillin g benzathine and
    procaine combined
RICKETS
  Vitamin D Analog
   Calciferol™ Injection
   Calciferol™ Oral
   Drisdol® Oral
   ergocalciferol
SKIN INFECTION (TOPICAL
  THERAPY)
  Antibacterial, Topical
   ACU-dyne® [OTC]
   Aeroaid® [OTC]
   Aerodine® [OTC]
   Betadine® [OTC]
   Biodine [OTC]
   Efodine® [OTC]
   hexachlorophene
   Iodex® [OTC]
   Iodex-p® [OTC]
   Mallisol® [OTC]
   Mersol® [OTC]
   Merthiolate® [OTC]
   Minidyne® [OTC]

Operand® [OTC]
pHisoHex®
Polydine® [OTC]
povidone-iodine
Septisol®
thimerosal
Antibiotic/Corticosteroid, Topical
  bacitracin, neomycin, polymyxin
   b, and hydrocortisone
  Cortisporin® Topical Cream
  Cortisporin® Topical Ointment
  Neo-Cortef®
  NeoDecadron® Topical
  neomycin and dexamethasone
  neomycin and hydrocortisone
  neomycin, polymyxin b, and
   hydrocortisone
Antibiotic, Topical
  Achromycin® Topical
  Akne-Mycin® Topical
  A/T/S® Topical
  Baciguent® Topical [OTC]
  bacitracin
  bacitracin and polymyxin b
  bacitracin, neomycin, and
   polymyxin b
  bacitracin, neomycin, polymyxin
   B, and lidocaine
  BactoShield® Topical [OTC]
  Bactroban®
  Betadine® First Aid Antibiotics
   + Moisturizer [OTC]
  Betasept® [OTC]
  chlorhexidine gluconate
  Clomycin® [OTC]
  Clorpactin® WCS-90
  Del-Mycin® Topical
  Dyna-Hex® Topical [OTC]
  Emgel™ Topical
  Eryderm® Topical
  Erygel® Topical
  Erymax® Topical
  erythromycin, topical

E-Solve-2® Topical
ETS-2%® Topical
Exidine® Scrub [OTC]
Flagyl®
Garamycin® Topical
gentamicin
G-myticin® Topical
Hibiclens® Topical [OTC]
Hibistat® Topical [OTC]
Medi-Quick® Topical Ointment
    [OTC]
MetroGel® Topical
metronidazole
mupirocin
Mycifradin® Sulfate Topical
Mycitracin® Topical [OTC]
Neomixin® Topical [OTC]
neomycin
neomycin and polymyxin b
Neosporin® Cream [OTC]
Neosporin® Topical Ointment
    [OTC]
Noritate® Cream
Ocutricin® Topical Ointment
oxychlorosene
Polysporin® Topical
Septa® Topical Ointment [OTC]
Staticin® Topical
tetracycline
Topicycline® Topical
Triple Antibiotic® Topical
T-Stat® Topical
Topical Skin Product
    Campho-Phenique® [OTC]
    camphor and phenol
    iodine
    merbromin
    Mercurochrome®
SKIN ULCER
    Enzyme
        Biozyme-C®
        collagenase
        Elase-Chloromycetin® Topical

Elase® Topical
fibrinolysin and
    desoxyribonuclease
Santyl®
Topical Skin Product
    Debrisan® [OTC]
    dextranomer
SPINAL CORD INJURY
    Skeletal Muscle Relaxant
        Dantrium®
        dantrolene
SUDECK'S ATROPHY
    Calcium Channel Blocker
        Adalat®
        Adalat® CC
        nifedipine
        Procardia®
        Procardia XL®
TINEA
    Antifungal Agent
        Absorbine® Antifungal [OTC]
        Absorbine® Antifungal Foot
            Powder [OTC]
        Absorbine® Jock Itch [OTC]
        Absorbine Jr.® Antifungal
            [OTC]
        Aftate® for Athlete's Foot [OTC]
        Aftate® for Jock Itch [OTC]
        benzoic acid and salicylic acid
        Blis-To-Sol® [OTC]
        Breezee® Mist Antifungal [OTC]
        butenafine
        Caldesene® Topical [OTC]
        carbol-fuchsin solution
        ciclopirox
        clioquinol
        clotrimazole
        Dr. Scholl's Athlete's Foot [OTC]
        Dr. Scholl's Maximum Strength
            Tritin [OTC]
        econazole
        Exelderm® Topical
        Femizole-7® [OTC]

Femizol-M® [OTC]
Fulvicin® P/G
Fulvicin-U/F®
Fungoid® AF Topical Solution [OTC]
Fungoid® Creme
Fungoid® Solution
Fungoid® Tincture
Genaspor® [OTC]
Grifulvin® V
Grisactin® Ultra
griseofulvin
Gris-PEG®
Gyne-Lotrimin® [OTC]
haloprogin
Halotex®
ketoconazole
Lamisil® Cream
Loprox®
Lotrimin®
Lotrimin® AF Cream [OTC]
Lotrimin® AF Lotion [OTC]
Lotrimin® AF Powder [OTC]
Lotrimin® AF Solution [OTC]
Lotrimin® AF Spray Liquid [OTC]
Lotrimin® AF Spray Powder [OTC]
Maximum Strength Desenex® Antifungal Cream [OTC]
Mentax®
Micatin® Topical [OTC]
miconazole
Monistat-Derm™ Topical
Mycelex®
Mycelex®-7
Mycelex®-G
M-Zole® 7 Dual Pack [OTC]

naftifine
Naftin®
Nizoral®
NP-27® [OTC]
Ony-Clear® Nail
Ony-Clear® Spray
oxiconazole
Oxistat® Topical
Pedi-Pro Topical [OTC]
Prescription Strength Desenex® [OTC]
Quinsana Plus® [OTC]
sodium thiosulfate
Spectazole™
sulconazole
terbinafine, topical
Tinactin® [OTC]
Tinactin® for Jock Itch [OTC]
Ting® [OTC]
tolnaftate
triacetin
undecylenic acid and derivatives
Vioform® [OTC]
Whitfield's Ointment [OTC]
Zeasorb-AF® Powder [OTC]
Antifungal/Corticosteroid
  betamethasone and clotrimazole
  Lotrisone®
Antiseborrheic Agent, Topical
  Exsel®
  Head & Shoulders® Intensive Treatment [OTC]
  selenium sulfide
  Selsun®
  Selsun Blue® [OTC]
  Selsun Gold® for Women [OTC]
Disinfectant
  sodium hypochlorite solution

Holistic Treatments by Indication

ARTHRALGIA
  acupuncture

ARTHRITIS
  aromatherapy
  Ayurveda
    medicated enema
  cell therapy
  chiropractic
  complementary alternative medicine
    (CAM)
  diet therapy
    Gerson diet
  herbal therapy
    alfalfa
    echinacea
    feverfew
    ginkgo biloba
    hawthorne
    kava root
    prickly ash bark
    St. John's Wort
  homeopathy
  hydrotherapy
  naturopathy
    glucosamine sulfate
  pancreatic enzyme therapy
  reflexology

ARTHRITIS, RHEUMATOID
  Ayurveda
  biofeedback
  hypnotherapy
  orthomolecular medicine/
    megavitamin therapy
    essential fatty acid
    zinc
    copper
    dietary modification

ARTHRITIS, SPINE (see also Arthritis)
  bodywork
  prolotherapy

ATHEROSCLEROSIS
  naturopathy

ATHLETIC INJURY
  pancreatic enzyme therapy

BURSITIS
  acupuncture
  chiropractic

CARPAL TUNNEL SYNDROME
  acupuncture
  chiropractic
  osteopathic manipulation

CENTRAL NERVOUS SYSTEM
DISEASES
  Ayurveda

CONTUSION, SOFT-TISSUE
  acupuncture

CURVATURE OF THE SPINE
  bodywork
  Rolfing

DECUBITUS ULCERS
  massage therapy

DEGENERATIVE DISK DISEASE
  acupuncture
  chiropractic

DISK HERNIATION
  bodywork
    prolotherapy
  chiropractic

FIBROMYALGIA
massage therapy
Trager method

FIBROSITIS
homeopathy
hydrotherapy

FRACTURE
magnetic therapy

FROZEN SHOULDER
acupuncture
Tui Na
osteopathic manipulation

GOUT
Ayurveda
medicated enema
bee venom therapy

HEADACHES (due to poor alignment
of the cervical spine)
chiropractic

HERNIATED DISK
See Disk Herniation

INSOMNIA
aromatherapy (lavender)
herbal therapy
alfalfa
chamomile
echinacea
ginkgo biloba
hawthorn
kava root
St. John's Wort
valerian
massage therapy
melatonin

MUSCLE SPASM
acupuncture
bodywork
Alexander technique
prolotherapy
chiropractic
hypnosis
magnetic therapy
massage
Shiatsu

MUSCLE TENSION
herbal therapy
echinacea
ginkgo biloba
hawthorn
kava root
St. John's Wort

MYOSITIS
hydrotherapy

NERVE INFLAMMATION
chiropractic

NERVE IMPINGEMENT
acupuncture
osteopathic manipulation

NEUROMUSCULAR DISORDERS
Feldenkrais method
Awareness Through Movement
(ATM)
Functional Integration (FI)
Tragerwork
yoga

OSTEOARTHRITIS
acupuncture
bee venom therapy
chiropractic
glucosamine sulfate
naturopathy

OSTEOMYELITIS
  hyperbaric oxygen therapy

OSTEOPOROSIS
  naturopathy
  orthomolecular medicine/
    megavitamin therapy
    copper
    dietary modification
    essential fatty acid
    zinc
  qigong

PAIN
  acupuncture
  biofeedback
  complementary alternative medicine
    (CAM)
  hypnosis
  osteopathic manipulation

PAIN, BACK
  acupuncture
  Ayurveda
    medicated enema
  bodywork
    Alexander technique
    prolotherapy
    Rolfing
  chiropractic
  complementary alternative medicine
    (CAM)
  craniosacral therapy
  herbal therapy
    black cohosh
    echinacea
    ginkgo biloba
    hawthorn
    kava root
    St. John's Wort
  homeopathy
  hydrotherapy
  hypnosis

massage therapy
meditation and mindfulness
mind-body therapy
Native American medicine
  acupuncture
  massage
  moxibustion
  osteopathic manipulation

PAIN, MUSCLE
  massage therapy

PAIN, MYOFASCIAL
  acupuncture
  biofeedback
  chiropractic
  hypnotherapy
  naturopathy
  orthomolecular medicine/
    megavitamin therapy
    copper
    dietary modification
    essential fatty acid
    zinc

PAIN, NECK
  acupuncture
  Ayurveda
    medicated enema
  bodywork
    Alexander technique
    Rolfing
  craniosacral therapy
  hypnosis
  mind-body therapy
  osteopathic manipulation

PAIN, POSTOPERATIVE
  acupuncture

PAIN, SHOULDER
  acupuncture
  chiropractic
  osteopathic manipulation

PARALYSIS
  hydrotherapy
    whirlpool

PLANTAR FASCIITIS
  acupuncture

REPETITIVE STRAIN INJURY (RSI)
  acupuncture

RHEUMATOID ARTHRITIS
  See Arthritis, Rheumatoid

SCIATICA
  Ayurveda
    medicated enema
  craniosacral therapy
  hydrotherapy
  reflexology

SPINAL INSTABILITY
  bodywork
    prolotherapy

SPINAL CORD INJURY
  acupuncture

SPONDYLOLISTHESIS
  chiropractic

SPRAIN/STRAIN,
MUSCULOTENDINOUS
  acupuncture
  chiropractic
  homeopathy
  Native American medicine
    acupuncture
    massage
    moxibustion
  osteopathic manipulation

STRAIN, BACK
  chiropractic

electrical modality
  high-volt galvanism
  interferential current
trigger point therapy

SUBLUXATION
  chiropractic

TENDINITIS
  chiropractic

TENNIS ELBOW
  acupuncture

THORACIC OUTLET SYNDROME
(TOS)
  osteopathic manipulation

TORTICOLLIS
  homeopathy
    strain-counterstrain

TRAUMA
  craniosacral therapy
  osteopathic manipulation
  spiritual healing

WARTS
  bee venom therapy
  hypnosis

WHIPLASH INJURY
  bodywork
    Alexander technique
    Rolfing
  chiropractic

WOUND HEALING
  herbal therapy
    echinacea
    ginkgo biloba
    hawthorn
    kava root
    St. John's Wort